Vital Statistics
of the United States
Births, Life Expectancy, Deaths, and Selected Health Data

Second Edition, 2006

Vital Statistics
of the United States
Births, Life Expectancy, Deaths, and Selected Health Data

Second Edition, 2004

Editors
Helmut F. Wendel
Christopher S. Wendel

Associate Editor
Mary Meghan Ryan

BERNAN PRESS

ISBN: 1-59888-010-1

ISSN: 1549-8603

Printed by United Book Press, Inc., Baltimore, MD, on acid-free paper that meets the American National Standards Institute Z39-48 standard.

2007 2006   4 3 2 1

BERNAN PRESS
4611-F Assembly Drive
Lanham, MD 20706
800-274-4447
email: info@bernan.com
www.bernanpress.com

CONTENTS

ABOUT THE EDITORS

Helmut F. Wendel, Ph.D. was the lead editor of the first edition of *Vital Statistics of the United States* and the second edition of *State Profiles: The Population and Economy of Each U.S. State*, also published by Bernan Press. Previously, he worked for many years as a monetary economist and macroeconomist at the Board of Governors of the Federal Reserve System, with one year on detail to the Congressional Budget Office. Dr. Wendel concluded his Federal Reserve career as Deputy Associate Director of Research. Since then, he has taught economics at Howard University in Washington, D.C., and at Mohyla Academy in Kiev, Ukraine. He has also served as a U.S. Treasury advisor at the Bulgarian National Bank.

Christopher S. Wendel, M.S., co-editor of the first edition of *Vital Statistics of the United States*, is an epidemiologist and biostatistician for the Health Services Research Center at the Southern Arizona VA Health Care System. His past work experience includes the National Research Council and the Arizona Cancer Center. He specializes in the design and analysis of studies of chronic diseases that are of particular relevance to veterans, such as diabetes, cancer, substance abuse, and post-traumatic stress disorder.

ACKNOWLEDGMENTS

Preparation of this book was very much a team activity. **Mary Meghan Ryan** skillfully and cheerfully assisted the editors with data research for this volume, and she capably compiled the tables and charts. **Shana Hertz** copyedited this edition, and **Rebecca Zayas** competently prepared the layout and graphics.

The principal data sources of this book and many of the analytic insights came from publications of the **National Center for Health Statistics**, a component of the Centers for Disease Control and Prevention (CDC). These publications, listed in the sources and definitions section, interpret the nation's birth and death certificates as well as many data on health. The editors are indebted to the authors of these publications.

Some of the tables on international comparisons, health insurance, and marriage and divorce were obtained from the **U.S. Census Bureau**. These authors are also gratefully acknowledged.

INTRODUCTION

Until 1993, the federal government published *Vital Statistics of the United States* in several thick-bound volumes. These volumes offered comprehensive data on births, deaths, and marriage and divorce, and can currently be found in libraries. However, there was nothing comparable published between 1993 and 2004, when the first edition of the present volume was published by Bernan Press. However, in the interim, the Centers for Disease Control and Prevention (CDC) and its National Center for Health Statistics (NCHS) continued to compile much of this information as periodical reports and news releases, which were available electronically on their Web site. A summary of these data can also be found in the *Statistical Abstract of the United States*, compiled by the U.S. Department of Commerce and published by Bernan Press. These circumstances gave Bernan Press the motivation to bring together a comprehensive collection of birth, death, health, marriage and divorce statistics into a single volume called *Vital Statistics of the United States*. The 2006 volume is the publication's second edition.

Each statistical table in this volume is complemented by descriptive or explanatory text, and a number of tables are illustrated by figures. Source information and references are cited at the end of the book in a sources and definitions section. Many tables provide historical background, and some give information for 2004. However, in view of the availability lags for vital statistics, many of the tables end at the years 2003 or 2002.

In light of long-term improvements in standards of living, including reduced disease risk factors and modernized medical care, favorable news has come to be expected from vital statistics. Indeed, in 2003, life expectancy at birth rose 0.2 years to an all-time high of 77.5 years, while age-adjusted death rates declined 3.5 percent for heart disease and 1.8 percent for cancer. However, the age-adjusted death rate for accidents rose 1.1 percent.

Chapter I, Births, provides information from preliminary data for 2004 and from final data for 2003 and earlier years on many aspects of natality, including birth and fertility rates, number of children, births to unmarried women, maternal health, methods of delivery, other characteristics of mothers, medical visits by pregnant women, and infant health status. The data were obtained from the National Center for Health Statistics.

Chapter II, Mortality, focuses on deaths and death rates, according to a number of medical, demographic, and social characteristics. Especially detailed are the tables on causes of death, which are shown by age, sex, Hispanic origin, race, and (to a lesser extent) state of residence. Death rates are also given by marital status and level of educational attainment, and special tables are provided for infant mortality. These tables were obtained from the National Center for Health Statistics, with most information coming from *Deaths: Final Data for 2002*. Other sources included *Deaths: Injuries, 2002; Deaths: Final Data for 2003* (issued Jan. 2006); and *Deaths: Preliminary Data for 2003*.

Chapter III, Health, offers a collection of statistics concerning health and disease in the United States. While health is not a traditional component of vital statistics, there are connections between health status and birth and death statistics. For example, a person analyzing death rates from cancer may also be interested in a table on the incidence rate of cancer. This chapter shows selected data on several topics, including determinants and measures of health, use of addictive substances, ambulatory care, inpatient care, health personnel, health expenditures, and health insurance. Data were obtained from different surveys conducted by the National Center for Health Statistics and the U.S. Census Bureau.

Chapter IV, Marriage and Divorce, presents the relatively limited data on these two events that are currently reported by states to the federal government, as well as an interesting collection of historical statistics and survey results. Reported marriage and divorce rates are shown by year, month, and state for the 2002–2004 period. An extensive survey of marital history in 2001 provided national estimates of marital status and duration of marriage by age, sex, race, and ethnicity, and birth cohort. Finally, the 2000 census provided demographic profiles of U.S. households maintained by couples, categorized as those shared by married couples, unmarried partners of the opposite sex, and unmarried partners of the same sex.

A **Sources and Definitions** section, at the end of the volume, provides information on source materials.

The **Glossary** defines particular terms used throughout the text.

It is of interest to view some of the vital statistics for the United States in the context of international experience. Tables A-1 to A-3, which comprise the **International Comparisons** tables shown on the following pages, compare selected vital statistics for various regions and countries. Data are provided for life expectancy, infant mortality, birth and death rates, and the natural rate of population increase in 2002. Among 37 selected countries, life expectancy in the United States ranked 25th for females and 26th for males. Hong Kong and Japan ranked first and second for life expectancy. The U.S. ranking in regard to infant mortality was similar to its ranking for life expectancy. The 2002 natural rate of population increase in the United States was 0.6 percent, as compared to 1.2 percent for Asia as a whole and -0.4 percent for Russia. (In addition, an international comparison of health expenditures is shown in Table III-63.)

Table A-1. Life Expectancy at Birth and at 65 Years of Age, According to Sex, Selected Countries, Selected Years, 1980–2001

(Number.)

Country	Male 2001 (rank)	Male — Life expectancy in years						Female 2001 (rank)	Female — Life expectancy in years					
		2001	2000	1999	1995	1990	1980		2001	2000	1999	1995	1990	1980
AT BIRTH														
Australia	7	77.0	76.6	76.2	75.0	73.9	71.0	7	82.4	82.0	81.8	80.8	80.1	78.1
Austria	14	75.6	75.1	74.8	73.3	72.2	69.0	11	81.5	81.1	80.8	79.9	78.8	76.1
Belgium	21	74.9	74.6	74.4	73.4	72.7	70.0	15	81.1	80.8	80.8	80.2	79.4	76.8
Bulgaria	34	68.6	68.5	68.4	67.4	68.3	68.5	35	75.4	75.1	75.1	74.9	75.0	73.9
Canada	5	77.1	76.7	76.3	75.1	74.4	71.7	8	82.2	82.0	81.7	81.1	80.8	78.9
Chile	29	72.7	72.6	72.4	71.8	71.1	. . .	30	78.7	78.6	78.4	77.8	76.9	. . .
Costa Rica	14	75.6	75.4	75.0	74.0	74.7	71.9	24	79.9	80.2	79.8	78.6	79.1	77.0
Cuba	22	74.7	74.7	73.3	75.4	74.6	72.2	28	79.2	79.0	77.5	77.7	76.9	. . .
Czech Republic [1]	30	72.1	71.7	71.4	69.7	67.6	66.8	31	78.5	78.4	78.2	76.6	75.4	73.9
Denmark	22	74.7	74.5	74.2	72.7	72.0	71.2	27	79.3	79.3	79.0	77.8	77.7	77.3
England and Wales	11	76.0	75.6	75.3	74.3	73.1	70.8	20	80.6	80.3	80.1	79.5	78.6	76.8
Finland	25	74.6	74.2	73.8	72.8	70.9	69.2	11	81.5	81.0	81.0	80.2	78.9	77.6
France	18	75.5	75.2	75.0	73.9	72.8	70.2	4	82.9	82.7	82.5	81.8	80.9	78.4
Germany [2]	14	75.6	75.0	74.7	73.3	72.0	69.6	14	81.3	81.0	80.7	79.7	78.4	76.1
Greece	19	75.4	75.5	75.5	75.0	74.6	72.2	18	80.7	80.6	80.6	80.3	79.5	76.8
Hong Kong	1	78.4	78.0	77.7	76.0	74.6	71.6	2	84.6	83.9	83.2	81.5	80.3	77.9
Hungary	35	68.1	67.4	66.4	65.3	65.1	65.5	34	76.4	75.9	75.2	74.5	73.7	72.7
Ireland	22	74.7	73.9	73.9	72.9	72.1	70.1	26	79.7	79.1	78.8	78.4	77.6	75.6
Israel	5	77.1	76.7	76.6	75.5	75.1	72.2	10	81.6	81.1	80.7	79.5	78.5	75.8
Italy	8	76.7	76.6	76.1	74.9	73.6	70.6	6	82.8	82.5	82.2	81.3	80.1	77.4
Japan	2	78.1	77.7	77.1	76.4	75.9	73.4	1	84.9	84.6	84.0	82.9	81.9	78.8
Netherlands	13	75.8	75.5	75.3	74.6	73.8	72.5	18	80.7	80.5	80.5	80.4	80.9	79.2
New Zealand	11	76.0	76.0	76.0	74.2	72.4	70.0	17	80.9	80.9	80.9	79.5	78.3	76.3
Northern Ireland	20	75.2	74.8	74.5	73.5	72.1	68.3	22	80.1	79.8	79.6	78.9	78.0	75.0
Norway	10	76.2	76.0	75.6	74.8	73.4	72.3	11	81.5	81.4	81.1	80.8	79.8	79.2
Poland	32	70.2	69.7	68.2	67.6	66.7	66.0	32	78.3	77.9	77.2	76.4	76.3	74.4
Portugal	27	73.5	73.2	72.6	71.6	70.4	67.7	21	80.3	80.0	79.5	78.7	77.4	75.2
Puerto Rico	31	71.0	70.8	70.7	69.6	69.1	70.8	23	80.0	79.9	79.8	78.9	77.2	76.9
Romania	36	67.7	67.8	67.2	65.5	66.6	66.6	36	75.0	74.8	74.2	73.5	73.1	71.9
Russian Federation	37	59.1	59.2	60.0	58.3	63.8	61.4	37	72.3	72.4	72.5	71.7	74.4	73.0
Scotland	28	73.3	73.1	72.8	72.1	71.1	69.0	29	78.8	78.6	78.4	77.7	76.7	75.2
Singapore	9	76.5	76.1	75.6	74.2	73.1	69.8	15	81.1	80.8	79.7	78.6	77.6	74.7
Slovakia [1]	33	69.6	69.2	69.0	68.4	66.6	66.8	33	77.7	77.4	77.2	76.3	75.4	74.3
Spain	14	75.6	75.7	75.1	74.3	73.3	72.5	4	82.9	82.5	82.1	81.5	80.3	78.6
Sweden	3	77.6	77.4	77.1	76.2	74.8	72.8	9	82.1	82.0	81.9	81.4	80.4	78.8
Switzerland	4	77.4	76.9	76.8	75.3	74.0	72.8	3	83.0	82.6	82.5	81.7	80.7	79.6
United States	26	74.4	74.1	73.9	72.5	71.8	70.0	25	79.8	79.5	79.4	78.9	78.8	77.4

Note: Rankings are from highest to lowest life expectancy (LE) for the most recent year available. Since calculation of LE estimates varies among countries, comparisons among them and subsequent interpretations should be made with caution.

[1] In 1993, Czechoslovakia was divided into two nations, the Czech Republic and Slovakia. Data for years prior to 1993 are from the Czech and Slovak regions of Czechoslovakia.
[2] Until 1990, estimates refer to the Federal Republic of Germany; from 1995 onward, data refer to Germany after reunification.
. . .= Not available.

Table A-1. Life Expectancy at Birth and at 65 Years of Age, According to Sex, Selected Countries, Selected Years, 1980–2001—Continued

(Number.)

Country	Male 2001 (rank)	Male Life expectancy in years 2001	2000	1999	1995	1990	1980	Female 2001 (rank)	Female Life expectancy in years 2001	2000	1999	1995	1990	1980
AT 65 YEARS OF AGE														
Australia	3	17.2	16.9	16.6	15.7	15.2	13.7	5	20.7	20.4	20.2	19.5	19.0	17.9
Austria	13	16.3	16.0	15.6	14.9	14.3	12.9	8	19.8	19.4	19.2	18.6	17.8	16.3
Belgium	18	15.8	15.5	15.4	14.8	14.3	13.0	12	19.7	19.5	19.4	19.1	18.5	16.9
Bulgaria	30	13.1	12.8	13.0	12.8	12.9	12.7	32	15.8	15.4	15.4	15.4	15.4	14.7
Canada	6	17.1	16.4	16.5	16.0	15.7	14.5	6	20.6	20.5	20.3	20.0	19.9	18.9
Chile	23	15.4	15.3	15.2	14.9	14.6	...	22	18.7	18.6	18.5	18.1	17.6	...
Costa Rica	6	17.1	17.2	17.1	16.7	17.1	16.1	15	19.4	19.6	19.3	18.6	19.3	18.1
Cuba	10	16.8	16.7	15.6	...	...	...	17	19.3	19.0	17.5	...	...	...
Czech Republic [1]	27	14.0	13.7	13.6	12.7	11.6	11.2	28	17.2	17.1	16.9	16.0	15.2	14.3
Denmark	24	15.2	15.2	14.9	14.1	14.0	13.6	24	18.4	18.3	18.1	17.5	17.8	17.6
England and Wales	14	16.1	15.8	15.5	14.8	14.1	12.9	19	19.2	19.0	18.8	18.3	17.9	16.9
Finland	19	15.7	15.5	15.1	14.5	13.7	12.5	13	19.6	19.3	19.2	18.6	17.7	16.5
France	8	16.9	16.7	16.5	16.1	15.5	13.6	3	21.3	21.2	20.9	20.6	19.8	18.2
Germany [2]	16	16.0	15.7	15.5	14.7	14.0	13.0	13	19.6	19.4	19.2	18.5	17.6	16.7
Greece	...	...	...	16.3	16.1	15.7	14.6	...	...	...	18.7	18.4	18.0	16.8
Hong Kong	2	17.7	17.3	17.2	16.2	15.3	13.9	2	22.1	21.5	21.0	19.5	18.8	13.9
Hungary	31	13.0	12.7	12.2	12.1	12.0	11.6	30	16.7	16.4	15.9	15.8	15.8	14.6
Ireland	25	15.0	14.6	14.1	13.6	13.3	12.6	25	18.3	17.8	17.5	17.3	16.9	15.7
Israel	3	17.2	16.9	16.6	16.0	15.9	14.4	8	19.8	19.3	19.0	18.0	17.8	15.8
Italy	...	...	16.6	16.2	15.8	15.1	13.3	...	...	20.4	20.1	19.6	18.8	17.1
Japan	1	17.8	17.5	17.0	16.5	16.2	14.6	1	22.7	22.4	21.9	20.9	20.0	17.7
Netherlands	22	15.5	15.3	15.1	14.7	14.4	13.7	17	19.3	19.2	19.1	19.0	18.9	18.0
New Zealand	11	16.5	16.5	16.5	15.4	14.7	13.2	8	19.8	19.8	19.8	19.0	18.3	17.0
Northern Ireland	19	15.7	15.3	15.0	14.4	13.7	11.9	22	18.7	18.5	18.4	18.0	17.5	15.8
Norway	14	16.1	16.0	15.6	15.1	14.6	14.3	8	19.8	19.7	19.5	19.1	18.5	18.0
Poland	28	13.9	13.6	13.2	12.9	12.7	12.0	27	17.6	17.3	17.0	16.6	16.9	15.5
Portugal	21	15.6	15.3	14.9	14.6	13.9	12.9	21	18.9	18.7	18.3	17.8	17.0	16.5
Puerto Rico	...	...	...	...	...	...	...	...	...	...	...	...	...	...
Romania	29	13.5	13.5	13.0	12.9	13.3	12.6	31	16.1	15.9	15.5	15.4	15.3	14.2
Russian Federation	33	11.1	11.1	11.2	10.9	12.1	11.6	33	15.3	15.2	15.2	15.1	15.9	15.6
Scotland	26	14.9	14.7	14.4	13.8	13.1	12.3	26	18.0	17.8	17.6	17.3	16.7	16.2
Singapore	16	16.0	15.8	15.4	14.6	14.5	12.6	19	19.2	19.0	17.9	17.3	16.9	15.4
Slovakia [1]	31	13.0	12.9	13.0	12.7	12.2	12.3	29	16.8	16.5	16.6	16.1	15.7	15.4
Spain	...	...	16.5	16.1	16.0	15.4	14.8	...	...	20.4	20.1	19.8	19.0	17.9
Sweden	8	16.9	16.7	16.4	16.0	15.3	14.3	7	20.1	20.0	19.9	19.6	19.0	17.9
Switzerland	3	17.2	16.9	16.8	16.1	15.3	14.4	4	21.0	20.7	20.6	20.2	19.4	17.9
United States	12	16.4	16.3	16.1	15.6	15.1	14.1	15	19.4	19.2	19.1	18.9	18.9	18.3

Note: Rankings are from highest to lowest life expectancy (LE) for the most recent year available. Since calculation of LE estimates varies among countries, comparisons among them and subsequent interpretations should be made with caution.

[1] In 1993, Czechoslovakia was divided into two nations, the Czech Republic and Slovakia. Data for years prior to 1993 are from the Czech and Slovak regions of Czechoslovakia.
[2] Until 1990, estimates refer to the Federal Republic of Germany; from 1995 onward, data refer to Germany after reunification.
. . . = Not available.

Table A-2. Infant Mortality Rates and International Rankings, Selected Countries, Selected Years, 1960–2002

(Number per 1,000 live births.)

Country[1]	International rankings[2]		2002	2001	2000	1990	1980	1970	1960
	2002	1960							
INFANT DEATHS PER 1,000 LIVE BIRTHS[3]									
Australia	17	5	5.0	5.3	5.2	8.2	10.7	17.9	20.2
Austria	8	24	4.1	4.8	4.8	7.8	14.3	25.9	37.5
Belgium	16	20	4.9	4.5	4.8	8.0	12.1	21.1	31.2
Bulgaria	36	30	13.3	14.4	13.3	14.8	20.2	27.3	45.1
Canada	23	14	5.4	5.2	5.3	6.8	10.4	18.8	27.3
Chile	32	36	7.8	8.3	11.7	16.0	33.0	82.2	120.3
Costa Rica	34	33	11.2	10.8	10.2	15.3	20.3	65.4	67.8
Cuba	27	23	6.5	6.2	7.2	10.7	19.6	38.7	37.3
Czech Republic	10	4	4.2	4.0	4.1	10.8	16.9	20.2	20.0
Denmark	12	8	4.4	4.9	5.3	7.5	8.4	14.2	21.5
England and Wales	21	9	5.2	5.5	5.6	7.9	12.1	18.5	22.4
Finland	4	6	3.0	3.2	3.8	5.6	7.6	13.2	21.0
France	8	15	4.1	4.5	4.6	7.3	10.0	18.2	27.5
Germany[4]	11	22	4.3	4.3	4.4	7.0	12.4	22.5	35.0
Greece	25	25	5.9	5.1	6.1	9.7	17.9	29.6	40.1
Hong Kong	1	26	2.3	2.6	3.0	6.2	11.2	19.2	41.5
Hungary	29	31	7.2	8.1	9.2	14.8	23.2	35.9	47.6
Ireland	20	17	5.1	5.7	6.2	8.2	11.1	19.5	29.3
Israel[5]	23	19	5.4	5.1	5.4	9.9	15.6	18.9	31.0
Italy	14	29	4.7	4.7	4.5	8.2	14.6	29.6	43.9
Japan	4	18	3.0	3.1	3.2	4.6	7.5	13.1	30.7
Netherlands	17	2	5.0	5.4	5.1	7.1	8.6	12.7	17.9
New Zealand	26	10	6.2	5.6	6.3	8.4	13.0	16.7	22.6
Northern Ireland	14	13	4.7	6.1	5.1	7.5	13.4	22.9	27.2
Norway	7	3	3.5	3.9	3.8	7.0	8.1	12.7	18.9
Poland	30	32	7.5	7.7	8.1	19.3	25.5	36.7	54.8
Portugal	17	35	5.0	5.0	5.5	11.0	24.3	55.5	77.5
Puerto Rico	33	27	9.8	9.2	9.9	13.4	18.5	27.9	43.3
Romania	37	34	17.3	18.4	18.6	26.9	29.3	49.4	75.7
Russian Federation[6]	35	. . .	13.2	14.6	15.2	17.6	22.0	. . .	. . .
Scotland	22	12	5.3	5.5	5.7	7.7	12.1	19.6	26.4
Singapore	3	21	2.9	2.2	2.5	6.7	11.7	21.4	34.8
Slovakia	31	16	7.6	6.2	8.6	12.0	20.9	25.7	28.6
Spain	6	28	3.4	3.5	3.9	7.6	12.3	28.1	43.7
Sweden	2	1	2.8	3.7	3.4	6.0	6.9	11.0	16.6
Switzerland	13	7	4.5	5.0	4.9	6.8	9.1	15.1	21.1
United States	28	11	7.0	6.8	6.9	9.2	12.6	20.0	26.0

[1]Refers to countries, territories, cities, or geographic areas with at least 1 million population and with "complete" counts of live births and infant deaths as indicated in the *United Nations Demographic Yearbook*.

[2]Rankings are from lowest to highest infant mortality rates (IMR). Countries with the same IMR receive the same rank. The country with the next highest IMR is assigned the rank it would have received had the lower-ranked countries not been tied, i.e., a rank is skipped. Some of the variation in IMRs is due to differences among countries in distinguishing between fetal and infant deaths.

[3]Under 1 year of age.

[4]Rates for 1990 and earlier years were calculated by combining information from the Federal Republic of Germany and the German Democratic Republic.

[5]Includes data for East Jerusalem and Israeli residents in certain other territories under occupation by Israeli military forces since June 1967.

[6]Excludes infants born alive after less than 28 weeks' gestation, of less than 1,000 grams in weight and 35 centimeters in length, who die within 7 days of birth.

. . .= Not available.

Table A-3. Population, Vital Events, and Rates, by Region and Country, 2002

(Population and events in thousands, except as noted. Figures may not add to totals because of rounding.)

Region and country or area	Population	Births	Deaths	Life expectancy at birth (years)		Births per 1,000 population	Deaths per 1,000 population	Annual rate of natural increase (percent)
				Male	Female			
WORLD	6 228 394	128 578	54 997	62	66	21	9	1.2
Less developed countries	5 029 539	115 120	42 794	61	64	23	9	1.4
More developed countries	1 198 856	13 458	12 203	73	80	11	10	0.1
AFRICA	838 720	30 133	12 097	49	51	36	14	2.2
Sub-Saharan Africa	686 522	26 538	11 285	46	48	39	16	2.2
Angola	10 554	486	272	36	38	46	26	2.0
Benin	6 835	299	93	50	52	44	14	3.0
Botswana	1 579	41	45	33	34	26	29	-0.2
Burkina Faso	12 887	581	242	43	46	45	19	2.6
Burundi	5 965	238	107	42	44	40	18	2.2
Cameroon	15 428	554	235	47	49	36	15	2.1
Cape Verde	409	11	3	66	73	28	7	2.1
Central African Republic	3 623	132	71	41	44	36	19	1.7
Chad	8 971	427	147	47	51	48	16	3.1
Comoros	614	24	6	59	63	39	9	3.0
Congo (Brazzaville)	2 908	88	41	50	51	30	14	1.6
Congo (Kinshasa)	55 042	2 509	832	47	51	46	15	3.0
Côte d'Ivoire	16 598	670	305	40	45	40	18	2.2
Djibouti	447	18	9	42	45	41	19	2.2
Equatorial Guinea	498	19	6	52	57	37	13	2.5
Eritrea	4 306	172	57	52	56	40	13	2.7
Ethiopia	65 254	2 634	1 304	41	42	40	20	2.0
Gabon	1 288	47	14	56	59	37	11	2.6
Gambia, The	1 456	60	18	52	56	41	13	2.9
Ghana	20 163	540	210	56	58	27	10	1.6
Guinea	8 816	377	140	48	51	43	16	2.7
Guinea-Bissau	1 333	52	22	45	49	39	17	2.2
Kenya	31 223	929	491	45	46	30	16	1.4
Lesotho	1 858	51	45	37	37	28	24	0.3
Liberia	3 262	150	58	47	50	46	18	2.8
Madagascar	16 473	699	200	53	58	42	12	3.0
Malawi	11 393	513	254	38	39	45	22	2.3
Mali	11 300	545	218	45	46	48	19	2.9
Mauritania	2 829	120	38	49	54	43	13	2.9
Mauritius	1 200	20	8	68	76	16	7	1.0
Mayotte	171	7	1	58	62	44	9	3.5
Mozambique	17 324	676	507	32	32	39	29	1.0
Namibia	1 897	66	33	46	44	35	18	1.7
Niger	10 760	540	236	42	42	50	22	2.8
Nigeria	130 500	5 120	1 771	51	52	39	14	2.6
Reunion	744	15	4	70	77	21	6	1.5
Rwanda	7 668	308	166	39	40	40	22	1.9
Saint Helena	7	*	*	74	80	13	6	0.7
São Tomé and Príncipe	170	7	1	64	67	42	7	3.5
Senegal	10 311	379	114	55	58	37	11	2.6
Seychelles	80	1	1	65	77	17	7	1.1
Sierra Leone	5 565	247	115	40	46	44	21	2.4
Somalia	7 753	363	139	45	49	47	18	2.9
South Africa	42 716	827	708	49	49	19	17	0.3
Sudan	37 090	1 380	364	56	59	37	10	2.7
Swaziland	1 150	35	22	43	40	30	19	1.1
Tanzania	35 302	1 411	612	43	46	40	17	2.3
Togo	5 299	191	60	52	56	36	11	2.5
Uganda	24 889	1 167	431	43	46	47	17	3.0
Zambia	10 149	407	246	35	35	40	24	1.6
Zimbabwe	12 463	382	260	42	39	31	21	1.0
North Africa	152 199	3 595	813	68	73	24	5	1.8
Algeria	32 278	721	166	69	72	22	5	1.7
Egypt	73 313	1 823	396	68	73	25	5	1.9
Libya	5 369	148	19	74	78	28	3	2.4
Morocco	31 168	738	183	67	72	24	6	1.8
Tunisia	9 816	165	49	73	76	17	5	1.2
Western Sahara	256	11	4	. . .	. . .	44	15	2.9
NEAR EAST	178 574	4 905	1 071	67	71	27	6	2.1
Bahrain	656	13	3	71	76	20	4	1.6
Cyprus	767	10	6	75	80	13	8	0.5
Gaza Strip	1 226	51	5	70	73	42	4	3.8
Iraq	24 002	821	144	66	69	34	6	2.8
Israel	6 030	114	37	77	81	19	6	1.3
Jordan	5 307	130	14	75	80	25	3	2.2
Kuwait	2 112	46	5	76	77	22	2	1.9
Lebanon	3 678	73	23	69	74	20	6	1.4
Oman	2 713	102	11	70	75	38	4	3.4
Qatar	793	13	3	70	75	16	4	1.1
Saudi Arabia	23 513	876	138	67	70	37	6	3.1
Syria	17 156	517	88	68	70	30	5	2.5
Turkey	67 309	1 208	400	69	74	18	6	1.2
United Arab Emirates	2 446	45	10	72	77	18	4	1.4
West Bank	2 164	76	9	71	74	35	4	3.1
Yemen	18 701	810	174	59	62	43	9	3.4

* = Between -500 and +500 for events and between -0.05 percent and +0.05 percent for rates.

. . . = Not available.

Table A-3. Population, Vital Events, and Rates, by Region and Country, 2002—*Continued*

(Population and events in thousands, except as noted. Figures may not add to totals because of rounding.)

Region and country or area	Population	Births	Deaths	Life expectancy at birth (years) Male	Female	Births per 1,000 population	Deaths per 1,000 population	Annual rate of natural increase (percent)
ASIA	3 517 862	68 104	26 671	65	68	19	8	1.2
Afghanistan	27 756	1 139	484	47	46	41	17	2.4
Bangladesh	135 657	4 025	1 186	61	61	30	9	2.1
Bhutan	2 094	74	29	54	53	35	14	2.2
Brunei	351	7	1	72	77	20	3	1.7
Burma	42 282	830	515	54	57	20	12	0.7
Cambodia	12 890	354	122	55	60	27	9	1.8
China	1 309 380	17 155	8 741	70	74	13	7	0.6
China, excl. Taiwan, Hong Kong S.A.R., and Macau S.A.R.	1 279 161	16 783	8 558	70	74	13	7	0.6
Hong Kong S.A.R.	7 303	80	45	77	83	11	6	0.5
Macau S.A.R.	462	6	2	79	85	12	4	0.8
Taiwan	22 454	287	137	74	80	13	6	0.7
East Timor	953	27	6	63	67	28	7	2.2
India	1 034 173	24 582	8 904	63	64	24	9	1.5
Indonesia	231 326	5 059	1 453	66	71	22	6	1.6
Iran	67 538	1 177	376	68	70	17	6	1.2
Japan	127 066	1 225	1 062	78	84	10	8	0.1
Korea, North	22 215	415	153	68	73	19	7	1.2
Korea, South	47 963	620	285	72	79	13	6	0.7
Laos	5 778	216	73	52	56	37	13	2.5
Malaysia	22 662	549	117	69	74	24	5	1.9
Maldives	320	12	3	62	64	37	8	3.0
Mongolia	2 674	57	19	61	66	21	7	1.4
Nepal	25 874	852	260	59	58	33	10	2.3
Pakistan	147 663	4 489	1 332	61	63	30	9	2.1
Philippines	82 995	2 223	471	66	72	27	6	2.1
Singapore	4 453	57	19	77	83	13	4	0.8
Sri Lanka	19 577	320	126	70	75	16	6	1.0
Thailand	63 645	1 062	432	69	73	17	7	1.0
Vietnam	80 577	1 579	501	67	72	20	6	1.3
LATIN AMERICA AND THE CARIBBEAN	538 680	11 282	3 256	68	74	21	6	1.5
Anguilla	12	*	*	74	80	15	6	0.9
Antigua and Barbuda	67	1	*	69	73	19	6	1.3
Argentina	38 331	679	291	71	79	18	8	1.0
Aruba	70	1	*	75	82	12	6	0.6
Bahamas, The	295	6	3	62	69	19	9	1.0
Barbados	276	4	2	70	74	13	9	0.4
Belize	260	8	2	65	69	31	6	2.5
Bolivia	8 445	223	68	62	67	26	8	1.8
Brazil	179 914	3 247	1 101	67	75	18	6	1.2
Cayman Islands	41	1	*	77	82	14	5	0.9
Chile	15 499	255	87	73	80	16	6	1.1
Colombia	41 008	902	232	67	75	22	6	1.6
Costa Rica	3 835	76	17	74	79	20	4	1.6
Cuba	11 224	136	82	74	79	12	7	0.5
Dominica	70	1	*	71	77	17	7	1.0
Dominican Republic	8 596	209	57	67	70	24	7	1.8
Ecuador	13 447	343	72	69	75	25	5	2.0
El Salvador	6 354	180	39	67	74	28	6	2.2
French Guiana	182	4	1	73	80	22	5	1.7
Grenada	89	2	1	63	66	23	8	1.5
Guadeloupe	436	7	3	74	81	17	6	1.0
Guatemala	13 542	481	92	64	66	36	7	2.9
Guyana	700	13	6	61	67	18	9	0.9
Haiti	7 405	255	100	50	53	34	14	2.1
Honduras	6 514	210	41	66	69	32	6	2.6
Jamaica	2 680	48	15	74	78	18	6	1.2
Martinique	422	6	3	79	78	15	6	0.9
Mexico	103 400	2 312	516	69	75	22	5	1.7
Montserrat	8	*	*	76	80	18	7	1.0
Netherlands Antilles	214	3	1	73	77	16	6	1.0
Nicaragua	5 024	136	24	67	71	27	5	2.2
Panama	2 920	62	18	70	75	21	6	1.5
Paraguay	5 884	179	28	72	77	31	5	2.6
Peru	27 950	653	160	68	73	23	6	1.8
Puerto Rico	3 863	59	29	73	81	15	8	0.8
Saint Kitts and Nevis	39	1	*	68	74	19	9	1.0
Saint Lucia	160	3	1	69	77	21	5	1.6
Saint Vincent and the Grenadines	116	2	1	71	75	18	6	1.1
Suriname	434	9	3	67	72	20	7	1.3
Trinidad and Tobago	1 112	14	9	67	73	13	8	0.4
Turks and Caicos Islands	19	*	*	72	76	24	4	2.0
Uruguay	3 387	59	30	72	79	17	9	0.8
Venezuela	24 288	491	119	71	77	20	5	1.5
Virgin Islands, British	21	*	*	75	77	15	4	1.1
Virgin Islands, U.S.	123	2	1	75	83	16	6	1.0
EUROPE AND THE NEW INDEPENDENT STATES	803 255	9 186	8 974	69	76	11	11	*
Western Europe	392 237	4 096	3 843	76	82	10	10	0.1
Andorra	68	1	*	81	87	10	6	0.4
Austria	8 170	78	79	75	81	10	10	*
Belgium	10 275	109	104	75	82	11	10	*
Denmark	5 369	63	58	74	80	12	11	0.1
Faroe Islands	46	1	*	75	82	14	9	0.5
Finland	5 184	55	51	74	82	11	10	0.1
France	59 925	763	542	75	83	13	9	0.4
Germany	82 351	723	844	75	81	9	10	-0.1
Gibraltar	28	*	*	76	82	11	9	0.2
Greece	10 645	105	104	76	81	10	10	*

* = Between -500 and +500 for events and between -0.05 percent and +0.05 percent for rates.

Table A-3. Population, Vital Events, and Rates, by Region and Country, 2002—Continued

(Population and events in thousands, except as noted. Figures may not add to totals because of rounding.)

Region and country or area	Population	Births	Deaths	Life expectancy at birth (years) Male	Female	Births per 1,000 population	Deaths per 1,000 population	Annual rate of natural increase (percent)
Western Europe—Continued								
Guernsey	65	1	1	77	83	10	10	*
Iceland	279	4	2	77	82	14	7	0.7
Ireland	3 883	57	31	74	80	15	8	0.7
Italy	57 927	538	581	76	82	9	10	-0.1
Jersey	90	1	1	76	81	11	9	0.2
Liechtenstein	33	*	*	75	83	11	7	0.4
Luxembourg	449	5	4	74	81	12	9	0.3
Malta	397	5	3	76	81	13	8	0.5
Man, Isle of	74	1	1	74	81	11	12	*
Monaco	32	*	*	75	83	10	13	-0.3
Netherlands	16 068	186	139	76	82	12	9	0.3
Norway	4 525	56	44	76	82	12	10	0.3
Portugal	10 084	116	103	73	80	12	10	0.1
San Marino	28	*	*	78	85	11	8	0.3
Spain	40 153	403	378	76	83	10	9	0.1
Sweden	8 877	87	94	77	83	10	11	-0.1
Switzerland	7 302	72	64	77	83	10	9	0.1
United Kingdom	59 912	666	612	76	81	11	10	0.1
Eastern Europe	120 864	1 296	1 314	69	77	11	11	*
Albania	3 545	66	23	69	75	19	6	1.2
Bosnia and Herzegovina	3 964	51	32	69	75	13	8	0.5
Bulgaria	7 621	61	110	68	75	8	14	-0.6
Croatia	4 391	56	50	71	78	13	11	0.1
Czech Republic	10 257	93	110	71	79	9	11	-0.2
Hungary	10 075	94	132	68	77	9	13	-0.4
Macedonia, The Former Yugoslav Republic of	2 055	27	16	72	77	13	8	0.6
Poland	38 625	397	385	70	78	10	10	*
Romania	22 318	241	274	67	74	11	12	-0.1
Slovakia	5 422	55	50	70	78	10	9	0.1
Slovenia	1 933	18	19	71	79	9	10	-0.1
Yugoslavia	10 658	136	113	71	77	13	11	0.2
New Independent States	290 154	3 794	3 818	61	71	13	13	*
Baltics	7 383	69	100	64	76	9	14	-0.4
Estonia	1 416	13	19	64	76	9	13	-0.4
Latvia	2 367	20	35	63	75	8	15	-0.6
Lithuania	3 601	37	46	64	76	10	13	-0.3
Commonwealth of Independent States	282 770	3 724	3 717	61	70	13	13	*
Armenia	3 330	40	33	62	71	12	10	0.2
Azerbaijan	7 798	147	75	59	68	19	10	0.9
Belarus	10 335	102	145	62	75	10	14	-0.4
Georgia	4 961	57	72	61	68	11	15	-0.3
Kazakhstan	16 742	299	179	58	69	18	11	0.7
Kyrgyzstan	4 822	126	44	59	68	26	9	1.7
Moldova	4 435	61	56	60	69	14	13	0.1
Russia	144 979	1 408	2 017	62	73	10	14	-0.4
Tajikistan	6 720	222	57	61	67	33	9	2.4
Turkmenistan	4 689	133	42	58	65	28	9	1.9
Ukraine	48 396	464	794	61	72	10	16	-0.7
Uzbekistan	25 563	667	204	60	68	26	8	1.8
NORTH AMERICA	319 705	4 432	2 701	74	80	14	8	0.5
Bermuda	64	1	*	75	79	12	7	0.5
Canada	31 902	354	241	76	83	11	8	0.4
Greenland	56	1	*	65	72	16	8	0.9
Saint Pierre and Miquelon	7	*	*	76	80	15	7	0.8
United States	287 676	4 076	2 460	74	80	14	9	0.6
OCEANIA	31 598	536	227	71	76	17	7	1.0
American Samoa	69	2	*	71	80	24	4	2.0
Australia	19 547	248	142	77	83	13	7	0.5
Cook Islands	21	*	*	*	*	22	5	1.7
Fiji	856	20	5	66	71	23	6	1.7
French Polynesia	258	5	1	73	78	18	4	1.4
Guam	161	4	1	76	81	24	4	2.0
Kiribati	96	3	1	58	64	32	9	2.3
Marshall Islands	55	2	*	67	71	34	5	2.9
Micronesia, Federated States of	136	4	1	. . .	. . .	27	6	2.1
Nauru	12	*	*	58	65	27	7	2.0
New Caledonia	208	4	1	70	76	20	6	1.4
New Zealand	3 908	56	30	75	81	14	8	0.7
Northern Mariana Islands	77	2	*	73	79	20	2	1.8
Palau	19	*	*	66	73	19	7	1.2
Papua New Guinea	5 172	163	40	62	66	32	8	2.4
Samoa	179	3	1	67	73	16	6	0.9
Solomon Islands	495	16	2	69	74	33	4	2.9
Tonga	106	3	1	66	71	24	6	1.8
Tuvalu	11	*	*	65	69	21	7	1.4
Vanuatu	196	5	2	60	63	25	8	1.7
Wallis and Futuna	16	*	*	. . .	. . .	20	4	1.6

* = Between -500 and +500 for events and between -0.05 percent and +0.05 percent for rates.
. . . = Not available.

CHAPTER I: BIRTHS

TABLE I-1. LIVE BIRTHS, BIRTH RATES, AND FERTILITY RATES, BY RACE, SELECTED YEARS, 1940–2003

Table I-1 provides data for every 5 years from 1940 to 1960, and annually for every year thereafter. Prior to 1980, some data on race were incomplete; prior to 1985, births in certain states were estimated from 50 percent samples. Beginning in 1980, births were tabulated by race of the mother, rather than by race of the child (as determined by the race of the parents on the birth certificate). This change provided a more uniform approach to the increasing incidence of interracial parentage and the large proportion of records in which the father's race is not reported.

Births totaled 4,090,000 in 2003, about 1.5 percent more than in 2002, representing the highest number of births since 1991. This increase reflected a higher level of 66.1 in the general fertility rate (that is, in the number of births per 1,000 women of childbearing age, here defined as 15–44 years old.) Also reflected is an increase in the crude birth rate (live births per 1,000 of the total population), up from 13.9 in 2002 to 14.1 in 2003.

Whites, including White Hispanics, accounted for 79 percent of total births; Blacks, including Black Hispanics, accounted for nearly 15 percent of total births. Asians and Pacific Islanders contributed over 5 percent of births, while American Indians added 1 percent to the total. Births to Asians or Pacific Islanders rose about 5 percent between 2002 and 2003, while other racial groups had increases of 1 to 1.5 percent in their numbers of births.

Despite the increases in the crude birth rate and the general fertility rate in 2003, measures were still historically low. For example, these rates were 16 and 7 percent lower, respectively, than rates in 1990. Historically, Blacks have had much higher birth rates than Whites, but this difference has been decreasing. The Black crude birth rate has fallen 30 percent since 1990, and the birth rate of American Indians has experienced a similar decline. In recent years, it reached a level closer to the lower rate for Whites.

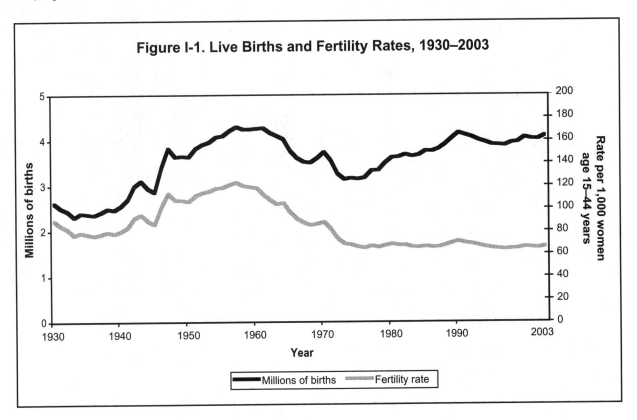

Figure I-1. Live Births and Fertility Rates, 1930–2003

Table I-1. Live Births, Birth Rates, and Fertility Rates, by Race, Selected Years, 1940–2003

(Number, live births per 1,000 population in specified group.)

Year	Number					Birth rate					Fertility rate				
	All races [1]	White	Black	American Indian [2]	Asian or Pacific Islander	All races [1]	White	Black	American Indian [2]	Asian or Pacific Islander	All races [1]	White	Black	American Indian [2]	Asian or Pacific Islander
Registered Births, Race of Mother															
2003	4 089 950	3 225 848	599 847	43 052	221 203	14.1	13.6	15.7	13.8	16.8	66.1	66.1	66.3	58.4	66.3
2002	4 021 726	3 174 760	593 691	42 368	210 907	13.9	13.5	15.7	13.8	16.5	64.8	64.8	65.8	58.0	64.1
2001	4 025 933	3 177 626	606 156	41 872	200 279	14.1	13.7	16.3	13.7	16.4	65.3	65.0	67.6	58.1	64.2
2000	4 058 814	3 194 005	622 598	41 668	200 543	14.4	13.9	17.0	14.0	17.1	65.9	65.3	70.0	58.7	65.8
1999	3 959 417	3 132 501	605 970	40 170	180 776	14.2	13.7	16.8	14.2	15.9	64.4	64.0	68.5	59.0	60.9
1998	3 941 553	3 118 727	609 902	40 272	172 652	14.3	13.8	17.1	14.8	15.9	64.3	63.6	69.4	61.3	60.1
1997	3 880 894	3 072 640	599 913	38 572	169 769	14.2	13.7	17.1	14.7	16.2	63.6	62.8	69.0	60.8	61.3
1996	3 891 494	3 093 057	594 781	37 880	165 776	14.4	13.9	17.3	14.9	16.5	64.1	63.3	69.2	61.8	62.3
1995	3 899 589	3 098 885	603 139	37 278	160 287	14.6	14.1	17.8	15.3	16.7	64.6	63.6	71.0	63.0	62.6
1994	3 952 767	3 121 004	636 391	37 740	157 632	15.0	14.3	19.1	16.0	17.1	65.9	64.2	75.9	65.8	63.9
1993	4 000 240	3 149 833	658 875	38 732	152 800	15.4	14.6	20.2	17.0	17.3	67.0	64.9	79.6	69.7	64.3
1992	4 065 014	3 201 678	673 633	39 453	150 250	15.8	15.0	21.1	17.9	17.9	68.4	66.1	82.4	73.1	66.1
1991	4 110 907	3 241 273	682 602	38 841	145 372	16.2	15.3	21.8	18.3	18.3	69.3	66.7	84.8	73.9	67.1
1990	4 158 212	3 290 273	684 336	39 051	141 635	16.7	15.8	22.4	18.9	19.0	70.9	68.3	86.8	76.2	69.6
1989	4 040 958	3 192 355	673 124	39 478	133 075	16.4	15.4	22.3	19.7	18.7	69.2	66.4	86.2	79.0	68.2
1988	3 909 510	3 102 083	638 562	37 088	129 035	16.0	15.0	21.5	19.3	19.2	67.3	64.5	82.6	76.8	70.2
1987	3 809 394	3 043 828	611 173	35 322	116 560	15.7	14.9	20.8	19.1	18.4	65.8	63.3	80.1	75.6	67.1
1986	3 756 547	3 019 175	592 910	34 169	107 797	15.6	14.8	20.5	19.2	18.0	65.4	63.1	78.9	75.9	66.0
1985	3 760 561	3 037 913	581 824	34 037	104 606	15.8	15.0	20.4	19.8	18.7	66.3	64.1	78.8	78.6	68.4
1984 [3]	3 669 141	2 967 100	568 138	33 256	98 926	15.6	14.8	20.1	20.1	18.8	65.5	63.2	78.2	79.8	69.2
1983 [3]	3 638 933	2 946 468	562 624	32 881	95 713	15.6	14.8	20.2	20.6	19.5	65.7	63.4	78.7	81.8	71.7
1982 [3]	3 680 537	2 984 817	568 506	32 436	93 193	15.9	15.1	20.7	21.1	20.3	67.3	64.8	80.9	83.6	74.8
1981 [3]	3 629 238	2 947 679	564 955	29 688	84 553	15.8	15.0	20.8	20.0	20.1	67.3	64.8	82.0	79.6	73.7
1980 [3]	3 612 258	2 936 351	568 080	29 389	74 355	15.9	15.1	21.3	20.7	19.9	68.4	65.6	84.7	82.7	73.2
Registered Births, Race of Child															
1980 [3]	3 612 258	2 898 732	589 616	36 797	. . .	15.9	14.9	22.1	. . .	. . .	68.4	64.7	88.1	. . .	. . .
1979 [3]	3 494 398	2 808 420	577 855	34 269	. . .	15.6	14.5	22.0	. . .	. . .	67.2	63.4	88.3	. . .	. . .
1978 [3]	3 333 279	2 681 116	551 540	33 160	. . .	15.0	14.0	21.3	. . .	. . .	65.5	61.7	86.7	. . .	. . .
1977 [3]	3 326 632	2 691 070	544 221	30 500	. . .	15.1	14.1	21.4	. . .	. . .	66.8	63.2	88.1	. . .	. . .
1976 [3]	3 167 788	2 567 614	514 479	29 009	. . .	14.6	13.6	20.5	. . .	. . .	65.0	61.5	85.8	. . .	. . .
1975 [3]	3 144 198	2 551 996	511 581	27 546	. . .	14.6	13.6	20.7	. . .	. . .	66.0	62.5	87.9	. . .	. . .
1974 [3]	3 159 958	2 575 792	507 162	26 631	. . .	14.8	13.9	20.8	. . .	. . .	67.8	64.2	89.7	. . .	. . .
1973 [3]	3 136 965	2 551 030	512 597	26 464	. . .	14.8	13.8	21.4	. . .	. . .	68.8	64.9	93.6	. . .	. . .
1972 [3]	3 258 411	2 655 558	531 329	27 368	. . .	15.6	14.5	22.5	. . .	. . .	73.1	68.9	99.9	. . .	. . .
1971 [4]	3 555 970	2 919 746	564 960	27 148	. . .	17.2	16.1	24.4	. . .	. . .	81.6	77.3	109.7	. . .	. . .
1970 [4]	3 731 386	3 091 264	572 362	25 864	. . .	18.4	17.4	25.3	. . .	. . .	87.9	84.1	115.4	. . .	. . .
1969 [4]	3 600 206	2 993 614	543 132	24 008	. . .	17.9	16.9	24.4	. . .	. . .	86.1	82.2	112.1	. . .	. . .
1968 [4]	3 501 564	2 912 224	531 152	24 156	. . .	17.6	16.6	24.2	. . .	. . .	85.2	81.3	112.7	. . .	. . .
1967 [5]	3 520 959	2 922 502	543 976	22 665	. . .	17.8	16.8	25.1	. . .	. . .	87.2	82.8	118.5	. . .	. . .
1966 [4]	3 606 274	2 993 230	558 244	23 014	. . .	18.4	17.4	26.2	. . .	. . .	90.8	86.2	124.7	. . .	. . .
1965 [4]	3 760 358	3 123 860	581 126	24 066	. . .	19.4	18.3	27.7	. . .	. . .	96.3	91.3	133.2	. . .	. . .
1964 [4]	4 027 490	3 369 160	607 556	24 382	. . .	21.1	20.0	30.0	. . .	. . .	104.7	99.8	142.6	. . .	. . .
1963 [4,6]	4 098 020	3 326 344	580 658	22 358	. . .	21.7	20.7	. . .	. . .	. . .	108.3	103.6	. . .	. . .	. . .
1962 [4,6]	4 167 362	3 394 068	584 610	21 968	. . .	22.4	21.4	. . .	. . .	. . .	112.0	107.5	. . .	. . .	. . .
1961 [4]	4 268 326	3 600 864	611 072	21 464	. . .	23.3	22.2	. . .	. . .	. . .	117.1	112.3	. . .	. . .	. . .
1960 [4]	4 257 850	3 600 744	602 264	21 114	. . .	23.7	22.7	31.9	. . .	. . .	118.0	113.2	153.5	. . .	. . .
Births Adjusted for Underregistration, Race of Child															
1955	4 097 000	3 485 000	. . .	. . .	. . .	25.0	23.8	. . .	. . .	. . .	118.3	113.7	. . .	. . .	. . .
1950	3 632 000	3 108 000	. . .	. . .	. . .	24.1	23.0	. . .	. . .	. . .	106.2	102.3	. . .	. . .	. . .
1945	2 858 000	2 471 000	. . .	. . .	. . .	20.4	19.7	. . .	. . .	. . .	85.9	83.4	. . .	. . .	. . .
1940	2 559 000	2 199 000	. . .	. . .	. . .	19.4	18.6	. . .	. . .	. . .	79.9	77.1	. . .	. . .	. . .

[1]For 1960–1991, includes births to races not shown separately. For 1992 and later years, unknown race of mother is imputed.
[2]Includes births to Aleuts and Eskimos.
[3]Based on 100 percent of births in selected states and on a 50 percent sample of births in all other states.
[4]Based on a 50 percent sample of births.
[5]Based on a 20 to 50 percent sample of births.
[6]Figures by race exclude New Jersey.
. . . = Not available.

TABLE I-1A. LIVE BIRTHS, BIRTH RATES, AND FERTILITY RATES, BY RACE AND HISPANIC ORIGIN OF MOTHER, FINAL 2003 AND PRELIMINARY 2004

The number of births increased, the crude birth rate dropped, and the general fertility rate rose slightly in 2004. There were 4.1 million births in 2004, nearly 1 percent more than in 2003. The number of births increased for Hispanic, Asian or Pacific Islander (API), and American Indian women; remained essentially unchanged for non-Hispanic Black women; and decreased for non-Hispanic White women. The 2004 crude birth rate (14.0

births per 1,000 total population) was 1 percent lower than that in 2003. However, the general fertility rate in 2004 rose to 66.3 births per 1,000 women age 15–44 years, a slight increase from the rate in 2003. The Total Fertility Rate (TFR) only increased for API and Hispanic women (each of which experienced a 1 percent increase). The TFR for non-Hispanic Black and non-Hispanic White women fell between 2003 and 2004, and the rate for American Indian women remained essentially unchanged. (For a definition of TFR, see the notes for Table I-4.)

Table I-1A. Live Births, Birth Rates, and Fertility Rates, by Race and Hispanic Origin of Mother, Final 2003 and Preliminary 2004

(Number, percent.)

Race and Hispanic origin of mother	Number		Birth rate		Fertility rate		Total fertility rate		Percent of births to unmarried women	
	2004	2003	2004	2003	2004	2003	2004	2003	2004	2003
All Races and Origins [1]	4 115 590	4 089 950	14.0	14.1	66.3	66.1	2 048.5	2 042.5	35.7	34.6
Non-Hispanic White [2]	2 304 181	2 321 904	11.7	11.8	58.5	58.5	1 852.5	1 856.5	24.5	23.6
Non-Hispanic Black [2]	576 105	576 033	15.1	15.9	66.7	67.1	2 010.5	2 027.5	69.2	68.5
American Indian [2,3]	43 931	43 052	14.0	13.8	58.9	58.4	1 735.0	1 731.5	62.3	61.3
Asian or Pacific Islander [2]	229 352	221 203	16.8	16.8	67.2	66.3	1 900.5	1 873.0	15.5	15.0
Hispanic [4]	944 993	912 329	22.9	22.9	97.7	96.9	2 820.5	2 785.5	46.4	45.0

Note: Data for 2004 are based on a continuous file of records received from the states. Birth rates are live births per 1,000 population in specified group. Fertility rates are live births per 1,000 women age 15–44 years in specified group. Total fertility rates are sums of birth rates for 5-year age groups in specified group multiplied by 5.

[1] Includes data for White and Black Hispanic women, not shown separately.
[2] Race and Hispanic origin are reported separately on the birth certificate. Race categories are consistent with the 1977 Office of Management and Budget (OMB) standards. The multiple-race data for these states were bridged to the single race categories of the 1977 OMB standards for comparability with other states. Data for persons of Hispanic origin are included in the data for each race group, according to the mother's reported race.
[3] Includes births to Aleuts and Eskimos.
[4] May be of any race.

TABLE I-2. LIVE BIRTHS, BY AGE OF MOTHER, LIVE-BIRTH ORDER, AND RACE OF MOTHER, 2003

This table classifies the number of births in 2003 by the age group of the mother. In addition, it shows the birth order (that is, whether the newborn was the mother's first child, second child, etc.). The mean age of mothers at the time of first birth was 25.2 years, slightly higher than the previous record age, which was set in 2002. Asian mothers had the highest mean age at the time of first birth, followed by non-Hispanic White mothers.

As expected, the percentage of firstborns tended to decrease as the age of the mother increased, while the

percentage of higher birth orders increased with the age of the mother. From age 30 to 44 years, a child was more likely to be second born than first born. From age 35 to 39 years, second children were the most frequent, while the numbers of first children and third children are almost the same. However, over the age of 45 years, the number of first and second children were almost the same, while third children were less frequent. There were 323 births to women age 50–54 years in 2003. Although the number of births to this age group has increased at an annual rate of 14 percent since 1997, it remains too small to compute the age-specific birth rates shown in Table I-3.

Table I-2. Live Births, by Age of Mother, Live-Birth Order, and Race of Mother, 2003

(Number of children born alive to mother.)

Live-birth order and race of mother	All ages	Under 15 years	15–19 years Total	15 years	16 years	17 years	18 years	19 years	20–24 years	25–29 years	30–34 years	35–39 years	40–44 years	45–49 years	50–54 years
All Races	4 089 950	6 661	414 580	18 238	41 344	74 802	117 750	162 446	1 032 305	1 086 366	975 546	467 642	101 005	5 522	323
1st child	1 633 987	6 511	330 160	17 520	38 152	64 671	93 595	116 222	481 624	394 295	288 323	109 377	22 212	1 391	94
2nd child	1 320 477	124	70 554	627	2 895	9 100	20 621	37 311	351 903	366 504	348 224	152 914	28 781	1 400	73
3rd child	684 296	4	11 224	28	165	769	2 878	7 384	142 104	202 610	198 580	107 847	20 956	924	47
4th child	267 683	1	1 322	5	12	56	269	980	40 751	78 656	82 663	51 291	12 379	582	38
5th child	97 308	1	162	1	1	5	37	118	10 037	27 041	31 136	21 997	6 527	383	24
6th child	38 816	-	22	1	-	1	5	15	2 223	9 194	13 040	10 411	3 659	249	18
7th child	17 347	-	4	-	1	-	3	-	501	3 327	5 784	5 455	2 113	155	8
8th child and over	18 081	-	7	-	-	-	2	5	181	1 690	5 083	6 745	3 945	412	18
Not stated	11 955	20	1 125	56	118	200	340	411	2 981	3 049	2 713	1 605	433	26	3
White	3 225 848	3 677	298 347	11 484	28 151	52 941	85 734	120 037	790 910	871 496	795 902	379 773	81 031	4 445	267
1st child	1 288 684	3 608	240 706	11 069	26 169	46 311	69 286	87 871	379 879	321 092	234 859	89 190	18 122	1 150	78
2nd child	1 057 829	54	48 971	355	1 822	5 976	14 274	26 544	273 145	300 418	286 948	124 099	22 996	1 132	66
3rd child	544 265	2	7 069	18	84	481	1 769	4 717	102 624	162 498	165 415	89 124	16 759	733	41
4th child	205 040	1	744	3	6	33	151	551	26 150	58 831	66 902	41 931	9 984	467	30
5th child	70 741	1	90	-	1	3	21	65	5 614	18 365	23 689	17 473	5 186	300	23
6th child	26 731	-	10	1	-	1	3	5	1 075	5 496	9 210	7 889	2 843	195	13
7th child	11 678	-	2	-	1	-	1	-	241	1 749	3 827	4 060	1 676	117	6
8th child and over	12 192	-	4	-	-	-	1	3	104	801	3 020	4 775	3 150	330	8
Not stated	8 688	11	751	38	68	136	228	281	2 078	2 246	2 032	1 232	315	21	2
Black	599 847	2 726	100 951	6 056	11 654	19 145	27 817	36 279	196 268	139 947	97 529	49 889	11 895	614	28
1st child	226 476	2 651	77 333	5 780	10 569	16 008	21 018	23 958	77 823	35 317	21 568	9 501	2 154	123	6
2nd child	174 614	65	18 968	250	960	2 799	5 588	9 371	65 234	43 567	29 781	13 881	2 976	138	4
3rd child	105 788	1	3 738	9	76	265	995	2 393	31 511	31 969	21 969	11 663	2 571	113	4
4th child	49 947	-	516	2	6	20	104	384	12 917	16 395	11 739	6 677	1 625	74	4
5th child	21 611	-	65	-	-	2	15	48	3 995	7 348	5 781	3 376	992	53	1
6th child	9 824	-	10	-	-	-	1	9	1 045	3 136	3 041	1 936	617	37	2
7th child	4 596	-	2	-	-	-	2	-	237	1 351	1 581	1 072	327	24	2
8th child and over	4 660	-	3	-	-	-	1	2	66	780	1 667	1 531	560	48	5
Not stated	2 331	9	316	15	43	51	93	114	733	542	402	252	73	4	-
American Indian[1]	43 052	154	7 690	411	815	1 449	2 115	2 900	14 645	10 524	6 423	2 906	666	41	3
1st child	15 237	150	5 955	392	744	1 253	1 648	1 918	5 488	2 169	1 048	360	62	5	-
2nd child	11 788	3	1 435	15	65	173	396	786	5 185	2 993	1 516	537	113	6	-
3rd child	7 738	1	234	1	2	13	55	163	2 709	2 624	1 441	603	121	5	-
4th child	4 152	-	35	-	-	2	7	26	932	1 534	1 048	489	106	5	3
5th child	1 992	-	2	-	-	-	1	1	229	691	621	361	82	6	-
6th child	1 022	-	1	-	-	-	-	1	47	300	381	233	57	3	-
7th child	486	-	-	-	-	-	-	-	8	117	176	140	42	3	-
8th child and over	477	-	-	-	-	-	-	-	5	45	169	173	77	8	-
Not stated	160	-	28	3	4	8	8	5	42	51	23	10	6	-	-
Asian or Pacific Islander	221 203	104	7 592	287	724	1 267	2 084	3 230	30 482	64 399	75 692	35 074	7 413	422	25
1st child	103 590	102	6 166	279	670	1 099	1 643	2 475	18 434	35 717	30 848	10 326	1 874	113	10
2nd child	76 246	2	1 180	7	48	152	363	610	8 339	19 526	29 979	14 397	2 696	124	3
3rd child	26 505	-	183	-	3	10	59	111	2 553	5 977	9 755	6 457	1 505	73	2
4th child	8 544	-	27	-	-	1	7	19	752	1 896	2 974	2 194	664	36	1
5th child	2 964	-	5	1	-	-	-	4	199	637	1 045	787	267	24	-
6th child	1 239	-	1	-	-	-	1	-	56	262	408	353	142	14	3
7th child	587	-	-	-	-	-	-	-	15	110	200	183	68	11	-
8th child and over	752	-	-	-	-	-	-	-	6	64	227	266	158	26	5
Not stated	776	-	30	-	3	5	11	11	128	210	256	111	39	1	1

[1]Includes births of Aleuts and Eskimos.

- = Quantity zero.

TABLE I-2A. LIVE BIRTHS AND BIRTH RATES, BY AGE, RACE, AND HISPANIC ORIGIN OF MOTHER, FINAL 2003 AND PRELIMINARY 2004

Teenage birth rates declined again in 2004, but at a much slower pace than observed since the declines began after 1991 (see also Table I-4A). The rate in 2004, a year in which teenage birth rates dropped to another record low, was 41.2 births per 1,000 females age 15–19 years, a 1 percent decrease from the rate in 2003. Rates declined modestly for teenagers age 15–17 and 18–19 years, but increased slightly for those 10–14 years old. Rates fell 2 to 3 percent for non-Hispanic White and non-Hispanic Black teenagers, and were unchanged for American Indian, Hispanic, and Asian or Pacific Islander teenagers. Childbearing by women in their early twenties showed a decline. The birth rate for women 20–24 years old decreased 1 percent to 101.8 births per 1,000 women in 2004, the lowest rate on record. The rate for women 25–29 years old was essentially unchanged in 2004 (115.5 per 1,000 women), but remained the highest birth rate among all age groups. Births to older women continued to increase. The birth rate for women 30–34 years old increased slightly (less than 0.5 percent) in 2004, while the rate for women 35–39 years old rose by 4 percent. The birth rate for women 40–44 years old increased 3 percent to 9.0, and the rate for women 45–49 years old increased in 0.6 births per 1,000 women.

Table 1-2A. Live Births and Birth Rates, by Age, Race, and Hispanic Origin of Mother, Final 2003 and Preliminary 2004

(Number, rate per 1,000 women in specified group.)

Age, race, and Hispanic origin of mother	2004 Number	2004 Rate	2003 Number	2003 Rate
All Races and Origins [1]				
Total [2]	4 115 590	66.3	4 089 950	66.1
10–14 years	6 789	0.7	6 661	0.6
15–19 years	415 408	41.2	414 580	41.6
15–17 years	133 987	22.1	134 384	22.4
18–19 years	281 421	70.0	280 196	70.7
20–24 years	1 034 834	101.8	1 032 305	102.6
25–29 years	1 105 297	115.5	1 086 366	115.6
30–34 years	967 008	95.5	975 546	95.1
35–39 years	476 123	45.4	467 642	43.8
40–44 years	103 917	9.0	101 005	8.7
45–54 years [3]	6 214	0.6	5 845	0.5
Non-Hispanic White [4]				
Total [2]	2 304 181	58.5	2 321 904	58.5
10–14 years	1 492	0.2	1 399	0.2
15–19 years	169 528	26.8	172 620	27.4
15–17 years	45 478	12.0	46 803	12.4
18–19 years	124 050	48.8	125 817	50.0
20–24 years	518 597	82.1	522 275	83.5
25–29 years	633 588	110.3	627 437	110.8
30–34 years	606 165	97.4	626 315	97.6
35–39 years	305 009	44.9	303 354	43.2
40–44 years	65 689	8.3	64 600	8.1
45–54 years [3]	4 112	0.5	3 904	0.5
Non-Hispanic Black [4]				
Total [2]	576 105	66.7	576 033	67.1
10–14 years	2 708	1.6	2 642	1.6
15–19 years	96 718	62.7	97 509	64.7
15–17 years	34 694	36.8	35 530	38.7
18–19 years	62 023	103.3	61 979	105.3
20–24 years	187 797	126.2	189 020	128.1
25–29 years	137 445	102.5	133 821	102.1
30–34 years	92 338	67.2	93 346	67.4
35–39 years	46 805	33.6	47 661	33.4
40–44 years	11 652	7.8	11 419	7.7
45–54 years [3]	643	0.5	615	0.5
American Indian [4, 5]				
Total [2]	43 931	58.9	43 052	58.4
10–14 years	139	0.9	154	1.0
15–19 years	7 699	52.5	7 690	53.1
15–17 years	2 669	30.1	2 675	30.6
18–19 years	5 030	86.8	5 015	87.3
20–24 years	15 130	109.7	14 645	110.0
25–29 years	10 726	92.8	10 524	93.5
30–34 years	6 506	58.2	6 423	57.4
35–39 years	2 984	26.7	2 906	25.4
40–44 years	726	6.0	666	5.5
45–54 years [3]	22	0.2	44	0.4
Asian or Pacific Islander [4]				
Total [2]	229 352	67.2	221 203	66.3
10–14 years	90	0.2	104	0.2
15–19 years	7 691	17.4	7 592	17.4
15–17 years	2 336	8.9	2 278	8.8
18–19 years	5 355	29.9	5 314	29.8
20–24 years	30 778	60.1	30 482	59.6
25–29 years	65 052	108.7	64 399	108.5
30–34 years	79 726	116.9	75 692	114.6
35–39 years	37 676	62.1	35 074	59.9
40–44 years	7 827	13.7	7 413	13.5
45–54 years [3]	512	1.0	447	0.9
Hispanic [6]				
Total [2]	944 993	97.7	912 329	96.9
10–14 years	2 364	1.3	2 356	1.3
15–19 years	132 983	82.6	128 524	82.3
15–17 years	48 644	49.7	46 955	49.7
18–19 years	84 339	133.4	81 569	132.0
20–24 years	279 566	165.2	273 311	163.4
25–29 years	253 980	145.4	246 361	144.4
30–34 years	177 330	103.8	169 054	102.0
35–39 years	80 765	52.7	75 801	50.8
40–44 years	17 215	12.4	16 172	12.2
45–54 years [3]	790	0.7	750	0.7

Note: Data for 2004 are based on a continuous file of records received from the states. Rates per 1,000 women in specified age and race and Hispanic origin group.

[1] Includes data for White and Black Hispanic women, not shown separately.
[2] The total number includes births to women age 10–54 years. The rate shown for all ages is the fertility rate, which is defined as the total number of births, regardless of age of mother, per 1,000 women age 15–44 years.
[3] The number of births shown is the total for women age 45–54 years. The birth rate is computed by relating the number of births to women age 45–54 years to women age 45–49 years, because most of the births in this group are to women age 45–49 years.
[4] Race and Hispanic origin are reported separately on the birth certificate. Race categories are consistent with the 1977 Office of Management and Budget (OMB) standards.
[5] Includes births to Aleuts and Eskimos.
[6] May be of any race.

TABLE I-3. FERTILITY RATES AND BIRTH RATES, BY AGE OF MOTHER, LIVE-BIRTH ORDER, AND RACE OF MOTHER, 2003

This table shows data from Table I-2 converted to general fertility rates (in the first column) and birth rates for mothers in specific age groups (in subsequent columns). These birth rates are computed separately for each age group by relating the number of births by mothers in the age bracket per 1,000 women of that same age bracket.

Birth rates for teenagers have declined over the last 12 years for all racial groups, but they remained relatively high for Blacks and American Indians. Asians and Pacific Islanders have very low teenage birth rates. (See Table I-8 for comparable statistics on Hispanics.) Beginning with age 25, Black birth rates became smaller than those of Whites. Birth rates for Asians or Pacific Islanders started exceeding the birth rates of White mothers after age 30.

The highest birth rate (115.6, for all races combined) occurred for mothers 25–29 years old. For mothers age 15–44 years, the general fertility rates for the different races showed remarkable convergence in 2003: Whites had a rate of 66.1, and Blacks and Asians both measured 66.3. The fertility rate of American Indians was lower at 58.4. In contrast, Black and American Indian fertility rates had been far above those of Whites during previous decades (such as the 1960s).

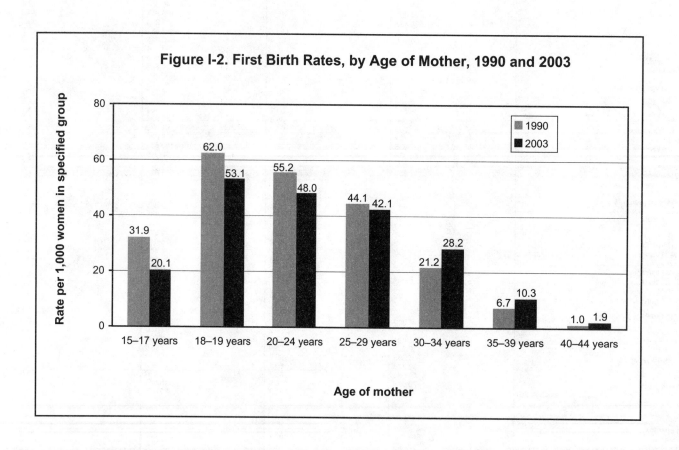

Figure I-2. First Birth Rates, by Age of Mother, 1990 and 2003

Table I-3. Fertility Rates and Birth Rates, by Age of Mother, Live-Birth Order, and Race of Mother, 2003

(Live births per 1,000 women in specified age and racial group.)

Live-birth order and race of mother	Fertility rate [1]	Age of mother									
		10–14 years	15–19 years			20–24 years	25–29 years	30–34 years	35–39 years	40–44 years	45–49 years [2]
			Total	15–17 years	18–19 years						
All Races	66.1	0.6	41.6	22.4	70.7	102.6	115.6	95.1	43.8	8.7	0.5
1st child	26.5	0.6	33.2	20.1	53.1	48.0	42.1	28.2	10.3	1.9	0.1
2nd child	21.4	0.0	7.1	2.1	14.7	35.1	39.1	34.1	14.4	2.5	0.1
3rd child	11.1	*	1.1	0.2	2.6	14.2	21.6	19.4	10.1	1.8	0.1
4th child	4.3	*	0.1	0.0	0.3	4.1	8.4	8.1	4.8	1.1	0.1
5th child	1.6	*	0.0	*	0.0	1.0	2.9	3.0	2.1	0.6	0.0
6th and 7th child	0.9	*	0.0	*	0.0	0.3	1.3	1.8	1.5	0.5	0.0
8th child and over	0.3	*	*	*	*	0.0	0.2	0.5	0.6	0.3	0.0
White	66.1	0.5	38.3	19.8	66.2	100.6	119.5	99.3	44.8	8.7	0.5
1st child	26.5	0.5	31.0	17.9	50.7	48.4	44.1	29.4	10.6	1.9	0.1
2nd child	21.7	0.0	6.3	1.7	13.2	34.8	41.3	35.9	14.7	2.5	0.1
3rd child	11.2	*	0.9	0.1	2.1	13.1	22.3	20.7	10.5	1.8	0.1
4th child	4.2	*	0.1	0.0	0.2	3.3	8.1	8.4	5.0	1.1	0.1
5th child	1.5	*	0.0	*	0.0	0.7	2.5	3.0	2.1	0.6	0.0
6th and 7th child	0.8	*	*	*	*	0.2	1.0	1.6	1.4	0.5	0.0
8th child and over	0.3	*	*	*	*	0.0	0.1	0.4	0.6	0.3	0.0
Black	66.3	1.6	63.8	38.2	103.7	126.1	100.4	66.5	33.2	7.7	0.5
1st child	25.1	1.5	49.0	33.6	73.0	50.2	25.4	14.8	6.4	1.4	0.1
2nd child	19.4	0.0	12.0	4.2	24.3	42.1	31.4	20.4	9.3	1.9	0.1
3rd child	11.7	*	2.4	0.4	5.5	22.1	22.7	15.0	7.8	1.7	0.1
4th child	5.5	*	0.3	0.0	0.8	8.3	11.8	8.0	4.5	1.1	0.1
5th child	2.4	*	0.0	*	0.1	2.6	5.3	4.0	2.3	0.6	0.0
6th and 7th child	1.6	*	*	*	*	0.8	3.2	3.2	2.0	0.6	0.0
8th child and over	0.5	*	*	*	*	0.0	0.6	1.1	1.0	0.4	0.0
American Indian [3]	58.4	1.0	53.1	30.6	87.3	110.0	93.5	57.4	25.4	5.5	0.4
1st child	20.7	1.0	41.2	27.5	62.2	41.3	19.4	9.4	3.2	0.5	*
2nd child	16.1	*	9.9	2.9	20.6	39.1	26.7	13.6	4.7	0.9	*
3rd child	10.5	*	1.6	*	3.8	20.4	23.4	12.9	5.3	1.0	*
4th child	5.7	*	0.2	*	0.6	7.0	13.7	9.4	4.3	0.9	*
5th child	2.7	*	*	*	*	1.7	6.2	5.6	3.2	0.7	*
6th and 7th child	2.1	*	*	*	*	0.4	3.7	5.0	3.3	0.8	*
8th child and over	0.6	*	*	*	*	*	0.4	1.5	1.5	0.6	*
Asian or Pacific Islander	66.3	0.2	17.4	8.8	29.8	59.6	108.5	114.6	59.9	13.5	0.9
1st child	31.1	0.2	14.2	8.0	23.2	36.2	60.4	46.9	17.7	3.4	0.2
2nd child	22.9	*	2.7	0.8	5.5	16.4	33.0	45.6	24.7	4.9	0.3
3rd child	8.0	*	0.4	*	1.0	5.0	10.1	14.8	11.1	2.7	0.1
4th child	2.6	*	0.1	*	0.1	1.5	3.2	4.5	3.8	1.2	0.1
5th child	0.9	*	*	*	*	0.4	1.1	1.6	1.3	0.5	0.0
6th and 7th child	0.5	*	*	*	*	0.1	0.6	0.9	0.9	0.4	0.1
8th child and over	0.2	*	*	*	*	*	0.1	0.3	0.5	0.3	0.1

Note: Figures for live-birth order not stated are distributed.

[1] Fertility rate computed by relating total births, regardless of age of mother, to women age 15–44 years.
[2] Birth rates computed by relating births to women age 45–54 years to women age 45–49 years.
[3] Includes births to Aleuts and Eskimos.
0.0 = Quantity more than zero but less than 0.05.
* = Figure does not meet standards of reliability or precision; based on fewer than 20 births in numerator.

TABLE I-4. TOTAL FERTILITY RATES AND BIRTH RATES, BY AGE AND RACE OF MOTHER, SELECTED YEARS, 1970–2003

This table introduces a different measure of fertility called the Total Fertility Rate (TFR). The objective of this rate is to show how many children would be born during the lifetime of a representative 1,000 women, provided that the current birth rates in each age bracket prevailed. In other words, the TFR shows the average number of children that would be born per 1,000 women. For 2003, the TFR was measured at 2,042.5. This is somewhat less than 2,100, the rate considered to be the replacement rate, or the rate at which a given generation can exactly replace itself. The TFR in the United States has been below the replacement rate for 32 consecutive years.

The 2003 rate suggests that there would be 2.04 births during the lifetime of a representative woman. To calculate the TFR, birth rates are added for the 5-year age groups between 10 and 49 years. The sum is then multiplied by 5, as each woman is assumed to pass through each year of these age groups.

Historically, the TFR dropped between 1970 and 1978. It then moved intermittently higher, reaching 2,056 in 2000 and 2,042.5 in 2003. The TFR for Blacks was considerably higher in the 1980s than that for Whites, but fell in subsequent years to a level slightly below the rate for Whites. The rate for American Indians has also fallen since 1989. The fertility rate for Whites has tended upward since 1980, and the influx of Hispanics (most of whom are classified as White) has also strengthened the fertility rates for Whites.

The teenage birthrate has fallen in every year since 1991 and it has seen an overall decline of 39 percent since 1970. The rate for teenagers 15–17 years old has dropped by 42 percent, and that for 18–19 year olds has dropped 38 percent. These declines occurred despite reported reductions in abortions. They are attributed to a steady decline in the proportion of teenagers who have had sexual intercourse, as well as to the increased use of both condoms and hormonal methods of contraception. (See the 2002 National Survey of Family Growth [NSFG] for more information.) Teenage birth rates by race and ethnicity continue to differ considerably (see Tables I-8 and I-9 for tabulation by ethnicity). The birth rate per 1,000 females age 15–19 years in 2003 was 17.4 for Asian or Pacific Islanders, 38.3 for Whites, 53.1 for American Indians, and 63.8 for Blacks.

Women in their twenties historically accounted for the largest share of births. However, the proportion of these births has declined in recent years, dropping from 65 percent of all births in 1980 to 52 percent of all births in 2003. This decline has been concentrated among women in their early twenties. Birth rates for women in their thirties have risen steadily since 1981, and the rate of increase was particularly large for those age 35–39 years old.

The birth rate for women in their forties has more than doubled since 1980. Still, only 9 of every 1,000 women age 40–44 years gave birth in 2003, compared to 44 per 1,000 for those 35 to 39 years old. The birth rate for women age 45 to 49 years old has remained unchanged at 0.5 since 2000, but it has risen from the level of 0.2 that was prevalent in the 1980s. Since the number of births to women age 50 years and older are too small to compute age-specific rates, these births are folded into the 45- to 49-year-old age bracket.

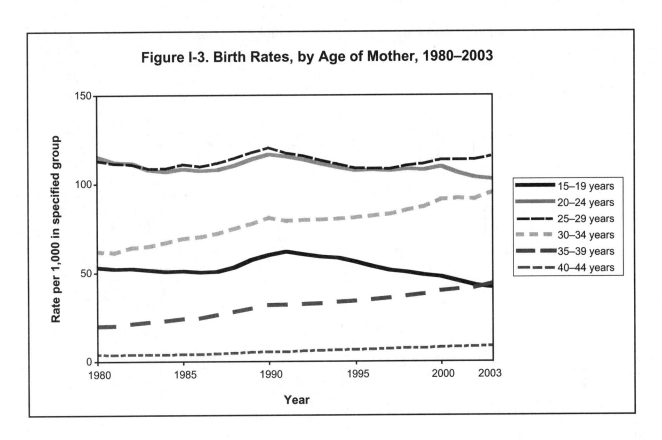

Figure I-3. Birth Rates, by Age of Mother, 1980–2003

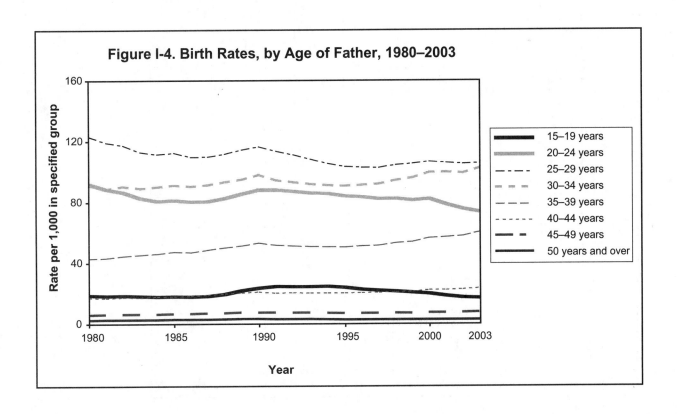

Figure I-4. Birth Rates, by Age of Father, 1980–2003

Table I-4. Total Fertility Rates and Birth Rates, by Age and Race of Mother, Selected Years, 1970–2003

(Live births per 1,000 women in specified group.)

Year and race	Total fertility rate [1]	10–14 years	15–19 years			20–24 years	25–29 years	30–34 years	35–39 years	40–44 years	45–49 years [2]
			Total	15–17 years	18–19 years						
All Races [3]											
2003	2 042.5	0.6	41.6	22.4	70.7	102.6	115.6	95.1	43.8	8.7	0.5
2002	2 013.0	0.7	43.0	23.2	72.8	103.6	113.6	91.5	41.4	8.3	0.5
2001	2 034.0	0.8	45.3	24.7	76.1	106.2	113.4	91.9	40.6	8.1	0.5
2000	2 056.0	0.9	47.7	26.9	78.1	109.7	113.5	91.2	39.7	8.0	0.5
1999	2 007.5	0.9	48.8	28.2	79.1	107.9	111.2	87.1	37.8	7.4	0.4
1998	1 999.0	1.0	50.3	29.9	80.9	108.4	110.2	85.2	36.9	7.4	0.4
1997	1 971.0	1.1	51.3	31.4	82.1	107.3	108.3	83.0	35.7	7.1	0.4
1996	1 976.0	1.2	53.5	33.3	84.7	107.8	108.6	82.1	34.9	6.8	0.3
1995	1 978.0	1.3	56.0	35.5	87.7	107.5	108.8	81.1	34.0	6.6	0.3
1994	2 001.5	1.4	58.2	37.2	90.2	109.2	111.0	80.4	33.4	6.4	0.3
1993	2 019.5	1.4	59.0	37.5	91.1	111.3	113.2	79.9	32.7	6.1	0.3
1992	2 046.0	1.4	60.3	37.6	93.6	113.7	115.7	79.6	32.3	5.9	0.3
1991	2 062.5	1.4	61.8	38.6	94.0	115.3	117.2	79.2	31.9	5.5	0.2
1990	2 081.0	1.4	59.9	37.5	88.6	116.5	120.2	80.8	31.7	5.5	0.2
1989	2 014.0	1.4	57.3	36.4	84.2	113.8	117.6	77.4	29.9	5.2	0.2
1988	1 934.0	1.3	53.0	33.6	79.9	110.2	114.4	74.8	28.1	4.8	0.2
1987	1 872.0	1.3	50.6	31.7	78.5	107.9	111.6	72.1	26.3	4.4	0.2
1986	1 837.5	1.3	50.2	30.5	79.6	107.4	109.8	70.1	24.4	4.1	0.2
1985	1 844.0	1.2	51.0	31.0	79.6	108.3	111.0	69.1	24.0	4.0	0.2
1984 [4]	1 806.5	1.2	50.6	31.0	77.4	106.8	108.7	67.0	22.9	3.9	0.2
1983 [4]	1 799.0	1.1	51.4	31.8	77.4	107.8	108.5	64.9	22.0	3.9	0.2
1982 [4]	1 827.5	1.1	52.4	32.3	79.4	111.6	111.0	64.1	21.2	3.9	0.2
1981 [4]	1 812.0	1.1	52.2	32.0	80.0	112.2	111.5	61.4	20.0	3.8	0.2
1980 [4]	1 839.5	1.1	53.0	32.5	82.1	115.1	112.9	61.9	19.8	3.9	0.2
1979 [4]	1 808.0	1.2	52.3	32.3	81.3	112.8	111.4	60.3	19.5	3.9	0.2
1978 [4]	1 760.0	1.2	51.5	32.2	79.8	109.9	108.5	57.8	19.0	3.9	0.2
1977 [4]	1 789.5	1.2	52.8	33.9	80.9	112.9	111.0	56.4	19.2	4.2	0.2
1976 [4]	1 738.0	1.2	52.8	34.1	80.5	110.3	106.2	53.6	19.0	4.3	0.2
1975 [4]	1 774.0	1.3	55.6	36.1	85.0	113.0	108.2	52.3	19.5	4.6	0.3
1974 [4]	1 835.0	1.2	57.5	37.3	88.7	117.7	111.5	53.8	20.2	4.8	0.3
1973 [4]	1 879.0	1.2	59.3	38.5	91.2	119.7	112.2	55.6	22.1	5.4	0.3
1972 [4]	2 010.0	1.2	61.7	39.0	96.9	130.2	117.7	59.8	24.8	6.2	0.4
1971 [5]	2 266.5	1.1	64.5	38.2	105.3	150.1	134.1	67.3	28.7	7.1	0.4
1970 [5]	2 480.0	1.2	68.3	38.8	114.7	167.8	145.1	73.3	31.7	8.1	0.5
White											
2003	2 061.0	0.5	38.3	19.8	66.2	100.6	119.5	99.3	44.8	8.7	0.5
2002	2 027.5	0.5	39.4	20.5	68.0	101.6	117.4	95.5	42.4	8.2	0.5
2001	2 040.0	0.5	41.2	21.4	70.8	103.7	117.0	95.8	41.3	8.0	0.5
2000	2 051.0	0.6	43.2	23.3	72.3	106.6	116.7	94.6	40.2	7.9	0.4
1999	2 007.5	0.6	44.0	24.4	73.0	105.0	114.9	90.7	38.5	7.4	0.4
1998	1 991.0	0.6	44.9	25.6	74.1	105.4	113.6	88.5	37.5	7.3	0.4
1997	1 955.0	0.7	45.5	26.6	75.0	104.5	111.3	85.7	36.1	6.9	0.3
1996	1 960.5	0.7	47.5	28.0	77.6	105.3	111.7	84.6	35.3	6.7	0.3
1995	1 954.5	0.8	49.5	29.6	80.2	104.7	111.7	83.3	34.2	6.4	0.3
1994	1 957.5	0.8	50.5	30.4	81.2	105.0	113.0	82.2	33.5	6.2	0.3
1993	1 961.5	0.8	50.6	30.0	81.5	106.1	114.7	81.3	32.6	5.9	0.3
1992	1 978.0	0.8	51.4	29.9	83.2	107.7	116.9	80.8	32.1	5.7	0.2
1991	1 988.0	0.8	52.6	30.5	83.3	108.8	118.0	80.2	31.8	5.2	0.2
1990	2 003.0	0.7	50.8	29.5	78.0	109.8	120.7	81.7	31.5	5.2	0.2
1989	1 931.0	0.7	47.9	28.1	72.9	106.9	117.8	78.1	29.7	4.9	0.2
1988	1 856.5	0.6	44.4	26.0	69.6	103.7	114.8	75.4	27.7	4.5	0.2
1987	1 804.5	0.6	42.5	24.6	68.9	102.3	112.3	73.0	25.9	4.1	0.2
1986	1 776.0	0.6	42.3	23.8	70.1	102.7	110.8	70.9	23.9	3.8	0.2
1985	1 787.0	0.6	43.3	24.4	70.4	104.1	112.3	69.9	23.3	3.7	0.2
1984 [4]	1 748.5	0.6	42.9	24.3	68.4	102.7	109.8	67.7	22.2	3.6	0.2
1983 [4]	1 740.5	0.6	43.9	25.0	68.8	103.8	109.4	65.3	21.3	3.6	0.2
1982 [4]	1 767.0	0.6	45.0	25.5	70.8	107.7	111.9	64.0	20.4	3.6	0.2
1981 [4]	1 748.0	0.5	44.9	25.4	71.5	108.3	112.3	61.0	19.0	3.4	0.2
1980 [4]	1 773.0	0.6	45.4	25.5	73.2	111.1	113.8	61.2	18.8	3.5	0.2
Black											
2003	1 999.0	1.6	63.8	38.2	103.7	126.1	100.4	66.5	33.2	7.7	0.5
2002	1 991.0	1.8	66.6	40.0	107.6	127.1	99.0	64.4	31.5	7.4	0.4
2001	2 051.0	2.0	71.8	43.9	114.0	133.2	99.2	64.8	31.6	7.2	0.4
2000	2 129.0	2.3	77.4	49.0	118.8	141.3	100.3	65.4	31.5	7.2	0.4
1999	2 082.5	2.5	79.1	50.5	120.6	137.9	97.3	62.7	30.2	6.5	0.3
1998	2 111.5	2.8	83.5	55.4	124.8	138.4	97.5	63.2	30.0	6.6	0.3
1997	2 091.5	3.1	86.3	59.3	127.7	135.2	95.0	62.6	29.3	6.5	0.3
1996	2 088.5	3.5	89.6	63.3	130.5	133.2	94.3	62.0	28.7	6.1	0.3
1995	2 127.5	4.1	94.4	68.5	135.0	133.7	95.6	63.0	28.4	6.0	0.3
1994	2 258.5	4.5	102.9	75.1	146.2	142.9	101.5	65.0	28.7	5.9	0.3
1993	2 351.0	4.5	107.3	78.9	150.2	150.2	106.4	66.6	29.0	5.9	0.3
1992	2 416.0	4.6	111.3	80.5	156.3	156.2	109.7	67.0	28.6	5.6	0.2
1991	2 462.0	4.7	114.8	83.5	157.6	159.7	112.0	67.3	28.2	5.5	0.2
1990	2 480.0	4.9	112.8	82.3	152.9	160.2	115.5	68.7	28.1	5.5	0.3
1989	2 432.5	5.1	111.5	81.9	151.9	156.8	114.4	66.3	26.7	5.4	0.3
1988	2 298.0	4.9	102.7	75.7	142.7	149.7	108.2	63.1	25.6	5.1	0.3
1987	2 198.0	4.8	97.6	72.1	135.8	142.7	104.3	60.6	24.6	4.8	0.2
1986	2 135.5	4.7	95.8	69.3	135.1	137.3	101.1	59.3	23.8	4.8	0.3
1985	2 109.0	4.5	95.4	69.3	132.4	135.0	100.2	57.9	23.9	4.6	0.3
1984 [4]	2 070.5	4.4	94.1	69.2	128.1	132.2	98.4	56.7	23.3	4.8	0.2
1983 [4]	2 066.0	4.1	93.9	69.6	127.1	131.9	98.4	56.2	23.3	5.1	0.3
1982 [4]	2 106.5	4.0	94.3	69.7	128.9	135.4	101.3	57.5	23.3	5.1	0.4
1981 [4]	2 117.5	4.0	94.5	69.3	131.0	136.5	102.3	57.4	23.1	5.4	0.3
1980 [4]	2 176.5	4.3	97.8	72.5	135.1	140.0	103.9	59.9	23.5	5.6	0.3

[1] Total fertility rates are sums of birth rates for 5-year age groups multiplied by 5.
[2] Beginning in 1997, rates computed by relating births to women age 45–54 years to women age 45–49 years.
[3] For 1970–1991, includes births to races not shown separately. For 1992 and later years, unknown race of mother is imputed.
[4] Based on 100 percent of births in selected states and on a 50 percent sample of births in all other states.
[5] Based on a 50 percent sample of births.

Table I-4. Total Fertility Rates and Birth Rates, by Age and Race of Mother, Selected Years, 1970–2003
—Continued

(Live births per 1,000 women in specified group.)

Year and race	Total fertility rate[1]	10–14 years	15–19 years			20–24 years	25–29 years	30–34 years	35–39 years	40–44 years	45–49 years[2]
			Total	15–17 years	18–19 years						
American Indian[6]											
2003	1 731.5	1.0	53.1	30.6	87.3	110.0	93.5	57.4	25.4	5.5	0.4
2002	1 735.0	0.9	53.8	30.7	89.2	112.6	91.8	56.4	25.4	5.8	0.3
2001	1 746.5	1.0	56.3	31.4	94.8	115.0	90.4	55.9	24.7	5.7	0.3
2000	1 772.5	1.1	58.3	34.1	97.1	117.2	91.8	55.5	24.6	5.7	0.3
1999	1 783.5	1.4	59.9	36.5	98.0	120.7	90.6	53.8	24.3	5.7	0.3
1998	1 851.0	1.5	64.7	39.7	106.9	125.1	92.0	56.8	24.6	5.3	*
1997	1 834.5	1.5	65.2	41.0	107.1	122.5	91.6	56.0	24.4	5.4	0.3
1996	1 855.0	1.6	68.2	42.7	113.3	123.5	91.1	56.5	24.4	5.5	*
1995	1 878.5	1.6	72.9	44.6	122.2	123.1	91.6	56.5	24.3	5.5	*
1994	1 950.0	1.8	76.4	48.4	123.7	126.5	98.2	56.6	24.8	5.4	0.3
1993	2 048.5	1.4	79.8	51.5	126.3	134.2	103.5	59.5	25.5	5.6	*
1992	2 135.5	1.6	82.4	52.3	130.5	142.3	107.0	61.0	26.7	5.9	*
1991	2 142.5	1.6	84.1	51.9	134.2	143.8	105.6	60.8	26.4	5.8	0.4
1990	2 184.5	1.6	81.1	48.5	129.3	148.7	110.3	61.5	27.5	5.9	*
1989	2 248.5	1.5	82.7	51.6	128.9	152.4	114.2	64.8	27.4	6.4	*
1988	2 155.0	1.7	77.5	49.7	121.1	145.2	110.9	64.5	25.6	5.3	*
1987	2 100.5	1.7	77.2	48.8	122.2	140.0	107.9	63.0	24.4	5.6	*
1986	2 083.0	1.8	78.1	48.7	125.3	138.8	107.9	60.7	23.8	5.3	*
1985	2 129.5	1.7	79.2	47.7	124.1	139.1	109.6	62.6	27.4	6.0	*
1984[4]	2 137.5	1.7	81.5	50.7	124.7	142.4	109.2	60.5	26.3	5.6	*
1983[4]	2 182.0	1.9	84.2	55.2	121.4	145.5	113.7	58.9	25.5	6.4	*
1982[4]	2 215.0	1.4	83.5	52.6	127.6	148.1	115.8	60.9	26.9	6.0	*
1981[4]	2 092.5	2.1	78.4	49.7	121.5	141.2	105.6	58.9	25.2	6.6	*
1980[4]	2 165.0	1.9	82.2	51.5	129.5	143.7	106.6	61.8	28.1	8.2	*
Asian or Pacific Islander											
2003	1 873.0	0.2	17.4	8.8	29.8	59.6	108.5	114.6	59.9	13.5	0.9
2002	1 819.5	0.3	18.3	9.0	31.5	60.4	105.4	109.6	56.5	12.5	0.9
2001	1 840.0	0.2	19.8	10.3	32.8	59.1	106.4	112.6	56.7	12.3	0.9
2000	1 892.0	0.3	20.5	11.6	32.6	60.3	108.4	116.5	59.0	12.6	0.8
1999	1 754.5	0.4	21.4	12.4	33.9	58.9	100.8	104.3	52.9	11.3	0.9
1998	1 731.5	0.5	22.2	13.8	34.5	59.2	98.7	101.6	51.4	11.8	0.9
1997	1 757.5	0.5	22.3	14.0	34.9	61.2	101.6	102.5	51.0	11.5	0.9
1996	1 787.0	0.6	23.5	14.7	36.8	63.5	102.8	104.1	50.2	11.9	0.8
1995	1 795.5	0.7	25.5	15.6	40.1	64.2	103.7	102.3	50.1	11.8	0.8
1994	1 834.0	0.7	26.6	16.3	41.3	66.4	108.0	102.2	50.4	11.5	1.0
1993	1 841.5	0.7	26.5	16.1	41.2	68.1	110.3	101.2	49.4	11.2	0.9
1992	1 894.5	0.7	26.5	15.4	41.9	71.7	114.6	102.7	50.7	11.1	0.9
1991	1 928.0	0.8	27.3	16.3	42.2	73.8	118.9	103.3	49.2	11.2	1.1
1990	2 002.5	0.7	26.4	16.0	40.2	79.2	126.3	106.5	49.6	10.7	1.1
1989	1 947.5	0.6	25.6	15.0	40.4	78.8	124.0	102.3	47.0	10.2	1.0
1988	1 983.5	0.6	24.2	13.6	39.6	80.7	128.0	104.4	47.5	10.3	1.0
1987	1 886.0	0.6	22.4	12.6	37.0	79.7	122.7	97.0	44.2	9.5	1.1
1986	1 836.0	0.5	22.8	12.1	38.8	79.2	119.9	92.6	41.9	9.3	1.0
1985	1 885.0	0.4	23.8	12.5	40.8	83.6	123.0	93.6	42.7	8.7	1.2
1984[4]	1 892.0	0.5	24.2	12.6	40.7	86.7	124.3	92.4	40.6	8.7	1.0
1983[4]	1 943.5	0.5	26.1	12.9	44.5	94.0	126.2	93.3	39.4	8.2	1.0
1982[4]	2 015.5	0.4	29.4	14.0	50.8	98.9	130.9	94.4	39.2	8.8	1.1
1981[4]	1 976.0	0.3	28.5	13.4	49.5	96.4	129.1	93.4	38.0	8.6	0.9
1980[4]	1 953.5	0.3	26.2	12.0	46.2	93.3	127.4	96.0	38.3	8.5	0.7

[1]Total fertility rates are sums of birth rates for 5-year age groups multiplied by 5.
[2]Beginning in 1997, rates computed by relating births to women age 45–54 years to women age 45–49 years.
[4]Based on 100 percent of births in selected states and on a 50 percent sample of births in all other states.
[6]Includes births to Aleuts and Eskimos.
* = Figure does not meet standards of reliability or precision; based on fewer than 20 births in the numerator.

TABLE I-4A. BIRTH RATES FOR WOMEN UNDER 20 YEARS OF AGE, BY AGE, RACE, AND HISPANIC ORIGIN, SELECTED YEARS, 1991–2003 AND PRELIMINARY 2004

Teenage birth rates by race and ethnicity differ considerably. All groups have experienced marked declines in their rates since 1991, with Hispanics showing the smallest declines. The teenage birth rate (age 15–19 years) declined by 33 percent between 1991 and 2004 for all races and ethnicities.

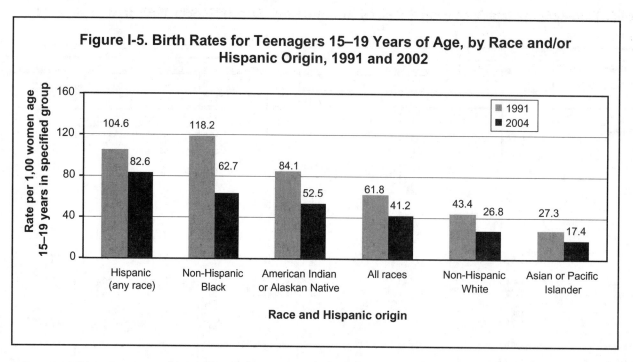

Figure I-5. Birth Rates for Teenagers 15–19 Years of Age, by Race and/or Hispanic Origin, 1991 and 2002

Table I-4A. Birth Rates for Women Under 20 Years of Age, by Age, Race, and Hispanic Origin, Selected Years, 1991–2003 and Preliminary 2004

(Rate per 1,000 women in specified group, percent change.)

Age, race, and Hispanic origin of mother	2004	2003	2002	1991	Percent change, 2003–2004	Percent change, 1991–2004
10–14 Years						
All races [1]	0.7	0.6	0.7	1.4	17	-50
Non-Hispanic White	0.2	0.2	0.2	0.5	0	-60
Non-Hispanic Black	1.6	1.6	1.9	4.9	0	-67
American Indian total [2,3]	0.9	1.0	0.9	1.6	-10	-44
Asian or Pacific Islander total [2]	0.2	0.2	0.3	0.8	0	-75
Hispanic [4]	1.3	1.3	1.4	2.4	0	-46
15–19 Years						
All races [1]	41.2	41.6	43.0	61.8	-1	-33
Non-Hispanic White	26.8	27.4	28.5	43.4	-2	-38
Non-Hispanic Black	62.7	64.7	68.3	118.2	-3	-47
American Indian total [2,3]	52.5	53.1	53.8	84.1	-1	-38
Asian or Pacific Islander total [2]	17.4	17.4	18.3	27.3	0	-36
Hispanic [4]	82.6	82.3	83.4	104.6	0	-21
15–17 Years						
All races [1]	22.1	22.4	23.2	38.6	-1	-43
Non-Hispanic White	12.0	12.4	13.1	23.6	-3	-49
Non-Hispanic Black	36.8	38.7	41.0	86.1	-5	-57
American Indian total [2,3]	30.1	30.6	30.7	51.9	-2	-42
Asian or Pacific Islander total [2]	8.9	8.8	9.0	16.3	1	-45
Hispanic [4]	49.7	49.7	50.7	69.2	0	-28
18–19 Years						
All races [1]	70.0	70.7	72.8	94.0	-1	-26
Non-Hispanic White	48.8	50.0	51.9	70.6	-2	-31
Non-Hispanic Black	103.3	105.3	110.3	162.2	-2	-36
American Indian total [2,3]	86.8	87.3	89.2	134.2	-1	-35
Asian or Pacific Islander total [2]	29.9	29.8	31.5	42.2	0	-29
Hispanic [4]	133.4	132.0	133.0	155.5	1	-14

[1]Includes races other than White and Black.
[2]Race and Hispanic origin are reported separately on the birth certificate. Data for persons of Hispanic origin are included in the data for each race group according to the mother's reported race.
[3]Includes births to Aleuts and Eskimos.
[4]May be of any race.

TABLE I-5. FERTILITY RATES AND BIRTH RATES, BY LIVE-BIRTH ORDER AND RACE OF MOTHER, 1980–2003

This table gives a history of general fertility rates since 1980 and birth rates by live-birth order; it also includes detail by race (White and Black only). The declines in fertility rates for Blacks and their convergence toward White rates are clearly shown. Each of the birth orders contributed to the overall declines in Black fertility rates. Fertility rates of Whites have been fairly stable since 1980. However, there has been a moderate tendency for the frequency of first-borns to decrease, while larger families—those with three or four children—have slightly increased in frequency.

Table I-5. Fertility Rates and Birth Rates, by Live-Birth Order and Race of Mother, 1980–2003

(Live births per 1,000 women age 15–44 years.)

Year and race of mother	Fertility rate	Live-birth order						
		1st	2nd	3rd	4th	5th	6th and 7th	8th and over
All Races [1]								
2003	66.1	26.5	21.4	11.1	4.3	1.6	0.9	0.3
2002	64.8	25.8	21.1	10.9	4.3	1.5	0.9	0.3
2001	65.3	26.0	21.3	11.0	4.3	1.6	0.9	0.3
2000	65.9	26.5	21.4	11.0	4.2	1.6	0.9	0.3
1999	64.4	26.0	21.0	10.7	4.1	1.5	0.9	0.3
1998	64.3	25.9	21.0	10.6	4.1	1.5	0.9	0.3
1997	63.6	25.9	20.7	10.4	4.0	1.5	0.9	0.3
1996	64.1	26.3	20.7	10.4	4.0	1.5	0.9	0.3
1995	64.6	26.9	20.7	10.3	4.0	1.5	0.9	0.3
1994	65.9	27.1	21.2	10.6	4.1	1.6	0.9	0.3
1993	67.0	27.3	21.7	10.9	4.3	1.6	1.0	0.3
1992	68.4	27.6	22.2	11.2	4.4	1.7	1.0	0.3
1991	69.3	28.2	22.3	11.4	4.4	1.7	1.0	0.3
1990	70.9	29.0	22.8	11.7	4.5	1.7	1.0	0.3
1989	69.2	28.4	22.4	11.3	4.3	1.6	0.9	0.3
1988	67.3	27.6	22.0	10.9	4.1	1.5	0.9	0.3
1987	65.8	27.2	21.6	10.5	3.9	1.4	0.8	0.3
1986	65.4	27.2	21.6	10.3	3.8	1.4	0.8	0.3
1985	66.3	27.6	22.0	10.4	3.8	1.4	0.8	0.3
1984 [2]	65.5	27.4	21.7	10.1	3.7	1.4	0.9	0.3
1983 [2]	65.7	27.8	21.5	10.1	3.7	1.4	0.9	0.3
1982 [2]	67.3	28.6	22.0	10.2	3.8	1.4	0.9	0.3
1981 [2]	67.3	29.0	21.6	10.1	3.8	1.5	0.9	0.4
1980 [2]	68.4	29.5	21.8	10.3	3.9	1.5	1.0	0.4
White								
2003	66.1	26.5	21.7	11.2	4.2	1.5	0.8	0.3
2002	64.8	25.7	21.5	11.0	4.1	1.4	0.8	0.2
2001	65.0	25.9	21.6	11.0	4.1	1.4	0.8	0.2
2000	65.3	26.3	21.5	11.0	4.0	1.4	0.8	0.2
1999	64.0	25.9	21.2	10.6	3.9	1.3	0.7	0.2
1998	63.6	25.7	21.2	10.5	3.9	1.3	0.7	0.2
1997	62.8	25.7	20.8	10.2	3.8	1.3	0.7	0.2
1996	63.3	26.2	20.9	10.2	3.8	1.3	0.7	0.2
1995	63.6	26.6	20.9	10.2	3.7	1.3	0.7	0.2
1994	64.2	26.7	21.2	10.3	3.8	1.3	0.7	0.2
1993	64.9	26.8	21.5	10.4	3.9	1.4	0.8	0.2
1992	66.1	27.1	21.9	10.7	4.0	1.4	0.8	0.2
1991	66.7	27.7	21.9	10.8	4.0	1.4	0.8	0.2
1990	68.3	28.4	22.4	11.1	4.0	1.4	0.8	0.2
1989	66.4	27.6	21.9	10.7	3.8	1.3	0.7	0.2
1988	64.5	26.8	21.6	10.4	3.6	1.2	0.7	0.2
1987	63.3	26.5	21.3	10.0	3.5	1.2	0.7	0.2
1986	63.1	26.6	21.3	9.8	3.4	1.2	0.7	0.2
1985	64.1	27.0	21.8	9.9	3.4	1.2	0.7	0.2
1984 [2]	63.2	26.8	21.4	9.6	3.3	1.2	0.7	0.2
1983 [2]	63.4	27.2	21.2	9.5	3.3	1.2	0.7	0.2
1982 [2]	64.8	28.0	21.6	9.6	3.4	1.2	0.7	0.3
1981 [2]	64.8	28.4	21.1	9.5	3.4	1.2	0.8	0.3
1980 [2]	65.6	28.8	21.3	9.6	3.4	1.3	0.8	0.3
Black								
2003	66.3	25.1	19.4	11.7	5.5	2.4	1.6	0.5
2002	65.8	24.8	19.2	11.7	5.5	2.4	1.6	0.5
2001	67.6	25.4	19.9	12.1	5.6	2.5	1.6	0.5
2000	70.0	26.2	20.8	12.5	5.8	2.5	1.7	0.6
1999	68.5	25.9	20.4	12.1	5.5	2.4	1.6	0.5
1998	69.4	26.5	20.6	12.0	5.6	2.5	1.7	0.6
1997	69.0	26.7	20.2	11.8	5.5	2.5	1.7	0.6
1996	69.2	27.0	20.1	11.7	5.5	2.5	1.7	0.6
1995	71.0	28.2	20.4	11.8	5.6	2.6	1.8	0.6
1994	75.9	29.4	21.9	12.9	6.2	2.9	2.0	0.6
1993	79.6	29.8	23.1	14.0	6.8	3.1	2.1	0.6
1992	82.4	30.3	24.1	14.8	7.1	3.3	2.1	0.6
1991	84.8	31.3	24.9	15.3	7.3	3.3	2.1	0.6
1990	86.8	32.4	25.6	15.6	7.4	3.2	2.0	0.6
1989	86.2	32.9	25.4	15.3	7.1	3.0	1.9	0.6
1988	82.6	31.8	24.6	14.4	6.6	2.8	1.8	0.5
1987	80.1	31.2	23.8	13.9	6.3	2.7	1.7	0.5
1986	78.9	31.0	23.4	13.5	6.1	2.6	1.7	0.5
1985	78.8	31.0	23.4	13.4	6.1	2.6	1.7	0.5
1984 [2]	78.1	30.9	23.0	13.2	6.0	2.6	1.7	0.6
1983 [2]	78.7	31.1	23.1	13.2	6.1	2.7	1.8	0.6
1982 [2]	80.9	31.7	23.9	13.8	6.3	2.7	1.8	0.7
1981 [2]	82.0	32.3	24.2	13.7	6.3	2.8	1.9	0.8
1980 [2]	84.9	33.7	24.7	14.0	6.5	2.9	2.1	0.9

Note: Figures for live-birth order not stated are distributed.

[1] Includes races other than White and Black.
[2] Based on 100 percent of births in selected states and on a 50 percent sample of births in all other states.

TABLE I-6. LIVE BIRTHS, BIRTH RATES, AND FERTILITY RATES, BY SPECIFIED HISPANIC ORIGIN AND RACE OF MOTHER, 1989–2003

In this table, births for Hispanic mothers are subdivided by country (or region) of origin, such as Mexico and Cuba. (See Table I-1A for preliminary data from 2004.) Birth rates and fertility rates were especially high among mothers from Mexico, Central America, and South America. Cuban-American fertility rates were much lower. In the 1990s, they were somewhat below those of non-Hispanic Whites; however, these rates have strengthened in the last three years. The birth rates for Puerto Ricans in the United States were similar to those of non-Hispanic Blacks. Altogether, Hispanic mothers accounted for about 22 percent of all births in 2003, an increase from 15 percent in 1990. During the last decade, the non-Hispanic Black birth rate has been well below the Hispanic average. It has been significantly above the rate for Whites—after the Hispanic component is removed from the group.

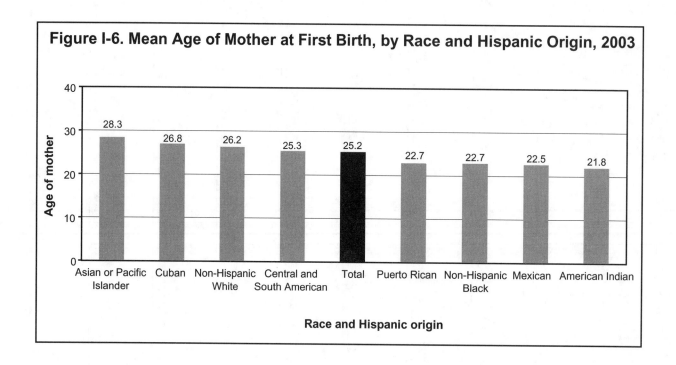

Figure I-6. Mean Age of Mother at First Birth, by Race and Hispanic Origin, 2003

Table I-6. Live Births, Birth Rates, and Fertility Rates, by Specified Hispanic Origin and Race of Mother, 1989–2003

(Number, live births per 1,000 population in specified group, live births per 1,000 women age 15–44 years in specified group.)

Measure and year	All origins [1]	Hispanic						Non-Hispanic		
		Total	Mexican	Puerto Rican	Cuban	Central and South American	Other and unknown Hispanic	Total [2]	White	Black
Number										
2003	4 089 950	912 329	654 504	58 400	14 867	135 586	48 972	3 149 034	2 321 904	576 033
2002	4 021 726	876 642	627 505	57 465	14 232	125 981	51 459	3 119 944	2 298 156	578 335
2001	4 025 933	851 851	611 000	57 568	14 017	121 365	47 901	3 149 572	2 326 578	589 917
2000	4 058 814	815 868	581 915	58 124	13 429	113 344	49 056	3 199 994	2 362 968	604 346
1999	3 959 417	764 339	540 674	57 138	13 088	103 307	50 132	3 147 580	2 346 450	588 981
1998	3 941 553	734 661	516 011	57 349	13 226	98 226	49 849	3 158 975	2 361 462	593 127
1997	3 880 894	709 767	499 024	55 450	12 887	97 405	45 001	3 115 174	2 333 363	581 431
1996	3 891 494	701 339	489 666	54 863	12 613	97 888	46 309	3 133 484	2 358 989	578 099
1995	3 899 589	679 768	469 615	54 824	12 473	94 996	47 860	3 160 495	2 382 638	587 781
1994	3 952 767	665 026	454 536	57 240	11 889	93 485	47 876	3 245 115	2 438 855	619 198
1993	4 000 240	654 418	443 733	58 102	11 916	92 371	48 296	3 295 345	2 472 031	641 273
1992 [3]	4 049 024	643 271	432 047	59 569	11 472	89 031	51 152	3 365 862	2 527 207	657 450
1991 [3]	4 094 566	623 085	411 233	59 833	11 058	86 908	54 053	3 434 464	2 589 878	666 758
1990 [4]	4 092 994	595 073	385 640	58 807	11 311	83 008	56 307	3 457 417	2 626 500	661 701
1989 [5]	3 903 012	532 249	327 233	56 229	10 842	72 443	65 502	3 297 493	2 526 367	611 269
Birth Rate										
2003 [6]	14.1	22.9	24.7	15.1	9.9	23.0	(6)	12.7	11.8	15.9
2002 [6]	13.9	22.6	24.2	16.5	10.0	22.4	(6)	12.6	11.7	16.1
2001 [6]	14.1	23.0	24.8	17.8	10.3	21.8	(6)	12.8	11.8	16.6
2000 [6]	14.4	23.1	25.0	18.1	9.7	21.8	(6)	13.2	12.2	17.3
1999 [6]	14.2	22.5	24.2	18.0	9.4	21.7	(6)	13.0	12.1	17.1
1998 [6]	14.3	22.7	24.6	17.9	9.7	21.7	(6)	13.2	12.2	17.5
1997 [6]	14.2	23.0	25.3	17.2	10.0	21.3	(6)	13.1	12.2	17.4
1996 [6]	14.4	23.8	26.2	17.2	10.6	22.5	(6)	13.3	12.3	17.6
1995 [6]	14.6	24.1	25.8	19.0	10.8	24.2	(6)	13.5	12.5	18.2
1994 [6]	15.0	24.7	26.1	20.8	10.7	24.9	(6)	13.9	12.8	19.5
1993 [6]	15.4	25.4	26.8	21.5	10.5	26.3	(6)	14.3	13.1	20.7
1992 [6,7]	15.8	26.1	27.4	22.9	10.1	27.5	(6)	14.8	13.4	21.6
1991 [6,7]	16.2	26.5	27.6	23.3	9.8	28.3	(6)	15.2	13.9	22.4
1990 [4,6]	16.7	26.7	28.7	21.6	10.9	27.5	(6)	15.7	14.4	23.0
1989 [5,6]	16.3	26.2	25.7	23.7	10.0	28.3	(6)	15.4	14.2	22.8
Fertility Rate										
2003 [6]	66.1	96.9	105.5	61.6	61.7	91.2	(6)	60.5	58.5	67.1
2002 [6]	64.8	94.4	102.8	65.4	59.0	86.1	(6)	59.6	57.4	67.4
2001 [6]	65.3	96.0	105.7	72.2	56.7	82.7	(6)	60.1	57.7	69.1
2000 [6]	65.9	95.9	105.1	73.5	49.3	85.1	(6)	61.1	58.5	71.4
1999 [6]	64.4	93.0	101.5	71.1	47.0	84.8	(6)	60.0	57.7	69.9
1998 [6]	64.3	93.2	103.2	69.7	46.5	83.5	(6)	60.0	57.6	70.9
1997 [6]	63.6	94.2	106.6	65.8	53.1	80.6	(6)	59.3	56.8	70.3
1996 [6]	64.1	97.5	110.7	66.5	55.1	84.2	(6)	59.6	57.1	70.7
1995 [6]	64.6	98.8	109.9	71.3	52.2	89.1	(6)	60.2	57.5	72.8
1994 [6]	65.9	100.7	109.9	78.2	53.6	93.2	(6)	61.6	58.2	77.5
1993 [6]	67.0	103.3	110.9	79.8	53.9	101.5	(6)	62.7	58.9	81.5
1992 [6,7]	68.4	106.1	113.3	87.9	49.4	104.7	(6)	64.2	60.0	84.5
1991 [6,7]	69.3	106.9	114.9	87.9	47.6	105.5	(6)	65.2	60.9	87.0
1990 [4,6]	71.0	107.7	118.9	82.9	52.6	102.7	(6)	67.1	62.8	89.0
1989 [5,6]	69.2	104.9	106.6	86.6	49.8	95.8	(6)	65.7	60.5	84.8

Note: Race and Hispanic origin are reported separately on birth certificates. Persons of Hispanic origin may be of any race. In this table, Hispanic women are classified only by place of origin; non-Hispanic women are classified by race.

[1] Includes origin not stated.
[2] Includes races other than White and Black.
[3] Excludes data for New Hampshire, which did not report Hispanic origin.
[4] Excludes data for New Hampshire and Oklahoma, which did not report Hispanic origin.
[5] Excludes data for Louisiana, New Hampshire, and Oklahoma, which did not report Hispanic origin.
[6] Rates for the Central and South American population includes other and unknown Hispanic.
[7] Rates are estimated for the United States based on birth data for 49 states and the District of Columbia. Births for New Hampshire, which did not report Hispanic origin, are included in the rates for non-Hispanic women.

TABLE I-7. LIVE BIRTHS, BY AGE, LIVE-BIRTH ORDER, SPECIFIED HISPANIC ORIGIN, AND RACE OF MOTHER, 2003

This table shows the number of births by mothers in various age and birth order categories. (See Table I-2A for preliminary data from 2004.) Detail is provided for countries of origin for Hispanics, and rates are given for non-Hispanic Whites and non-Hispanic Blacks. The organization of the data is similar to that in Table I-2. The ethnic and racial categories reflect those in Table I-6.

Table I-7. Live Births, by Age, Live-Birth Order, Specified Hispanic Origin, and Race of Mother, 2003

(Number of children born alive to mother, includes births with stated origin of mother only.)

Live-birth order and origin of mother	All ages	Under 15 years	15–19 years Total	15 years	16 years	17 years	18 years	19 years	20–24 years	25–29 years	30–34 years	35–39 years	40–44 years	45–49 years	50–54 years
HISPANIC															
Total	912 329	2 356	128 524	6 818	15 151	24 986	35 927	45 642	273 311	246 361	169 054	75 801	16 172	738	12
1st child	330 032	2 299	98 961	6 519	13 784	20 918	27 208	30 532	117 279	64 418	33 173	11 638	2 141	122	1
2nd child	280 462	47	24 661	257	1 264	3 627	7 431	12 082	98 707	85 060	49 833	18 733	3 296	122	3
3rd child	175 225	1	3 993	16	66	341	1 059	2 511	41 204	60 095	46 009	20 158	3 618	146	1
4th child	76 317	1	484	2	4	26	105	347	11 768	24 359	24 007	12 700	2 887	108	3
5th child	28 959	-	53	-	1	2	9	41	2 812	8 148	9 527	6 568	1 771	78	2
6th child	10 928	-	8	1	-	1	2	4	598	2 452	3 678	3 071	1 053	67	1
7th child	4 489	-	1	-	1	-	-	-	128	840	1 416	1 457	613	33	1
8th child and over	3 545	-	2	-	-	-	-	2	58	374	1 031	1 279	740	61	-
Not stated	2 372	8	361	23	31	71	113	123	757	615	380	197	53	1	-
Mexican	654 504	1 842	98 396	5 274	11 741	19 252	27 538	34 591	203 314	177 499	115 033	48 120	9 858	435	7
1st child	227 447	1 799	74 989	5 043	10 643	15 986	20 603	22 714	84 114	41 396	18 402	5 732	966	48	1
2nd child	198 082	34	19 483	200	1 010	2 910	5 902	9 461	74 905	60 948	31 196	9 884	1 569	61	2
3rd child	130 702	1	3 224	13	57	278	863	2 013	31 767	46 404	33 855	13 232	2 143	75	1
4th child	58 997	1	393	2	4	23	85	279	9 143	19 114	18 942	9 384	1 955	64	1
5th child	22 709	-	45	-	1	2	8	34	2 202	6 368	7 589	5 132	1 317	56	-
6th child	8 509	-	8	1	-	1	2	4	485	1 883	2 876	2 412	794	50	1
7th child	3 600	-	1	-	1	-	-	-	112	678	1 123	1 181	477	27	1
8th child and over	2 819	-	2	-	-	-	-	2	47	288	794	1 030	604	54	-
Not stated	1 639	7	251	15	25	52	75	84	539	420	256	133	33	-	-
Puerto Rican	58 400	191	10 239	579	1 203	2 038	2 804	3 615	19 004	14 169	9 301	4 515	934	47	-
1st child	22 913	189	7 980	558	1 105	1 740	2 137	2 440	7 697	3 727	2 255	872	184	9	-
2nd child	18 020	2	1 890	18	96	269	569	938	6 672	4 734	3 043	1 406	261	12	-
3rd child	10 222	-	288	1	2	20	73	192	3 210	3 291	2 113	1 114	199	7	-
4th child	4 262	-	48	-	-	2	12	34	1 038	1 466	1 000	562	142	6	-
5th child	1 629	-	1	-	-	-	1	-	266	546	466	277	65	8	-
6th child	705	-	-	-	-	-	-	-	48	246	222	146	42	1	-
7th child	260	-	-	-	-	-	-	-	11	77	96	59	16	1	-
8th child and over	220	-	-	-	-	-	-	-	3	44	82	67	22	2	-
Not stated	169	-	32	2	-	7	12	11	59	38	24	12	3	1	-
Cuban	14 867	15	1 162	36	104	209	339	474	2 608	3 966	4 298	2 283	511	24	-
1st child	6 969	14	990	35	99	193	286	377	1 585	1 966	1 623	652	131	8	-
2nd child	5 283	1	148	1	5	12	43	87	760	1 404	1 835	951	178	6	-
3rd child	1 885	-	18	-	-	3	8	7	207	440	639	465	109	7	-
4th child	493	-	1	-	-	-	-	1	41	120	146	130	53	2	-
5th child	130	-	1	-	-	-	-	1	10	20	33	45	20	1	-
6th child	54	-	-	-	-	-	-	-	1	8	13	23	9	-	-
7th child	20	-	-	-	-	-	-	-	-	4	5	6	5	-	-
8th child and over	15	-	-	-	-	-	-	-	-	2	-	8	5	-	-
Not stated	18	-	4	-	-	1	2	1	4	2	4	3	1	-	-
Central and South American	135 586	152	11 119	440	1 140	2 009	3 204	4 326	33 588	38 505	31 448	16 629	3 960	183	2
1st child	53 522	148	9 096	422	1 050	1 761	2 599	3 264	17 692	13 780	8 615	3 462	689	40	-
2nd child	43 849	4	1 749	16	84	223	532	894	11 133	13 816	10 794	5 269	1 051	33	-
3rd child	23 856	-	227	-	1	21	63	142	3 663	7 279	7 339	4 306	996	46	-
4th child	8 940	-	19	-	-	-	3	16	822	2 464	2 951	2 058	595	30	1
5th child	3 205	-	3	-	-	-	-	3	168	807	1 072	850	292	12	1
6th child	1 170	-	-	-	-	-	-	-	27	203	399	372	155	14	-
7th child	430	-	-	-	-	-	-	-	3	43	131	157	92	4	-
8th child and over	335	-	-	-	-	-	-	-	7	21	97	124	82	4	-
Not stated	279	-	25	2	5	4	7	7	73	92	50	31	8	-	-
Other and Unknown Hispanic	48 972	156	7 608	489	963	1 478	2 042	2 636	14 797	12 222	8 974	4 254	909	49	3
1st child	19 181	149	5 906	461	887	1 238	1 583	1 737	6 191	3 549	2 278	920	171	17	-
2nd child	15 228	6	1 391	22	69	213	385	702	5 237	4 158	2 965	1 223	237	10	1
3rd child	8 560	-	236	2	6	19	52	157	2 357	2 681	2 063	1 041	171	11	-
4th child	3 625	-	23	-	-	1	5	17	724	1 195	968	566	142	6	1
5th child	1 286	-	3	-	-	-	-	3	166	407	367	264	77	1	1
6th child	490	-	-	-	-	-	-	-	37	112	168	118	53	2	-
7th child	179	-	-	-	-	-	-	-	2	38	61	54	23	1	-
8th child and over	156	-	-	-	-	-	-	-	1	19	58	50	27	1	-
Not stated	267	1	49	4	1	7	17	20	82	63	46	18	8	-	-

Note: Race and Hispanic origin are reported separately on birth certificates. Persons of Hispanic origin may be of any race. In this table, Hispanic women are classified only by place of origin; non-Hispanic women are classified by race.

- = Quantity zero.

Table I-7. Live Births, by Age, Live-Birth Order, Specified Hispanic Origin, and Race of Mother, 2003
—Continued

(Number of children born alive to mother, includes births with stated origin of mother only.)

Live-birth order and origin of mother	All ages	Under 15 years	15–19 years						20–24 years	25–29 years	30–34 years	35–39 years	40–44 years	45–49 years	50–54 years
			Total	15 years	16 years	17 years	18 years	19 years							
NON-HISPANIC															
Total [1]	3 149 034	4 258	283 602	11 317	25 956	49 350	81 111	115 868	752 607	832 783	799 179	387 807	83 812	4 689	297
1st child	1 292 838	4 171	229 334	10 910	24 164	43 361	65 861	85 038	361 482	327 158	252 813	96 684	19 849	1 257	90
2nd child	1 031 628	74	45 498	368	1 614	5 425	13 054	25 037	251 100	279 333	296 055	133 018	25 224	1 258	68
3rd child	504 732	3	7 148	10	98	423	1 800	4 817	100 098	141 324	151 304	86 893	17 162	756	44
4th child	189 495	-	832	3	8	30	164	627	28 719	53 773	58 077	38 211	9 387	464	32
5th child	67 577	-	107	1	-	3	26	77	7 150	18 696	21 369	15 251	4 687	296	21
6th child	27 525	-	14	-	-	-	3	11	1 608	6 660	9 237	7 252	2 561	178	15
7th child	12 679	-	3	-	-	-	3	-	370	2 456	4 305	3 947	1 473	119	6
8th child and over	14 337	-	5	-	-	-	2	3	123	1 303	4 005	5 385	3 155	343	18
Not stated	8 223	10	661	25	72	108	198	258	1 957	2 080	2 014	1 166	314	18	3
White	2 321 904	1 399	172 620	4 878	13 375	28 550	50 484	75 333	522 275	627 437	626 315	303 354	64 600	3 660	244
1st child	961 897	1 384	144 011	4 754	12 743	25 917	42 636	57 961	264 696	256 719	200 974	77 145	15 872	1 022	74
2nd child	780 026	12	24 817	111	585	2 424	6 958	14 739	62 118	103 249	119 674	69 039	13 142	573	38
3rd child	370 971	1	3 137	3	17	144	725	2 248	14 613	34 879	43 045	29 324	7 106	352	26
4th child	129 615	-	270	1	2	7	49	211	2 879	14 269	14 269	10 930	3 404	218	20
5th child	42 120	-	36	-	-	1	11	24	496	3 093	5 580	4 833	1 789	128	11
6th child	15 932	-	2	-	-	-	1	1	112	927	2 430	2 597	1 048	82	4
7th child	7 201	-	1	-	-	-	1	-	49	439	2 006	3 481	2 391	267	8
8th child and over	8 643	-	2	-	-	-	1	1	1 197	1 413	1 434	875	218	14	2
Not stated	5 499	2	344	9	28	57	102	148	1 197	1 413	1 434	875	218	14	2
Black	576 033	2 642	97 509	5 852	11 247	18 431	26 915	35 064	189 020	133 821	93 346	47 661	11 419	588	27
1st child	217 190	2 572	74 576	5 590	10 193	15 383	20 298	23 112	74 504	33 589	20 636	9 106	2 084	117	6
2nd child	167 441	61	18 414	240	931	2 723	5 437	9 083	62 774	41 512	28 434	13 263	2 849	130	4
3rd child	101 657	1	3 648	7	76	259	976	2 330	33 281	30 174	20 938	11 055	2 446	110	4
4th child	48 203	-	509	2	6	20	104	377	12 602	15 816	11 272	6 368	1 560	72	4
5th child	20 934	-	64	-	-	2	14	48	3 902	7 124	5 590	3 242	960	51	1
6th child	9 547	-	10	-	-	-	1	9	1 019	3 062	2 947	1 878	595	35	1
7th child	4 488	-	2	-	-	-	2	-	235	1 316	1 539	1 051	319	24	2
8th child and over	4 555	-	3	-	-	-	1	2	64	762	1 633	1 497	545	46	5
Not stated	2 018	8	283	13	41	44	82	103	639	466	357	201	61	3	-

Note: Race and Hispanic origin are reported separately on birth certificates. Persons of Hispanic origin may be of any race. In this table, Hispanic women are classified only by place of origin; non-Hispanic women are classified by race.

[1] Includes races other than White and Black.
- = Quantity zero.

TABLE I-8. FERTILITY RATES AND BIRTH RATES, BY AGE, LIVE-BIRTH ORDER, SPECIFIED HISPANIC ORIGIN, AND RACE OF MOTHER, 2003

This table converts the number of births shown in Table I-7 into general fertility and birth rates. It highlights the high fertility rate (105.5) of Mexican-origin mothers. This can be compared to a rate of 58.5 for non-Hispanic White mothers. The fertility rate of all Hispanics averaged 96.9 in 2003, well exceeding rates for non-Hispanic Whites and non-Hispanic Blacks. Hispanic birth rates were especially high for mothers under 25 years old. The average birth rates for non-Hispanic Whites prior to age 25 averaged less than half the rate for Hispanics of the same age; those of non-Hispanic Black mothers fell in between the two. For those age 25 years old and over, these differences narrowed considerably. The birth rates for non-Hispanic Whites, although below those of Hispanic mothers, peaked at 25 to 29 years old—making them somewhat higher than those of non-Hispanic Blacks.

Table I-8. Fertility Rates and Birth Rates, by Age, Live-Birth Order, Specified Hispanic Origin, and Race of Mother, 2003

(Live births per 1,000 women in specified age and racial group.)

Live-birth order and race of mother	Fertility rate [1]	10–14 years	15–19 years Total	15–17 years	18–19 years	20–24 years	25–29 years	30–34 years	35–39 years	40–44 years	45–49 years [2]
HISPANIC											
Total	96.9	1.3	82.3	49.7	132.0	163.4	144.4	102.0	50.8	12.2	0.7
1st child	35.2	1.3	63.5	43.8	93.7	70.3	37.8	20.1	7.8	1.6	0.1
2nd child	29.9	0.0	15.8	5.5	31.7	59.2	50.0	30.1	12.6	2.5	0.1
3rd child	18.7	*	2.6	0.4	5.8	24.7	35.3	27.8	13.5	2.7	0.1
4th child	8.1	*	0.3	0.0	0.7	7.1	14.3	14.5	8.5	2.2	0.1
5th child	3.1	*	0.0	*	0.1	1.7	4.8	5.8	4.4	1.3	0.1
6th and 7th child	1.6	*	*	*	*	0.4	1.9	3.1	3.0	1.3	0.1
8th child and over	0.4	*	*	*	*	0.0	0.2	0.6	0.9	0.6	0.1
Mexican	105.5	1.5	93.2	56.9	148.8	176.9	151.5	104.7	50.2	12.8	0.7
1st child	36.8	1.4	71.2	49.8	104.0	73.4	35.4	16.8	6.0	1.3	0.1
2nd child	32.0	0.0	18.5	6.5	36.9	65.3	52.1	28.5	10.3	2.0	0.1
3rd child	21.1	*	3.1	0.5	6.9	27.7	39.7	30.9	13.8	2.8	0.1
4th child	9.5	*	0.4	0.0	0.9	8.0	16.3	17.3	9.8	2.6	0.1
5th child	3.7	*	0.0	*	0.1	1.9	5.4	6.9	5.4	1.7	0.1
6th and 7th child	2.0	*	*	*	*	0.5	2.2	3.6	3.8	1.7	0.1
8th child and over	0.5	*	*	*	*	0.0	0.2	0.7	1.1	0.8	0.1
Puerto Rican	61.6	1.0	60.8	35.9	*	127.9	86.6	55.6	29.5	6.4	0.4
1st child	24.3	1.0	47.5	32.1	*	52.0	22.8	13.5	5.7	1.3	*
2nd child	19.1	*	11.3	3.6	*	45.1	29.0	18.3	9.2	1.8	*
3rd child	10.8	*	1.7	0.2	*	21.7	20.2	12.7	7.3	1.4	*
4th child	4.5	*	0.3	*	*	7.0	9.0	6.0	3.7	1.0	*
5th child	1.7	*	*	*	*	1.8	3.3	2.8	1.8	0.4	*
6th and 7th child	1.0	*	*	*	*	0.4	2.0	1.9	1.3	0.4	*
8th child and over	0.2	*	*	*	*	*	0.3	0.5	0.4	0.1	*
Cuban	61.7	*	*	*	*	*	*	*	*	*	*
1st child	29.0	*	*	*	*	*	*	*	*	*	*
2nd child	22.0	*	*	*	*	*	*	*	*	*	*
3rd child	7.8	*	*	*	*	*	*	*	*	*	*
4th child	2.1	*	*	*	*	*	*	*	*	*	*
5th child	0.5	*	*	*	*	*	*	*	*	*	*
6th and 7th child	0.3	*	*	*	*	*	*	*	*	*	*
8th child and over	*	*	*	*	*	*	*	*	*	*	*
Other Hispanic [3]	91.2	1.0	60.4	36.4	93.1	142.2	152.8	112.3	63.2	13.9	0.8
1st child	36.0	1.0	48.6	32.6	70.3	70.4	52.3	30.3	13.3	2.5	0.2
2nd child	29.3	*	10.2	3.5	19.2	48.3	54.3	38.3	19.7	3.7	0.2
3rd child	16.1	*	1.5	0.3	3.2	17.7	30.1	26.2	16.2	3.3	0.2
4th child	6.2	*	0.1	*	0.3	4.6	11.1	10.9	8.0	2.1	0.1
5th child	2.2	*	*	*	*	1.0	3.7	4.0	3.4	1.1	*
6th and 7th child	1.1	*	*	*	*	0.2	1.2	2.1	2.1	0.9	0.1
8th child and over	0.2	*	*	*	*	*	0.1	0.4	0.5	0.3	*
NON-HISPANIC [4]											
Total [5]	60.5	0.5	34.1	17.3	59.4	90.5	109.2	93.8	42.6	8.3	0.5
1st child	24.9	0.5	27.6	15.7	45.6	43.5	43.0	29.8	10.7	2.0	0.1
2nd child	19.9	0.0	5.5	1.5	11.5	30.3	36.7	34.8	14.7	2.5	0.1
3rd child	9.7	*	0.9	0.1	2.0	12.1	18.6	17.8	9.6	1.7	0.1
4th child	3.7	*	0.1	0.0	0.2	3.5	7.1	6.8	4.2	0.9	0.1
5th child	1.3	*	0.0	*	0.0	0.9	2.5	2.5	1.7	0.5	0.0
6th and 7th child	0.8	*	*	*	*	0.2	1.2	1.6	1.2	0.4	0.0
8th child and over	0.3	*	*	*	*	0.0	0.2	0.5	0.6	0.3	0.0
White	58.5	0.2	27.4	12.4	50.0	83.5	110.8	97.6	43.2	8.1	0.5
1st child	24.3	0.2	22.9	11.5	40.1	42.4	45.5	31.4	11.0	2.0	0.1
2nd child	19.7	*	4.0	0.8	8.7	28.2	38.3	37.0	15.0	2.5	0.1
3rd child	9.4	*	0.5	0.0	1.2	10.0	18.3	18.7	9.9	1.6	0.1
4th child	3.3	*	0.0	*	0.1	2.3	6.2	6.7	4.2	0.9	0.0
5th child	1.1	*	0.0	*	0.0	0.5	1.8	2.2	1.6	0.4	0.0
6th and 7th child	0.6	*	*	*	*	0.1	0.7	1.3	1.1	0.4	0.0
8th child and over	0.2	*	*	*	*	0.0	0.1	0.3	0.5	0.3	0.0
Black	67.1	1.6	64.7	38.7	105.3	128.1	102.1	67.4	33.4	7.7	0.5
1st child	25.4	1.6	49.7	34.1	74.0	50.7	25.7	15.0	6.4	1.4	0.1
2nd child	19.6	0.0	12.2	4.3	24.7	42.7	31.7	20.6	9.3	1.9	0.1
3rd child	11.9	*	2.4	0.4	5.6	22.6	23.1	15.2	7.8	1.7	0.1
4th child	5.6	*	0.3	0.0	0.8	8.6	12.1	8.2	4.5	1.1	0.1
5th child	2.5	*	0.0	*	0.1	2.7	5.5	4.1	2.3	0.7	0.0
6th and 7th child	1.6	*	*	*	*	0.9	3.4	3.3	2.1	0.6	0.0
8th child and over	0.5	*	*	*	*	0.0	0.6	1.2	1.1	0.4	0.0

Note: Race and Hispanic origin are reported separately on birth certificates. Persons of Hispanic origin may be of any race. In this table, Hispanic women are classified only by place of origin; non-Hispanic women are classified by race. Figures for live-birth order not stated are distributed.

[1] Fertility rates computed by relating total births, regardless of age of mother, to women age 15–44 years.
[2] Birth rates computed by relating births to women age 45–54 years to women age 45–49 years.
[3] Includes Central and South American and other and unknown Hispanic.
[4] Includes origin not stated.
[5] Includes races other than White and Black.
0.0 = Quantity more than zero but less than 0.05.
* = Figure does not meet standards of reliability or precision; based on fewer than 20 births in the numerator or, for the Hispanic subgroups, fewer than 75,000 women in the denominator.

TABLE I-9. TOTAL FERTILITY RATES, FERTILITY RATES, AND BIRTH RATES, BY AGE, SPECIFIED HISPANIC ORIGIN, AND RACE OF MOTHER, 1989–2003

This table is similar in organization to Table I-4; it shows the Total Fertility rate, or TFR (see comment for Table I-4 for definition), the general fertility rate, and birth rates by age of mother. (See Table I-2A for preliminary data from 2004.) Time series from 1989 onward are presented, in contrast to Table I-4's starting date of 1970. The focus of Table I-9 is on Hispanics (and subgroups of Hispanics); these groups are compared to non-Hispanic Whites and Blacks. As would be expected, the TFR of Hispanics in 2003 was high, at 2,786 per 1,000 women over the course of their childbearing years. This can be compared to averages of 2,028 for non-Hispanic Blacks and 1,856 for non-Hispanic Whites. Although the TFR for most groups was below the "replacement rate," it was above the replacement rate (2,100 births per 1,000 women) for Mexican and "other" Hispanics (mostly those from Central and South America).

The TFR of Hispanics has declined moderately since the early 1990s, although the Cuban subgroup has experienced an upward trend. The TFR of non-Hispanic Blacks also declined, but the rate for non-Hispanic Whites stayed roughly the same.

The drop in teenage birth rates, previously noted in Table I-4, occurred widely among both race and ethnic groups. The data since 1989 have shown the drop to be especially pronounced among non-Hispanic teenagers. Although Hispanics also contributed to the overall decline, the birth rate for Hispanic teenagers has remained considerably higher than those for other groups. This was partly caused by the very high teenage birth rates among Mexicans. Large declines in birth rates occurred among the 15- to 17-year-old subgroup. The decline in this age group was large for non-Hispanics and particularly for non-Hispanic Blacks.

As indicated in Table I-4, the birth rates for women in their thirties and forties have been increasing since 1989, while the birth rates for women in the twenties have moderated. Non-Hispanic Blacks and Whites and Hispanics all experienced these trends.

Table I-9. Total Fertility Rates, Fertility Rates, and Birth Rates, by Age, Specified Hispanic Origin, and Race of Mother, 1989–2003

(Live births per 1,000 women in specified age and racial group.)

Year and origin/race of mother	Total fertility rate[1]	Fertility rate[2]	Age of mother									
			10–14 years	15–19 years			20–24 years	25–29 years	30–34 years	35–39 years	40–44 years	45–49 years[3]
				Total	15–17 years	18–19 years						
ALL ORIGINS												
2003	2 042.5	66.1	0.6	41.6	22.4	70.7	102.6	115.6	95.1	43.8	8.7	0.5
2002	2 013.0	64.8	0.7	43.0	23.2	72.8	103.6	113.6	91.5	41.4	8.3	0.5
2001	2 034.0	65.3	0.8	45.3	24.7	76.1	106.2	113.4	91.9	40.6	8.1	0.5
2000	2 056.0	65.9	0.9	47.7	26.9	78.1	109.7	113.5	91.2	39.7	8.0	0.5
1999	2 007.5	64.4	0.9	48.8	28.2	79.1	107.9	111.2	87.1	37.8	7.4	0.4
1998	1 999.0	64.3	1.0	50.3	29.9	80.9	108.4	110.2	85.2	36.9	7.4	0.4
1997	1 971.0	63.6	1.1	51.3	31.4	82.1	107.3	108.3	83.0	35.7	7.1	0.4
1996	1 976.0	64.1	1.2	53.5	33.3	84.7	107.8	108.6	82.1	34.9	6.8	0.3
1995	1 978.0	64.6	1.3	56.0	35.5	87.7	107.5	108.8	81.1	34.0	6.6	0.3
1994	2 001.5	65.9	1.4	58.2	37.2	90.2	109.2	111.0	80.4	33.4	6.4	0.3
1993	2 019.5	67.0	1.4	59.0	37.5	91.1	111.3	113.2	79.9	32.7	6.1	0.3
1992	2 046.0	68.4	1.4	60.3	37.6	93.6	113.7	115.7	79.6	32.3	5.9	0.3
1991	2 062.5	69.3	1.4	61.8	38.6	94.0	115.3	117.2	79.2	31.9	5.5	0.2
1990	2 081.0	70.9	1.4	59.9	37.5	88.6	116.5	120.2	80.8	31.7	5.5	0.2
1989	2 014.0	69.2	1.4	57.3	36.4	84.2	113.8	117.6	77.4	29.9	5.2	0.2
HISPANIC												
Total												
2003	2 785.5	96.9	1.3	82.3	49.7	132.0	163.4	144.4	102.0	50.8	12.2	0.7
2002	2 718.0	94.4	1.4	83.4	50.7	133.0	164.3	139.4	95.1	47.8	11.5	0.7
2001	2 748.5	96.0	1.6	86.4	52.8	135.5	163.5	140.4	97.6	47.9	11.6	0.7
2000	2 730.0	95.9	1.7	87.3	55.5	132.6	161.3	139.9	97.1	46.6	11.5	0.6
1999	2 649.0	93.0	1.9	86.8	56.9	129.5	157.3	135.8	92.3	44.5	10.6	0.6
1998	2 652.5	93.2	1.9	87.9	58.5	131.5	159.3	136.1	90.5	43.4	10.8	0.6
1997	2 680.5	94.2	2.1	89.6	61.1	132.4	162.6	137.5	89.6	43.4	10.7	0.6
1996	2 772.0	97.5	2.4	94.6	64.2	140.0	170.2	140.7	91.3	43.9	10.7	0.6
1995	2 798.5	98.8	2.6	99.3	68.3	145.4	171.9	140.4	90.5	43.7	10.7	0.6
1994	2 839.0	100.7	2.6	101.3	69.9	147.5	175.7	142.4	91.1	43.4	10.7	0.6
1993	2 894.5	103.3	2.6	101.8	68.5	151.1	180.0	146.0	93.2	44.1	10.6	0.6
1992 [4]	2 957.5	106.1	2.5	103.3	68.9	153.9	185.2	148.8	94.8	45.3	11.0	0.6
1991 [4]	2 963.5	106.9	2.4	104.6	69.2	155.5	184.6	150.0	95.1	44.7	10.7	0.6
1990 [5]	2 959.5	107.7	2.4	100.3	65.9	147.7	181.0	153.0	98.3	45.3	10.9	0.7
1989 [6]	2 903.5	104.9	2.3	100.8	. . .	. . .	184.4	146.6	92.1	43.5	10.4	0.6
Mexican												
2003	2 957.5	105.5	1.5	93.2	56.9	148.8	176.9	151.5	104.7	50.2	12.8	0.7
2002	2 879.5	102.8	1.5	94.5	58.6	147.5	176.9	144.5	97.9	47.5	12.3	0.8
2001	2 928.5	105.7	1.7	95.4	59.3	147.0	177.0	146.4	101.9	50.0	12.6	0.7
2000	2 906.5	105.1	1.9	95.4	60.6	146.7	174.9	144.7	102.3	49.2	12.2	0.7
1999	2 823.0	101.5	2.1	94.3	60.8	145.6	170.8	141.4	97.4	47.2	10.7	0.7
1998	2 878.0	103.2	2.1	96.4	62.9	149.2	176.5	147.4	94.9	46.9	10.8	0.6
1997	2 957.0	106.6	2.3	103.4	71.3	151.6	180.9	150.0	95.3	47.4	11.5	0.6
1996	3 052.0	110.7	2.6	112.2	77.7	161.6	185.3	154.7	96.5	46.4	12.0	0.7
1995	3 033.5	109.9	2.7	115.9	79.1	170.7	190.4	146.6	93.0	45.5	11.9	0.7
1994	3 024.0	109.9	2.7	109.2	73.6	163.3	189.1	153.6	92.5	45.3	11.7	0.7
1993	3 041.5	110.9	2.5	103.6	68.4	156.6	187.9	159.5	97.2	45.5	11.3	0.8
1992 [4]	3 107.0	113.3	2.4	105.1	. . .	. . .	196.6	160.2	97.1	47.4	11.8	0.8
1991 [4]	3 103.5	114.9	2.5	108.3	70.0	164.7	192.4	156.1	99.7	49.1	11.9	0.7
1990 [5]	3 214.0	118.9	2.5	108.0	69.7	162.2	200.3	165.3	104.4	49.1	12.4	0.8
1989 [6]	2 916.5	106.6	2.0	94.5	. . .	. . .	184.3	153.7	96.1	41.0	11.1	0.6

Note: Race and Hispanic origin are reported separately on birth certificates. Persons of Hispanic origin may be of any race. In this table, Hispanic women are classified only by place of origin; non-Hispanic women are classified by race.

[1]Total fertility rates are sums of birth rates for 5-year age groups multiplied by 5.
[2]Fertility rates computed by relating total births, regardless of age of mother, to women 15–44 years old.
[3]Beginning in 1997, rates computed by relating births to women age 45–54 years to women 45–49 years old.
[4]Excludes data for New Hampshire, which did not report Hispanic origin.
[5]Excludes data for New Hampshire and Oklahoma, which did not report Hispanic origin.
[6]Excludes data for Louisiana, New Hampshire, and Oklahoma, which did not report Hispanic origin.
. . . = Not available.

Table I-9. Total Fertility Rates, Fertility Rates, and Birth Rates, by Age, Specified Hispanic Origin, and Race of Mother, 1989–2003—Continued

(Live births per 1,000 women in specified age and racial group.)

Year and origin/race of mother	Total fertility rate[1]	Fertility rate[2]	10–14 years	15–19 years Total	15–17 years	18–19 years	20–24 years	25–29 years	30–34 years	35–39 years	40–44 years	45–49 years[3]
Puerto Rican												
2003	1 841.0	61.6	1.0	60.8	35.9	*	127.9	86.6	55.6	29.5	6.4	0.4
2002	1 947.5	65.4	1.4	61.4	39.7	*	136.5	90.6	61.5	31.3	6.3	0.5
2001	2 165.0	72.2	1.7	82.2	*	*	147.2	93.6	70.5	30.7	6.7	0.4
2000	2 178.5	73.5	1.7	82.9	54.7	120.4	149.5	101.6	61.1	32.0	6.6	0.3
1999	2 104.5	71.1	1.6	74.0	49.4	*	146.0	106.5	58.0	27.3	7.2	0.3
1998	2 043.5	69.7	1.8	76.2	51.7	*	146.7	88.7	61.9	25.8	7.2	0.4
1997	1 931.5	65.8	1.7	68.9	45.0	*	136.0	92.9	54.1	26.1	6.2	0.4
1996	1 965.0	66.5	1.9	76.5	48.6	*	133.7	95.6	54.3	25.2	5.6	*
1995	2 078.0	71.3	2.9	82.8	57.3	*	138.1	97.9	61.2	26.9	5.5	0.3
1994	2 341.5	78.2	3.1	99.6	68.8	*	169.0	103.8	59.5	27.5	5.6	0.2
1993	2 416.0	79.8	3.1	104.9	70.1	*	184.6	102.8	54.4	26.7	6.2	*
1992[4]	2 568.5	87.9	3.4	106.5	. . .	. . .	199.1	102.6	65.3	29.9	6.6	*
1991[4]	2 573.5	87.9	2.7	111.0	*	*	193.3	108.9	68.1	23.9	6.5	*
1990[5]	2 301.0	82.9	2.9	101.6	71.6	141.6	150.1	109.9	62.8	26.2	6.2	0.5
1989[6]	2 421.0	86.6	3.8	112.7	. . .	. . .	171.0	98.0	65.2	26.9	6.3	*
Cuban												
2003	2 059.5	61.7	*	*	*	*	*	*	*	*	*	*
2002	1 940.5	59.0	*	*	*	*	*	*	*	*	*	*
2001	1 792.5	56.7	*	*	*	*	*	*	*	*	*	*
2000	1 528.0	49.3	*	23.5	14.2	43.4	64.2	104.0	68.1	37.3	7.9	*
1999	1 388.5	47.0	*	*	*	*	*	*	*	*	*	*
1998	1 402.5	46.5	*	*	*	*	*	*	*	*	*	*
1997	1 619.5	53.1	*	*	*	*	*	*	*	*	*	*
1996	1 617.0	55.1	*	*	*	*	*	*	*	*	*	*
1995	1 584.0	52.2	*	*	*	*	*	*	*	*	*	*
1994	1 587.0	53.6	*	*	*	*	*	*	*	*	*	*
1993	1 570.0	53.9	*	*	*	*	*	*	*	*	*	*
1992[4]	1 453.5	49.4	*	*	. . .	. . .	*	*	*	*	*	*
1991[4]	1 352.5	47.6	*	*	*	*	*	*	*	*	*	*
1990[5]	1 459.5	52.6	*	30.3	18.2	46.1	64.6	95.4	67.6	28.2	4.9	*
1989[6]	1 479.0	49.8	*	*	. . .	. . .	*	*	*	*	*	*
Other Hispanic[7]												
2003	2 733.0	91.2	1.0	60.4	36.4	93.1	142.2	152.8	112.3	63.2	13.9	0.8
2002	2 610.5	86.1	1.1	63.0	34.7	110.3	143.3	147.2	98.4	56.1	12.2	0.8
2001	2 519.5	82.7	1.1	65.3	35.6	115.2	136.0	143.3	95.4	50.3	11.6	0.9
2000	2 563.5	85.1	1.2	69.9	44.4	102.0	133.2	143.9	103.6	47.7	12.5	0.7
1999	2 517.0	84.8	1.5	75.5	53.1	100.5	130.2	138.4	98.3	46.5	12.3	0.7
1998	2 448.5	83.5	1.8	75.0	53.3	100.3	122.7	133.6	97.8	45.4	12.8	0.6
1997	2 376.5	80.6	1.8	66.4	44.5	98.0	129.3	125.8	95.6	43.9	11.8	0.7
1996	2 516.5	84.2	2.2	64.8	43.4	95.6	149.6	127.9	98.0	49.1	11.0	0.7
1995	2 629.5	89.1	2.3	72.1	51.3	99.4	144.3	147.7	97.9	49.4	11.6	0.6
1994	2 693.0	93.2	2.5	82.6	62.7	105.0	151.2	137.0	104.4	48.4	11.9	0.6
1993	2 914.5	101.5	2.6	102.0	74.7	134.6	167.5	139.4	106.7	51.7	12.5	0.5
1992[4]	2 989.0	104.7	2.4	108.2	. . .	. . .	168.0	151.9	104.4	49.9	12.5	0.5
1991[4]	3 064.5	105.5	2.2	100.7	67.3	145.6	184.1	164.5	100.2	49.2	11.4	0.6
1990[5]	2 877.0	102.7	2.1	86.0	57.2	123.8	162.9	155.8	106.9	49.4	11.6	0.7
1989[6]	2 683.0	95.8	1.7	66.4	. . .	. . .	159.2	150.4	85.1	60.3	12.7	0.8

Note: Race and Hispanic origin are reported separately on birth certificates. Persons of Hispanic origin may be of any race. In this table, Hispanic women are classified only by place of origin; non-Hispanic women are classified by race.

[1]Total fertility rates are sums of birth rates for 5-year age groups multiplied by 5.
[2]Fertility rates computed by relating total births, regardless of age of mother, to women 15–44 years old.
[3]Beginning in 1997, rates computed by relating births to women age 45–54 years to women 45–49 years old.
[4]Excludes data for New Hampshire, which did not report Hispanic origin.
[5]Excludes data for New Hampshire and Oklahoma, which did not report Hispanic origin.
[6]Excludes data for Louisiana, New Hampshire, and Oklahoma, which did not report Hispanic origin.
[7]Includes Central and South American and other and unknown Hispanic.
* = Figure does not meet standards of reliability or precision; based on fewer than 20 births in the numerator or, for the Hispanic subgroups, fewer than 50 women for census years and 75,000 women for noncensus years in the denominator.
. . . = Not available.

Table I-9. Total Fertility Rates, Fertility Rates, and Birth Rates, by Age, Specified Hispanic Origin, and Race of Mother, 1989–2003—Continued

(Live births per 1,000 women in specified age and racial group.)

Year and origin/race of mother	Total fertility rate [1]	Fertility rate [2]	10–14 years	15–19 years			20–24 years	25–29 years	30–34 years	35–39 years	40–44 years	45–49 years[3]
				Total	15–17 years	18–19 years						
NON-HISPANIC [8]												
Total [9]												
2003	1 897.5	60.5	0.5	34.1	17.3	59.4	90.5	109.2	93.8	42.6	8.3	0.5
2002	1 877.0	59.6	0.6	35.5	18.2	61.8	91.8	107.9	90.8	40.4	7.9	0.5
2001	1 898.5	60.1	0.6	37.9	19.6	65.2	94.9	107.7	90.9	39.5	7.7	0.5
2000	1 931.5	61.1	0.7	40.7	21.9	68.2	99.5	108.4	90.2	38.8	7.6	0.4
1999	1 894.0	60.0	0.8	42.2	23.3	70.2	98.4	106.7	86.2	37.0	7.1	0.4
1998	1 887.5	60.0	0.8	44.0	25.2	72.4	98.9	105.8	84.4	36.2	7.0	0.4
1997	1 853.0	59.3	0.9	45.0	26.7	73.7	97.4	103.5	82.0	34.8	6.7	0.3
1996	1 852.0	59.6	1.0	47.0	28.4	75.8	97.3	103.6	80.8	33.9	6.5	0.3
1995	1 856.5	60.2	1.1	49.3	30.5	78.6	97.4	104.1	79.9	33.0	6.2	0.3
1994	1 883.5	61.6	1.2	51.7	32.3	81.4	99.5	106.5	79.1	32.4	6.0	0.3
1993	1 901.5	62.7	1.2	52.7	32.9	82.3	101.7	108.7	78.4	31.6	5.7	0.3
1992 [4]	1 929.0	64.2	1.2	54.3	33.2	85.3	104.3	111.4	77.9	31.1	5.4	0.3
1991 [4]	1 953.0	65.2	1.3	56.1	34.4	86.1	106.5	113.1	77.5	30.8	5.1	0.2
1990 [5]	1 979.5	67.1	1.3	54.8	33.8	81.4	108.1	116.5	79.2	30.7	5.1	0.2
1989 [6]	1 921.0	65.7	1.3	53.4	. . .	. . .	107.8	113.4	74.7	28.6	4.8	0.2
White												
2003	1 856.5	58.5	0.2	27.4	12.4	50.0	83.5	110.8	97.6	43.2	8.1	0.5
2002	1 828.5	57.4	0.2	28.5	13.1	51.9	84.3	109.3	94.4	40.9	7.6	0.5
2001	1 843.0	57.7	0.3	30.3	14.0	54.8	87.1	108.9	94.3	39.8	7.5	0.4
2000	1 866.0	58.5	0.3	32.6	15.8	57.5	91.2	109.4	93.2	38.8	7.3	0.4
1999	1 838.5	57.7	0.3	34.1	17.1	59.4	90.6	108.6	89.5	37.3	6.9	0.4
1998	1 825.0	57.6	0.3	35.3	18.3	60.9	91.2	107.4	87.2	36.4	6.8	0.4
1997	1 785.5	56.8	0.4	36.0	19.3	62.1	90.0	104.8	84.3	34.8	6.5	0.3
1996	1 781.0	57.1	0.4	37.6	20.6	64.0	90.1	104.9	82.8	33.9	6.2	0.3
1995	1 777.5	57.5	0.4	39.3	22.0	66.2	90.2	105.1	81.5	32.8	5.9	0.3
1994	1 782.5	58.2	0.5	40.4	22.7	67.6	90.9	106.6	80.2	32.0	5.7	0.2
1993	1 786.0	58.9	0.5	40.7	22.7	67.7	92.2	108.2	79.0	31.0	5.4	0.2
1992 [4]	1 803.5	60.0	0.5	41.7	22.7	69.8	93.9	110.6	78.3	30.4	5.1	0.2
1991 [4]	1 822.5	60.9	0.5	43.4	23.6	70.6	95.7	112.1	77.7	30.2	4.7	0.2
1990 [5]	1 850.5	62.8	0.5	42.5	23.2	66.6	97.5	115.3	79.4	30.0	4.7	0.2
1989 [6]	1 770.0	60.5	0.4	39.9	. . .	. . .	94.7	111.7	75.0	27.8	4.3	0.2
Black												
2003	2 027.5	67.1	1.6	64.7	38.7	105.3	128.1	102.1	67.4	33.4	7.7	0.5
2002	2 047.0	67.4	1.9	68.3	41.0	110.3	131.0	102.1	66.1	32.1	7.5	0.4
2001	2 104.5	69.1	2.1	73.5	44.9	116.7	137.2	102.1	66.2	32.1	7.3	0.4
2000	2 178.5	71.4	2.4	79.2	50.1	121.9	145.4	102.8	66.5	31.8	7.2	0.4
1999	2 134.0	69.9	2.6	81.0	51.7	123.9	142.1	99.8	63.9	30.6	6.5	0.3
1998	2 164.0	70.9	2.9	85.7	56.8	128.2	142.5	99.9	64.4	30.4	6.7	0.3
1997	2 137.5	70.3	3.2	88.3	60.7	131.0	138.8	97.2	63.6	29.6	6.5	0.3
1996	2 140.0	70.7	3.6	91.9	64.8	134.1	137.0	96.7	63.2	29.1	6.2	0.3
1995	2 186.5	72.8	4.2	97.2	70.4	139.2	137.8	98.5	64.4	28.8	6.1	0.3
1994	2 314.5	77.5	4.6	105.7	77.0	150.4	146.8	104.1	66.3	29.1	6.0	0.3
1993	2 412.5	81.5	4.6	110.5	81.1	154.6	154.5	109.2	68.1	29.4	5.9	0.3
1992 [4]	2 482.5	84.5	4.8	114.7	82.9	161.1	160.8	112.8	68.4	29.1	5.7	0.2
1991 [4]	2 532.0	87.0	4.9	118.2	86.1	162.2	164.8	115.1	68.9	28.7	5.6	0.2
1990 [5]	2 547.5	89.0	5.0	116.2	84.9	157.5	165.1	118.4	70.2	28.7	5.6	0.3
1989 [6]	2 424.0	84.8	5.2	111.9	. . .	. . .	156.3	113.8	65.7	26.3	5.3	0.3

Note: Race and Hispanic origin are reported separately on birth certificates. Persons of Hispanic origin may be of any race. In this table, Hispanic women are classified only by place of origin; non-Hispanic women are classified by race.

[1] Total fertility rates are sums of birth rates for 5-year age groups multiplied by 5.
[2] Fertility rates computed by relating total births, regardless of age of mother, to women 15–44 years old.
[3] Beginning in 1997, rates computed by relating births to women age 45–54 years to women 45–49 years old.
[4] Excludes data for New Hampshire, which did not report Hispanic origin.
[5] Excludes data for New Hampshire and Oklahoma, which did not report Hispanic origin.
[6] Excludes data for Louisiana, New Hampshire, and Oklahoma, which did not report Hispanic origin.
[8] Includes origin not stated.
[9] Includes races other than White and Black.
. . . = Not available.

TABLE I-10. NUMBER OF BIRTHS, BIRTH RATES, FERTILITY RATES, TOTAL FERTILITY RATES, AND BIRTH RATES FOR TEENAGERS 15–19 YEARS OLD, FOR EACH STATE AND TERRITORY, 2003

The largest number of births, 540,000 in 2003, took place in California, followed by 380,000 in Texas and 250,000 in New York. The highest Total Fertility Rate (or TFR, see comment for Table I-4 for definition), almost 2,600, was found in Utah. TFRs above 2,300 occurred in Alaska,

Arizona, Idaho, and Texas. The lowest TFRs were recorded in the District of Columbia, Maine, Massachusetts, and Vermont.

Fertility tends to be higher for states in the western half of the country. In 2003, as in previous years, the majority of states in the western part of the country reported TFRs well above the national rate, while the majority of eastern states reported TFRs well below the national rate. The greater presence of Hispanic women in some western states partly contributed to this result. In the U.S. territories, American Samoa experienced only 1,600 births, but its TFR was an astounding 3,852.

Since 1991, teenage birth rates have declined significantly for all reporting areas (see Table I-4). In 2003, the birth rate per 1,000 female teenagers was lowest in the New England states (18.2 in New Hampshire and 18.9 in Vermont). The rate exceeded 60 in Texas, New Mexico,

Table I-10. Number of Births, Birth Rates, Fertility Rates, Total Fertility Rates, and Birth Rates for Teenagers 15–19 Years Old, for Each State and Territory, 2003

(Number, rate.)

State	Number of births	Birth rate [1]	Fertility rate [2]	Total fertility rate [3]	Teenage birth rate [4] 15–19 years Total	15–17 years	18–19 years
UNITED STATES [5]	4 089 950	14.1	66.1	2 042.5	41.6	22.4	70.7
Alabama	59 552	13.2	62.5	1 918.0	52.4	28.9	87.1
Alaska	10 086	15.5	72.5	2 374.5	38.6	19.3	68.2
Arizona	90 967	16.3	79.2	2 385.0	61.1	35.5	102.0
Arkansas	37 784	13.9	67.4	2 055.0	59.0	30.5	101.1
California	540 997	15.2	69.9	2 131.5	40.1	21.8	68.1
Colorado	69 339	15.2	69.5	2 119.5	43.9	24.9	73.2
Connecticut	42 873	12.3	59.6	1 915.5	24.8	12.9	43.6
Delaware	11 329	13.9	64.6	2 009.5	44.9	23.7	77.7
District of Columbia	7 619	13.5	53.9	1 593.5	60.3	39.4	84.9
Florida	212 250	12.5	63.4	2 005.0	42.5	22.2	74.2
Georgia	135 979	15.7	69.3	2 121.5	53.5	29.0	91.3
Hawaii	18 100	14.4	72.2	2 242.5	37.3	18.7	63.9
Idaho	21 800	16.0	76.0	2 319.0	39.3	17.4	70.7
Illinois	182 495	14.4	67.0	2 052.5	40.4	22.9	66.6
Indiana	86 434	14.0	66.4	2 054.0	43.5	21.6	77.2
Iowa	38 174	13.0	63.3	1 986.5	31.9	15.2	55.5
Kansas	39 476	14.5	69.5	2 152.0	41.2	20.2	71.3
Kentucky	55 236	13.4	63.1	1 951.5	49.6	24.7	86.5
Louisiana	65 040	14.5	66.1	2 001.5	56.0	30.1	92.9
Maine	13 855	10.6	52.0	1 746.0	24.9	12.4	43.6
Maryland	74 930	13.6	62.4	1 977.5	33.3	18.2	56.9
Massachusetts	80 184	12.5	57.2	1 735.5	23.0	12.0	39.9
Michigan	131 094	13.0	61.7	1 939.0	34.4	18.2	59.3
Minnesota	70 050	13.8	64.1	2 024.5	26.6	13.4	46.0
Mississippi	42 380	14.7	67.9	2 030.0	62.5	35.3	101.9
Missouri	77 045	13.5	64.1	1 994.0	43.2	21.5	75.4
Montana	11 422	12.4	62.6	2 029.0	35.0	16.5	61.4
Nebraska	25 917	14.9	71.4	2 209.0	36.0	18.5	61.0
Nevada	33 647	15.0	72.2	2 208.0	53.0	29.1	91.2
New Hampshire	14 393	11.2	52.7	1 771.5	18.2	7.1	35.9
New Jersey	116 983	13.5	64.9	2 051.0	25.5	13.8	44.1
New Mexico	27 821	14.8	71.4	2 200.5	62.7	37.4	100.5
New York	253 714	13.2	61.0	1 866.0	28.2	14.9	48.1
North Carolina	118 323	14.1	65.8	2 018.0	49.0	26.6	84.4
North Dakota	7 972	12.6	61.6	1 933.5	26.8	12.1	46.6
Ohio	149 679	13.1	62.7	1 964.0	39.4	20.2	68.1
Oklahoma	50 981	14.5	69.9	2 110.5	55.9	28.8	94.8
Oregon	45 953	12.9	62.5	1 901.5	34.4	17.1	60.4
Pennsylvania	145 959	11.8	58.1	1 855.0	31.2	17.5	52.3
Rhode Island	13 209	12.3	56.6	1 763.0	31.3	18.8	50.1
South Carolina	55 649	13.4	62.9	1 929.5	51.5	28.7	86.2
South Dakota	11 027	14.4	70.8	2 241.5	34.7	17.5	59.4
Tennessee	78 890	13.5	63.1	1 950.5	53.5	28.2	91.1
Texas	377 476	17.1	77.5	2 346.5	62.9	37.2	102.1
Utah	49 860	21.2	92.2	2 566.5	34.6	16.4	60.7
Vermont	6 589	10.6	51.1	1 683.0	18.9	6.7	37.1
Virginia	101 254	13.7	63.3	1 973.5	36.1	17.4	64.6
Washington	80 489	13.1	61.2	1 899.5	31.5	15.5	55.5
West Virginia	20 935	11.6	58.1	1 798.5	44.8	21.1	79.7
Wisconsin	70 040	12.8	60.7	1 943.0	31.3	15.7	54.5
Wyoming	6 700	13.4	65.6	2 058.5	40.8	19.3	71.1
Puerto Rico	50 696	13.1	59.4	1 756.5	59.5	41.0	87.2
Virgin Islands	1 522	14.0	66.8	2 157.0	50.9	25.2	106.1
Guam	3 281	20.1	89.4	2 678.5	64.3	36.4	109.5
American Samoa	1 608	27.8	124.7	3 852.0	40.4	15.8	87.6
Northern Marianas	1 349	17.7	45.1	1 290.5	42.3	33.1	53.5

[1]Birth rates are live births per 1,000 estimated total population in each area.
[2]Fertility rates are live births per 1,000 women age 15–44 years estimated in each area.
[3]Total fertility rates are sums of birth rates for 5-year age groups multiplied by 5.
[4]Live births per 1,000 women in specified group.
[5]Excludes data for the territories.

Mississippi, Arizona, and the District of Columbia. States reporting teenage birth rates above 60 also had TFRs above 2,000, with the exception of the District of Columbia, whose TFR was an unusually low 1,594. This indicates low birth rates among white-collar adult workers with relatively high incomes. A birth rate of over 60 births per 1,000 female teenagers also occurred in Guam. A rate of 59.5 was reported for Puerto Rico.

TABLE I-10A. BIRTH RATES FOR TEENAGERS 15–19 YEARS, FOR EACH STATE AND TERRITORY, 1991 AND 2003

This table shows the drop in teenage birth rates by state over a little more than a decade. California, New Hampshire, Vermont, and the District of Columbia had declines of 45 percent or more. Nebraska, Texas, and New Mexico had the least amount of change. The highest absolute rates in 2003 were found in Texas (62.9 per 1,000 women age 15–19 years), New Mexico (62.7), Mississippi (62.5), and Arizona (61.1).

Table I-10A. Birth Rates for Teenagers 15–19 Years, for Each State and Territory, 1991 and 2003

(Birth rates per 1,000 estimated female population age 15–19 years in each area.)

State	2003	1991	Percent change, 1991–2003
UNITED STATES [1]	41.6	61.8	-33
Alabama	52.4	73.6	-29
Alaska	38.6	66.0	-42
Arizona	61.1	79.7	-23
Arkansas	59.0	79.5	-26
California	40.1	73.8	-46
Colorado	43.9	58.3	-25
Connecticut	24.8	40.1	-38
Delaware	44.9	60.4	-26
District of Columbia	60.3	109.6	-45
Florida	42.5	67.9	-37
Georgia	53.5	76.0	-30
Hawaii	37.3	59.2	-37
Idaho	39.3	53.9	-27
Illinois	40.4	64.5	-37
Indiana	43.5	60.4	-28
Iowa	31.9	42.5	-25
Kansas	41.2	55.4	-26
Kentucky	49.6	68.8	-28
Louisiana	56.0	76.0	-26
Maine	24.9	43.5	-43
Maryland	33.3	54.1	-38
Massachusetts	23.0	37.5	-39
Michigan	34.4	58.9	-42
Minnesota	26.6	37.3	-29
Mississippi	62.5	85.3	-27
Missouri	43.2	64.4	-33
Montana	35.0	46.8	-25
Nebraska	36.0	42.4	-15
Nevada	53.0	74.5	-29
New Hampshire	18.2	33.1	-45
New Jersey	25.5	41.3	-38
New Mexico	62.7	79.5	-21
New York	28.2	45.5	-38
North Carolina	49.0	70.0	-30
North Dakota	26.8	35.5	-25
Ohio	39.4	60.5	-35
Oklahoma	55.9	72.1	-22
Oregon	34.4	54.8	-37
Pennsylvania	31.2	46.7	-33
Rhode Island	31.3	44.7	-30
South Carolina	51.5	72.5	-29
South Dakota	34.7	47.6	-27
Tennessee	53.5	74.8	-28
Texas	62.9	78.4	-20
Utah	34.6	48.0	-28
Vermont	18.9	39.2	-52
Virginia	36.1	53.4	-32
Washington	31.5	53.7	-41
West Virginia	44.8	58.0	-23
Wisconsin	31.3	43.7	-28
Wyoming	40.8	54.3	-25
Puerto Rico	59.5	72.4	-18
Virgin Islands	50.9	77.9	-35
Guam	64.3	95.7	-33
American Samoa	40.4	. . .	. . .
Northern Marianas	42.3	. . .	. . .

[1]Excludes data for the territories.
. . . = Not available.

TABLE I-11. LIVE BIRTHS, BY RACE OF MOTHER, FOR EACH STATE AND TERRITORY, 2003

The three states that had the largest number of births—California, Texas, and New York—also led in the number of births to Whites. The highest number of Black births took place in New York, followed by Florida, Georgia, and Texas. The largest number of American Indian births took place in Arizona, followed by Oklahoma and New Mexico. By far, the largest number of Asian or Pacific Islander births took place in California—about 30 percent of the total of such births in this group—followed by New York, Texas, and Hawaii.

Table I-11. Live Births, by Race of Mother, for Each State and Territory, 2003

(Number.)

State	Number				
	All races	White	Black	American Indian [1]	Asian or Pacific Islander
UNITED STATES [2]	4 089 950	3 225 848	599 847	43 052	221 203
Alabama	59 552	40 868	17 931	146	607
Alaska	10 086	6 493	404	2 477	712
Arizona	90 967	78 940	3 261	6 068	2 698
Arkansas	37 784	29 750	7 236	259	539
California	540 997	438 374	32 349	2 916	67 358
Colorado	69 339	63 166	2 937	564	2 672
Connecticut	42 873	35 388	5 187	262	2 036
Delaware	11 329	7 941	2 907	32	449
District of Columbia	7 619	2 108	5 250	5	256
Florida	212 250	158 026	47 341	1 088	5 795
Georgia	135 979	88 125	43 099	319	4 436
Hawaii	18 100	5 086	583	71	12 360
Idaho	21 800	20 974	106	369	351
Illinois	182 495	141 820	31 565	260	8 850
Indiana	86 434	75 541	9 375	136	1 382
Iowa	38 174	35 688	1 287	260	939
Kansas	39 476	35 007	2 763	480	1 226
Kentucky	55 236	49 416	4 851	101	868
Louisiana	65 040	37 312	26 224	403	1 101
Maine	13 855	13 365	183	99	208
Maryland	74 930	44 704	25 515	188	4 523
Massachusetts	80 184	66 009	8 596	184	5 395
Michigan	131 094	103 166	22 567	639	4 722
Minnesota	70 050	59 404	5 362	1 416	3 868
Mississippi	42 380	23 251	18 553	284	292
Missouri	77 045	63 816	11 166	366	1 697
Montana	11 422	9 848	50	1 400	124
Nebraska	25 917	23 376	1 468	470	603
Nevada	33 647	27 700	2 900	520	2 527
New Hampshire	14 393	13 646	243	35	469
New Jersey	116 983	85 858	20 200	188	10 737
New Mexico	27 821	23 284	532	3 603	402
New York	253 714	183 829	48 025	637	21 223
North Carolina	118 323	86 407	27 171	1 637	3 108
North Dakota	7 972	6 890	109	858	115
Ohio	149 679	123 617	22 678	298	3 086
Oklahoma	50 981	39 959	4 625	5 320	1 077
Oregon	45 953	41 574	1 018	867	2 494
Pennsylvania	145 959	118 394	22 056	333	5 176
Rhode Island	13 209	11 225	1 258	163	563
South Carolina	55 649	36 270	18 334	152	893
South Dakota	11 027	8 903	122	1 875	127
Tennessee	78 890	60 972	16 249	180	1 489
Texas	377 476	321 542	41 885	902	13 147
Utah	49 860	47 328	383	617	1 532
Vermont	6 589	6 411	53	7	118
Virginia	101 254	71 918	22 607	178	6 551
Washington	80 489	66 581	4 015	2 051	7 842
West Virginia	20 935	20 043	721	25	146
Wisconsin	70 040	60 244	6 494	1 054	2 248
Wyoming	6 700	6 291	53	290	66
Puerto Rico	50 696	46 067	4 605	. . .	22
Virgin Islands	1 522	351	1 147	2	. . .
Guam	3 281	276	39	5	2 961
American Samoa	1 608	2	-	-	1 606
Northern Marianas	1 349	13	-	-	1 336

[1]Includes births to Aleuts and Eskimos.
[2]Excludes data for the territories.
- = Quantity zero.
. . . = Not available.

TABLE I-12. LIVE BIRTHS, BY SPECIFIED HISPANIC ORIGIN AND RACE OF MOTHER, FOR EACH STATE AND TERRITORY, 2003

In California and Texas, Hispanic births accounted for almost one-half of total births; in Arizona, their share was 44 percent. The mothers were predominantly of Mexican origin. In New Mexico, 53 percent of births were to Hispanics, but many families in this state traced their origin to Spanish settlers rather than to Mexico. In Florida, about one-quarter of all births came from Hispanic mothers, whose origin was most frequently Central or South America, followed by Mexico and Cuba. Cuban mothers accounted for 19 percent of Florida's Hispanic births. Outside of Florida, New Jersey had the highest number of births to mothers of Cuban origin. In New York, 22 percent of births were to Hispanic mothers. Almost half of these mothers were Central and South American, and almost a quarter were Puerto Rican.

Table I-12. Live Births, by Specified Hispanic Origin and Race of Mother, for Each State and Territory, 2003

(Number.)

State	All origins	Origin of mother									Not stated
		Hispanic						Non-Hispanic			
		Total	Mexican	Puerto Rican	Cuban	Central and South American	Other and unknown Hispanic	Total [1]	White	Black	
UNITED STATES [2]	4 089 950	912 329	654 504	58 400	14 867	135 586	48 972	3 149 034	2 321 904	576 033	28 587
Alabama	59 552	2 904	2 163	82	20	231	408	56 603	37 996	17 887	45
Alaska	10 086	770	286	61	12	80	331	7 546	4 917	264	1 770
Arizona	90 967	39 780	37 398	276	63	788	1 255	49 547	39 222	2 636	1 640
Arkansas	37 784	3 278	2 752	35	5	444	42	34 425	26 480	7 190	81
California	540 997	269 705	235 975	1 975	729	25 577	5 449	265 467	166 764	30 925	5 825
Colorado	69 339	21 387	17 003	272	71	796	3 245	47 942	42 348	2 807	10
Connecticut	42 873	7 547	897	4 261	94	2 034	261	35 096	28 047	4 812	230
Delaware	11 329	1 380	791	309	5	271	4	9 907	6 584	2 848	42
District of Columbia	7 619	962	101	12	3	803	43	6 641	1 844	4 570	16
Florida	212 250	54 857	13 355	9 514	10 558	20 187	1 243	157 083	104 289	46 295	310
Georgia	135 979	18 262	14 372	586	137	3 057	110	115 449	68 900	42 038	2 268
Hawaii	18 100	2 617	503	760	12	88	1 254	15 453	4 275	483	30
Idaho	21 800	2 939	2 349	26	4	65	495	18 714	17 923	103	147
Illinois	182 495	42 460	35 891	2 701	192	1 864	1 812	139 935	99 565	31 303	100
Indiana	86 434	6 779	5 861	298	23	465	132	79 301	68 511	9 327	354
Iowa	38 174	2 519	2 012	60	3	361	83	35 588	33 185	1 264	67
Kansas	39 476	5 442	4 489	102	18	319	514	33 612	29 230	2 725	422
Kentucky	55 236	1 959	1 465	104	91	259	40	53 234	47 568	4 812	43
Louisiana	65 040	1 675	673	95	84	160	663	63 315	35 726	26 140	50
Maine	13 855	166	29	30	4	38	65	13 630	13 153	176	59
Maryland	74 930	6 976	1 599	375	63	4 543	396	67 883	39 234	24 125	71
Massachusetts	80 184	9 800	499	4 334	78	4 708	181	69 975	57 884	6 579	409
Michigan	131 094	7 670	6 221	382	91	499	477	120 886	93 630	22 312	2 538
Minnesota	70 050	4 932	3 684	100	29	717	402	64 472	54 074	5 251	646
Mississippi	42 380	543	252	16	3	59	213	41 780	22 664	18 542	57
Missouri	77 045	3 483	2 631	117	41	390	304	73 490	60 488	11 012	72
Montana	11 422	379	174	10	7	22	166	10 851	9 299	49	192
Nebraska	25 917	3 453	2 693	28	15	528	189	21 884	19 404	1 444	580
Nevada	33 647	12 198	10 172	247	203	1 197	379	21 151	15 612	2 752	298
New Hampshire	14 393	528	133	130	16	181	68	13 261	12 590	173	604
New Jersey	116 983	26 534	5 300	6 758	739	13 537	200	90 251	61 911	17 601	198
New Mexico	27 821	14 843	7 220	70	42	108	7 403	12 968	8 606	476	10
New York	253 714	55 281	9 366	12 512	405	24 529	8 469	197 562	132 088	43 796	871
North Carolina	118 323	16 080	12 222	670	128	2 932	128	102 155	70 473	26 983	88
North Dakota	7 972	168	97	9	-	13	49	7 637	6 571	106	167
Ohio	149 679	5 352	2 985	1 250	54	659	404	143 952	118 304	22 326	375
Oklahoma	50 981	5 733	5 229	124	18	276	86	45 152	34 349	4 556	96
Oregon	45 953	8 439	7 827	82	35	327	168	37 219	33 074	977	295
Pennsylvania	145 959	10 832	2 374	5 703	159	1 575	1 021	133 218	109 259	18 974	1 909
Rhode Island	13 209	2 483	186	706	18	1 516	57	9 023	7 251	1 117	1 703
South Carolina	55 649	3 662	2 636	194	22	619	191	51 924	32 677	18 250	63
South Dakota	11 027	340	207	20	2	85	26	10 677	8 616	116	10
Tennessee	78 890	4 934	3 711	199	61	816	147	73 931	56 119	16 170	25
Texas	377 476	183 139	164 422	1 090	324	10 238	7 065	193 266	138 194	41 252	1 071
Utah	49 860	7 069	5 224	113	15	724	993	42 571	40 154	341	220
Vermont	6 589	59	24	13	2	9	11	6 486	6 311	52	44
Virginia	101 254	10 401	2 967	675	77	5 960	722	90 667	62 347	21 838	186
Washington	80 489	13 320	11 024	282	52	608	1 354	65 008	53 848	3 072	2 161
West Virginia	20 935	104	39	15	2	16	32	20 747	19 874	713	84
Wisconsin	70 040	5 539	4 428	606	38	294	173	64 487	54 845	6 421	14
Wyoming	6 700	667	593	11	-	14	49	6 012	5 627	52	21
Puerto Rico	50 696	. . .	. . .	. . .	. . .	. . .	. . .	. . .	. . .	. . .	50 696
Virgin Islands	1 522	344	1	79	-	50	214	1 038	104	914	140
Guam	3 281	54	27	11	1	7	8	3 150	241	35	77
American Samoa	1 608	. . .	. . .	. . .	. . .	. . .	. . .	. . .	. . .	. . .	1 608
Northern Marianas	1 349	. . .	. . .	. . .	. . .	. . .	. . .	. . .	. . .	. . .	1 349

Note: Race and Hispanic origin are reported separately on birth certificates. Persons of Hispanic origin may be of any race. In this table, Hispanic women are classified only by place of origin; non-Hispanic women are classified by race.

[1]Includes races other than White and Black.
[2]Excludes data for the territories.
- = Quantity zero.
. . . = Not available.

TABLE I-13. TOTAL NUMBER OF BIRTHS, RATES (BIRTH, FERTILITY, AND TOTAL FERTILITY), AND PERCENT OF BIRTHS WITH SELECTED DEMOGRAPHIC CHARACTERISTICS, BY DETAILED RACE AND PLACE OF BIRTH OF MOTHER, 2003

This table summarizes the birth rate, the fertility rate, and the TFR for the major races: White, Black, American Indian, and Asian or Pacific Islander. It also shows the ratio of male to female births, which averaged 1.049 in 2003. The ratio exceeded 1 for each of the races. It was highest at 1.067 for Asians or Pacific Islanders. The overall ratio has fluctuated narrowly over the past 60 years, ranging from 1.046 to 1.059.

Demographic data are shown separately for mothers born in the United States and those born outside the country. Births to teenagers were more frequent for native-born mothers. Foreign-born Whites more frequently gave birth to four children or more. Native-born mothers, especially Black and American Indian mothers, were more frequently unmarried than foreign-born mothers. Native-born White mothers tended to have more education than foreign-born mothers. For Asian or Pacific Islanders, only 17 percent of mothers were born in the United States.

TABLE I-14. TOTAL NUMBER OF BIRTHS, RATES (BIRTH, FERTILITY, AND TOTAL FERTILITY), AND PERCENT OF BIRTHS WITH SELECTED DEMOGRAPHIC CHARACTERISTICS, BY SPECIFIED HISPANIC ORIGIN, RACE, AND PLACE OF BIRTH OF MOTHER, 2003

This table replicates the information of Table I-13, but focuses on Hispanics by major countries of origin. It also shows data for non-Hispanic Whites and Blacks. Once again, this table highlights the large size of the Hispanic birth rate relative to the rate for non-Hispanics (particularly the rate for non-Hispanic Whites). It also shows the moderate proportion of Hispanic mothers in 2003 that were born in the United States (36.7 percent), in contrast to the proportion of native-born, non-Hispanic White mothers (94.2 percent). About 88.5 percent of non-Hispanic White mothers completed 12 years or more of school, but only 52.5 percent of Hispanic mothers and 76.2 percent of non-Hispanic Blacks had similar levels of educational attainment. Hispanic mothers born in the United States had substantially more educational achievement than foreign-born Hispanic mothers. However, to a lesser extent, foreign-born non-Hispanic Whites and Blacks, as well as Cubans, had a somewhat greater high school completion rate than their native-born counterparts.

Table I-13. Total Number of Births, Rates (Birth, Fertility, and Total Fertility), and Percent of Births with Selected Demographic Characteristics, by Detailed Race and Place of Birth of Mother, 2003

(Number, live births per 1,000 population.)

Characteristic	All races	White	Black	American Indian [1]	Asian or Pacific Islander
Births (Number)	4 089 950	3 225 848	599 847	43 052	221 203
Birth rate	14.1	13.6	15.7	13.8	16.8
Fertility rate [2]	66.1	66.1	66.3	58.4	66.3
Total fertility rate [3]	2 043.0	2 061.0	1 999.0	1 732.0	1 873.0
Sex ratio [4]	1 049	1 050	1 036	1 047	1 067
All Births (Percent)					
Births to mothers under 20 years	10.3	9.4	17.3	18.2	3.5
4th- and higher-order births	10.8	10.1	15.2	19.0	6.4
Births to unmarried mothers	34.6	29.4	68.2	61.3	15.0
Mothers completing 12 years or more of school	78.4	78.2	76.0	69.5	90.1
Mothers born in the 50 states and DC	76.3	78.3	86.0	94.4	17.0
Mothers Born in the 50 States and DC (Percent)					
Births to mothers under 20 years	11.2	9.4	19.2	18.8	11.5
4th- and higher-order births	10.3	9.2	15.5	19.3	7.6
Births to unmarried mothers	35.4	27.5	72.4	62.9	31.6
Mothers completing 12 years or more of school	83.8	85.8	75.0	69.9	89.9
Mothers Born Outside the 50 States and DC (Percent)					
Births to mothers under 20 years	7.5	9.2	5.2	8.8	1.8
4th- and higher-order births	12.2	13.6	13.2	13.2	6.1
Births to unmarried mothers	31.9	36.0	41.9	34.4	11.6
Mothers completing 12 years or more of school	61.2	51.3	82.3	62.8	90.2

Note: Race and Hispanic origin are reported separately on birth certificates. In this table, all women (including Hispanic women) are classified only according to their race.

[1] Includes births to Aleuts and Eskimos.
[2] Fertility rates are computed by relating total births, regardless of age of mother, to women age 15–44 years.
[3] Total fertility rates are sums of birth rates for 5-year age groups multiplied by 5.
[4] Male live births per 1,000 female live births.

Table I-14. Total Number of Births, Rates (Birth, Fertility, and Total Fertility), and Percent of Births with Selected Demographic Characteristics, by Specified Hispanic Origin, Race, and Place of Birth of Mother, 2003

(Live births per 1,000 population.)

Characteristic	All origins [1]	Hispanic						Non-Hispanic		
		Total	Mexican	Puerto Rican	Cuban	Central and South American	Other and unknown Hispanic	Total [2]	White	Black
Births (Number)	4 089 950	912 329	654 504	58 400	14 867	135 586	48 972	3 149 034	2 321 904	576 033
Birth rate [3]	14.1	22.9	24.7	15.1	9.9	23.0	(3)	12.7	11.8	15.9
Fertility rate [3,4]	66.1	96.9	105.5	61.6	61.7	91.2	(3)	60.5	58.5	67.1
Total fertility rate [3,5]	2 042.5	2 785.5	2 957.5	1 841.0	2 059.5	2 733.0	(3)	1 897.5	1 856.5	2 027.5
Sex ratio [6]	1 049	1 041	1 040	1 043	1 035	1 044	1 036	1 051	1 053	1 036
All Births (Percent)										
Births to mothers under 20 years	10.3	14.3	15.3	17.9	7.9	8.3	15.9	9.1	7.5	17.4
4th- and higher-order births	10.8	13.7	14.8	12.2	4.8	10.4	11.8	9.9	8.8	15.3
Births to unmarried mothers	34.6	45.0	43.7	59.8	31.4	46.0	46.7	31.6	23.6	68.5
Mothers completing 12 years or more of school	78.4	52.5	46.4	70.1	88.5	64.7	69.9	86.1	88.5	76.2
Mothers born in the 50 states and DC	76.3	36.7	36.2	66.6	47.2	12.1	73.0	87.8	94.2	87.6
Mothers Born in the 50 States and DC (Percent)										
Births to mothers under 20 years	11.2	20.6	21.4	19.5	11.8	18.8	18.8	10.0	7.8	19.2
4th- and higher-order births	10.3	12.1	12.8	11.6	5.2	5.3	11.8	10.1	8.7	15.5
Births to unmarried mothers	35.4	49.6	48.3	62.1	30.1	47.1	49.0	33.7	24.3	72.6
Mothers completing 12 years or more of school	83.8	69.3	67.4	70.0	86.9	81.2	73.0	85.7	88.4	75.0
Mothers Born Outside the 50 States and DC (Percent)										
Births to mothers under 20 years	7.5	10.7	11.8	14.4	4.4	6.9	7.6	2.6	2.9	4.5
4th- and higher-order births	12.2	14.6	15.9	13.3	4.4	11.1	11.8	8.6	9.4	13.5
Births to unmarried mothers	31.9	42.3	41.0	55.0	32.5	45.9	39.2	16.4	11.2	39.5
Mothers completing 12 years or more of school	61.2	42.6	34.3	70.3	89.8	62.4	61.1	89.7	90.9	85.4

Note: Race and Hispanic origin are reported separately on birth certificates. Persons of Hispanic origin may be of any race. In this table Hispanic women are classified only by place of origin; non-Hispanic women are classified by race.

[1]Includes origin not stated.
[2]Includes races other than White and Black.
[3]Rates for Central and South American include other and unknown Hispanic.
[4]Fertility rates are computed by relating total births, regardless of age of mother, to women age 15–44 years.
[5]Total fertility rates are sums of birth rates for 5-year age groups multiplied by 5.
[6]Male live births per 1,000 female live births.

Table I-15. Live Births, by Race of Mother and Observed and Seasonally Adjusted Birth and Fertility Rates, by Month, 2003

(Number, rates on annual basis per 1,000 population for specified month.)

Month	Number			Observed		Seasonally adjusted	
	All races [1]	White	Black	Birth rate	Fertility rate [2]	Birth rate	Fertility rate [2]
Total	4 089 950	3 225 848	599 847	14.1	66.1	X	X
January	329 803	257 667	50 803	13.4	62.5	14.7	66.0
February	307 248	241 252	46 156	13.8	64.5	14.7	66.0
March	336 920	266 258	48 714	13.7	63.8	14.7	66.1
April	330 106	262 671	46 252	13.8	64.6	14.6	65.6
May	346 754	276 206	47 990	14.0	65.7	14.6	66.0
June	337 425	267 731	48 114	14.1	66.0	14.6	65.9
July	364 226	288 949	52 553	14.7	68.9	14.6	65.7
August	360 103	283 960	53 094	14.5	68.1	14.6	66.0
September	359 644	284 332	52 494	15.0	70.3	14.6	66.0
October	354 048	279 270	51 704	14.3	66.9	14.6	66.0
November	320 094	249 416	49 197	13.3	62.5	14.7	66.4
December	343 579	268 136	52 776	13.8	64.9	14.5	65.6

Note: Monthly populations estimated as of the first of each month.

[1]Includes races other than White and Black.
[2]Fertility rates are live births per 1,000 women age 15–44 years.
X = Not applicable.

TABLE I-15. LIVE BIRTHS, BY RACE OF MOTHER AND OBSERVED AND SEASONALLY ADJUSTED BIRTH AND FERTILITY RATES, BY MONTH, 2003

The monthly average number of births in 2003 was 340,829. The actual number of births per month ranged from about 307,000 (February) to 364,000 (July). Historically, the number of births tends to peak during the summer months and dip toward the end of the year and into winter. This tendency is taken into account in the table's seasonally adjusted birth and fertility rates. Rates remained largely unchanged from month to month, indicating that the variations in the unadjusted data reflect a seasonal pattern. Note that the observed birth rates, as shown in the table, have been adjusted for the different number of days in each month.

TABLE I-16. LIVE BIRTHS, BY DAY OF WEEK AND INDEX OF OCCURRENCE, BY METHOD OF DELIVERY, DAY OF WEEK, AND RACE OF MOTHER, 2003

In 2003, there were an average of 11,205 births per day. The number of births varied considerably according to the day of the week, as it did in previous years. The highest number of average births (13,001) occurred on Tuesdays in 2003. The two days with the fewest births were Sundays and Saturdays, which averaged 7,563 and 8,605 births, respectively.

An index of occurrence is shown in Table I-16. For each category, such as race of mother or method of delivery, the average number of daily births is expressed as 100, and births on the days of the week are shown as percentages of this average. For all races, the index was 116.0 on Tuesdays, 67.5 on Sundays, and 76.8 on Saturdays. The results are different according to the method of delivery. The weekend birth deficit was particularly large for cesarean deliveries, for which Sunday births have an index number of 49.0 (59.5 for primary cesareans and 32.5 for repeat cesareans); vaginal deliveries have a Sunday index number of 74.7. The weekend birth deficit for all cesarean births has grown noticeably since such data became available in 1989; at that time, the Sunday index number was 60.7 percent (data not shown). This trend was not unexpected, as cesarean deliveries—especially repeat cesareans—are surgeries that are decided on prior to labor.

TABLE I-17. NUMBER, BIRTH RATE, AND PERCENT OF BIRTHS TO UNMARRIED WOMEN, BY AGE, RACE, AND HISPANIC ORIGIN OF MOTHER, 2003

Unmarried mothers accounted for 34.6 percent of all births in the United States in 2003. This percentage was highest for teenagers (81.3 percent for births at 15–19 years of age) and lowest for mothers in their thirties (about 15 percent). Unmarried mothers, age 40 years and over, accounted for a somewhat higher percentage of total births (17.9 percent) than those in their thirties, perhaps reflecting a higher level of income or a push to beat the biological clock.

Births to unmarried mothers (as a percentage of total births) were lowest for Asians or Pacific Islanders (15.0 percent), and they were relatively low for non-Hispanic Whites (23.6 percent). For non-Hispanic Blacks, the percentage of births to unmarried mothers was 68.5 (with the proportion remaining quite high into the mid-twenties age bracket). For Hispanics, the rate was 45 percent.

Table I-16. Live Births, by Day of Week and Index of Occurrence, by Method of Delivery, Day of the Week, and Race of Mother, 2003

(Number, ratio.)

Day of week and race of mother	Average number of births	Index of occurrence [1]				
		Total [2]	Method of delivery			
			Vaginal	Cesarean		
				Total	Primary	Repeat
All Races [3]	11 205	100.0	100.0	100.0	100.0	100.0
Sunday	7 563	67.5	74.7	49.0	59.5	32.5
Monday	11 733	104.7	101.7	112.4	101.7	129.4
Tuesday	13 001	116.0	113.2	123.4	120.2	128.5
Wednesday	12 598	112.4	110.3	117.9	116.4	120.2
Thursday	12 514	111.7	109.7	116.8	114.8	120.0
Friday	12 396	110.6	106.5	121.2	114.9	131.0
Saturday	8 605	76.8	83.7	59.0	72.3	38.0
White	8 838	100.0	100.0	100.0	100.0	100.0
Sunday	5 818	65.8	73.0	47.1	57.7	30.7
Monday	9 326	105.5	102.4	113.6	102.6	130.6
Tuesday	10 320	116.8	113.9	124.2	121.1	128.8
Wednesday	9 995	113.1	111.0	118.5	117.3	120.3
Thursday	9 918	112.2	110.3	117.2	115.1	120.4
Friday	9 834	111.3	106.9	122.5	115.7	133.0
Saturday	6 634	75.1	82.2	56.6	70.1	35.9
Black	1 643	100.0	100.0	100.0	100.0	100.0
Sunday	1 189	72.4	79.6	55.1	65.0	39.1
Monday	1 676	102.0	99.1	108.6	98.3	125.5
Tuesday	1 878	114.3	111.4	121.2	117.4	127.3
Wednesday	1 821	110.8	108.5	116.2	113.6	120.4
Thursday	1 808	110.0	107.7	115.5	113.6	118.6
Friday	1 773	107.9	104.5	116.1	112.1	122.5
Saturday	1 356	82.5	89.0	67.0	79.8	46.1

[1]Index is the ratio of the average number of births by a specified method of delivery on a given day of the week to the average daily number of births by a specified method of delivery for the year, multiplied by 100.
[2]Includes method of delivery not stated.
[3]Includes races other than White and Black.

Table I-17. Number, Birth Rate, and Percent of Births to Unmarried Women, by Age, Race, and Hispanic Origin of Mother, 2003

(Number, percent.)

Measure and age of mother	All races [1]	White		Black		American Indian [2,3]	Asian or Pacific Islander [2]	Hispanic [4]
		Total [2]	Non-Hispanic	Total [2]	Non-Hispanic			
Number								
All ages	1 415 995	947 012	546 991	409 333	394 831	26 401	33 249	410 620
Under 15 years	6 469	3 499	1 353	2 715	2 633	152	103	2 224
15–19 years	337 201	227 879	132 482	97 000	93 918	6 778	5 544	97 925
15 years	17 331	10 647	4 627	6 020	5 820	398	266	6 226
16 years	37 666	24 727	11 980	11 535	11 150	778	626	13 105
17 years	65 574	44 380	24 454	18 823	18 154	1 365	1 006	20 473
18 years	96 105	65 850	39 516	26 831	26 028	1 849	1 575	26 946
19 years	120 525	82 275	51 905	33 791	32 766	2 388	2 071	31 175
20–24 years	549 353	367 924	224 941	160 312	155 153	10 002	11 115	146 729
25–29 years	287 205	190 605	101 454	83 421	80 087	5 293	7 886	91 644
30–34 years	147 555	97 957	52 167	41 692	39 926	2 668	5 238	46 995
35–39 years	69 071	46 038	26 352	19 260	18 400	1 193	2 580	20 158
40 years and over	19 141	13 110	8 242	4 933	4 714	315	783	4 945
Rate per 1,000 Unmarried Women in Specified Group								
15–44 years [5]	44.9	40.4	28.6	66.3	...	...	22.2	92.2
15–19 years	34.8	30.1	21.5	62.2	...	...	13.1	66.6
15–17 years	20.3	17.2	11.0	38.1	...	...	7.5	43.0
18–19 years	57.6	50.4	37.9	100.4	...	...	21.4	107.0
20–24 years	71.2	63.0	47.2	118.0	...	...	26.6	133.7
25–29 years	65.7	60.8	40.8	90.4	...	...	30.7	136.0
30–34 years	44.0	42.0	27.8	51.2	...	...	31.5	99.2
35–39 years	22.3	21.2	14.7	25.3	...	...	19.8	54.7
40–44 years [6]	5.8	5.5	4.1	6.5	...	...	7.9	13.3
Percent of Births to Unmarried Women								
All ages	34.6	29.4	23.6	68.2	68.5	61.3	15.0	45.0
Under 15 years	97.1	95.2	96.7	99.6	99.7	98.7	99.0	94.4
15–19 years	81.3	76.4	76.7	96.1	96.3	88.1	73.0	76.2
15 years	95.0	92.7	94.9	99.4	99.5	96.8	92.7	91.3
16 years	91.1	87.8	89.6	99.0	99.1	95.5	86.5	86.5
17 years	87.7	83.8	85.7	98.3	98.5	94.2	79.4	81.9
18 years	81.6	76.8	78.3	96.5	96.7	87.4	75.6	75.0
19 years	74.2	68.5	68.9	93.1	93.4	82.3	64.1	68.3
20–24 years	53.2	46.5	43.1	81.7	82.1	68.3	36.5	53.7
25–29 years	26.4	21.9	16.2	59.6	59.8	50.3	12.2	37.2
30–34 years	15.1	12.3	8.3	42.7	42.8	41.5	6.9	27.8
35–39 years	14.8	12.1	8.7	38.6	38.6	41.1	7.4	26.6
40 years and over	17.9	15.3	12.0	39.3	39.2	44.4	10.0	29.2

Note: For 48 states and the District of Columbia, marital status is reported on the birth certificate; for Michigan and New York, mother's marital status is inferred. Rates cannot be computed for unmarried non-Hispanic Black or American Indian women because the necessary populations are not available.

[1] Includes races other than White and Black and origin not stated.
[2] Race and Hispanic origin are reported separately on the birth certificate. Race categories are consistent with the 1977 Office of Management and Budget (OMB) guidelines. Data for persons of Hispanic origin are included in the data for each race group according to the mother's reported race.
[3] Includes births to Aleuts and Eskimos.
[4] May be of any race.
[5] Birth rates computed by relating total births to unmarried mothers, regardless of age of mother, to unmarried women age 15–44 years.
[6] Birth rates computed by relating births to unmarried mothers age 40 years and over to unmarried women age 40–44 years.
. . . = Not available.

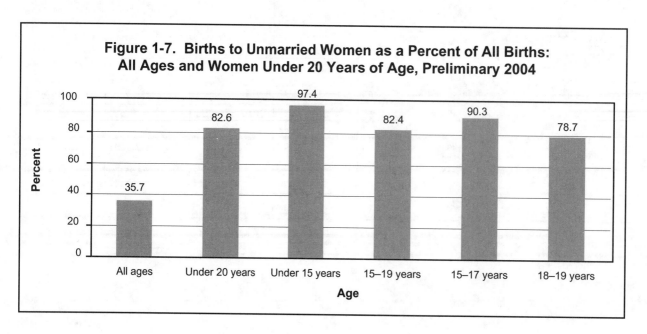

Figure 1-7. Births to Unmarried Women as a Percent of All Births: All Ages and Women Under 20 Years of Age, Preliminary 2004

TABLE I-17A. NUMBER AND PERCENT OF BIRTHS TO UNMARRIED WOMEN, ALL AGES AND BY AGE FOR TEENAGERS, FINAL 2003 AND PRELIMINARY 2004

Childbearing by unmarried women reached a record high of almost 1.5 million births in 2004, up 4 percent from 2003. More than four-fifths of births to teenagers were nonmarital. Over half of births to women in their early twenties and nearly 30 percent of births to women age 25 to 29 years old were to unmarried women. In 2004, 35.7 percent of all births were to unmarried women. The percentages increased for all age, race, and Hispanic origin subgroups. (See Table I-1A for a breakdown by race and ethnicity.) The birth rate increased 3 percent to 46.1 births per 1,000 unmarried women age 15–44 years. (See Table I-18A.)

Table I-17A. Number and Percent of Births to Unmarried Women, All Ages and by Age for Teenagers, Final 2003 and Preliminary 2004

(Number, percent.)

Age of mother	Number		Percent	
	2004	2003	2004	2003
All Ages	1 470 152	1 415 995	35.7	34.6
Under 20 years	348 934	343 670	82.6	81.6
Under 15 years	6 614	6 469	97.4	97.1
15–19 years	342 320	337 201	82.4	81.3
15–17 years	120 972	120 571	90.3	89.7
18–19 years	221 348	216 630	78.7	77.3

Note: Data for 2004 are based on a continuous file of records received from the states. Figures from 2004 are based on weighted data rounded to the nearest individual.

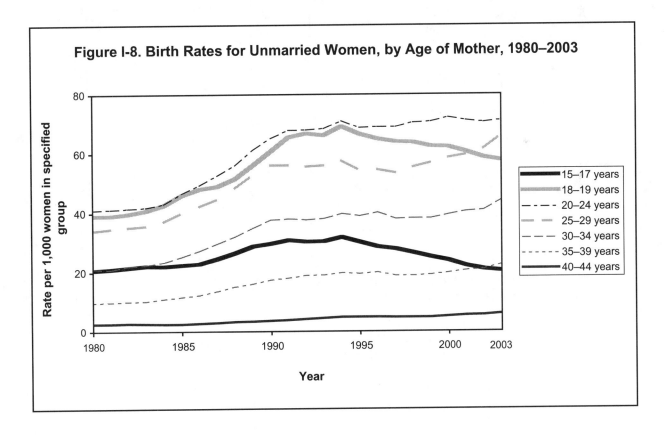

Figure I-8. Birth Rates for Unmarried Women, by Age of Mother, 1980–2003

TABLE I-18. BIRTH RATES FOR UNMARRIED WOMEN, BY AGE, RACE, AND HISPANIC ORIGIN OF MOTHER, SELECTED YEARS, 1970–2003

This table shows the birth rates of unmarried women in specified age, race, and Hispanic origin groups. For childbearing ages across all races, the rate was 44.9 births per 1,000 unmarried women in 2003. By comparison, the birth rate for married women was 88.1. The birth rate for unmarried women rose sharply between 1970 and 1990, but has remained fairly stable since then. However, the percent age of total births to unmarried women increased by 1 percent between 2003 and 2004, according to preliminary data for 2004. (See Table I-17A.)

Table I-18. Birth Rates for Unmarried Women, by Age, Race, and Hispanic Origin of Mother, Selected Years, 1970–2003

(Live births to unmarried women per 1,000 unmarried women.)

Year, race, and Hispanic origin	15–44 years [1]	Age of mother			20–24 years	25–29 years	30–34 years	35–39 years	40–44 years [2]
		15–19 years							
		Total	15–17 years	18–19 years					
All Races [3]									
2003 [4]	44.9	34.8	20.3	57.6	71.2	65.7	44.0	22.3	5.8
2002 [4]	43.7	35.4	20.8	58.6	70.5	61.5	40.8	20.8	5.4
2001 [4]	43.8	37.0	22.0	60.6	71.3	59.5	40.4	20.4	5.3
2000 [4]	44.1	39.0	23.9	62.2	72.2	58.5	39.3	19.7	5.0
1999 [4]	43.3	39.7	25.0	62.3	70.8	56.9	38.1	19.0	4.6
1998 [4]	43.3	40.9	26.5	63.6	70.4	55.4	38.1	18.7	4.6
1997 [4]	42.9	41.4	27.7	63.9	68.9	53.4	37.9	18.7	4.6
1996 [4]	43.8	42.2	28.5	64.9	68.9	54.5	40.2	19.9	4.8
1995 [4]	44.3	43.8	30.1	66.5	68.7	54.3	38.9	19.3	4.7
1994 [4]	46.2	45.8	31.7	69.1	70.9	57.4	39.6	19.7	4.7
1993 [4]	44.8	44.0	30.3	66.2	68.5	55.9	38.0	18.9	4.4
1992 [4]	44.9	44.2	30.2	66.7	67.9	55.6	37.6	18.8	4.1
1991 [4]	45.0	44.6	30.8	65.4	67.8	56.0	37.9	17.9	3.8
1990 [4]	43.8	42.5	29.6	60.7	65.1	56.0	37.6	17.3	3.6
1989 [4]	41.6	40.1	28.7	56.0	61.2	52.8	34.9	16.0	3.4
1988 [4]	38.5	36.4	26.4	51.5	56.0	48.5	32.0	15.0	3.2
1987 [4]	36.0	33.8	24.5	48.9	52.6	44.5	29.6	13.5	2.9
1986 [4]	34.2	32.3	22.8	48.0	49.3	42.2	27.2	12.2	2.7
1985 [4]	32.8	31.4	22.4	45.9	46.5	39.9	25.2	11.6	2.5
1984 [4,5]	31.0	30.0	21.9	42.5	43.0	37.1	23.3	10.9	2.5
1983 [4,5]	30.3	29.5	22.0	40.7	41.8	35.5	22.4	10.2	2.6
1982 [4,5]	30.0	28.7	21.5	39.6	41.5	35.1	21.9	10.0	2.7
1981 [4,5]	29.5	27.9	20.9	39.0	41.1	34.5	20.8	9.8	2.6
1980 [4,5]	29.4	27.6	20.6	39.0	40.9	34.0	21.1	9.7	2.6
1980 [5,6]	28.4	27.5	20.7	38.7	39.7	31.4	18.5	8.4	2.3
1975 [5,6]	24.5	23.9	19.3	32.5	31.2	27.5	17.9	9.1	2.6
1970 [6,7]	26.4	22.4	17.1	32.9	38.4	37.0	27.1	13.6	3.5
White Total									
2003 [4]	40.4	30.1	17.2	50.4	63.0	60.8	42.0	21.2	5.5
2002 [4]	38.9	30.4	17.5	51.0	61.6	56.8	38.3	19.4	5.0
2001 [4]	38.5	31.3	18.1	52.1	61.8	54.6	37.2	18.6	4.9
2000 [4]	38.2	32.7	19.7	53.1	61.7	52.9	35.9	17.9	4.5
1999 [4]	37.4	33.2	20.6	52.9	60.2	50.8	34.9	17.4	4.1
1998 [4]	36.9	33.6	21.5	53.1	59.5	48.6	34.1	16.9	4.1
1997 [4]	36.3	33.6	22.0	52.9	57.9	47.0	33.6	16.6	3.9
1996 [4]	37.0	34.0	22.3	53.5	57.9	48.1	35.4	17.7	4.3
1995 [4]	37.0	35.0	23.3	54.7	57.2	47.4	33.7	16.8	4.2
1994 [4]	37.8	35.8	23.9	55.8	57.5	48.6	33.8	17.2	4.3
1993 [4]	35.6	33.3	21.9	52.0	53.8	46.0	31.9	16.3	3.9
1992 [4]	35.0	32.7	21.4	51.2	52.4	44.8	31.3	16.1	3.6
1991 [4]	34.5	32.7	21.7	49.4	51.4	44.3	30.9	15.2	3.2
1990 [4]	32.9	30.6	20.4	44.9	48.2	43.0	29.9	14.5	3.2
1989 [4]	30.2	28.0	19.3	40.2	43.8	39.1	26.8	13.1	2.9
1988 [4]	27.4	25.3	17.6	36.8	39.2	35.4	24.2	12.1	2.7
1987 [4]	25.3	23.2	16.2	34.5	36.6	32.0	22.3	10.7	2.4
1986 [4]	23.9	21.8	14.9	33.5	34.2	30.5	20.1	9.7	2.2
1985 [4]	22.5	20.8	14.5	31.2	31.7	28.5	18.4	9.0	2.0
1984 [4,5]	20.6	19.3	13.7	27.9	28.5	25.5	16.8	8.4	2.0
1983 [4,5]	19.8	18.7	13.6	26.4	27.1	23.8	15.9	7.8	2.0
1982 [4,5]	19.3	18.0	13.1	25.3	26.5	23.1	15.3	7.4	2.1
1981 [4,5]	18.6	17.2	12.6	24.6	25.8	22.3	14.2	7.2	1.9
1980 [4,5]	18.1	16.5	12.0	24.1	25.1	21.5	14.1	7.1	1.8

Note: Race and Hispanic origin are reported separately on the birth certificate. Data for persons of Hispanic origin are included in the data for each race group according to the mother's reported race. Rates cannot be computed for unmarried non-Hispanic Black or American Indian women because the necessary populations are not available.

[1]Fertility rates computed by relating total births to unmarried mothers, regardless of age of mother, to unmarried women age 15–44 years.
[2]Rates computed by relating births to unmarried mothers age 40 years and over to unmarried women age 40–44 years.
[3]Includes races other than White, Black, and Asian or Pacific Islander.
[4]Data for states in which marital status was not reported have been inferred and included with data from the remaining states.
[5]Based on 100 percent of births in selected states and on a 50 percent sample of births in all other states.
[6]Births to unmarried women are estimated for the United States from data for registration areas in which marital status of mother was reported.
[7]Based on a 50 percent sample of births.

Table I-18. Birth Rates for Unmarried Women, by Age, Race, and Hispanic Origin of Mother, Selected Years, 1970–2003—Continued

(Live births to unmarried women per 1,000 unmarried women.)

Year, race, and Hispanic origin	15–44 years [1]	15–19 years Total	15–17 years	18–19 years	20–24 years	25–29 years	30–34 years	35–39 years	40–44 years [2]
Non-Hispanic White									
2003 [4]	28.6	21.5	11.0	37.9	47.2	40.8	27.8	14.7	4.1
2002 [4]	27.8	22.1	11.5	38.8	46.1	38.5	26.0	13.5	3.7
2001 [4]	27.8	23.1	12.1	40.3	46.4	37.5	25.4	13.2	3.6
2000 [4]	28.0	24.7	13.6	42.1	47.0	36.9	24.8	12.9	3.3
1999 [4]	27.9	25.6	14.6	42.7	46.3	36.2	24.8	13.0	3.1
1998 [4]	27.9	26.2	15.5	43.1	46.3	35.4	25.0	13.1	3.1
1997 [4]	27.5	26.4	16.2	43.3	44.8	34.4	24.9	12.7	2.9
1996 [4]	28.2	27.0	16.9	43.9	44.5	35.0	26.4	13.8	3.3
1995 [4]	28.1	27.7	17.6	44.6	43.9	34.4	25.1	12.9	3.2
1994 [4]	28.4	28.1	17.9	45.0	43.8	34.7	24.6	12.8	3.1
1993 [4]	...	...	...	...	...	...	...	...	...
1992 [4]	...	...	...	...	...	...	...	...	...
1991 [4]	...	...	...	...	...	...	...	...	...
1990 [4,8]	24.4	25.0	16.2	37.0	36.4	30.3	20.5	6.1	...
Black Total									
2003 [4]	66.3	62.2	38.1	100.4	118.0	90.4	51.2	25.3	6.5
2002 [4]	66.2	64.8	39.9	104.1	119.2	85.9	49.9	24.9	6.3
2001 [4]	68.1	69.9	43.8	110.2	122.8	84.1	51.1	25.4	6.3
2000 [4]	70.5	75.0	48.3	115.0	129.0	85.9	50.2	25.4	6.3
1999 [4]	69.7	76.5	50.0	115.8	126.8	85.5	49.0	24.2	5.8
1998 [4]	71.6	81.5	55.0	121.5	127.8	86.5	50.5	24.3	6.0
1997 [4]	71.5	84.5	59.0	124.8	124.2	81.4	51.0	24.3	6.5
1996 [4]	72.8	87.5	62.6	127.2	122.6	81.2	53.4	25.2	6.1
1995 [4]	74.5	91.2	67.4	129.2	124.6	82.3	53.3	25.3	6.0
1994 [4]	80.8	99.3	73.9	139.6	135.2	91.3	56.5	26.0	5.9
1993 [4]	83.0	101.2	75.9	140.0	139.9	92.8	56.7	25.7	5.8
1992 [4]	85.7	104.8	77.2	146.4	142.6	96.8	57.3	25.6	5.4
1991 [4]	89.0	107.8	79.9	147.7	146.4	100.0	59.8	25.5	5.4
1990 [4]	90.5	106.0	78.8	143.7	144.8	105.3	61.5	25.5	5.1
1989 [4]	90.7	104.5	78.9	140.9	142.4	102.9	60.5	24.9	5.0
1988 [4]	86.5	96.1	73.5	130.5	133.6	97.2	57.4	24.1	5.0
1987 [4]	82.6	90.9	69.9	123.0	126.1	91.6	53.1	22.4	4.7
1986 [4]	79.0	88.5	67.0	121.1	118.0	84.6	50.0	20.6	4.4
1985 [4]	77.0	87.6	66.8	117.9	113.1	79.3	47.5	20.4	4.3
1984 [4,5]	75.2	86.1	66.5	113.6	107.9	77.8	43.8	19.4	4.3
1983 [4,5]	76.2	85.5	66.8	111.9	107.2	79.7	43.8	19.4	4.8
1982 [4,5]	77.9	85.1	66.3	112.7	109.3	82.7	44.1	19.5	5.2
1981 [4,5]	79.4	85.0	65.9	114.2	110.7	83.1	45.5	19.6	5.6
1980 [4,5]	81.1	87.9	68.8	118.2	112.3	81.4	46.7	19.0	5.5
Asian or Pacific Islander Total									
2003 [4]	22.2	13.1	7.5	21.4	26.6	30.7	31.5	19.8	7.9
2002 [4]	21.3	13.4	7.5	22.2	26.5	27.5	28.6	18.7	6.8
2001 [4]	21.2	14.6	8.7	23.0	25.2	26.7	29.4	19.7	6.3
2000 [4]	20.9	15.2	9.6	23.2	24.2	25.4	29.7	18.4	6.9
Hispanic [9]									
2003 [4]	92.2	66.6	43.0	107.0	133.7	136.0	99.2	54.7	13.3
2002 [4]	87.9	66.1	43.0	105.3	131.4	123.1	88.1	51.3	12.6
2001 [4]	87.8	67.1	44.2	104.3	132.3	120.7	91.4	49.7	12.2
2000 [4]	87.3	68.5	47.0	102.2	130.5	121.6	89.4	46.1	12.2
1999 [4]	84.9	68.6	48.7	99.9	126.1	119.6	84.2	42.4	11.2
1998 [4]	82.8	69.3	49.8	101.2	120.6	115.9	78.2	38.8	12.0
1997 [4]	83.2	69.2	50.7	100.6	122.8	114.8	78.8	40.5	12.1
1996 [4]	86.2	69.3	49.7	102.3	131.6	122.0	84.6	41.2	12.3
1995 [4]	88.8	73.2	52.8	108.6	135.8	122.3	84.1	42.2	12.1
1994 [4]	95.8	77.7	55.7	115.4	144.5	131.7	91.2	47.4	13.9
1993 [4]	91.4	71.1	49.6	108.8	134.3	130.4	87.8	47.1	14.1
1992 [4]	92.8	70.3	49.2	106.6	138.2	133.4	89.9	47.8	14.6
1991 [4]	92.5	71.0	49.5	107.5	134.2	135.1	88.2	47.6	14.1
1990 [4,8]	89.6	65.9	45.9	98.9	129.8	131.7	88.1	50.8	13.7

Note: Race and Hispanic origin are reported separately on the birth certificate. Data for persons of Hispanic origin are included in the data for each race group according to the mother's reported race. Rates cannot be computed for unmarried non-Hispanic Black or American Indian women because the necessary populations are not available.

[1] Fertility rates computed by relating total births to unmarried mothers, regardless of age of mother, to unmarried women age 15–44 years.
[2] Rates computed by relating births to unmarried mothers age 40 years and over to unmarried women age 40–44 years.
[4] Data for states in which marital status was not reported have been inferred and included with data from the remaining states.
[5] Based on 100 percent of births in selected states and on a 50 percent sample of births in all other states.
[8] Rates for 1990 based on data for 48 states and the District of Columbia that reported Hispanic origin on the birth certificate. Rates shown for 1990 for age 35–39 years are based on births to unmarried women age 35–44 years.
[9] May be of any race.
. . . = Not available.

Typically, the birth rate is highest for unmarried women in their early twenties, and tends to peak in the 25- to 29-year-old age group. (See Table I-4.) In 2003, the birth rate for unmarried women was 71.2 for women 20–24 years of age. It declined to 65.7 for women age 25–29 years, and it dropped down to 22.3 for women 35–39 years old. For 18- and 19-year-old women, the rate was 57.6.

Since 1990, the birth rate for unmarried mothers has developed differently for the major population groups. For non-Hispanic Whites, it has increased moderately; for Hispanics, it appears to have remained stable; and for Blacks, there has been a considerable decrease. This decrease has been concentrated in the sharp drop in the birth rate for unmarried Black teenagers that began in 1991. The older Black age groups have also shown declines since the early 1990s, offsetting the increases that occurred in the 1980s.

TABLE I-18A. NUMBER, RATE, AND PERCENT OF BIRTHS TO UNMARRIED WOMEN, AND BIRTH RATE FOR MARRIED WOMEN, SELECTED YEARS, 1980–2003 AND PRELIMINARY 2004

Between 1980 and 2003, the number of births to unmarried women increased from 666,000 to 1,416,000. The share of these births to total births has increased from 18.4 percent to 34.6 percent. Preliminary data for 2004 indicated the proportion of total births to unmarried women will have increased further to 35.7 percent. Much of this increase took place by the mid-1990s, when the rate of birth by unmarried women reached a peak. The 13 percent increase in nonmarital births since 1995 is mainly due to the increasing number of unmarried women of childbearing age. In 2003, the birth rate—that is, births to unmarried women per 1,000 unmarried women age 15–44 years—was 44.9, while the comparable rate for married women stood at 88.1.

Table I-18A. Number, Rate, and Percent of Births to Unmarried Women, and Birth Rate for Married Women, Selected Years, 1980–2003 and Preliminary 2004

(Number, rate, and percent.)

| Year | Births to unmarried women | | | Birth rate for married women [3] |
	Number	Rate [1]	Percent [2]	
2004	1 470 152	46.1	35.7	87.6
2003	1 415 995	44.9	34.6	88.1
2002	1 365 966	43.7	34.0	86.3
2001	1 349 249	43.8	33.5	86.7
2000	1 347 043	44.0	33.2	87.4
1999	1 308 560	43.3	33.0	84.8
1998	1 293 567	43.3	32.8	84.2
1997	1 257 444	42.9	32.4	82.7
1996	1 260 306	43.8	32.4	82.3
1995	1 253 976	44.3	32.2	82.6
1994	1 289 592	46.2	32.6	82.9
1993	1 240 172	44.8	31.0	86.1
1992	1 224 876	44.9	30.1	88.5
1991	1 213 769	45.0	29.5	89.6
1990	1 165 384	43.8	28.0	93.2
1989	1 094 169	41.6	27.1	91.9
1988	1 005 299	38.5	25.7	90.8
1987	933 013	36.0	24.5	90.0
1986	878 477	34.2	23.4	90.7
1985	828 174	32.8	22.0	93.3
1980	665 747	29.4	18.4	97.0

[1]Births to unmarried women per 1,000 unmarried women age 15–44 years.
[2]Percent of all births to unmarried women.
[3]Births to married women per 1,000 married women age 15–44 years.

TABLE I-19. NUMBER AND PERCENT OF BIRTHS TO UNMARRIED WOMEN, BY RACE AND HISPANIC ORIGIN OF MOTHER, FOR EACH STATE AND TERRITORY, 2003

For all races and origins of mothers, the proportion of births to unmarried mothers in the United States was 34.6 percent for 2003 and 35.7 percent in the preliminary data for 2004. The three states with the highest percentages of births by non-Hispanic White unmarried mothers were Maine (33.5 percent), West Virginia (33.2 percent), and Indiana (31.0 percent). For all states, the average share of births to non-Hispanic White unmarried mothers was 23.6 percent in 2003 and 24.5 percent in preliminary data for 2004. For non-Hispanic Black mothers, the highest percentages were 82.4 percent in Wisconsin, 76.5 percent in Illinois, and 76.3 percent in Indiana. The national average for non-Hispanic Blacks was 68.5 percent (69.2 percent in preliminary data for 2004). For Hispanics, the highest relative count occurred in the northeastern states, where immigration from Puerto Rico has been impor-

tant: Massachusetts (62.4 percent), Connecticut (62.1 percent), and New York (60.5 percent). The average percent of births to unmarried mothers for all Hispanics was 45.0 percent (46.4 percent in preliminary data for 2004).

Table I-19. Number and Percent of Births to Unmarried Women, by Race and Hispanic Origin of Mother, for Each State and Territory, 2003

(Number, percent.)

State	Births to unmarried mothers						Percent unmarried					
	All races[1]	White		Black		Hispanic[3]	All races[1]	White		Black		Hispanic[3]
		Total[2]	Non-Hispanic	Total[2]	Non-Hispanic			Total[2]	Non-Hispanic	Total[2]	Non-Hispanic	
UNITED STATES[4]	1 415 995	947 012	546 991	409 333	394 831	410 620	34.6	29.4	23.6	68.2	68.5	45.0
Alabama	20 827	8 274	7 577	12 434	12 409	707	35.0	20.2	19.9	69.3	69.4	24.3
Alaska	3 487	1 556	1 154	187	115	311	34.6	24.0	23.5	46.3	43.6	40.4
Arizona	37 762	30 833	9 968	2 028	1 628	21 017	41.5	39.1	25.4	62.2	61.8	52.8
Arkansas	14 358	8 682	7 331	5 483	5 462	1 355	38.0	29.2	27.7	75.8	76.0	41.3
California	181 364	150 305	33 916	20 099	19 287	116 468	33.5	34.3	20.3	62.1	62.4	43.2
Colorado	18 519	16 311	7 722	1 530	1 456	8 827	26.7	25.8	18.2	52.1	51.9	41.3
Connecticut	12 874	9 214	4 713	3 420	3 196	4 685	30.0	26.0	16.8	65.9	66.4	62.1
Delaware	4 747	2 666	1 880	2 032	1 985	810	41.9	33.6	28.6	69.9	69.7	58.7
District of Columbia	4 084	223	102	3 810	3 381	560	53.6	10.6	5.5	72.6	74.0	58.2
Florida	84 762	51 729	29 943	31 695	31 095	22 477	39.9	32.7	28.7	67.0	67.2	41.0
Georgia	51 854	22 950	14 824	28 244	27 781	8 154	38.1	26.0	21.5	65.5	66.1	44.7
Hawaii	6 058	1 287	993	143	122	1 134	33.5	25.3	23.2	24.5	25.3	43.3
Idaho	4 865	4 554	3 437	41	41	1 072	22.3	21.7	19.2	38.7	39.8	36.5
Illinois	64 439	39 609	21 000	24 117	23 942	18 774	35.3	27.9	21.1	76.4	76.5	44.2
Indiana	32 100	24 714	21 207	7 148	7 117	3 398	37.1	32.7	31.0	76.2	76.3	50.1
Iowa	11 395	10 084	9 017	959	944	1 076	29.9	28.3	27.2	74.5	74.7	42.7
Kansas	12 475	10 197	7 712	1 892	1 870	2 452	31.6	29.1	26.4	68.5	68.6	45.1
Kentucky	18 683	14 925	14 109	3 557	3 542	859	33.8	30.2	29.7	73.3	73.6	43.8
Louisiana	30 922	10 608	10 072	19 922	19 883	573	47.5	28.4	28.2	76.0	76.1	34.2
Maine	4 642	4 468	4 400	63	58	55	33.5	33.4	33.5	34.4	33.0	33.1
Maryland	26 084	10 661	8 241	14 917	14 182	3 214	34.8	23.8	21.0	58.5	58.8	46.1
Massachusetts	22 263	16 360	11 425	5 003	3 741	6 118	27.8	24.8	19.7	58.2	56.9	62.4
Michigan	45 386	27 865	24 058	16 646	16 522	3 362	34.6	27.0	25.7	73.8	74.0	43.8
Minnesota	19 425	14 202	11 679	3 035	2 961	2 471	27.7	23.9	21.6	56.6	56.4	50.1
Mississippi	19 926	5 740	5 491	13 945	13 941	242	47.0	24.7	24.2	75.2	75.2	44.6
Missouri	27 426	18 383	16 912	8 598	8 497	1 585	35.6	28.8	28.0	77.0	77.2	45.5
Montana	3 677	2 670	2 440	27	26	161	32.2	27.1	26.2	54.0	53.1	42.5
Nebraska	7 687	6 250	4 605	1 033	1 019	1 503	29.7	26.7	23.7	70.4	70.6	43.5
Nevada	13 172	10 159	4 580	2 022	1 930	5 627	39.1	36.7	29.3	69.7	70.1	46.1
New Hampshire	3 571	3 429	3 028	102	73	210	24.8	25.1	24.1	42.0	42.2	39.8
New Jersey	34 313	20 870	8 240	12 801	11 341	14 093	29.3	24.3	13.3	63.4	64.4	53.1
New Mexico	13 479	10 377	2 380	326	281	8 113	48.4	44.6	27.7	61.3	59.0	54.7
New York	92 597	56 594	25 739	31 946	29 071	33 424	36.5	30.8	19.5	66.5	66.4	60.5
North Carolina	41 802	22 491	14 579	18 001	17 899	7 995	35.3	26.0	20.7	66.3	66.3	49.7
North Dakota	2 276	1 599	1 490	32	30	56	28.5	23.2	22.7	29.4	28.3	33.3
Ohio	54 130	36 551	33 925	17 096	16 846	2 719	36.2	29.6	28.7	75.4	75.5	50.8
Oklahoma	18 915	12 721	10 349	3 291	3 243	2 466	37.1	31.8	30.1	71.2	71.2	43.0
Oregon	14 586	13 017	9 360	652	627	3 645	31.7	31.3	28.3	64.0	64.2	43.2
Pennsylvania	49 547	32 134	27 166	16 460	14 148	6 408	33.9	27.1	24.9	74.6	74.6	59.2
Rhode Island	4 728	3 616	1 871	815	731	1 411	35.8	32.2	25.8	64.8	65.4	56.8
South Carolina	22 857	9 380	7 832	13 269	13 224	1 574	41.1	25.9	24.0	72.4	72.5	43.0
South Dakota	3 768	2 193	2 071	56	52	166	34.2	24.6	24.0	45.9	44.8	48.8
Tennessee	29 367	17 141	14 854	11 934	11 889	2 338	37.2	28.1	26.5	73.4	73.5	47.4
Texas	129 484	101 812	30 629	26 256	25 902	71 229	34.3	31.7	22.2	62.7	62.8	38.9
Utah	8 590	7 794	5 062	181	165	2 726	17.2	16.5	12.6	47.3	48.4	38.6
Vermont	1 978	1 929	1 896	28	27	17	30.0	30.1	30.0	52.8	51.9	*
Virginia	30 816	16 164	12 154	14 080	13 706	4 420	30.4	22.5	19.5	62.3	62.8	42.5
Washington	23 207	18 225	13 193	2 064	1 592	5 653	28.8	27.4	24.5	51.4	51.8	42.4
West Virginia	7 235	6 665	6 598	538	533	35	34.6	33.3	33.2	74.6	74.8	33.7
Wisconsin	21 300	14 881	12 444	5 347	5 291	2 542	30.4	24.7	22.7	82.3	82.4	45.9
Wyoming	2 186	1 950	1 623	28	27	333	32.6	31.0	28.8	52.8	51.9	49.9
Puerto Rico	26 962	23 825	. . .	3 125	. . .	. . .	53.2	51.7	. . .	67.9	. . .	. . .
Virgin Islands	1 047	183	28	859	684	226	68.8	52.1	26.9	74.9	74.8	65.7
Guam	1 821	39	33	12	12	17	55.5	14.1	13.7	*	*	*
American Samoa	609	-	. . .	-	. . .	. . .	37.9	*	. . .	*	. . .	. . .
Northern Marianas	780	4	. . .	-	. . .	. . .	57.8	*	. . .	*	. . .	. . .

[1]Includes races other than White and Black and origin not stated.
[2]Race and Hispanic origin are reported separately on the birth certificate. Data for persons of Hispanic origin are included in the data for each race group according to the mother's reported race.
[3]May be of any race.
[4]Excludes data for the territories.
* = Figure does not meet standards of reliability or precision; based on fewer than 20 births in numerator.
- = Quantity zero.
. . . = Not available.

TABLE I-19A. WOMEN 15–44 YEARS OF AGE WHO HAVE NOT HAD AT LEAST 1 LIVE BIRTH, BY AGE, SELECTED YEARS, 1960–2002

Almost 16 percent of women age 40–44 years have not had at least one live birth (essentially a measure of lifetime nulliparity for a birth cohort of women). This percentage declined between 1960 and 1975, rose to a plateau in the late 1990s, and fell slightly in the early 2000s. The percentage of childless teenage women has increased slowly but steadily from 91.4 percent in 1960 to 94.4 percent in 2002. The pattern in the intervening age categories demonstrates that by 2002, American women had delayed having their first child—sometimes by 5 or more years, as compared to 1960.

Table I-19A. Women 15–44 Years of Age Who Have Not Had At Least 1 Live Birth, by Age, Selected Years, 1960–2002

(Percent.)

Year[1]	15–19 years	20–24 years	25–29 years	30–34 years	35–39 years	40–44 years
2002	94.4	66.8	41.5	24.9	17.3	15.8
2001	94.0	66.6	41.7	25.5	17.6	16.0
2000	93.7	66.0	42.1	25.9	17.9	16.2
1999	93.4	65.5	42.5	26.1	18.1	16.4
1998	93.1	65.1	43.0	26.1	18.2	16.5
1997	92.8	64.9	43.5	26.2	18.4	16.6
1996	92.5	65.0	43.8	26.2	18.5	16.6
1995	92.5	65.5	44.0	26.2	18.6	16.5
1994	92.6	66.1	43.9	26.2	18.7	16.2
1993	92.6	66.7	43.8	26.1	18.8	15.8
1992	92.7	67.3	43.7	26.0	18.8	15.2
1991	93.0	67.9	43.6	26.0	18.7	14.5
1990	93.3	68.3	43.5	25.9	18.5	13.9
1989	93.7	68.4	43.3	25.9	18.2	13.5
1988	93.8	68.4	43.0	25.7	17.7	13.0
1987	93.8	68.2	42.5	25.5	16.9	12.6
1986	93.8	68.0	42.0	25.1	16.1	12.2
1985	93.7	67.7	41.5	24.6	15.4	11.7
1980	93.4	66.2	38.9	19.7	12.5	9.0
1975	92.6	62.5	31.1	15.2	9.6	8.8
1970	93.0	57.0	24.4	11.8	9.4	10.6
1965	92.7	51.4	19.7	11.7	11.4	11.0
1960	91.4	47.5	20.0	14.2	12.0	15.1

[1]As of January 1.

TABLE I-20. BIRTH RATES, BY AGE AND RACE OF FATHER, 1980–2003

The rate of 48.9 in 2003 shows total births per 1,000 men, age 15 to 54 years. The rate was smaller than the fertility rate of women (66.1), because the population of women was included only to age 44, while the population of men was included for 10 years further. This table measures the frequency with which men in various age groups became fathers of a newborn.

Similar to the female fertility rate, the male rate has been declining since 1990. It was the highest in the 25- to 34-year-old age bracket. In comparison with the birth rates of mothers, the fathers' rates were low for men under 30 years of age, but they exceeded the mothers' birth rates for age 30 and over. For Whites in 2003, the fathers' birth rate between 20 and 24 years was 69.2, and peaked at 106.1 between the ages of 25 and 29 years. Blacks had higher fathers' birth rates at all ages, except in their thirties. The overall Black fathers' birth rate in 2003 was 61.0, substantially smaller than in 1990, but higher than the overall rate for White fathers.

Information on the age of the father is often missing on birth certificates of children born to mothers under 25 years old and to unmarried mothers. Such missing data are estimated according to the most prevalent age patterns reported by mothers in each age group.

TABLE I-21. LIVE BIRTHS, BY EDUCATIONAL ATTAINMENT, AGE, RACE, AND HISPANIC ORIGIN OF MOTHER: UNITED STATES EXCLUDING PENNSYLVANIA AND WASHINGTON STATE, 2003

As many as 78.4 percent of mothers had completed at least 12 years of education in 2003, and 26.6 percent had 16 years or more of schooling. These percentages were notably higher for non-Hispanic White mothers. Approximately 52.5 percent of Hispanic mothers had 12 years or more of schooling, and 8.7 percent of the group had at least 16 years of education. The educational attainment of non-Hispanic Black mothers was considerably higher than that of Hispanics, but below that of non-Hispanic Whites: 76.2 percent had completed 12 years of school or more, and 13.4 percent were college graduates or more. Educational achievement has been positively correlated with timely prenatal care, behavior conducive to a healthy pregnancy, and a smaller number of children.

Table I-20. Birth Rates, by Age and Race of Father, 1980–2003

(Live births per 1,000 men in specified group.)

Year and race of father	15–54 years [1]	Age of father								
		15–19 years [2]	20–24 years	25–29 years	30–34 years	35–39 years	40–44 years	45–49 years	50–54 years	55 years and over
All Races [3]										
2003	48.9	16.9	73.5	105.7	102.2	60.2	23.4	7.6	2.5	0.3
2002	48.4	17.4	75.6	105.0	99.1	57.7	22.6	7.4	2.4	0.3
2001	49.0	18.5	78.5	105.8	99.6	57.0	22.3	7.3	2.4	0.3
2000	50.0	19.8	82.1	106.5	99.5	56.3	22.2	7.3	2.5	0.3
1999	49.2	20.6	81.1	105.3	95.9	53.9	21.1	7.0	2.4	0.3
1998	49.6	21.3	82.3	104.4	94.4	53.1	21.0	7.1	2.5	0.3
1997	49.4	21.9	82.1	102.6	92.0	51.5	20.7	7.0	2.5	0.3
1996	50.2	22.7	83.4	102.8	91.3	51.1	20.5	6.9	2.5	0.3
1995	51.0	23.9	83.9	103.2	90.7	50.4	20.3	7.0	2.5	0.3
1994	52.4	24.6	85.6	105.3	91.1	50.5	20.3	7.2	2.6	0.3
1993	53.7	24.4	86.0	108.1	91.7	50.7	20.2	7.3	2.7	0.4
1992	55.3	24.4	87.1	111.1	93.0	51.1	20.4	7.3	2.7	0.4
1991	56.8	24.7	87.9	113.5	94.3	51.6	20.2	7.4	2.7	0.4
1990	58.4	23.5	88.0	116.4	97.8	53.0	21.0	7.5	2.8	0.4
1989	57.2	21.9	85.4	114.3	94.8	51.3	20.4	7.4	2.7	0.6
1988	55.8	19.6	82.4	111.6	93.2	49.9	19.9	7.1	2.7	0.4
1987	55.0	18.3	80.5	109.9	91.2	48.6	19.0	6.9	2.6	0.4
1986	54.8	17.9	80.3	109.6	90.3	46.8	18.3	6.7	2.6	0.4
1985	55.6	18.0	81.2	112.3	91.1	47.3	18.1	6.6	2.5	0.4
1984 [4]	55.0	17.8	80.7	111.4	89.9	46.0	17.8	6.3	2.4	0.4
1983 [4]	55.1	18.2	82.6	113.0	89.1	45.2	17.4	6.4	2.3	0.4
1982 [4]	56.4	18.6	86.5	117.3	90.3	44.5	17.5	6.4	2.3	0.4
1981 [4]	56.3	18.4	88.4	119.1	88.7	43.3	17.0	6.2	2.3	0.4
1980 [4]	57.0	18.8	92.0	123.1	91.0	42.8	17.1	6.1	2.2	0.3
White										
2003	47.1	14.3	69.2	106.1	102.8	58.9	21.9	6.7	2.1	0.3
2002	46.4	14.8	70.8	104.8	99.4	56.4	21.0	6.6	2.0	0.3
2001	46.9	15.5	73.1	105.4	99.9	55.7	20.8	6.5	2.0	0.3
2000	47.6	16.6	75.8	105.4	99.5	54.7	20.7	6.5	2.1	0.3
1999	46.9	17.3	74.7	104.1	96.2	52.7	19.8	6.3	2.1	0.3
1998	47.1	17.7	75.6	102.7	94.3	51.9	19.6	6.3	2.1	0.3
1997	46.8	18.0	75.3	100.9	91.7	50.2	19.3	6.2	2.1	0.3
1996	47.7	18.7	76.7	101.4	91.1	49.9	19.2	6.1	2.1	0.2
1995	48.4	19.4	77.0	101.7	90.4	49.1	19.1	6.2	2.1	0.2
1994	49.3	19.5	77.4	103.1	90.4	48.9	18.9	6.3	2.2	0.3
1993	50.3	18.9	77.2	105.5	90.7	48.9	18.7	6.4	2.2	0.2
1992	51.8	18.8	77.8	108.2	91.9	49.1	18.8	6.4	2.2	0.3
1991	53.1	19.0	78.4	110.2	92.8	49.6	18.5	6.5	2.2	0.3
1990	54.6	18.1	78.3	113.2	96.1	50.9	19.2	6.5	2.2	0.3
1989	53.3	16.7	75.9	110.8	93.0	49.1	18.7	6.3	2.1	0.4
1988	52.2	14.8	73.7	108.3	91.2	47.6	18.1	6.1	2.1	0.3
1987	51.6	13.9	72.8	107.0	89.5	46.2	17.3	5.9	2.0	0.3
1986	51.7	13.8	73.3	107.0	88.7	44.4	16.6	5.7	2.0	0.3
1985	52.6	14.0	74.7	109.9	89.5	44.8	16.3	5.6	1.9	0.3
1984 [4]	51.8	14.0	74.3	108.8	87.9	43.5	16.0	5.3	1.9	0.3
1983 [4]	52.0	14.4	76.3	110.2	86.8	42.6	15.5	5.3	1.8	0.3
1982 [4]	53.1	14.9	80.1	114.2	87.5	41.7	15.6	5.3	1.9	0.3
1981 [4]	52.9	15.0	81.7	115.8	85.8	40.3	15.0	5.2	1.8	0.3
1980 [4]	53.4	15.4	84.9	119.4	87.8	39.7	15.0	5.1	1.8	0.3
Black										
2003	61.0	32.5	111.9	122.3	96.2	59.9	29.6	12.4	4.9	0.9
2002	61.2	33.3	116.2	123.6	94.0	57.8	28.5	12.0	4.7	0.9
2001	63.3	36.5	124.5	125.9	95.6	57.1	28.2	11.8	4.7	1.0
2000	66.2	39.6	135.5	131.0	95.2	56.9	28.4	11.7	5.0	1.0
1999	65.4	41.0	133.8	129.6	91.6	54.3	26.5	11.2	4.9	1.0
1998	66.8	42.8	137.0	130.3	90.9	54.0	26.7	11.6	5.0	1.0
1997	66.7	45.1	136.3	126.3	88.8	52.6	26.1	11.4	5.2	1.0
1996	67.2	46.7	137.6	123.9	87.0	51.8	25.7	11.3	5.3	1.1
1995	69.1	49.9	139.2	123.9	87.7	52.0	25.7	11.9	5.4	1.1
1994	74.0	54.1	149.1	129.6	91.4	53.8	26.4	12.8	5.8	1.1
1993	77.6	56.2	152.7	134.2	94.0	56.3	27.7	13.4	6.3	1.3
1992	80.4	57.0	157.1	138.6	95.8	56.7	28.4	13.7	6.1	1.4
1991	83.0	57.8	158.5	142.0	99.2	58.5	29.4	14.1	6.7	1.4
1990	84.9	55.2	158.2	144.9	103.2	60.4	31.1	15.0	7.1	1.4
1989	84.1	52.9	153.4	143.5	101.4	59.9	31.1	14.9	6.9	2.7
1988	80.7	48.1	144.1	137.9	100.0	58.0	30.6	14.3	6.9	1.4
1987	78.3	44.6	136.1	133.9	97.4	58.0	30.0	13.8	6.6	1.3
1986	77.2	42.6	131.4	131.6	97.4	58.0	29.1	13.5	6.7	1.3
1985	77.2	41.8	129.5	132.7	97.3	59.4	29.5	13.3	6.5	1.2
1984 [4]	76.7	40.9	128.0	132.2	98.3	58.4	29.3	13.3	6.1	1.2
1983 [4]	77.2	40.7	129.1	134.4	99.0	59.6	29.6	13.5	6.0	1.2
1982 [4]	79.5	40.3	133.4	141.2	103.6	61.1	29.6	13.9	6.0	1.2
1981 [4]	80.4	38.9	138.4	145.6	104.3	61.3	29.7	13.3	5.7	1.2
1980 [4]	83.0	40.1	145.3	152.8	109.6	62.0	31.2	13.6	5.9	1.1

Note: Race and Hispanic origin are reported separately on birth certificates. In this table, all men (including Hispanic men) are classified only according to their race. Age of father was not stated for 13 percent of births in 2002. Figures for age of father not stated are distributed.

[1] Rates computed by relating total births, regardless of age of father, to men age 15–54 years.
[2] Rates computed by relating births of fathers under 20 years of age to men age 15–19 years.
[3] Includes races other than White and Black.
[4] Based on 100 percent of births in selected states and on a 50 percent sample of births in all other states.

Table I-21. Live Births, by Educational Attainment, Age, Race, and Hispanic Origin of Mother: United States Excluding Pennsylvania and Washington State, 2003

(Number, percent.)

Age and race of mother	Total	Years of school completed by mother						Percent 12 years or more	Percent 16 years or more
		0–8 years	9–11 years	12 years	13–15 years	16 years or more	Not stated		
All Races [1]									
All ages	3 863 502	233 840	588 283	1 162 697	811 985	1 012 730	53 967	78.4	26.6
Under 15 years	6 341	4 884	1 298	-	-	-	159	*	*
15–19 years	394 919	33 508	196 889	137 333	21 114	-	6 075	40.7	*
15 years	17 344	5 129	11 735	-	-	-	480	*	*
16 years	39 332	4 963	32 475	1 119	-	-	775	2.9	*
17 years	71 353	5 913	52 278	11 741	241	-	1 180	17.1	*
18 years	112 293	7 972	50 769	48 493	3 516	-	1 543	47.0	*
19 years	154 597	9 531	49 632	75 980	17 357	-	2 097	61.2	*
20–24 years	980 514	63 057	204 945	423 305	220 117	56 387	12 703	72.3	5.8
25–29 years	1 025 666	61 487	104 139	299 115	258 304	288 933	13 688	83.6	28.6
30–34 years	916 840	42 846	54 016	190 800	199 543	417 131	12 504	89.3	46.1
35–39 years	438 771	21 643	22 032	90 951	91 675	205 602	6 868	89.9	47.6
40 years and over	100 451	6 415	4 964	21 193	21 232	44 677	1 970	88.4	45.4
White Total [2]									
All ages	3 040 873	210 711	443 337	879 194	629 732	837 720	40 179	78.2	27.9
Under 15 years	3 512	2 654	770	-	-	-	88	*	*
15–19 years	284 360	28 528	139 800	97 463	14 252	-	4 317	39.9	*
15 years	10 963	3 350	7 299	-	-	-	314	*	*
16 years	26 861	3 952	21 584	768	-	-	557	2.9	*
17 years	50 615	5 226	36 181	8 201	174	-	833	16.8	*
18 years	81 801	7 218	37 295	33 847	2 335	-	1 106	44.8	*
19 years	114 120	8 782	37 441	54 647	11 743	-	1 507	59.0	*
20–24 years	750 290	58 793	157 422	316 774	163 806	43 939	9 556	70.8	5.9
25–29 years	821 227	57 145	82 021	231 504	203 379	236 883	10 295	82.8	29.2
30–34 years	745 992	38 746	42 990	147 820	159 135	348 034	9 267	88.9	47.2
35–39 years	355 111	19 271	16 739	69 768	72 446	171 685	5 202	89.7	49.1
40 years and over	80 381	5 574	3 595	15 865	16 714	37 179	1 454	88.4	47.1
Non-Hispanic White									
All ages	2 158 797	33 454	212 021	620 663	513 666	760 496	18 497	88.5	35.5
Under 15 years	1 316	1 042	250	-	-	-	24	*	*
15–19 years	161 828	8 148	76 711	65 249	10 172	-	1 548	47.1	*
15 years	4 548	1 364	3 088	-	-	-	96	*	*
16 years	12 496	1 391	10 536	409	-	-	160	3.3	*
17 years	26 846	1 574	20 006	4 869	112	-	285	18.8	*
18 years	47 441	1 882	21 483	22 104	1 566	-	406	50.3	*
19 years	70 497	1 937	21 598	37 867	8 494	-	601	66.3	*
20–24 years	488 194	10 422	83 319	224 817	128 393	37 466	3 777	80.6	7.7
25–29 years	582 914	6 599	31 320	161 587	166 223	212 531	4 654	93.4	36.8
30–34 years	580 329	4 249	13 443	105 645	133 308	318 774	4 910	96.9	55.4
35–39 years	280 645	2 217	5 519	51 239	61 266	157 579	2 825	97.2	56.7
40 years and over	63 571	777	1 459	12 126	14 304	34 146	759	96.4	54.4
Black Total [2]									
All ages	573 776	14 570	121 098	220 995	132 461	75 613	9 039	76.0	13.4
Under 15 years	2 588	2 059	464	-	-	-	65	*	*
15–19 years	96 294	4 206	50 240	34 553	5 826	-	1 469	42.6	*
15 years	5 744	1 627	3 972	-	-	-	145	*	*
16 years	11 047	877	9 689	291	-	-	190	2.7	*
17 years	18 180	575	14 211	3 055	59	-	280	17.4	*
18 years	26 567	587	11 849	12 782	975	-	374	52.5	*
19 years	34 756	540	10 519	18 425	4 792	-	480	67.7	*
20–24 years	187 923	2 698	40 520	88 414	45 546	8 306	2 439	76.7	4.5
25–29 years	133 853	2 254	17 335	50 587	38 799	22 803	2 075	85.1	17.3
30–34 years	93 416	1 855	7 815	29 141	26 379	26 455	1 771	89.4	28.9
35–39 years	47 722	1 112	3 761	14 602	12 886	14 429	932	89.6	30.8
40 years and over	11 980	386	963	3 698	3 025	3 620	288	88.5	31.0
Non-Hispanic Black									
All ages	553 987	12 376	117 279	214 309	128 458	73 396	8 169	76.2	13.4
Under 15 years	2 531	2 019	450	-	-	-	62	*	*
15–19 years	93 623	3 940	48 944	33 691	5 678	-	1 370	42.7	*
15 years	5 595	1 577	3 880	-	-	-	138	*	*
16 years	10 741	845	9 441	275	-	-	180	2.6	*
17 years	17 640	528	13 842	2 953	56	-	261	17.3	*
18 years	25 875	529	11 574	12 490	938	-	344	52.6	*
19 years	33 772	461	10 207	17 973	4 684	-	447	68.0	*
20–24 years	182 032	2 133	39 330	86 037	44 230	8 043	2 259	76.9	4.5
25–29 years	128 686	1 642	16 608	48 887	37 574	22 138	1 837	85.6	17.5
30–34 years	89 775	1 425	7 432	28 098	25 557	25 695	1 568	90.0	29.1
35–39 years	45 795	887	3 589	14 003	12 486	14 012	818	90.0	31.2
40 years and over	11 545	330	926	3 593	2 933	3 508	255	88.9	31.1
Hispanic [3]									
All ages	888 177	179 657	234 793	263 657	118 461	75 687	15 922	52.5	8.7
Under 15 years	2 250	1 653	538	-	-	-	59	*	*
15–19 years	124 616	20 695	64 310	33 008	4 227	-	2 376	30.5	*
15 years	6 569	2 048	4 319	-	-	-	202	*	*
16 years	14 645	2 597	11 321	381	-	-	346	2.7	*
17 years	24 201	3 706	16 513	3 433	63	-	486	14.7	*
18 years	34 864	5 411	16 053	12 006	807	-	587	37.4	*
19 years	44 337	6 933	16 104	17 188	3 357	-	755	47.1	*
20–24 years	265 614	49 087	75 075	93 818	36 383	6 567	4 684	52.4	2.5
25–29 years	239 989	51 257	51 384	71 223	37 833	24 022	4 270	56.5	10.2
30–34 years	165 152	34 900	29 919	42 897	26 180	28 455	2 801	60.1	17.5
35–39 years	74 008	17 231	11 402	18 912	11 397	13 688	1 378	60.6	18.8
40 years and over	16 548	4 834	2 165	3 799	2 441	2 955	354	56.8	18.2

Note: Excludes data for Pennsylvania and Washington, which implemented a forthcoming revision in the standard birth certificate and thus impaired comparability with the data from other states.

[1] Includes races other than White and Black.
[2] Race and Hispanic origin are reported separately on the birth certificate. Data for persons of Hispanic origin are included in the data for each race group according to the mother's reported race.
[3] May be of any race.
* = Figure does not meet standards of reliability or precision; based on fewer than 20 births in numerator.
- = Quantity zero.

TABLE I-21A. MATERNAL EDUCATION FOR LIVE BIRTHS, ACCORDING TO DETAILED RACE AND HISPANIC ORIGIN OF MOTHER, SELECTED YEARS, 1970–2003

Educational achievement has been increasing substantially since 1970 among all racial groups and ethnicities. However, progress was relatively slow among Hispanic mothers, especially those of Mexican origin.

TABLE I-22. NUMBER OF LIVE BIRTHS AND PERCENT DISTRIBUTION, BY WEIGHT GAIN OF MOTHER DURING PREGNANCY AND MEDIAN WEIGHT GAIN, ACCORDING TO PERIOD OF GESTATION, RACE, AND HISPANIC ORIGIN OF MOTHER: UNITED STATES EXCLUDING CALIFORNIA, 2003

The median weight gain of mothers during pregnancy was 30.5 pounds, a figure that has remained unchanged for 6 years. Non-Hispanic Blacks had a slightly smaller median weight gain of 29.8 pounds, and Hispanics had a median weight gain of 28.7 pounds. To some extent, weight gain is related to the duration of gestation. Among mothers with a gestation period of 40 weeks or more, 14.2 percent had a weight gain of 46 pounds or more, while for those with a gestation period under 37 weeks, only 11.6 percent had this large of a weight gain. Conversely, among mothers with a gestation period under 37 weeks, 18.1 percent (but 25.0 percent of non-Hispanic Black mothers) had weight gains of less than 16 pounds. For mothers with a gestation period of 40 weeks or more, this small weight gain occurred in only 10.8 percent of cases. In 2003, almost a third of mothers had weight gains outside the guidelines recommended by the Institute of Medicine; this represented a sizable increase since 1989. A weight gain of less than 16 pounds is generally considered inadequate for most women, whereas a weight gain of more than 40 pounds is considered excessive in most cases (underweight women are recommended to gain more weight, while overweight women are recommended to gain less weight).

Table I-21A. Maternal Education for Live Births, According to Detailed Race and Hispanic Origin of Mother, Selected Years, 1970–2003

(Percent.)

Education, race, and Hispanic origin of mother	2003	2002	2001	2000	1999	1998	1995	1990	1985	1980	1975	1970
PERCENT OF LIVE BIRTHS [1]												
Less than 12 Years of Education												
All races	21.6	21.5	21.7	21.7	21.7	21.9	22.6	23.8	20.6	23.7	28.6	30.8
White	21.8	21.6	21.7	21.4	21.3	21.2	21.6	22.4	17.8	20.8	25.1	27.1
Black or African American	24.0	24.4	24.9	25.5	26.0	26.9	28.7	30.2	32.6	36.4	45.3	51.2
American Indian or Alaska Native	30.5	30.8	31.0	31.6	32.2	32.7	33.0	36.4	39.0	44.2	52.7	60.5
Asian or Pacific Islander	9.9	10.3	10.8	11.6	12.4	12.9	16.1	20.0	19.4	21.0	...	...
Chinese	...	11.3	11.9	11.7	12.0	11.4	12.9	15.8	15.5	15.2	16.5	23.0
Japanese	...	2.2	1.8	2.1	2.0	2.4	2.6	3.5	4.8	5.0	9.1	11.8
Filipino	...	5.3	6.0	6.2	6.3	6.9	8.0	10.3	13.9	16.4	22.3	26.4
Hawaiian	...	14.3	15.4	16.7	16.8	18.5	17.6	19.3	18.7	20.7	...	...
Other Asian or Pacific Islander	...	11.6	12.2	13.5	14.8	15.9	21.2	26.8	24.3	27.6	...	...
Hispanic or Latino [2]	47.5	48.1	48.8	48.9	49.1	49.3	52.1	53.9	44.5	51.1	...	...
Mexican	53.6	54.2	55.0	55.0	55.2	55.2	58.6	61.4	59.0	62.8	...	...
Puerto Rican	29.9	31.5	32.3	33.4	34.4	35.9	38.6	42.7	46.6	55.3	...	...
Cuban	11.5	11.8	11.8	11.9	12.3	13.0	14.4	17.8	21.1	24.1	...	...
Central and South American	35.3	35.8	36.5	37.2	37.9	38.5	41.7	44.2	37.0	41.2	...	...
Other and unknown Hispanic or Latino	30.1	31.7	30.4	31.4	32.5	33.6	33.8	33.3	36.5	40.1	...	...
Not Hispanic or Latino [2]												
White	11.5	11.7	12.0	12.2	12.6	12.8	13.3	15.2	15.7	18.1	...	...
Black or African American	23.8	24.3	24.8	25.3	25.9	26.7	28.6	30.0	33.4	37.3	...	...
16 Years or More of Education												
All races	26.6	25.9	25.2	24.7	24.1	23.4	21.4	17.5	16.7	14.0	11.4	8.6
White	27.9	27.3	26.7	26.3	25.7	25.1	23.1	19.3	18.6	15.5	12.7	9.6
Black or African American	13.4	12.7	12.1	11.7	11.4	11.0	9.5	7.2	7.0	6.2	4.3	2.8
American Indian or Alaska Native	8.5	8.7	8.2	7.8	7.2	6.8	6.2	4.4	3.7	3.5	2.2	2.7
Asian or Pacific Islander	47.1	45.7	44.0	42.8	40.9	39.7	35.0	31.0	30.3	30.8	...	...
Chinese	...	57.3	55.9	55.6	54.3	53.8	49.0	40.3	35.2	41.5	37.8	34.0
Japanese	...	53.5	52.0	51.1	49.5	49.1	46.2	44.1	38.1	36.8	30.6	20.7
Filipino	...	43.3	41.8	40.5	39.6	39.2	36.7	34.5	35.2	37.1	36.6	28.1
Hawaiian	...	14.6	13.2	13.5	12.7	11.0	9.7	6.8	6.5	7.9	...	...
Other Asian or Pacific Islander	...	44.4	42.6	40.7	38.5	36.7	30.5	27.3	30.2	29.2	...	...
Hispanic or Latino [2]	8.7	8.3	7.9	7.6	7.4	7.0	6.1	5.1	6.0	4.2	...	...
Mexican	5.9	5.5	5.3	5.1	5.0	4.7	4.0	3.3	3.0	2.2	...	...
Puerto Rican	12.9	11.8	11.1	10.4	10.3	9.5	8.7	6.5	4.6	3.0	...	...
Cuban	31.3	30.5	30.8	31.0	29.9	28.6	26.5	20.4	15.0	11.6	...	...
Central and South American	16.0	15.5	14.8	14.1	13.2	12.5	10.3	8.6	8.1	6.1	...	...
Other and unknown Hispanic or Latino	14.4	13.2	13.2	12.5	12.0	11.5	10.5	8.5	7.2	5.5	...	...
Not Hispanic or Latino [2]												
White	35.5	34.3	33.3	32.5	31.4	30.4	27.7	22.6	19.4	16.6	...	...
Black or African American	13.4	12.7	12.2	11.7	11.4	11.0	9.5	7.3	6.7	5.8	...	...

[1]Excludes live births for whom education of mother is unknown.
[2]Prior to 1993, data shown only for states with an Hispanic-origin item and education of mother item on the birth certificate.
. . . = Not available.

Inadequate maternal weight gain has been associated with an increased risk of intrauterine growth retardation, shortened period of gestation, low birthweight, and perinatal mortality. High weight gain has been linked with an elevated risk of a large-for-gestational-age infant, cesarean delivery, and long-term maternal weight retention.

The weight gain most often reported, with an overall frequency of 17.5 percent, was 26 to 30 pounds. Mothers with gestation periods under 37 weeks most frequently gained less than 16 pounds, with a frequency of 18.1 percent among all races and a frequency of 25.0 percent for non-Hispanic Blacks.

Table I-22. Number of Live Births and Percent Distribution, by Weight Gain of Mother During Pregnancy and Median Weight Gain, According to Period of Gestation, Race, and Hispanic Origin of Mother: United States Excluding California, 2003

(Number, percent.)

Period of gestation [1] and race and Hispanic origin of mother	All births	Less than 16 pounds	16–20 pounds	21–25 pounds	26–30 pounds	31–35 pounds	36–40 pounds	41–45 pounds	46 pounds or more	Not stated	Median weight gain in pounds
NUMBER											
All Gestation Periods [2]											
All races [3]	3 548 953	410 229	357 405	458 300	585 514	454 516	418 727	228 945	428 973	206 344	X
White total [4]	2 787 474	297 601	270 105	360 388	467 186	371 152	339 605	187 293	344 316	149 828	X
Non-Hispanic White	2 155 140	209 691	191 953	273 520	364 606	301 256	276 213	155 532	288 331	94 038	X
Black total [4]	567 498	92 425	65 566	69 982	83 575	57 462	57 291	30 703	68 200	42 294	X
Non-Hispanic Black	545 108	89 567	63 330	67 261	80 128	54 794	54 955	29 358	65 593	40 122	X
Hispanic [5]	642 624	89 493	79 745	88 603	104 476	71 213	64 337	32 378	57 131	55 248	X
Under 37 Weeks											
All races [3]	446 127	74 658	54 205	58 190	65 791	45 957	42 005	23 039	47 909	34 373	X
White total [4]	323 512	48 655	37 925	42 906	49 059	35 270	32 146	17 939	36 835	22 777	X
Non-Hispanic White	245 822	34 007	27 164	32 544	37 889	28 240	25 827	14 801	31 057	14 293	X
Black total [4]	100 594	22 643	13 279	12 078	13 313	8 379	7 940	4 103	9 307	9 552	X
Non-Hispanic Black	97 637	22 095	12 934	11 716	12 913	8 118	7 670	3 980	9 030	9 181	X
Hispanic [5]	79 155	14 951	11 001	10 606	11 437	7 172	6 481	3 185	5 924	8 398	X
37–39 Weeks											
All races [3]	1 840 887	206 842	187 372	244 844	313 404	241 613	218 550	116 542	212 395	99 325	X
White total [4]	1 453 012	152 418	142 680	193 129	250 810	197 615	177 547	95 375	170 584	72 854	X
Non-Hispanic White	1 132 187	108 662	102 628	147 745	197 456	161 398	145 178	79 633	143 168	46 319	X
Black total [4]	285 044	44 031	32 885	36 383	43 419	29 983	29 633	15 521	33 735	19 454	X
Non-Hispanic Black	273 918	42 660	31 749	34 956	41 644	28 572	28 466	14 863	32 538	18 470	X
Hispanic [5]	325 928	44 501	40 890	46 283	54 296	36 926	32 799	16 034	27 880	26 319	X
40 Weeks and Over											
All races [3]	1 255 561	128 090	115 499	154 873	205 866	166 612	157 852	89 183	168 291	69 295	X
White total [4]	1 006 388	96 115	89 267	124 055	166 970	138 004	129 669	73 837	136 636	51 835	X
Non-Hispanic White	774 234	66 768	62 008	93 030	129 014	111 458	105 044	60 990	113 905	32 017	X
Black total [4]	180 423	25 553	19 326	21 447	26 773	19 047	19 662	11 044	25 062	12 509	X
Non-Hispanic Black	172 228	24 625	18 574	20 517	25 502	18 052	18 768	10 484	23 930	11 776	X
Hispanic [5]	236 120	29 887	27 779	31 618	38 640	27 016	24 979	13 122	23 275	19 804	X
PERCENT DISTRIBUTION											
All Gestation Periods [2]											
All races [3]	100.0	12.3	10.7	13.7	17.5	13.6	12.5	6.8	12.8	X	30.5
White total [4]	100.0	11.3	10.2	13.7	17.7	14.1	12.9	7.1	13.1	X	30.7
Non-Hispanic White	100.0	10.2	9.3	13.3	17.7	14.6	13.4	7.5	14.0	X	31.0
Black total [4]	100.0	17.6	12.5	13.3	15.9	10.9	10.9	5.8	13.0	X	29.9
Non-Hispanic Black	100.0	17.7	12.5	13.3	15.9	10.9	10.9	5.8	13.0	X	29.8
Hispanic [5]	100.0	15.2	13.6	15.1	17.8	12.1	11.0	5.5	9.7	X	28.7
Under 37 Weeks											
All races [3]	100.0	18.1	13.2	14.1	16.0	11.2	10.2	5.6	11.6	X	28.3
White total [4]	100.0	16.2	12.6	14.3	16.3	11.7	10.7	6.0	12.2	X	29.4
Non-Hispanic White	100.0	14.7	11.7	14.1	16.4	12.2	11.2	6.4	13.4	X	30.2
Black total [4]	100.0	24.9	14.6	13.3	14.6	9.2	8.7	4.5	10.2	X	25.6
Non-Hispanic Black	100.0	25.0	14.6	13.2	14.6	9.2	8.7	4.5	10.2	X	25.6
Hispanic [5]	100.0	21.1	15.5	15.0	16.2	10.1	9.2	4.5	8.4	X	25.7
37–39 Weeks											
All races [3]	100.0	11.9	10.8	14.1	18.0	13.9	12.5	6.7	12.2	X	30.5
White total [4]	100.0	11.0	10.3	14.0	18.2	14.3	12.9	6.9	12.4	X	30.6
Non-Hispanic White	100.0	10.0	9.5	13.6	18.2	14.9	13.4	7.3	13.2	X	30.9
Black total [4]	100.0	16.6	12.4	13.7	16.3	11.3	11.2	5.8	12.7	X	30.0
Non-Hispanic Black	100.0	16.7	12.4	13.7	16.3	11.2	11.1	5.8	12.7	X	30.0
Hispanic [5]	100.0	14.9	13.6	15.4	18.1	12.3	10.9	5.4	9.3	X	28.6
40 Weeks and Over											
All races [3]	100.0	10.8	9.7	13.1	17.4	14.0	13.3	7.5	14.2	X	30.9
White total [4]	100.0	10.1	9.4	13.0	17.5	14.5	13.6	7.7	14.3	X	31.1
Non-Hispanic White	100.0	9.0	8.4	12.5	17.4	15.0	14.2	8.2	15.3	X	32.3
Black total [4]	100.0	15.2	11.5	12.8	15.9	11.3	11.7	6.6	14.9	X	30.4
Non-Hispanic Black	100.0	15.3	11.6	12.8	15.9	11.3	11.7	6.5	14.9	X	30.4
Hispanic [5]	100.0	13.8	12.8	14.6	17.9	12.5	11.5	6.1	10.8	X	30.0

Note: Excludes data for California, which did not require this information.

[1] Expressed in completed weeks.
[2] Includes births with period of gestation not stated.
[3] Includes races other than White and Black and origin not stated.
[4] Race and Hispanic origin are reported separately on the birth certificate. Data for persons of Hispanic origin are included in the data for each race group according to the mother's reported race.
[5] May be of any race.
X = Not applicable.

TABLE I-23. PERCENT LOW BIRTHWEIGHT, BY WEIGHT GAIN OF MOTHER DURING PREGNANCY, PERIOD OF GESTATION, AND RACE AND HISPANIC ORIGIN OF MOTHER: UNITED STATES EXCLUDING CALIFORNIA, 2003

This table focuses on the percentage of newborns with low birthweight, defined as less than 5.5 pounds. The dominant factor is the length of the gestation period. For a gestation period under 37 weeks, 43.6 percent of births have low birthweight. For gestation periods of 37–39 weeks and of 40 weeks or over, this percentage falls to 4.0 and 1.6 percent, respectively. In addition to the length of gestation, maternal weight gain has a positive relationship to infant birthweight (although the trend begins to reverse for weight gains above 40 pounds). Blacks have a markedly higher risk of low birthweight than non-Hispanic Whites and Hispanics.

TABLE I-24. PERCENT OF BIRTHS WITH SELECTED MEDICAL OR HEALTH CHARACTERISTICS, BY DETAILED RACE AND PLACE OF BIRTH OF MOTHER, 2003

According to birth certificates, 10.7 percent of new mothers in 2003 were smokers and 0.7 percent were drinkers. The National Center for Health Statistics, on the basis of national surveys of pregnant women, has concluded that alcohol use is substantially underreported (perhaps more than tenfold) on birth certificates. The lowest prevalence of smoking and drinking was reported for Asian or Pacific Islander mothers. The highest prevalence occurred for American Indians, with 18.1 percent listed as smokers and 2.2 percent listed as drinkers. (The allegedly high incidence of fetal alcohol syndrome in American Indian children suggests that this percentage of drinkers may also be an underestimate.)

Table I-23. Percent Low Birthweight, by Weight Gain of Mother During Pregnancy, Period of Gestation, and Race and Hispanic Origin of Mother: United States Excluding California, 2003

(Percent low birthweight.)

Period of gestation [1] and race and Hispanic origin of mother	Total	Weight gain during pregnancy							
		Less than 16 pounds	16–20 pounds	21–25 pounds	26–30 pounds	31–35 pounds	36–40 pounds	41–45 pounds	46 pounds or more	Not stated
All Gestation Periods [2]										
All races [3]	8.1	13.9	10.7	8.3	6.9	5.9	5.6	5.7	6.1	12.2
White total [4]	7.1	11.8	9.3	7.4	6.1	5.3	5.1	5.3	5.7	10.4
Non-Hispanic White	7.1	12.2	9.8	7.6	6.2	5.4	5.1	5.3	5.9	11.0
Black total [4]	13.4	20.9	16.3	13.4	11.7	10.0	9.1	8.6	8.3	18.8
Non-Hispanic Black	13.6	21.1	16.5	13.5	11.9	10.2	9.2	8.7	8.3	19.0
Hispanic [5]	7.0	10.9	8.2	6.8	5.8	5.2	4.8	4.9	4.9	9.5
Mexican	6.5	10.0	7.5	6.2	5.4	4.8	4.3	4.5	4.5	8.5
Puerto Rican	10.1	17.3	13.2	10.4	8.5	7.4	7.1	6.8	6.2	17.5
Cuban	7.0	14.1	10.6	7.9	6.1	6.5	5.5	3.8	4.4	12.0
Central and South American	6.6	11.5	8.2	6.8	5.8	4.5	4.2	4.9	4.9	9.7
Other and unknown Hispanic	8.2	12.6	9.9	7.7	6.8	6.7	6.5	5.2	5.7	13.7
Under 37 Weeks										
All races [3]	43.6	55.5	47.8	42.6	39.1	37.1	36.0	37.1	37.0	53.4
White total [4]	41.3	52.1	45.6	40.6	37.2	35.6	35.1	36.4	36.6	50.6
Non-Hispanic White	42.8	54.9	48.3	42.4	38.8	36.7	36.6	37.4	37.8	54.6
Black total [4]	51.4	62.9	54.6	49.9	46.3	44.0	40.6	40.9	39.3	61.0
Non-Hispanic Black	51.6	63.0	54.8	50.1	46.6	44.3	40.6	41.2	39.3	61.1
Hispanic [5]	36.6	45.7	38.6	35.1	31.8	31.0	29.5	31.3	29.7	43.4
37–39 Weeks										
All races [3]	4.0	5.9	5.1	4.4	3.7	3.3	3.0	3.1	3.2	5.0
White total [4]	3.4	5.0	4.3	3.8	3.2	2.9	2.6	2.8	2.9	4.2
Non-Hispanic White	3.4	5.0	4.3	3.8	3.1	2.8	2.6	2.8	2.9	4.1
Black total [4]	6.7	8.9	8.2	7.2	6.4	5.4	5.2	4.8	4.6	7.7
Non-Hispanic Black	6.7	9.0	8.3	7.2	6.5	5.5	5.3	4.8	4.6	7.8
Hispanic [5]	3.7	5.0	4.3	3.8	3.5	3.2	2.7	2.9	2.9	4.4
40 Weeks and Over										
All races [3]	1.6	2.8	2.3	1.8	1.5	1.3	1.2	1.1	1.1	2.1
White total [4]	1.3	2.3	1.9	1.5	1.3	1.1	1.0	0.9	1.0	1.6
Non-Hispanic White	1.3	2.3	2.0	1.5	1.2	1.1	0.9	0.9	0.9	1.5
Black total [4]	3.0	4.6	4.0	3.4	2.9	2.3	2.3	1.9	1.7	3.8
Non-Hispanic Black	3.1	4.7	4.0	3.4	3.0	2.3	2.3	1.9	1.8	3.8
Hispanic [5]	1.5	2.6	1.9	1.6	1.4	1.1	1.1	1.0	1.1	1.9

Note: Low birthweight is defined as weight of less than 2,500 grams (5 lb 8 oz). Excludes data for California, which did not require this information.

[1]Expressed in completed weeks.
[2]Includes births with period of gestation not stated.
[3]Includes races other than White and Black and origin not stated.
[4]Race and Hispanic origin are reported separately on the birth certificate. Data for persons of Hispanic origin are included in the data for each race group according to the mother's reported race.
[5]May be of any race.

While prenatal smoking is also believed to be somewhat underreported on birth certificates, the patterns of maternal smoking based on birth certificates have been largely corroborated by nationally representative surveys. (See Tables I-29 through I-32 for more detail on maternal smoking.)

The cesarean delivery rate averaged 27.5 percent in 2003, with a somewhat higher rate for Blacks. This table also shows an early beginning for prenatal care for most prospective White and Asian mothers, with lower proportions of prenatal care for American Indians and Blacks. Data are given on birthweight, percentages of preterm births, and 5-minute Apgar scores (an index of birth asphyxia of the newborn). Blacks and American Indians show higher proportions of inadequate maternal weight gain. Black infants are at higher risk for preterm delivery, low birthweight, and a 5-minute Apgar score of less than 7.

Table I-24. Percent of Births with Selected Medical or Health Characteristics, by Detailed Race and Place of Birth of Mother, 2003

(Percent.)

Characteristic	All races	White	Black	American Indian[1]	Asian or Pacific Islander
ALL BIRTHS					
Mother					
Prenatal care beginning in the first trimester	84.1	85.7	75.9	70.8	85.4
Late or no prenatal care	3.5	3.0	6.0	7.6	3.1
Smoker[2]	10.7	11.6	8.1	18.1	2.2
Drinker[3]	0.7	0.8	0.7	2.2	0.3
Weight gain of less than 16 lbs[4]	12.3	11.3	17.6	17.3	9.6
Median weight gain[4]	30.5	30.7	29.9	29.8	30.2
Cesarean delivery rate	27.5	27.3	29.1	24.1	26.6
Infant					
Preterm births[5]	12.3	11.5	17.6	13.5	10.5
Birthweight					
Very low birthweight[6]	1.4	1.2	3.1	1.3	1.1
Low birthweight[7]	7.9	6.9	13.4	7.4	7.8
4,000 grams or more[8]	8.9	9.8	4.9	10.9	5.3
5-minute Apgar score of less than 7[9]	1.4	1.3	2.3	1.5	1.0
MOTHERS BORN IN THE 50 STATES AND DC					
Mother					
Prenatal care beginning in the first trimester	85.7	88.0	75.9	70.5	83.7
Late or no prenatal care	3.0	2.4	5.8	7.7	3.2
Smoker[2]	13.1	13.9	9.3	19.0	7.3
Drinker[3]	0.9	0.8	0.8	2.3	0.6
Weight gain of less than 16 lbs[4]	11.9	10.6	17.9	17.4	9.4
Median weight gain[4]	30.7	30.9	30.0	30.0	30.8
Cesarean delivery rate	27.7	27.6	28.8	24.0	23.6
Infant					
Preterm births[5]	12.7	11.6	18.2	13.6	12.2
Birthweight					
Very low birthweight[6]	1.5	1.2	3.1	1.3	1.3
Low birthweight[7]	8.3	7.2	13.9	7.3	8.8
4,000 grams or more[8]	9.1	10.0	4.5	11.1	6.3
5-minute Apgar score of less than 7[9]	1.5	1.3	2.3	1.5	1.2
MOTHERS BORN OUTSIDE THE 50 STATES AND DC					
Mother					
Prenatal care beginning in the first trimester	79.1	77.8	76.2	76.2	85.8
Late or no prenatal care	5.1	5.4	6.8	6.2	3.1
Smoker[2]	1.5	1.7	1.0	2.6	1.1
Drinker[3]	0.3	0.3	0.2	*	0.3
Weight gain of less than 16 lbs[4]	13.8	14.6	15.6	16.0	9.7
Median weight gain[4]	28.9	28.6	28.8	27.6	30.1
Cesarean delivery rate	26.9	26.3	31.0	26.6	27.2
Infant					
Preterm births[5]	11.0	10.9	13.9	12.4	10.1
Birthweight					
Very low birthweight[6]	1.1	1.0	2.4	1.1	1.0
Low birthweight[7]	6.6	6.0	9.6	8.2	7.6
4,000 grams or more[8]	8.2	9.0	7.7	6.8	5.1
5-minute Apgar score of less than 7[9]	1.1	1.0	1.8	1.4	1.0

Note: Race and Hispanic origin are reported separately on birth certificates. In this table, all women (including Hispanic women) are classified only according to their race.

[1]Includes births to Aleuts and Eskimos.
[2]Excludes data for California, which did not report tobacco use on the birth certificate.
[3]Excludes data for California, which did not report alcohol use on the birth certificate.
[4]Excludes data for California, which did not report weight gain on the birth certificate. Median weight shown in pounds.
[5]Born prior to 37 completed weeks of gestation.
[6]Birthweight of less than 1,500 grams (3 lb 4 oz).
[7]Birthweight of less than 2,500 grams (5 lb 8 oz).
[8]Equivalent to 8 lb 14 oz.
[9]Excludes data for California and Texas, which did not report 5-minute Apgar score on the birth certificate.
* = Figure does not meet standards of reliability or precision; based on fewer than 20 births in numerator.

TABLE I-25. PERCENT OF BIRTHS WITH SELECTED MEDICAL OR HEALTH CHARACTERISTICS, BY SPECIFIED HISPANIC ORIGIN, RACE, AND PLACE OF BIRTH OF MOTHER, 2003

Smoking and drinking rates were low among Hispanic mothers and particularly low for those originating in Central and South America. Non-Hispanic White mothers, however, had a relatively high smoking rate of 14.3 percent. Preterm births—babies born prior to 37 weeks

Table I-25. Percent of Births with Selected Medical or Health Characteristics, by Specified Hispanic Origin, Race, and Place of Birth of Mother, 2003

(Percent.)

Characteristic	All origins [1]	Origin of mother								
		Hispanic						Non-Hispanic		
		Total	Mexican	Puerto Rican	Cuban	Central and South American	Other and unknown Hispanic	Total [2]	White	Black
ALL BIRTHS										
Mother										
Prenatal care beginning in the first trimester	84.1	77.5	76.5	81.2	92.1	79.2	77.0	86.1	89.0	75.9
Late or no prenatal care	3.5	5.3	5.6	3.7	1.3	4.7	5.4	3.0	2.1	6.0
Smoker [3]	10.7	2.7	2.0	7.9	2.4	1.1	6.6	12.6	14.3	8.3
Drinker [4]	0.7	0.4	0.4	0.6	0.3	0.3	0.9	0.8	0.9	0.8
Weight gain of less than 16 lbs [5]	12.3	15.2	16.9	12.8	7.8	12.3	13.2	11.6	10.2	17.7
Median weight gain [5]	30.5	28.7	27.3	30.7	31.9	30.1	30.3	30.7	31.0	29.8
Cesarean delivery rate	27.5	26.5	25.8	27.6	39.8	28.4	25.9	27.8	27.6	29.2
Infant										
Preterm births [6]	12.3	11.9	11.7	13.8	11.8	11.4	12.6	12.5	11.3	17.8
Birthweight										
Very low birthweight [7]	1.4	1.2	1.1	2.0	1.4	1.2	1.3	1.5	1.2	3.1
Low birthweight [8]	7.9	6.7	6.3	10.0	7.0	6.7	8.0	8.3	7.0	13.6
4,000 grams or more [9]	8.9	8.2	8.5	6.2	8.3	8.0	7.0	9.0	10.4	4.8
5-minute Apgar score of less than 7 [10]	1.4	1.1	1.1	1.5	0.8	0.9	1.2	1.5	1.3	2.3
MOTHERS BORN IN THE 50 STATES AND DC										
Mother										
Prenatal care beginning in the first trimester	85.7	80.8	80.6	80.7	91.5	84.2	77.8	86.3	89.1	75.9
Late or no prenatal care	3.0	4.1	4.1	3.9	1.4	3.1	5.2	2.9	2.1	5.8
Smoker [3]	13.1	5.8	4.7	9.1	3.5	3.5	8.7	13.8	14.9	9.3
Drinker [4]	0.9	0.8	0.8	0.6	0.5	0.5	1.1	0.9	0.9	0.8
Weight gain of less than 16 lbs [5]	11.9	13.6	14.7	12.2	7.9	9.0	13.1	11.7	10.2	18.0
Median weight gain [5]	30.7	30.3	30.1	30.8	32.6	31.0	30.5	30.8	31.0	30.0
Cesarean delivery rate	27.7	26.8	26.6	27.0	35.8	26.8	25.6	27.8	27.7	28.9
Infant										
Preterm births [6]	12.7	13.0	13.0	13.6	12.4	11.6	13.3	12.7	11.4	18.3
Birthweight										
Very low birthweight [7]	1.5	1.4	1.3	2.0	1.7	1.6	1.3	1.5	1.2	3.2
Low birthweight [8]	8.3	7.8	7.4	10.0	7.8	7.6	8.7	8.4	7.1	14.0
4,000 grams or more [9]	9.1	7.3	7.6	6.3	7.3	7.4	6.8	9.3	10.4	4.4
5-minute Apgar score of less than 7 [10]	1.5	1.2	1.2	1.4	0.9	1.0	1.2	1.5	1.3	2.4
MOTHERS BORN OUTSIDE THE 50 STATES AND DC										
Mother										
Prenatal care beginning in the first trimester	79.1	75.6	74.1	82.3	92.6	78.5	75.2	84.5	86.9	76.5
Late or no prenatal care	5.1	5.9	6.5	3.4	1.1	4.9	5.8	3.8	3.1	6.9
Smoker [3]	1.5	0.9	0.5	5.7	1.5	0.8	1.5	2.4	4.5	1.0
Drinker [4]	0.3	0.2	0.2	0.4	*	0.3	0.3	0.5	0.8	0.2
Weight gain of less than 16 lbs [5]	13.8	16.2	18.2	13.9	7.7	12.7	13.3	10.7	9.0	15.9
Median weight gain [5]	28.9	27.3	25.9	30.3	31.0	29.8	29.8	30.3	30.7	28.5
Cesarean delivery rate	26.9	26.4	25.3	28.9	43.3	28.6	26.8	27.6	26.0	31.7
Infant										
Preterm births [6]	11.0	11.2	11.0	14.2	11.3	11.4	10.5	10.7	9.5	14.2
Birthweight										
Very low birthweight [7]	1.1	1.0	0.9	2.0	1.1	1.1	0.9	1.3	1.0	2.6
Low birthweight [8]	6.6	6.0	5.7	10.0	6.3	6.6	5.9	7.5	6.2	10.0
4,000 grams or more [9]	8.2	8.7	9.0	6.1	9.2	8.1	7.4	7.4	10.4	7.7
5-minute Apgar score of less than 7 [10]	1.1	1.0	1.1	1.6	0.8	0.9	1.0	1.2	0.9	1.9

Note: Race and Hispanic origin are reported separately on birth certificates. Persons of Hispanic origin may be of any race. In this table, Hispanic women are classified only by place of origin; non-Hispanic women are classified by race.

[1] Includes origin not stated.
[2] Includes races other than White and Black.
[3] Excludes data for California, which did not report tobacco use on the birth certificate.
[4] Excludes data for California, which did not report alcohol use on the birth certificate.
[5] Excludes data for California, which did not report weight gain on the birth certificate. Median weight gain shown in pounds.
[6] Born prior to 37 completed weeks of gestation.
[7] Birthweight of less than 1,500 grams (3 lb 4 oz).
[8] Birthweight of less than 2,500 grams (5 lb 8 oz).
[9] Equivalent to 8 lb 14 oz.
[10] Excludes data for California and Texas, which did not report 5-minute Apgar score on the birth certificate.
* = Figure does not meet standards of reliability or precision; based on fewer than 20 births in numerator.

of gestation—averaged 12.3 percent for all mothers, but rates were especially high for non-Hispanic Blacks (17.8 percent). This group also had a relatively high frequency (3.1 percent) of births with very low birthweight (less than 3.25 pounds). Compared to non-Hispanic Whites, Hispanic infants had lower risks of low birthweight and low Apgar scores.

The cesarean delivery rate was particularly high among Cuban mothers; it amounted to 35.8 percent for Cuban mothers born in the United States and 43.3 percent for foreign-born Cuban mothers.

TABLE I-26. LIVE BIRTHS TO MOTHERS WITH SELECTED MEDICAL RISK FACTORS AND RATES, BY AGE AND RACE OF MOTHER, 2003

Medical risk factors during pregnancy can contribute to serious complications and to maternal and infant morbid-ity and mortality if not treated properly. Sixteen medical risk factors that can affect pregnancy outcome have been separately identified on birth certificates since 1989. The most frequently reported risk factors in 2003 were preg-nancy-associated hypertension (37.4 per 1,000 births), diabetes (32.8 per 1,000 births), and anemia (23.8 per 1,000 births). The last two rates have risen nearly 40 per-cent since the early 1990s.

Chronic hypertension, which is high blood pressure prior to pregnancy or before the 20th week of gestation, has increased about 35 percent since 1990. Occurrences of eclampsia, coma and/or convulsions associated with hyper-tension, edema, and proteinuria of unclear origin, have declined 25 percent since 1990. This is most likely due to increased first trimester prenatal care (see Table I-33A) and improved treatment of pre-eclampsia symptoms. The rate of hydramnios/oligohydramnios (the excess or shortage of amniotic fluid) per 1,000 births more than

Table I-26. Live Births to Mothers with Selected Medical Risk Factors and Rates, by Age and Race of Mother, 2003

(Number, rate of live births with specified medical risk factor per 1,000 live births in specified group.)

Medical risk factor and race of mother	All births [1]	Medical risk factor reported	Rate by age of mother							Not stated [2]
			All ages	Under 20 years	20–24 years	25–29 years	30–34 years	35–39 years	40–54 years	
All Races [3]										
Anemia [4]	3 863 502	91 535	23.8	33.0	28.3	22.1	19.6	19.1	19.6	21 412
Cardiac disease [4]	3 863 502	18 639	4.9	2.6	3.4	4.5	6.1	7.4	8.9	21 412
Acute or chronic lung disease [4]	3 863 502	46 356	12.1	14.5	12.6	11.6	11.2	11.5	12.5	21 412
Diabetes	4 089 950	133 547	32.8	9.9	18.6	31.1	43.0	58.0	75.9	21 150
Genital herpes [4,5]	3 486 026	31 567	9.1	6.3	8.0	8.3	10.2	12.6	13.1	19 121
Hydramnios/oligohydramnios [4]	3 863 502	53 141	13.8	14.5	13.8	13.3	13.6	14.4	17.0	21 412
Hemoglobinopathy [4]	3 863 502	3 112	0.8	1.0	0.9	0.7	0.8	0.8	0.7	21 412
Hypertension, chronic	4 089 950	35 953	8.8	2.9	5.0	8.0	10.9	16.3	26.1	21 150
Hypertension, pregnancy-associated	4 089 950	152 268	37.4	41.2	36.9	36.9	35.5	37.9	47.8	21 150
Eclampsia	4 089 950	12 059	3.0	4.1	3.1	2.6	2.6	3.0	3.7	21 150
Incompetent cervix [4]	3 863 502	11 464	3.0	1.5	2.1	2.9	3.8	4.6	5.1	21 412
Previous infant 4,000+ grams [4]	3 863 502	36 422	9.5	1.1	5.3	9.8	13.2	16.0	18.5	21 412
Previous preterm or small-for-gestational-age infant [4]	3 863 502	44 671	11.6	4.1	11.1	12.3	12.9	14.6	15.9	21 412
Renal disease [4]	3 863 502	11 668	3.0	3.2	3.3	3.2	2.8	2.5	2.5	21 412
Rh sensitization [4,6]	3 824 026	26 040	6.8	5.4	6.2	6.7	7.7	7.8	7.4	21 401
Uterine bleeding [4,5]	3 486 026	18 494	5.3	4.0	4.7	5.3	5.8	6.5	8.0	19 121
White										
Anemia [4]	3 040 873	63 274	20.9	29.0	24.6	19.4	17.9	17.4	17.8	17 412
Cardiac disease [4]	3 040 873	15 582	5.2	2.6	3.5	4.8	6.5	7.8	9.4	17 412
Acute or chronic lung disease [4]	3 040 873	34 801	11.5	12.6	11.7	11.2	11.1	11.3	12.4	17 412
Diabetes	3 225 848	100 954	31.5	10.0	18.3	29.3	40.3	53.8	70.2	16 400
Genital herpes [4,5]	2 719 331	24 126	8.9	5.6	7.0	7.8	10.5	13.3	14.3	15 506
Hydramnios/oligohydramnios [4]	3 040 873	40 374	13.4	13.8	13.3	12.9	13.1	13.9	15.9	17 412
Hemoglobinopathy [4]	3 040 873	1 229	0.4	0.3	0.3	0.4	0.5	0.6	0.5	17 412
Hypertension, chronic	3 225 848	24 422	7.6	2.5	4.3	7.0	9.4	13.3	21.0	16 400
Hypertension, pregnancy-associated	3 225 848	121 834	38.0	40.4	37.4	38.4	36.2	37.9	46.9	16 400
Eclampsia	3 225 848	8 772	2.7	3.6	2.9	2.5	2.5	2.7	3.6	16 400
Incompetent cervix [4]	3 040 873	7 660	2.5	1.3	1.7	2.3	3.2	4.0	4.5	17 412
Previous infant 4,000+ grams [4]	3 040 873	32 403	10.7	1.3	5.8	10.8	14.7	17.9	20.8	17 412
Previous preterm or small-for-gestational-age infant [4]	3 040 873	34 285	11.3	3.8	10.4	11.9	12.7	14.4	15.4	17 412
Renal disease [4]	3 040 873	10 098	3.3	3.6	3.7	3.5	3.0	2.7	2.8	17 412
Rh sensitization [4,6]	3 005 866	23 384	7.8	6.3	7.1	7.6	8.8	9.0	8.4	17 402
Uterine bleeding [4,5]	2 719 331	15 207	5.6	4.2	5.0	5.6	6.0	6.8	8.1	15 506
Black										
Anemia [4]	573 776	22 222	38.9	42.5	41.3	38.5	35.1	32.2	32.6	2 525
Cardiac disease [4]	573 776	2 221	3.9	2.6	3.0	3.9	5.1	6.4	8.0	2 525
Acute or chronic lung disease [4]	573 776	9 167	16.0	19.4	16.4	15.2	14.1	14.4	14.3	2 525
Diabetes	599 847	18 352	30.7	9.0	18.2	33.0	49.7	67.2	89.4	2 655
Genital herpes [4,5]	531 891	6 290	11.9	8.5	12.1	13.4	12.7	12.5	9.9	2 247
Hydramnios/oligohydramnios [4]	573 776	9 305	16.3	16.6	15.2	15.5	17.2	18.7	23.7	2 525
Hemoglobinopathy [4]	573 776	1 708	3.0	3.0	3.2	2.9	3.1	2.6	2.3	2 525
Hypertension, chronic	599 847	9 921	16.6	4.3	8.2	16.2	27.4	43.5	64.6	2 655
Hypertension, pregnancy-associated	599 847	24 003	40.2	43.7	37.0	36.4	42.7	46.7	58.2	2 655
Eclampsia	599 847	2 751	4.6	5.7	4.2	3.9	4.6	5.8	5.1	2 655
Incompetent cervix [4]	573 776	3 228	5.7	1.9	3.7	6.6	9.4	10.3	9.2	2 525
Previous infant 4,000+ grams [4]	573 776	2 371	4.2	0.6	2.8	5.2	6.7	7.8	8.2	2 525
Previous preterm or small-for-gestational-age infant [4]	573 776	8 000	14.0	4.8	13.7	16.9	17.8	17.6	19.3	2 525
Renal disease [4]	573 776	1 073	1.9	1.9	1.9	1.9	1.9	1.8	*	2 525
Rh sensitization [4,6]	571 013	2 129	3.7	3.1	3.7	3.8	4.2	4.0	4.6	2 525
Uterine bleeding [4,5]	531 891	2 253	4.3	3.4	3.7	4.1	5.4	5.3	8.2	2 247

[1]Total number of births to residents of areas reporting specified medical risk factor.
[2]No response reported for the medical risk factor item.
[3]Includes races other than White and Black.
[4]Excludes data for Pennsylvania and Washington State, which implemented the 2003 Revision to the U.S. Standard Certificate of Live Birth for data year 2003.
[5]Texas does not report this risk factor.
[6]Kansas does not report this risk factor.
* = Figure does not meet standards of reliability or precision; based on fewer than 20 births in the numerator.

doubled between 1990 and 2003 (from 5.9 to 13.8); this condition is associated with maternal diabetes. Acute or chronic lung diseases, such as asthma and tuberculosis, also rose rapidly during this period (more than quadrupled), with the most notable increases occurring in younger women.

The risk of having a medical condition during pregnancy often differs by maternal age. Anemia is more frequent at a young age, with teenagers especially susceptible. Diabetes (like most other chronic conditions) occurred more frequently in the older age groups, with an incidence rate of 75.9 per 1,000 pregnancies among women over 40 years old. When Whites and Blacks were compared, Blacks reported higher rates of chronic hypertension for all age groups and higher rates of pregnancy-associated hypertension for teenage mothers and mothers over 30 years old, higher rates of diabetes for older age groups, and higher rates of anemia for all age groups.

TABLE I-27. NUMBER AND RATE OF LIVE BIRTHS TO MOTHERS WITH SELECTED MEDICAL RISK FACTORS, COMPLICATIONS OF LABOR, AND OBSTETRIC PROCEDURES, BY DETAILED RACE OF MOTHER, 2003

American Indian women had the highest rates of anemia and pregnancy-associated hypertension. They also had a high rate of diabetes, but this was surpassed by the rate of diabetes in Asian or Pacific Islander mothers (particularly Filipinos and native Hawaiians). Blacks have higher rates of anemia than Whites.

Blacks also had higher rates of meconium staining and fetal distress, but lower rates of cephalopelvic disproportion and breech/malpresentation (leading risk factors for cesarean delivery) than Whites.

In regard to obstetric procedures, most mothers (854 out of 1,000 pregnancies) received electronic fetal monitoring (EFM). Despite some controversy over routine use of

Table I-27. Number and Rate of Live Births to Mothers with Selected Medical Risk Factors, Complications of Labor, and Obstetric Procedures, by Detailed Race of Mother, 2003

(Number, rate of live births with specified risk factors, complications, or procedures per 1,000 live births in specified group.)

Medical risk factor, complication, and obstetric procedure	All races	White	Black	American Indian [1]	Asian or Pacific Islander
NUMBER					
Medical Risk Factors					
Anemia	91 535	63 274	22 222	2 113	3 926
Diabetes	133 547	100 954	18 352	2 139	12 102
Hypertension, pregnancy-associated	152 268	121 834	24 003	2 120	4 311
Uterine bleeding [2]	18 494	15 207	2 253	263	771
Complications of Labor and/or Delivery					
Meconium, moderate/heavy	197 865	146 301	38 349	2 098	11 117
Premature rupture of membrane	83 103	62 759	14 401	1 331	4 612
Dysfunctional labor	109 836	85 039	16 027	1 515	7 255
Breech/malpresentation	156 804	127 933	19 075	1 499	8 297
Cephalopelvic disproportion	56 111	45 314	6 074	588	4 135
Fetal distress [3]	132 377	98 501	25 049	1 372	7 455
Obstetric Procedures					
Amniocentesis	66 901	54 686	6 092	435	5 688
Electronic fetal monitoring	3 289 703	2 591 505	493 605	34 831	169 762
Induction of labor	840 137	696 703	104 123	8 501	30 810
Ultrasound	2 592 258	2 069 050	355 001	24 983	143 224
Stimulation of labor	645 075	512 549	89 024	6 553	36 949
RATE					
Medical Risk Factors					
Anemia	23.8	20.9	38.9	52.4	19.0
Diabetes	32.8	31.5	30.7	50.1	55.1
Hypertension, pregnancy-associated	37.4	38.0	40.2	49.7	19.6
Uterine bleeding [2]	5.3	5.6	4.3	6.7	4.0
Complications of Labor and/or Delivery					
Meconium, moderate/heavy	48.6	45.5	64.1	49.1	50.6
Premature rupture of membrane	21.6	20.7	25.2	33.0	22.2
Dysfunctional labor	28.5	28.1	28.0	37.5	35.0
Breech/malpresentation	38.5	39.8	31.9	35.2	37.8
Cephalopelvic disproportion	14.6	15.0	10.6	14.6	19.9
Fetal distress [3]	38.1	36.4	47.2	34.8	38.4
Obstetric Procedures					
Amniocentesis	17.4	18.0	10.6	10.8	27.4
Electronic fetal monitoring	854.2	855.1	862.1	861.7	817.6
Induction of labor	206.0	216.6	174.0	198.8	140.0
Ultrasound	673.1	682.7	620.1	618.0	689.8
Stimulation of labor	167.5	169.1	155.5	162.1	177.9

[1]Includes births to Aleuts and Eskimos.
[2]Texas does not report this risk factor.
[3]Texas does not report this complication.

EFM, this rate has climbed continually since 1989. The use of ultrasound has leveled out in recent years; it was received by 673 out of 1,000 mothers in 2003. Advances in this technology allow early screening and detection of fetal abnormalities. In comparison, amniocentesis was rarely used (17 out of 1,000 pregnancies), and its use has declined somewhat since 1989. Amniocentesis was obtained most frequently by Asians.

TABLE I-28. NUMBER AND RATE OF LIVE BIRTHS TO MOTHERS WITH SELECTED MEDICAL RISK FACTORS, COMPLICATIONS OF LABOR, AND OBSTETRIC PROCEDURES, BY SPECIFIED HISPANIC ORIGIN AND RACE OF MOTHER, 2003

Compared to non-Hispanic White women, Hispanic mothers had a substantially less risk of pregnancy-induced hypertension, a somewhat greater risk of anemia, and virtually the same frequency of diabetes. Hispanics—especially Mexicans—seldom obtained amniocentesis (less than one percent of births) and experienced a lower frequency of induced labor than non-Hispanic Whites. Puerto Rican women had greater rates of medical risk factors and of complications of labor and/or delivery than Mexican women. Cuban women had high rates of dysfunctional labor and breech/malpresentation. (Cubans also had high rates of cesarean delivery, as shown in Table I-25.)

Non-Hispanic Blacks had higher rates of anemia than non-Hispanic Whites. In regard to complications of labor and/or delivery, Blacks had a greater frequency of meconium staining and of fetal distress.

Table I-28. Number and Rate of Live Births to Mothers with Selected Medical Risk Factors, Complications of Labor, and Obstetric Procedures, by Specified Hispanic Origin and Race of Mother, 2003

(Number, rate of live births with specified risk factors, complications, or procedures per 1,000 live births in specified group.)

Medical risk factor, complication, and obstetric procedure	All origins [1]	Origin of mother								
		Hispanic						Non-Hispanic		
		Total	Mexican	Puerto Rican	Cuban	Central and South American	Other and unknown Hispanic	Total [2]	White	Black
NUMBER										
Medical Risk Factors										
Anemia	91 535	21 217	14 476	1 713	299	2 727	2 002	69 831	42 710	21 438
Diabetes	133 547	29 022	20 329	2 372	367	4 258	1 696	103 717	72 492	17 508
Hypertension, pregnancy-associated	152 268	23 569	15 982	1 847	479	3 576	1 685	127 766	98 511	23 229
Uterine bleeding [3]	18 494	2 697	1 525	241	42	454	435	15 691	12 565	2 143
Complications of Labor and/or Delivery										
Meconium, moderate/heavy	197 865	48 400	34 326	3 088	453	7 949	2 584	148 180	98 960	36 727
Premature rupture of membrane	83 103	14 667	9 897	1 151	215	2 367	1 037	67 889	48 231	13 985
Dysfunctional labor	109 836	22 822	14 880	1 796	591	3 953	1 602	86 477	62 538	15 442
Breech/malpresentation	156 804	26 967	18 008	2 122	595	4 470	1 772	128 684	101 192	18 166
Cephalopelvic disproportion	56 111	9 239	6 479	646	140	1 439	535	46 495	36 034	5 901
Fetal distress [4]	132 377	19 509	11 896	1 922	360	4 028	1 303	112 108	79 272	24 346
Obstetric Procedures										
Amniocentesis	66 901	7 831	3 934	843	305	2 075	674	58 579	46 892	5 763
Electronic fetal monitoring	3 289 703	726 986	517 951	45 579	12 777	110 643	40 036	2 546 356	1 873 108	476 993
Induction of labor	840 137	125 518	84 986	9 564	2 864	18 105	9 999	709 690	571 669	100 473
Ultrasound	2 592 258	537 689	371 064	35 760	9 561	87 677	33 627	2 040 502	1 537 340	341 764
Stimulation of labor	645 075	131 642	91 306	9 797	1 590	22 064	6 885	510 148	382 310	85 797
RATE										
Medical Risk Factors										
Anemia	23.8	24.0	22.7	32.8	20.4	20.6	43.1	23.8	19.9	38.9
Diabetes	32.8	31.9	31.2	40.8	24.7	31.6	34.8	33.1	31.4	30.5
Hypertension, pregnancy-associated	37.4	25.9	24.5	31.7	32.3	26.5	34.5	40.8	42.6	40.5
Uterine bleeding [3]	5.3	3.8	3.2	4.7	2.9	3.7	11.0	5.7	6.3	4.2
Complications of Labor and/or Delivery										
Meconium, moderate/heavy	48.6	53.2	52.5	53.0	30.5	58.8	52.9	47.2	42.8	63.9
Premature rupture of membrane	21.6	16.5	15.5	22.0	14.7	17.8	22.3	23.1	22.5	25.3
Dysfunctional labor	28.5	25.7	23.2	34.4	40.4	29.7	34.5	29.4	29.1	28.0
Breech/malpresentation	38.5	29.6	27.6	36.4	40.1	33.1	36.4	41.1	43.8	31.6
Cephalopelvic disproportion	14.6	10.4	10.1	12.4	9.6	10.8	11.5	15.8	16.8	10.7
Fetal distress [4]	38.1	27.7	25.0	37.6	25.2	32.8	33.1	40.9	39.4	47.6
Obstetric Procedures										
Amniocentesis	17.4	8.8	6.1	16.1	20.8	15.6	14.5	19.9	21.8	10.4
Electronic fetal monitoring	854.2	819.6	808.6	872.4	872.7	831.2	861.2	866.0	871.2	862.8
Induction of labor	206.0	137.8	130.0	164.1	192.9	133.9	204.7	226.1	247.0	174.8
Ultrasound	673.1	606.2	579.3	684.4	653.0	658.7	723.4	694.0	715.0	618.2
Stimulation of labor	167.5	148.4	142.5	187.5	108.6	165.8	148.1	173.5	177.8	155.2

Note: Race and Hispanic origin are reported separately on birth certificates. Persons of Hispanic origin may be of any race. In this table, Hispanic women are classified only by place of origin; non-Hispanic women are classified by race.

[1] Includes origin not stated.
[2] Includes races other than White and Black.
[3] Texas does not report this risk factor.
[4] Texas does not report this complication.

TABLE I-29. NUMBER OF LIVE BIRTHS BY SMOKING STATUS DURING PREGNANCY, PERCENT SMOKERS, AND CIGARETTE CONSUMPTION, ACCORDING TO AGE AND RACE OF MOTHER: UNITED STATES EXCLUDING CALIFORNIA, PENNSYLVANIA, AND WASHINGTON STATE, 2003

The negative consequences of prenatal smoking on birth outcomes are well documented. They include risks of low birthweight, intrauterine growth retardation, miscarriage, and infant mortality, as well as future negative impacts on child health and development. The impact of low birthweight is more severe with greater cigarette consumption, but studies show that there is no safe level of smoking for expectant mothers.

Occurrences of smoking during pregnancy declined in 2003 to 10.7 percent of pregnant women, down from 11.2 percent in 2002 (when measured for the same 47 states and the District of Columbia) and 19.5 percent in 1989 (measured for the entire United States, excluding California), the first year this information became avail-

Table I-29. Number of Live Births by Smoking Status During Pregnancy, Percent Smokers, and Cigarette Consumption, According to Age and Race of Mother: United States Excluding California, Pennsylvania, and Washington State, 2003

(Number, percent.)

Smoking status, smoking measure, and race of mother	Age of mother									
	All ages	Under 15 years	15–19 years			20–24 years	25–29 years	30–34 years	35–39 years	40–54 years
			Total	15–17 years	18–19 years					
NUMBER										
All Races [1]										
Total	3 322 505	5 629	345 580	111 832	233 748	856 641	885 042	781 987	366 092	81 534
Smoker	354 586	297	53 056	13 289	39 767	137 255	82 482	50 173	24 890	6 433
Nonsmoker	2 948 476	5 296	290 759	97 957	192 802	714 848	797 511	726 854	338 777	74 431
Not stated	19 443	36	1 765	586	1 179	4 538	5 049	4 960	2 425	670
White										
Total	2 602 499	2 919	241 936	74 469	167 467	644 521	706 918	642 021	298 724	65 460
Smoker	301 069	241	45 649	11 252	34 397	117 011	69 662	42 757	20 568	5 181
Nonsmoker	2 285 689	2 661	194 980	62 795	132 185	523 983	633 134	595 112	276 101	59 718
Not stated	15 741	17	1 307	422	885	3 527	4 122	4 152	2 055	561
Black										
Total	541 427	2 506	91 881	33 516	58 365	178 617	126 098	87 215	44 107	11 003
Smoker	43 739	44	5 741	1 569	4 172	16 661	10 479	6 045	3 686	1 083
Nonsmoker	495 364	2 444	85 852	31 848	54 004	161 241	115 054	80 712	40 203	9 858
Not stated	2 324	18	288	99	189	715	565	458	218	62
PERCENT SMOKERS										
Total [1]	10.7	5.3	15.4	11.9	17.1	16.1	9.4	6.5	6.8	8.0
White	11.6	8.3	19.0	15.2	20.6	18.3	9.9	6.7	6.9	8.0
Black	8.1	1.8	6.3	4.7	7.2	9.4	8.3	7.0	8.4	9.9
PERCENT DISTRIBUTION [2]										
All Races [1]										
Smoker	100.0	100.0	100.0	100.0	100.0	100.0	100.0	100.0	100.0	100.0
1–5 cigarettes	33.2	52.3	41.1	45.6	39.6	34.4	30.5	29.1	28.8	27.6
6–10 cigarettes	42.4	34.9	42.3	40.4	42.9	43.5	42.7	41.3	39.6	38.4
11–15 cigarettes	5.2	*	3.8	2.9	4.1	4.8	5.6	6.4	6.9	7.1
16–20 cigarettes	16.8	9.3	11.6	9.9	12.1	15.5	18.6	20.0	20.9	21.9
21–30 cigarettes	1.7	*	1.0	1.0	1.0	1.4	1.9	2.3	2.7	3.3
31–40 cigarettes	0.5	*	0.2	0.2	0.3	0.4	0.6	0.9	1.0	1.4
41 cigarettes or more	0.1	*	0.1	*	0.1	0.1	0.1	0.1	0.1	*
White										
Smoker	100.0	100.0	100.0	100.0	100.0	100.0	100.0	100.0	100.0	100.0
1–5 cigarettes	30.0	47.8	37.5	41.5	36.1	30.7	27.4	26.5	26.0	24.2
6–10 cigarettes	43.7	37.8	44.5	43.4	44.9	45.2	43.6	41.6	39.5	38.5
11–15 cigarettes	5.7	*	4.1	3.2	4.4	5.2	6.1	6.9	7.5	7.9
16–20 cigarettes	18.1	11.0	12.5	10.7	13.1	16.9	20.1	21.4	22.7	23.8
21–30 cigarettes	1.8	*	1.1	1.0	1.1	1.5	2.1	2.5	3.1	3.8
31–40 cigarettes	0.6	*	0.3	0.2	0.3	0.4	0.6	0.9	1.1	1.6
41 cigarettes or more	0.1	*	0.1	*	0.1	0.1	0.1	0.1	0.2	*
Black										
Smoker	100.0	100.0	100.0	100.0	100.0	100.0	100.0	100.0	100.0	100.0
1–5 cigarettes	52.8	73.7	66.1	70.6	64.5	56.8	48.9	44.7	41.8	42.7
6–10 cigarettes	34.5	*	26.1	22.3	27.6	32.8	36.9	38.9	40.0	37.9
11–15 cigarettes	2.5	*	1.6	1.6	1.7	2.1	2.7	3.2	4.1	3.7
16–20 cigarettes	8.9	*	5.2	4.7	5.4	7.4	10.1	11.6	12.5	14.0
21–30 cigarettes	0.8	*	0.6	*	0.5	0.6	0.9	1.0	1.0	*
31–40 cigarettes	0.3	*	*	*	*	0.2	0.4	0.6	*	*
41 cigarettes or more	0.1	*	*	*	*	*	*	*	*	*

Note: Excludes data for California, which did not require reporting of tobacco use during pregnancy, and for Pennsylvania and Washington State, which implemented a forthcoming revision in the standard birth certificate and thus impaired comparability with the data from other states.

[1] Includes races other than White and Black.
[2] Excludes data for Indiana and New York State (but includes New York City), and for South Dakota, which did not report average number of cigarettes smoked per day in standard categories.
* = Figure does not meet standards of reliability or precision; based on fewer than 20 births in numerator.

able on birth certificates. The highest prevalence of smoking in 2003 was a 17.1 percent occurence rate among mothers 18 to 19 years old. The frequency of smoking declined for age groups through the mid-thirties, with a low of 6.5 percent in the 30- to 34-year-old age group. However, as age increases, women who smoke are more likely to be heavier smokers. Smoking by Blacks was considerably less frequent than smoking by Whites under 30 years old, but became more frequent in older age groups.

The trends and variations of smoking, as reported from birth certificates, are corroborated by data from comparable surveys. However, the extent of maternal smoking is believed to be somewhat underreported on birth certificates. The results are partly affected by the stigma associated with tobacco use, particularly in cases of poor birth outcome. The most frequent daily consumptions of cigarettes by smokers were 6 to 10 cigarettes for Whites and 1 to 5 cigarettes for Blacks. The proportion of smokers who smoked 11 cigarettes or more per day has fallen from 41 percent in 1989 to 24 percent in 2003.

TABLE I-30. NUMBER OF LIVE BIRTHS BY SMOKING STATUS DURING PREGNANCY AND PERCENT SMOKERS, BY AGE, SPECIFIED HISPANIC ORIGIN, AND RACE OF MOTHER: UNITED STATES EXCLUDING CALIFORNIA, PENNSYLVANIA, AND WASHINGTON STATE, 2003

This table details the smoking patterns of Hispanic mothers, by country of origin; rates are also given for non-Hispanic Whites and Blacks. Compared to other groups, Hispanic mothers smoked very little. Only 2.7 percent of Hispanic mothers were smokers in 2003, compared to 8.3 percent of non-Hispanic Blacks and 14.3 percent of non-Hispanic Whites. Smoking in the 18- to 19-year-old age group was reported by 3.6 percent of Hispanic mothers, compared to 29.1 percent of non-Hispanic Whites. Among Hispanics, occurrences of smoking were highest for Puerto Ricans and Cubans.

Table I-30. Number of Live Births by Smoking Status During Pregnancy and Percent Smokers, by Age, Specified Hispanic Origin, and Race of Mother: United States Excluding California, Pennsylvania, and Washington State, 2003

(Number, percent.)

Origin of mother	Smoking status (number)				Age of mother (percent smokers)									
	Total births	Smoker	Nonsmoker	Not stated	All ages	Under 15 years	15–19 years			20–24 years	25–29 years	30–34 years	35–39 years	40–54 years
							Total	15–17 years	18–19 years					
All Origins [1]	3 322 505	354 586	2 948 476	19 443	10.7	5.3	15.4	11.9	17.1	16.1	9.4	6.5	6.8	8.0
Hispanic	618 472	16 401	599 698	2 373	2.7	1.8	3.3	2.8	3.6	3.3	2.2	1.9	2.2	2.7
Mexican	405 131	8 231	395 286	1 614	2.0	2.0	2.4	2.0	2.7	2.5	1.6	1.5	1.8	2.1
Puerto Rican	50 440	3 989	46 318	133	7.9	*	7.6	5.9	8.7	9.3	8.0	6.2	6.6	8.2
Cuban	13 927	334	13 574	19	2.4	*	5.5	*	6.4	3.4	1.9	1.5	2.2	*
Central and South American	107 826	1 158	106 399	269	1.1	*	1.5	1.3	1.7	1.3	1.0	0.8	1.0	1.3
Other and unknown Hispanic	41 148	2 689	38 121	338	6.6	*	7.9	7.6	8.1	8.5	5.7	4.3	4.8	6.2
Non-Hispanic [2]	2 685 341	335 794	2 333 575	15 972	12.6	6.9	19.7	15.9	21.5	19.7	11.0	7.2	7.6	8.7
White	1 992 033	283 663	1 695 771	12 599	14.3	16.8	27.9	24.8	29.1	24.2	12.2	7.7	7.8	9.0
Black	523 062	43 068	477 853	2 141	8.3	1.8	6.3	4.7	7.2	9.5	8.6	7.2	8.6	10.1

Note: Excludes data for California, which did not require reporting of tobacco use during pregnancy, and for Pennsylvania and Washington State, which implemented a forthcoming revision in the standard birth certificate and thus impaired comparability with the data from other states. Race and Hispanic origin are reported separately on birth certificates. Persons of Hispanic origin may be of any race. In this table, Hispanic women are classified only by place of origin; non-Hispanic women are classified by race.

[1]Includes origin not stated.
[2]Includes races other than White and Black.
* = Figure does not meet standards of reliability or precision; based on fewer than 20 births in numerator.

TABLE I-31. NUMBER OF LIVE BIRTHS, PERCENT SMOKERS DURING PREGNANCY, AND CIGARETTE CONSUMPTION, ACCORDING TO EDUCATIONAL ATTAINMENT, RACE, AND HISPANIC ORIGIN OF MOTHER: UNITED STATES EXCLUDING CALIFORNIA, PENNSYLVANIA, AND WASHINGTON STATE, 2003

Mothers who completed only 9 to 11 years of education were most likely to be smokers, a pattern which held true for non-Hispanic Whites, Blacks, and Hispanics. For non-Hispanic Whites, 41.9 percent of those with this level of educational attainment were smokers. This rate was 16.5 percent for non-Hispanic Blacks, and 4.2 percent for Hispanics. As educational attainment increased, the prevalence of smoking fell. Only 1.8 percent of non-Hispanic White mothers with 16 or more years of education were reported smokers. For those who were smokers, the number of cigarettes smoked per day did not change considerably according to educational attainment. Most smokers reported using half a pack per day or less. On average, non-Hispanic Whites smoked more cigarettes per day than the other groups.

Table I-31. Number of Live Births, Percent Smokers During Pregnancy, and Cigarette Consumption, According to Educational Attainment, Race, and Hispanic Origin of Mother: United States Excluding California, Pennsylvania, and Washington State, 2003

(Number, percent.)

Smoking measure and race and Hispanic origin of mother	Total	Years of school completed by mother					
		0–8 years	9–11 years	12 years	13–15 years	16 years or more	Not stated
ALL BIRTHS							
All races [1]	3 322 505	175 122	498 587	1 012 812	709 728	885 116	41 140
White total [2]	2 602 499	154 199	362 569	756 306	552 072	747 611	29 742
Non-Hispanic White	1 992 033	32 235	202 124	578 389	472 654	689 864	16 767
Black total [2]	541 427	14 277	116 208	208 564	123 642	70 565	8 171
Non-Hispanic Black	523 062	12 111	112 612	202 330	119 981	68 522	7 506
Hispanic [3]	618 472	124 347	163 545	182 241	81 246	56 079	11 014
PERCENT SMOKERS							
Total	10.7	7.6	22.8	15.0	8.4	1.6	9.3
White total [2]	11.6	7.5	25.3	17.4	9.5	1.7	9.9
Non-Hispanic White	14.3	31.0	41.9	21.7	10.7	1.8	15.6
Black total [2]	8.1	9.2	16.2	7.9	4.6	1.2	9.1
Non-Hispanic Black	8.3	10.5	16.5	8.1	4.7	1.2	9.3
Hispanic [3]	2.7	1.2	4.2	3.0	2.3	0.8	2.2
PERCENT DISTRIBUTION [4]							
All Races [1]							
Smoker	100.0	100.0	100.0	100.0	100.0	100.0	100.0
10 cigarettes or less	75.7	70.5	75.6	75.3	77.0	80.5	75.7
11–20 cigarettes	22.0	25.7	21.8	22.5	21.1	18.0	22.0
21 cigarettes or more	2.3	3.8	2.6	2.2	1.9	1.5	2.3
White Total [2]							
Smoker	100.0	100.0	100.0	100.0	100.0	100.0	100.0
10 cigarettes or less	73.7	68.5	72.9	73.4	75.6	79.8	74.0
11–20 cigarettes	23.8	27.4	24.2	24.2	22.4	18.6	23.4
21 cigarettes or more	2.5	4.0	2.9	2.4	2.1	1.5	2.6
Non-Hispanic White							
Smoker	100.0	100.0	100.0	100.0	100.0	100.0	100.0
10 cigarettes or less	73.0	65.5	71.7	72.9	75.2	79.6	73.2
11–20 cigarettes	24.4	30.1	25.2	24.7	22.7	18.8	24.0
21 cigarettes or more	2.6	4.5	3.0	2.4	2.1	1.6	2.8
Black Total [2]							
Smoker	100.0	100.0	100.0	100.0	100.0	100.0	100.0
10 cigarettes or less	87.3	84.6	87.0	88.0	87.7	88.6	80.9
11–20 cigarettes	11.5	13.3	11.7	10.9	11.3	10.7	17.5
21 cigarettes or more	1.2	2.1	1.3	1.1	1.0	*	*
Non-Hispanic Black							
Smoker	100.0	100.0	100.0	100.0	100.0	100.0	100.0
10 cigarettes or less	87.4	84.4	87.0	88.0	87.7	88.8	80.9
11–20 cigarettes	11.4	13.5	11.7	10.9	11.4	10.5	17.4
21 cigarettes or more	1.2	2.1	1.3	1.1	0.9	*	*
Hispanic [3]							
Smoker	100.0	100.0	100.0	100.0	100.0	100.0	100.0
10 cigarettes or less	86.7	88.4	87.2	86.4	85.3	86.1	83.1
11–20 cigarettes	12.2	10.3	11.6	12.8	13.5	13.4	16.3
21 cigarettes or more	1.0	*	1.2	0.7	1.2	*	*

Note: Excludes data for California, which did not require reporting of tobacco use during pregnancy, and for Pennsylvania and Washington State, which implemented a forthcoming revision in the standard birth certificate and thus impaired comparability with the data from other states.

[1] Includes races other than White and Black and origin not stated.
[2] Race and Hispanic origin are reported separately on the birth certificate. Data for persons of Hispanic origin are included in the data for each race group according to the mother's reported race.
[3] May be of any race.
[4] Excludes data for Indiana, New York State (but includes New York City), and for South Dakota, which did not report average number of cigarettes smoked per day in standard categories.
* = Figure does not meet standards of reliability or precision; based on fewer than 20 births in numerator.

TABLE I-32. PERCENT LOW BIRTHWEIGHT, BY SMOKING STATUS DURING PREGNANCY, AGE, RACE, AND HISPANIC ORIGIN OF MOTHER: UNITED STATES EXCLUDING CALIFORNIA, PENNSYLVANIA, AND WASHINGTON STATE, 2003

In 2003, the rate of low birthweight (less than 5.5 pounds) for babies born to smokers was 12.4 percent, compared to 7.7 percent for nonsmokers. The gap between smokers and nonsmokers tended to widen with advancing maternal age; for mothers 35–39 years old,

smokers had a 17.4 percent incidence of low birthweight, while babies of nonsmokers in the same age group had a low birthweight frequency of 8.3 percent. Apart from the influence of age, this could reflect the fact that maternal smokers in the older age brackets tend to be somewhat heavier smokers (see Table I-29). Black nonsmokers have roughly double the frequency of low birthweight as non-Hispanic White or Hispanic nonsmokers, reflecting other risk factors. However, the additional effects of smoking in Blacks are comparable to those for the other racial and ethnic groups.

Table I-32. Percent Low Birthweight, by Smoking Status During Pregnancy, Age, Race, and Hispanic Origin of Mother: United States Excluding California, Pennsylvania, and Washington State, 2003

(Percent.)

Smoking status and race of mother	All ages	Age of mother								
		Under 15 years	15–19 years			20–24 years	25–29 years	30–34 years	35–39 years	40–54 years
			Total	15–17 years	18–19 years					
All Races [1]										
Total	8.2	13.0	10.0	10.8	9.7	8.3	7.3	7.6	8.9	11.4
Smoker	12.4	12.2	11.8	12.8	11.5	11.1	11.9	13.8	17.4	20.7
Nonsmoker	7.7	13.0	9.7	10.5	9.3	7.7	6.8	7.1	8.3	10.5
Not stated	11.9	*	13.8	12.6	14.4	11.8	10.6	11.3	12.8	16.4
White Total [2]										
Total	7.1	10.2	8.6	9.2	8.3	7.0	6.4	6.8	8.0	10.4
Smoker	11.3	12.9	11.2	12.2	10.9	10.2	10.8	12.5	15.3	18.3
Nonsmoker	6.5	9.8	7.9	8.7	7.5	6.2	5.9	6.3	7.4	9.7
Not stated	10.9	*	12.8	11.2	13.6	10.5	10.0	10.4	11.6	15.6
Non-Hispanic White										
Total	7.2	10.3	8.8	9.6	8.5	7.2	6.4	6.7	8.0	10.3
Smoker	11.2	11.9	11.2	12.2	10.8	10.1	10.7	12.3	15.2	18.1
Nonsmoker	6.5	9.9	7.8	8.8	7.5	6.2	5.8	6.2	7.3	9.5
Not stated	11.0	*	14.4	12.6	15.1	10.5	10.0	10.2	12.0	15.9
Black Total [2]										
Total	13.4	16.3	14.2	14.4	14.0	13.1	12.3	13.4	15.5	17.1
Smoker	20.2	*	17.5	17.4	17.5	17.4	19.2	23.9	30.1	31.9
Nonsmoker	12.8	16.4	13.9	14.2	13.7	12.6	11.7	12.6	14.2	15.4
Not stated	19.1	*	17.7	*	17.2	18.5	15.4	22.3	22.9	*
Non-Hispanic Black										
Total	13.6	16.4	14.3	14.5	14.1	13.3	12.5	13.6	15.8	17.2
Smoker	20.3	*	17.6	17.5	17.6	17.5	19.3	24.0	30.2	31.9
Nonsmoker	13.0	16.4	14.0	14.3	13.8	12.8	11.8	12.8	14.4	15.6
Not stated	18.9	*	17.8	*	17.3	18.5	15.5	21.7	22.4	*
Hispanic [3]										
Total	7.0	10.0	8.1	8.7	7.8	6.6	6.2	6.9	8.1	10.9
Smoker	13.0	*	12.1	12.5	11.9	12.2	12.7	14.0	16.7	21.1
Nonsmoker	6.8	9.7	8.0	8.6	7.6	6.4	6.1	6.8	7.9	10.6
Not stated	9.7	*	8.7	*	*	9.0	8.9	10.8	11.0	*

Note: Low birthweight defined as weight of less than 2,500 grams (5 lb 8 oz). Excludes data for California, which did not require reporting of tobacco use during pregnancy and for Pennsylvania and Washington State, which implemented a forthcoming revision in the standard birth certificate and thus impaired comparability with the data from other states.

[1]Includes races other than White and Black and origin not stated.
[2]Race and Hispanic origin are reported separately on the birth certificate. Data for persons of Hispanic origin are included in the data for each race group according to the mother's reported race.
[3]May be of any race.
* = Figure does not meet standards of reliability or precision; based on fewer than 20 births in numerator.

TABLE I-33. LIVE BIRTHS BY MONTH OF PREGNANCY WHEN PRENATAL CARE BEGAN, PERCENT OF MOTHERS BEGINNING CARE IN THE FIRST TRIMESTER, AND PERCENT WITH LATE OR NO CARE, BY AGE, RACE, AND HISPANIC ORIGIN OF MOTHER: UNITED STATES EXCLUDING PENNSYLVANIA AND WASHINGTON STATE, 2003

Prenatal care began in the first trimester for 89.0 percent of non-Hispanic White mothers, 75.9 percent of non-Hispanic Black mothers, and 77.5 percent of Hispanic mothers. Young mothers, particularly teenagers, had lower rates of medical care during the first trimester than those 25 years old and over. For all three racial/ethnic groups, the frequency of first trimester care increased with age until age 34, then decreased slightly in older age brackets. The frequency of late care (beginning in the third trimester) or no care was 2.1 percent for non-Hispanic Whites, 6.0 percent for non-Hispanic Blacks, and 5.3 percent for Hispanics.

First trimester care has increased by an average of 11 percent since 1990, and gains for Blacks, American Indians, and Hispanics were more than 20 percent. (See Table I-33A.) Recent studies suggest that the expansion of Medicaid for pregnant women in the late 1980s contributed to these increases.

Table I-33. Live Births by Month of Pregnancy When Prenatal Care Began, Percent of Mothers Beginning Care in the First Trimester, and Percent with Late or No Care, by Age, Race, and Hispanic Origin of Mother: United States Excluding Pennsylvania and Washington State, 2003

(Number, percent.)

Age, race, and Hispanic origin of mother	All births	Month of pregnancy prenatal care began							Not stated	Percent	
		1st trimester			2nd trimester	Late or no care				1st trimester	Late or no care
		Total	1st and 2nd months	3rd month	4th–6th months	Total	7th–9th months	No care			
All Races [1]											
All ages	3 863 502	3 189 794	2 475 340	714 454	469 649	134 057	94 601	39 456	70 002	84.1	3.5
Under 15 years	6 341	3 030	1 841	1 189	2 174	944	660	284	193	49.3	15.4
15–19 years	394 919	273 266	187 884	85 382	88 202	24 681	17 774	6 907	8 770	70.8	6.4
15 years	17 344	9 841	6 257	3 584	5 279	1 768	1 263	505	456	58.3	10.5
16 years	39 332	24 502	16 090	8 412	10 741	3 120	2 297	823	969	63.9	8.1
17 years	71 353	47 805	32 343	15 462	17 086	4 821	3 479	1 342	1 641	68.6	6.9
18 years	112 293	78 836	54 512	24 324	24 398	6 618	4 693	1 925	2 441	71.8	6.0
19 years	154 597	112 282	78 682	33 600	30 698	8 354	6 042	2 312	3 263	74.2	5.5
20–24 years	980 514	759 481	562 335	197 146	157 910	44 162	31 506	12 656	18 961	79.0	4.6
25–29 years	1 025 666	872 030	688 793	183 237	106 103	30 065	21 249	8 816	17 468	86.5	3.0
30–34 years	916 840	810 907	656 825	154 082	70 583	20 604	14 399	6 205	14 746	89.9	2.3
35–39 years	438 771	385 989	310 514	75 475	34 663	10 452	6 947	3 505	7 667	89.5	2.4
40 years and over	100 451	85 091	67 148	17 943	10 014	3 149	2 066	1 083	2 197	86.6	3.2
White Total [2]											
All ages	3 040 873	2 562 458	2 001 335	561 123	336 407	91 183	65 011	26 172	50 825	85.7	3.0
Under 15 years	3 512	1 847	1 138	709	1 106	465	319	146	94	54.0	13.6
15–19 years	284 861	202 977	140 494	62 483	59 211	16 214	11 768	4 446	5 958	72.9	5.8
15 years	10 963	6 656	4 304	2 352	3 014	1 024	719	305	269	62.2	9.6
16 years	26 861	17 549	11 691	5 858	6 760	1 932	1 425	507	620	66.9	7.4
17 years	50 615	34 997	23 871	11 126	11 288	3 225	2 367	858	1 105	70.7	6.5
18 years	81 801	58 994	40 990	18 004	16 727	4 376	3 138	1 238	1 704	73.7	5.5
19 years	114 120	84 781	59 638	25 143	21 422	5 657	4 119	1 538	2 260	75.8	5.1
20–24 years	750 290	592 950	440 831	152 119	113 198	30 583	22 093	8 490	13 559	80.5	4.2
25–29 years	821 214	709 352	563 020	146 332	78 104	20 883	14 789	6 094	12 888	87.8	2.6
30–34 years	745 992	668 973	544 438	124 535	52 039	13 990	9 861	4 129	10 990	91.0	1.9
35–39 years	355 111	317 145	256 476	60 669	25 332	6 929	4 762	2 167	5 705	90.8	2.0
40 years and over	80 381	69 214	54 938	14 276	7 417	2 119	1 419	700	1 631	87.9	2.7
Non-Hispanic White											
All ages	2 158 797	1 892 768	1 501 689	391 079	189 306	45 721	33 333	12 388	31 002	89.0	2.1
Under 15 years	1 316	723	467	256	387	176	130	46	30	56.2	13.7
15–19 years	161 828	121 256	83 790	37 466	30 699	6 967	5 358	1 609	2 906	76.3	4.4
15 years	4 548	2 861	1 832	1 029	1 208	367	270	97	112	64.5	8.3
16 years	12 496	8 501	5 666	2 835	3 023	728	577	151	244	69.4	5.9
17 years	26 846	19 489	13 138	6 351	5 505	1 336	1 032	304	516	74.0	5.1
18 years	47 441	35 792	24 727	11 065	8 878	1 915	1 458	457	856	76.8	4.1
19 years	70 497	54 613	38 427	16 186	12 085	2 621	2 021	600	1 178	78.8	3.8
20–24 years	488 194	401 428	300 829	100 599	63 988	15 201	11 329	3 872	7 577	83.5	3.2
25–29 years	582 914	522 461	421 324	101 137	42 478	10 231	7 378	2 853	7 744	90.8	1.8
30–34 years	580 329	534 305	440 425	93 880	30 869	7 644	5 381	2 263	7 511	93.3	1.3
35–39 years	280 645	256 513	209 861	46 652	15 938	4 138	2 851	1 287	4 056	92.7	1.5
40 years and over	63 571	56 082	44 993	11 089	4 947	1 364	906	458	1 178	89.9	2.2
Black Total [2]											
All ages	573 776	425 303	318 287	107 016	101 347	33 528	22 089	11 439	13 598	75.9	6.0
Under 15 years	2 588	1 075	638	437	992	430	306	124	91	43.1	17.2
15–19 years	96 294	61 815	41 936	19 879	24 865	7 223	5 057	2 166	2 391	65.8	7.7
15 years	5 744	2 901	1 789	1 112	2 031	654	478	176	158	51.9	11.7
16 years	11 047	6 233	3 958	2 275	3 492	1 021	750	271	301	58.0	9.5
17 years	18 180	11 379	7 539	3 840	4 986	1 364	928	436	451	64.2	7.7
18 years	26 567	17 494	12 014	5 480	6 535	1 905	1 301	604	633	67.5	7.3
19 years	34 756	23 808	16 636	7 172	7 821	2 279	1 600	679	848	70.2	6.7
20–24 years	187 923	136 035	99 971	36 064	36 443	11 101	7 457	3 644	4 344	74.1	6.0
25–29 years	133 853	104 614	80 760	23 854	19 523	6 697	4 419	2 278	3 019	80.0	5.1
30–34 years	93 416	74 937	58 777	16 160	11 669	4 627	2 912	1 715	2 183	82.1	5.1
35–39 years	47 722	37 704	29 281	8 423	6 146	2 665	1 487	1 178	1 207	81.1	5.7
40 years and over	11 980	9 123	6 924	2 199	1 709	785	451	334	363	78.5	6.8

Note: Excludes data for Pennsylvania and Washington State, which implemented a forthcoming revision in the standard birth certificate and thus impaired comparability with the data from the other states.

[1] Includes races other than White and Black and origin not stated.
[2] Race and Hispanic origin are reported separately on the birth certificate. Data for persons of Hispanic origin are included in the data for each race group according to the mother's reported race.

Table I-33. Live Births by Month of Pregnancy When Prenatal Care Began, Percent of Mothers Beginning Care in the First Trimester, and Percent with Late or No Care, by Age, Race, and Hispanic Origin of Mother: United States Excluding Pennsylvania and Washington State, 2003—*Continued*

(Number, percent.)

Age, race, and Hispanic origin of mother	All births	Month of pregnancy prenatal care began							Not stated	Percent	
		1st trimester			2nd trimester	Late or no care				1st trimester	Late or no care
		Total	1st and 2nd months	3rd month	4th–6th months	Total	7th–9th months	No care			
Non-Hispanic Black											
All ages	553 987	411 013	307 917	103 096	97 826	32 406	21 258	11 148	12 742	75.9	6.0
Under 15 years	2 531	1 058	627	431	977	413	292	121	83	43.2	16.9
15–19 years	93 623	60 117	40 793	19 324	24 202	7 031	4 925	2 106	2 273	65.8	7.7
15 years	5 595	2 820	1 749	1 071	1 992	630	459	171	153	51.8	11.6
16 years	10 741	6 058	3 846	2 212	3 402	996	735	261	285	57.9	9.5
17 years	17 640	11 036	7 300	3 736	4 844	1 331	912	419	429	64.1	7.7
18 years	25 875	17 049	11 711	5 338	6 366	1 859	1 268	591	601	67.5	7.4
19 years	33 772	23 154	16 187	6 967	7 598	2 215	1 551	664	805	70.2	6.7
20–24 years	182 032	131 924	97 046	34 878	35 261	10 744	7 200	3 544	4 103	74.1	6.0
25–29 years	128 686	100 767	77 924	22 843	18 699	6 397	4 186	2 211	2 823	80.1	5.1
30–34 years	89 775	72 175	56 694	15 481	11 125	4 465	2 789	1 676	2 010	82.2	5.1
35–39 years	45 795	36 191	28 161	8 030	5 901	2 590	1 428	1 162	1 113	81.0	5.8
40 years and over	11 545	8 781	6 672	2 109	1 661	766	438	328	337	78.3	6.8
Hispanic [3]											
All ages	888 177	673 271	501 115	172 156	150 083	45 894	32 179	13 715	18 929	77.5	5.3
Under 15 years	2 250	1 142	685	457	734	305	201	104	69	52.4	14.0
15–19 years	124 616	83 053	57 576	25 477	29 156	9 384	6 514	2 870	3 023	68.3	7.7
15 years	6 569	3 882	2 515	1 367	1 853	676	464	212	158	60.6	10.5
16 years	14 645	9 228	6 143	3 085	3 808	1 235	871	364	374	64.7	8.7
17 years	24 201	15 775	10 922	4 853	5 932	1 908	1 345	563	586	66.8	8.1
18 years	34 864	23 542	16 493	7 049	7 999	2 484	1 704	780	839	69.2	7.3
19 years	44 337	30 626	21 503	9 123	9 564	3 081	2 130	951	1 066	70.8	7.1
20–24 years	265 614	193 954	141 562	52 392	50 259	15 556	10 933	4 623	5 845	74.7	6.0
25–29 years	239 989	187 974	142 265	45 709	36 343	10 773	7 562	3 211	4 899	80.0	4.6
30–34 years	165 152	134 008	103 173	30 835	21 561	6 348	4 530	1 818	3 235	82.8	3.9
35–39 years	74 008	60 201	46 119	14 082	9 545	2 785	1 925	860	1 477	83.0	3.8
40 years and over	16 548	12 939	9 735	3 204	2 485	743	514	229	381	80.0	4.6

Note: Excludes data for Pennsylvania and Washington State, which implemented a forthcoming revision in the standard birth certificate and thus impaired comparability with the data from the other states.

[3]May be of any race.

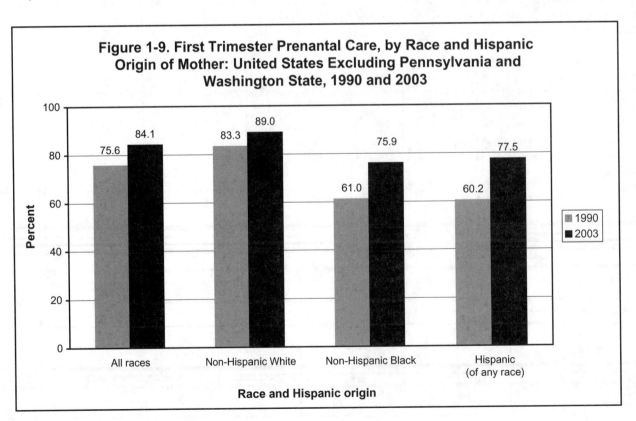

Figure 1-9. First Trimester Prenantal Care, by Race and Hispanic Origin of Mother: United States Excluding Pennsylvania and Washington State, 1990 and 2003

TABLE I-33A. FIRST TRIMESTER PRENATAL CARE, BY RACE AND HISPANIC ORIGIN OF MOTHER: UNITED STATES EXCLUDING PENNSYLVANIA AND WASHINGTON STATE, SELECTED YEARS, 1990–2003

Timely initiation of prenatal care has improved slowly but steadily in recent years, rising more than 11 percent since 1990 (up from 75.6 percent in reporting states). Disparities in the frequency of care among listed minorities were pronounced in 1990, but gains of 24 percent for non-Hispanic Blacks and 29 percent for Hispanics have been posted since then. (See Tables I-24 and I-25 for the percentage of mothers of other races and origins receiving first trimester prenatal care in 2003.)

Table I-33A. First Trimester Prenatal Care, by Race and Hispanic Origin of Mother: United States Excluding Pennsylvania and Washington State, Selected Years, 1990–2003

(Percent.)

Year	All races [1]	Non-Hispanic [1]		Hispanic [2]
		White	Black	
2003	84.1	89.0	75.9	77.5
2002	83.7	88.7	75.3	76.8
2001	83.3	88.6	74.5	75.8
2000	83.1	88.6	74.3	74.5
1995	81.2	87.1	70.6	70.8
1990	75.6	83.3	61.0	60.2

Note: Excludes data for Pennsylvania and Washington State, which implemented a forthcoming revision in the standard birth certificate and thus impaired comparability with the data from other states.

[1]Includes races other than White and Black and origin not stated.
[2]May be of any race.

TABLE I-34. PERCENT OF MOTHERS BEGINNING PRENATAL CARE IN THE FIRST TRIMESTER VERSUS LATE OR NO PRENATAL CARE, BY RACE AND HISPANIC ORIGIN OF MOTHER, FOR EACH STATE AND TERRITORY, 2003

Three states in New England (New Hampshire, Rhode Island, and Vermont) reported levels of first trimester care above 90 percent and levels of late or no prenatal care of less than 2 percent. Conditions were least favorable in New Mexico, where only 68.9 of all mothers and 66.2 percent of Hispanic mothers obtained first trimester care. Approximately 8.1 percent of all mothers and 9.2 percent of Hispanic mothers sought late or no prenatal care. Another state with a low percentage of early care was Nevada (75.8 percent), where 6.4 percent of all mothers and 9.9 percent of Hispanic mothers sought late or no prenatal care. These data were not much different for the District of Columbia, where 9.1 percent of non-Hispanic Blacks received late or no care.

Table I-34. Percent of Mothers Beginning Prenatal Care in the First Trimester Versus Late or No Prenatal Care, by Race and Hispanic Origin of Mother, for Each State and Territory, 2003

(Percent.)

State	Percent beginning care in first trimester						Percent late [1] or no care					
	All races [2]	White		Black		Hispanic [4]	All races [2]	White		Black		Hispanic [4]
		Total [3]	Non-Hispanic	Total [3]	Non-Hispanic			Total [3]	Non-Hispanic	Total [3]	Non-Hispanic	
UNITED STATES [5]	84.1	85.7	89.0	75.9	75.9	77.5	3.5	3.0	2.1	6.0	6.0	5.3
Alabama	83.8	87.3	90.0	75.7	75.7	52.0	3.5	3.0	1.6	4.8	4.8	21.6
Alaska	79.8	83.7	82.9	81.8	81.0	79.6	5.2	4.7	5.1	*	*	5.2
Arizona	76.6	76.9	88.0	76.0	79.5	66.7	7.3	7.3	2.7	8.2	5.5	11.1
Arkansas	81.3	83.2	84.6	73.5	73.4	71.5	4.3	3.7	3.2	6.9	6.9	7.6
California	87.3	87.4	90.8	84.1	84.1	85.2	2.5	2.5	1.8	3.2	3.2	3.0
Colorado	79.3	79.8	86.1	70.9	70.7	67.0	4.4	4.3	2.8	6.8	6.8	7.4
Connecticut	88.7	89.8	92.7	81.0	81.4	78.2	1.5	1.3	0.9	3.0	2.9	2.8
Delaware	84.4	86.2	88.8	78.8	79.6	71.9	4.4	3.4	2.9	7.3	7.1	6.8
District of Columbia	76.1	86.4	89.6	71.1	71.0	69.6	6.6	2.5	2.0	8.5	9.1	4.7
Florida	85.8	88.1	90.1	77.9	77.8	84.2	2.8	2.3	1.8	4.8	4.8	3.1
Georgia	84.0	86.2	90.5	79.1	79.1	69.1	3.8	3.3	2.0	4.8	4.8	8.3
Hawaii	82.4	85.5	86.3	89.3	89.1	80.8	3.6	2.1	1.9	*	*	3.0
Idaho	81.4	81.6	83.9	87.8	87.4	68.3	3.4	3.4	2.8	*	*	6.9
Illinois	85.4	87.7	91.0	74.2	74.1	80.0	2.8	2.0	1.5	6.7	6.7	3.2
Indiana	81.5	83.0	84.7	69.3	69.3	66.0	3.8	3.3	2.9	8.1	8.1	7.7
Iowa	88.9	89.5	90.6	76.8	76.8	74.8	2.0	1.8	1.7	5.5	5.5	4.1
Kansas	87.8	88.5	90.5	80.1	80.2	77.2	2.3	2.1	1.7	4.4	4.5	4.7
Kentucky	87.0	87.7	88.2	80.7	80.7	74.0	2.6	2.4	2.2	4.8	4.8	6.4
Louisiana	84.1	90.0	90.3	75.5	75.5	83.3	3.4	1.7	1.6	5.8	5.8	3.8
Maine	87.5	87.9	87.9	74.9	75.6	80.7	1.7	1.6	1.6	*	*	*
Maryland	83.7	88.7	91.0	74.6	75.3	70.1	3.9	2.3	1.8	6.7	6.7	6.4
Massachusetts	90.0	91.4	92.4	81.5	80.3	83.9	2.0	1.6	1.4	5.2	6.0	2.6
Michigan	86.1	89.0	89.8	72.8	72.7	77.6	3.1	2.2	2.0	7.3	7.4	4.7
Minnesota	86.5	88.8	90.5	72.3	72.3	71.0	2.2	1.6	1.3	5.4	5.4	5.0
Mississippi	84.9	90.7	91.0	77.8	77.8	79.6	2.9	1.6	1.5	4.4	4.4	6.9
Missouri	88.4	89.7	90.2	81.0	80.9	81.0	2.2	1.8	1.6	4.4	4.4	3.9
Montana	84.4	86.9	87.4	86.0	87.8	80.6	2.7	2.0	1.9	*	*	*
Nebraska	83.4	84.4	86.9	72.7	72.8	69.8	2.8	2.6	2.0	3.8	3.6	6.3
Nevada	75.8	75.8	84.6	70.7	70.6	64.1	6.4	6.3	3.4	8.6	8.8	9.9
New Hampshire	92.8	93.0	93.4	85.1	85.5	84.4	1.1	1.0	0.9	*	*	*
New Jersey	80.2	83.4	89.2	64.4	63.5	68.6	4.7	3.6	2.3	10.6	11.2	6.8
New Mexico	68.9	70.2	77.0	68.7	69.1	66.2	8.1	7.5	5.0	5.9	5.5	9.1
New York	82.4	85.2	88.6	73.1	72.8	76.2	4.5	3.5	2.7	8.3	8.5	5.5
North Carolina	84.5	86.9	90.8	76.8	76.8	69.6	2.9	2.4	1.5	4.9	4.9	6.0
North Dakota	87.3	89.7	90.0	85.2	84.8	79.5	2.7	1.9	1.8	*	*	*
Ohio	87.7	89.3	89.8	78.8	78.8	79.0	3.0	2.4	2.3	6.1	6.1	4.6
Oklahoma	77.8	79.6	82.0	69.8	69.8	65.5	4.8	4.2	3.8	7.1	7.1	6.7
Oregon	81.2	81.5	84.5	78.0	77.6	70.0	4.0	3.9	3.3	5.5	5.6	6.2
Pennsylvania	76.0	79.2	80.4	57.2	57.4	61.2	5.6	4.5	4.2	12.6	12.7	8.8
Rhode Island	90.9	92.2	93.5	82.8	82.1	86.9	1.1	1.0	0.9	2.3	2.2	1.4
South Carolina	77.5	81.0	83.6	70.5	70.6	56.9	4.9	3.9	3.2	6.7	6.7	11.0
South Dakota	78.4	82.8	83.4	64.8	65.5	64.0	3.9	2.2	2.0	*	*	9.4
Tennessee	83.4	86.2	88.1	73.0	73.0	63.7	3.8	3.0	2.2	7.2	7.2	12.4
Texas	80.9	81.1	88.4	77.0	77.0	75.5	4.7	4.7	2.5	5.5	5.5	6.3
Utah	80.3	81.2	83.9	63.2	61.8	65.1	4.4	4.0	3.2	13.6	14.3	8.6
Vermont	90.6	90.8	90.8	74.0	73.5	81.5	1.6	1.6	1.5	*	*	*
Virginia	85.3	87.9	90.4	76.9	77.3	71.2	3.6	2.8	2.0	5.8	5.8	7.7
Washington	74.0	75.0	77.6	67.9	68.9	63.1	5.8	5.4	4.8	8.2	8.0	8.0
West Virginia	85.8	86.2	86.4	73.5	73.5	69.3	2.3	2.3	2.2	3.7	3.8	*
Wisconsin	84.9	86.9	88.5	73.6	73.7	70.7	3.1	2.6	2.3	6.4	6.3	5.9
Wyoming	86.4	87.0	87.9	96.2	96.2	80.1	2.5	2.3	2.2	*	*	*
Puerto Rico	82.4	83.2	. . .	74.7	. . .	. . .	2.6	2.4	. . .	4.6	. . .	. . .
Virgin Islands	63.4	71.1	76.0	60.8	60.5	65.8	11.4	8.3	*	12.5	12.4	9.4
Guam	62.2	87.2	86.7	89.7	91.4	87.0	12.0	*	*	*	*	. . .
American Samoa	. . .	. . .	. . .	. . .	. . .	. . .	. . .	. . .	. . .	. . .	. . .	. . .
Northern Marianas	29.9	*	. . .	*	. . .	. . .	27.8	*	. . .	*	. . .	. . .

[1]Care beginning in third trimester.
[2]Includes races other than White and Black and origin not stated.
[3]Race and Hispanic origin are reported separately on the birth certificate. Data for persons of Hispanic origin are included in the data for each race group according to the mother's reported race.
[4]May be of any race.
[5]Excludes data for the territories.
* = Figure does not meet standards of reliability or precision; based on fewer than 20 births in numerator.
. . . = Not available.

TABLE I-34A. PRENATAL CARE FOR LIVE BIRTHS, ACCORDING TO DETAILED RACE AND HISPANIC ORIGIN OF MOTHER, SELECTED YEARS, 1970–2003

The percentage of mothers receiving prenatal care in the first trimester of pregnancy has continued to edge upward, increasing from 76 percent in 1990 to 84 percent in 2003. This upward trend reflects increases experienced during the 1970s and the 1990s. Increases in the use of prenatal care during the 1990s were greatest for those with the lowest rates of care: Hispanic, non-Hispanic Black, and American Indian mothers. Although gains occurred for all racial and ethnic groups, the percentage of mothers with early prenatal care in 2002 still varied substantially, from 70 percent for American Indian mothers to between 91–92 percent for mothers of Japanese and Cuban origin. Attitudes toward pregnancy, lifestyle factors, and cultural beliefs have been suggested as reasons for delaying recommended prenatal care. Financial and health insurance problems are among the most important barriers to such care. Expansion of Medicaid coverage for pregnancy-related services has increased the availability and use of prenatal care by low-income women.

TABLE I-35. LIVE BIRTHS BY MONTH OF PREGNANCY PRENATAL CARE BEGAN, NUMBER OF PRENATAL VISITS, AND MEDIAN NUMBER OF VISITS, BY RACE AND HISPANIC ORIGIN OF MOTHER: UNITED STATES EXCLUDING PENNSYLVANIA AND WASHINGTON STATE, 2003

This table summarizes the number of prenatal care visits by expectant mothers and classifies them according to the time when care began. It also shows details by race and ethnicity. The median number of prenatal visits for all births was 12.3, and it was 12.8 for mothers who started care during the first two months of pregnancy. The frequency of visits dropped for those who began later; the median was 5.5 visits for women who began care in the 7th to 9th month. The median number of visits by non-Hispanic Black and Hispanic mothers was 11.7 and 11.8, respectively—somewhat less than the 12.3 median for non-Hispanic Whites.

Table I-34A. Prenatal Care for Live Births, According to Detailed Race and Hispanic Origin of Mother, Selected Years, 1970–2003

(Percent.)

Prenatal care, race and Hispanic origin of mother	2003	2002	2001	2000	1999	1998	1995	1990	1985	1980	1975	1970
PERCENT OF LIVE BIRTHS [1]												
Prenatal Care Began During 1st Trimester												
All races	84.1	83.7	83.4	83.2	83.2	82.8	81.3	75.8	76.2	76.3	72.4	68.0
White	85.7	85.4	85.2	85.0	85.1	84.8	83.6	79.2	79.3	79.2	75.8	72.3
Black or African American	75.9	75.2	74.5	74.3	74.1	73.3	70.4	60.6	61.5	62.4	55.5	44.2
American Indian or Alaska Native	70.8	69.8	69.3	69.3	69.5	68.8	66.7	57.5	57.5	55.8	45.4	38.2
Asian or Pacific Islander	85.4	84.8	84.0	84.0	83.7	83.1	79.9	75.1	74.1	73.7	. . .	. . .
Chinese	. . .	87.2	87.0	87.6	88.5	88.5	85.7	81.3	82.0	82.6	76.7	71.8
Japanese	. . .	90.5	90.1	91.0	90.7	90.2	89.7	87.0	84.7	86.1	82.7	78.1
Filipino	. . .	85.4	85.0	84.9	84.2	84.2	80.9	77.1	76.5	77.3	70.6	60.6
Hawaiian	. . .	78.1	79.1	79.9	79.6	78.8	75.9	65.8	67.7	68.8	. . .	. . .
Other Asian or Pacific Islander	. . .	83.9	82.7	82.5	81.8	80.9	77.0	71.9	69.9	67.4	. . .	. . .
Hispanic or Latino [2]	77.5	76.7	75.7	74.4	74.4	74.3	70.8	60.2	61.2	60.2	. . .	. . .
Mexican	76.5	75.7	74.6	72.9	73.1	72.8	69.1	57.8	60.0	59.6	. . .	. . .
Puerto Rican	81.2	79.9	79.1	78.5	76.9	76.9	74.0	63.5	58.3	55.1	. . .	. . .
Cuban	92.1	92.0	91.8	91.7	91.4	91.8	89.2	84.8	82.5	82.7	. . .	. . .
Central and South American	79.2	78.7	77.4	77.6	77.6	78.0	73.2	61.5	60.6	58.8	. . .	. . .
Other and unknown Hispanic or Latino	77.0	76.7	77.3	75.8	74.8	74.8	74.3	66.4	65.8	66.4	. . .	. . .
Not Hispanic or Latino [2]												
White	89.0	88.6	88.5	88.5	88.4	87.9	87.1	83.3	81.4	81.2	. . .	. . .
Black or African American	75.9	75.2	74.5	74.3	74.1	73.3	70.4	60.7	60.2	60.8	. . .	. . .
Prenatal Care Began During 3rd Trimester or No Prenatal Care												
All races	3.5	3.6	3.7	3.9	3.8	3.9	4.2	6.1	5.7	5.1	6.0	7.9
White	3.0	3.1	3.2	3.3	3.2	3.3	3.5	4.9	4.8	4.3	5.0	6.3
Black or African American	6.0	6.2	6.5	6.7	6.6	7.0	7.6	11.3	10.2	8.9	10.5	16.6
American Indian or Alaska Native	7.6	8.0	8.2	8.6	8.2	8.5	9.5	12.9	12.9	15.2	22.4	28.9
Asian or Pacific Islander	3.1	3.1	3.4	3.3	3.5	3.6	4.3	5.8	6.5	6.5	. . .	. . .
Chinese	. . .	2.1	2.4	2.2	2.0	2.2	3.0	3.4	4.4	3.7	4.4	6.5
Japanese	. . .	2.1	2.0	1.8	2.1	2.1	2.3	2.9	3.1	2.1	2.7	4.1
Filipino	. . .	2.8	3.0	3.0	2.8	3.1	4.1	4.5	4.8	4.0	4.1	7.2
Hawaiian	. . .	4.7	4.8	4.2	4.0	4.7	5.1	8.7	7.4	6.7	. . .	. . .
Other Asian or Pacific Islander	. . .	3.5	3.8	3.8	4.1	4.2	5.0	7.1	8.2	9.3	. . .	. . .
Hispanic or Latino [2]	5.3	5.5	5.9	6.3	6.3	6.3	7.4	12.0	12.4	12.0	. . .	. . .
Mexican	5.6	5.8	6.2	6.9	6.7	6.8	8.1	13.2	12.9	11.8	. . .	. . .
Puerto Rican	3.7	4.1	4.6	4.5	5.0	5.1	5.5	10.6	15.5	16.2	. . .	. . .
Cuban	1.3	1.3	1.3	1.4	1.4	1.2	2.1	2.8	3.7	3.9	. . .	. . .
Central and South American	4.7	4.9	5.7	5.4	5.2	4.9	6.1	10.9	12.5	13.1	. . .	. . .
Other and unknown Hispanic or Latino	5.4	5.3	5.4	5.9	6.3	6.0	6.0	8.5	9.4	9.2	. . .	. . .
Not Hispanic or Latino [2]												
White	2.1	2.2	2.2	2.3	2.3	2.4	2.5	3.4	4.0	3.5	. . .	. . .
Black or African American	6.0	6.2	6.5	6.7	6.6	7.0	7.6	11.2	10.9	9.7	. . .	. . .

Note: Data are based on birth certificates.

[1] Excludes live births for whom trimester when prenatal care began is unknown.
[2] Prior to 1993, data from states lacking an Hispanic-origin item on the birth certificate were excluded.
. . . = Not available.

Table I-35. Live Births by Month of Pregnancy Prenatal Care Began, Number of Prenatal Visits, and Median Number of Visits, by Race and Hispanic Origin of Mother: United States Excluding Pennsylvania and Washington State, 2003

(Number.)

Number of prenatal visits and race and Hispanic origin of mother	All births	Month of pregnancy prenatal care began							Not stated
		1st trimester			2nd trimester	Late or no care			
		Total	1st and 2nd months	3rd month	4th–6th months	Total	7th–9th months	No care	
All Races [1]	3 863 502	3 189 794	2 475 340	714 454	469 649	134 057	94 601	39 456	70 002
No visits	39 537	X	X	X	X	39 456	X	39 456	81
1–2 visits	37 687	10 642	7 193	3 449	8 987	16 836	16 836	X	1 222
3–4 visits	76 376	24 488	14 677	9 811	26 761	23 485	23 485	X	1 642
5–6 visits	168 879	75 954	45 404	30 550	67 135	23 319	23 319	X	2 471
7–8 visits	321 019	202 657	127 146	75 511	101 612	13 504	13 504	X	3 246
9–10 visits	767 280	622 517	430 248	192 269	130 441	8 130	8 130	X	6 192
11–12 visits	1 027 397	943 826	733 402	210 424	75 703	3 470	3 470	X	4 398
13–14 visits	640 635	609 678	507 357	102 321	26 999	1 576	1 576	X	2 382
15–16 visits	453 807	434 410	379 868	54 542	16 884	1 138	1 138	X	1 375
17–18 visits	98 043	93 962	81 341	12 621	3 367	296	296	X	418
19 visits or more	139 116	132 828	118 201	14 627	5 233	437	437	X	618
Not stated	93 726	38 832	30 503	8 329	6 527	2 410	2 410	X	45 957
Median number of visits	12.3	12.6	12.8	11.5	9.6	5.5	5.5	X	10.3
White Total [2]	3 040 873	2 562 458	2 001 335	561 123	336 407	91 183	65 011	26 172	50 825
No visits	26 242	X	X	X	X	26 172	X	26 172	70
1–2 visits	24 920	7 418	5 110	2 308	5 614	11 031	11 031	X	857
3–4 visits	50 620	16 595	10 083	6 512	17 072	15 778	15 778	X	1 175
5–6 visits	117 974	54 079	32 260	21 819	45 963	16 173	16 173	X	1 759
7–8 visits	239 346	154 402	97 266	57 136	72 903	9 546	9 546	X	2 495
9–10 visits	594 969	490 312	340 664	149 648	94 878	5 811	5 811	X	3 968
11–12 visits	832 463	769 803	600 818	168 985	56 462	2 604	2 604	X	3 594
13–14 visits	526 824	503 244	419 726	83 518	20 419	1 188	1 188	X	1 973
15–16 visits	367 482	353 012	309 187	43 825	12 505	818	818	X	1 147
17–18 visits	79 797	76 824	66 915	9 909	2 416	221	221	X	336
19 visits or more	111 978	107 482	96 135	11 347	3 681	317	317	X	498
Not stated	68 258	29 287	23 171	6 116	4 494	1 524	1 524	X	32 953
Median number of visits	12.3	12.6	12.8	11.6	9.7	5.6	5.6	X	10.5
Non-Hispanic White	2 158 797	1 892 768	1 501 689	391 079	189 306	45 721	33 333	12 388	31 002
No visits	12 449	X	X	X	X	12 388	X	12 388	61
1–2 visits	12 474	3 898	2 772	1 126	2 679	5 407	5 407	X	490
3–4 visits	26 664	9 845	6 145	3 700	8 570	7 597	7 597	X	652
5–6 visits	67 295	34 393	21 438	12 955	23 704	8 086	8 086	X	1 112
7–8 visits	151 199	104 571	67 779	36 792	39 918	5 081	5 081	X	1 629
9–10 visits	406 077	346 412	245 705	100 707	53 617	3 251	3 251	X	2 797
11–12 visits	627 661	588 479	464 577	123 902	34 862	1 596	1 596	X	2 724
13–14 visits	402 527	387 025	324 008	63 017	13 209	731	731	X	1 562
15–16 visits	267 029	258 718	228 341	30 377	6 974	450	450	X	887
17–18 visits	62 221	60 218	52 488	7 730	1 618	120	120	X	265
19 visits or more	86 458	83 593	75 594	7 999	2 298	201	201	X	366
Not stated	36 743	15 616	12 842	2 774	1 857	813	813	X	18 457
Median number of visits	12.5	12.6	12.8	11.9	9.9	5.8	5.8	X	10.8
Black Total [2]	573 776	425 303	318 287	107 016	101 347	33 528	22 089	11 439	13 598
No visits	11 447	X	X	X	X	11 439	X	11 439	8
1–2 visits	10 054	2 507	1 584	923	2 774	4 486	4 486	X	287
3–4 visits	20 020	6 183	3 593	2 590	7 578	5 919	5 919	X	340
5–6 visits	37 971	15 983	9 640	6 343	16 076	5 370	5 370	X	542
7–8 visits	57 620	32 639	19 993	12 646	21 569	2 883	2 883	X	529
9–10 visits	120 374	90 069	60 430	29 639	26 782	1 679	1 679	X	1 844
11–12 visits	126 893	111 531	83 781	27 750	14 315	546	546	X	501
13–14 visits	76 350	70 948	58 028	12 920	4 912	228	228	X	262
15–16 visits	60 834	56 904	49 134	7 770	3 560	210	210	X	160
17–18 visits	12 817	11 958	9 908	2 050	756	51	51	X	52
19 visits or more	20 370	18 895	16 318	2 577	1 285	92	92	X	98
Not stated	19 026	7 686	5 878	1 808	1 740	625	625	X	8 975
Median number of visits	11.7	12.4	12.6	11.0	9.2	5.1	5.1	X	10.1
Non-Hispanic Black	553 987	411 013	307 917	103 096	97 826	32 406	21 258	11 148	12 742
No visits	11 156	X	X	X	X	11 148	X	11 148	8
1–2 visits	9 745	2 427	1 541	886	2 697	4 342	4 342	X	279
3–4 visits	19 441	6 019	3 492	2 527	7 369	5 731	5 731	X	322
5–6 visits	36 638	15 427	9 301	6 126	15 538	5 157	5 157	X	516
7–8 visits	55 410	31 403	19 266	12 137	20 745	2 754	2 754	X	508
9–10 visits	115 300	86 443	58 007	28 436	25 743	1 605	1 605	X	1 509
11–12 visits	122 353	107 542	80 807	26 735	13 824	519	519	X	468
13–14 visits	73 892	68 710	56 272	12 438	4 729	212	212	X	241
15–16 visits	59 256	55 431	47 899	7 532	3 481	197	197	X	147
17–18 visits	12 506	11 670	9 662	2 008	741	45	45	X	50
19 visits or more	19 934	18 492	15 968	2 524	1 261	89	89	X	92
Not stated	18 356	7 449	5 702	1 747	1 698	607	607	X	8 602
Median number of visits	11.7	12.4	12.6	11.1	9.2	5.1	5.1	X	10.0
Hispanic [3]	888 177	673 271	501 115	172 156	150 083	45 894	32 179	13 715	18 929
No visits	13 722	X	X	X	X	13 715	0	13 715	7
1–2 visits	12 659	3 573	2 363	1 210	2 992	5 727	5 727	X	367
3–4 visits	24 428	6 838	3 984	2 854	8 705	8 368	8 368	X	517
5–6 visits	51 848	20 127	11 068	9 059	22 778	8 292	8 292	X	651
7–8 visits	89 820	50 603	29 921	20 682	33 781	4 572	4 572	X	864
9–10 visits	192 173	145 849	96 151	49 698	42 266	2 597	2 597	X	1 461
11–12 visits	205 724	181 967	136 392	45 575	21 903	989	989	X	865
13–14 visits	124 882	116 700	95 969	20 731	7 320	443	443	X	419
15–16 visits	100 162	94 047	80 550	13 497	5 511	334	334	X	270
17–18 visits	17 489	16 537	14 353	2 184	804	76	76	X	72
19 visits or more	25 109	23 479	20 155	3 324	1 398	96	96	X	136
Not stated	30 161	13 551	10 209	3 342	2 625	685	685	X	13 300
Median number of visits	11.8	12.4	12.7	11.1	9.4	5.4	5.4	X	9.9

Note: Excludes data for Pennsylvania and Washington State, which implemented a forthcoming revision in the standard birth certificate and thus impaired comparability with the data from other states.

[1] Includes races other than White and Black and origin not stated.
[2] Race and Hispanic origin are reported separately on the birth certificate. Data for persons of Hispanic origin are included in the data for each race group according to the mother's reported race.
[3] May be of any race.
X = Not applicable.

TABLE I-35A. ADEQUACY OF PRENATAL CARE UTILIZATION INDEX, BY RACE AND HISPANIC ORIGIN OF MOTHER: UNITED STATES EXCLUDING PENNSYLVANIA AND WASHINGTON STATE, 2003

The Adequacy of Prenatal Care Utilization Index (APNCU) is a measure based on recommendations from the American College of Obstetricians and Gynecologists. The APNCU incorporates the month in which prenatal care began, the number of prenatal visits by the mother, and the mother's gestational age. It categorizes prenatal care utilization as follows: intensive, adequate, intermediate, and inadequate. According to the APNCU, about one-third (32.5 percent) of all women had intensive utilization of prenatal care in 2003, or more than the recommended amount of care. Eleven percent of mothers received inadequate care. This compares with levels of 25 and 18 percent, respectively, in 1990 (data not shown). Wide differences in utilization by race and Hispanic origin were also observed in the APNCU. In 2003, 7 percent of non-Hispanic White mothers received inadequate care, compared with between 16 and 17 percent of Hispanic and non-Hispanic Black women.

TABLE I-36. LIVE BIRTHS TO MOTHERS WITH SELECTED OBSTETRIC PROCEDURES AND RATES, BY AGE AND RACE OF MOTHER, 2003

Electronic fetal monitoring was the most frequently used obstetric procedure in 2003, despite being somewhat controversial; for both Whites and Blacks, electronic fetal monitoring was used in 86 percent of pregnancies. The use of ultrasound averaged 67 percent and was somewhat more frequently used by Whites than Blacks. Induction of labor was applied in 22 percent of White pregnancies, compared to 17 percent of Black pregnancies. These rates have more than doubled since 1990, when they averaged 9.5 percent. A study of variation in labor induction rates among hospitals and clinicians suggested that 25 percent of inductions had no apparent medical indication. (Glantz, J.C. 2003. Labor induction rate variation in upstate New York: What is the difference? *Birth* 30 (3): 168-74)

Amniocentesis can uncover birth defects that are more prevalent in older mothers. Testing rises sharply in the 35- to 39-year-old age bracket and again for mothers between 40 and 54 years of age, especially for White mothers in this group. However, the rate for amniocentesis has declined considerably since 1989, as noninvasive

Table I-35A. Adequacy of Prenatal Care Utilization Index, by Race and Hispanic Origin of Mother: United States Excluding Pennsylvania and Washington State, 2003

(Percent.)

All races and Hispanic origin	Intensive use	Adequate	Intermediate	Inadequate
Total	32.5	42.9	13.6	11.0
Non-Hispanic White	34.0	46.0	12.7	7.2
Non-Hispanic Black	33.3	35.7	13.6	17.4
Hispanic [1]	29.3	39.2	15.5	16.0

Note: Excludes data for Pennsylvania and Washington State, which implemented a forthcoming revision in the standard birth certificate and thus impaired comparability with the data from other states.

[1]May be of any race.

Table I-36. Live Births to Mothers with Selected Obstetric Procedures and Rates, by Age and Race of Mother, 2003

(Number, rate of live births with specified procedure per 1,000 live births in specified group.)

Obstetric procedure and race of mother	All births [1]	Obstetric procedure reported	Rate by age of mother							Not stated [2]
			All ages	Under 20 years	20–24 years	25–29 years	30–34 years	35–39 years	40–54 years	
All Races [3]										
Amniocentesis	3 863 502	66 901	17.4	4.8	5.8	7.7	13.2	66.8	101.3	12 272
Electronic fetal monitoring	3 863 502	3 289 703	854.2	866.6	862.5	856.6	848.0	837.8	825.6	12 272
Induction of labor	4 089 950	840 137	206.0	203.2	210.2	213.9	203.7	190.7	184.4	12 294
Stimulation of labor	3 863 502	645 075	167.5	186.9	175.5	170.6	160.9	146.2	132.6	12 272
Tocolysis	4 089 950	85 961	21.1	23.7	22.7	21.0	19.7	18.7	19.0	12 348
Ultrasound	3 863 502	2 592 258	673.1	639.6	658.2	676.2	689.2	693.2	686.2	12 272
White										
Amniocentesis	3 040 873	54 686	18.0	5.0	5.9	7.7	13.3	68.4	105.8	10 235
Electronic fetal monitoring	3 040 873	2 591 505	855.1	865.3	862.7	858.1	850.6	839.9	826.6	10 235
Induction of labor	3 225 848	696 703	216.6	213.8	222.2	224.9	213.7	199.7	192.6	9 491
Stimulation of labor	3 040 873	512 549	169.1	191.0	178.8	171.6	161.9	148.2	134.0	10 235
Tocolysis	3 225 848	68 200	21.2	24.2	22.9	21.3	19.8	18.6	18.8	9 538
Ultrasound	3 040 873	2 069 050	682.7	652.8	670.5	684.2	695.7	699.9	692.2	10 235
Black										
Amniocentesis	573 776	6 092	10.6	4.1	5.5	7.1	11.0	40.8	62.3	1 248
Electronic fetal monitoring	573 776	493 605	862.1	874.6	868.1	860.1	853.4	842.3	836.5	1 248
Induction of labor	599 847	104 123	174.0	180.1	174.3	176.4	171.1	161.8	162.4	1 382
Stimulation of labor	573 776	89 024	155.5	175.7	162.7	154.8	141.2	124.9	117.5	1 248
Tocolysis	599 847	12 651	21.1	21.2	21.5	20.7	21.4	20.7	19.8	1 377
Ultrasound	573 776	355 001	620.1	602.2	610.7	625.6	635.5	642.5	641.8	1 248

[1]Total number of births to residents of areas reporting specified obstetric procedures.
[2]No response reported for the obstetric procedures item.
[3]Includes races other than White and Black.

screening tests, such as ultrasound and measurement of serum markers, have found increasing popularity.

The frequency of most obstetric procedures, other than amniocentesis, does not change substantially as the age of the mother increases. However, induction of labor, stimulation of labor, and tocolysis (medications to avoid early contractions and pre-term birth) show declines as the age of the mother advances. (See also notes to Table I-27 and I-28 for racial and ethnic data.)

TABLE I-37. LIVE BIRTHS TO MOTHERS WITH SELECTED COMPLICATIONS OF LABOR AND/OR DELIVERY AND RATES, BY AGE AND RACE OF MOTHER, 2003

Depending on the severity of the condition, certain complications of labor and delivery may affect the health outcome of the infant. Many of these conditions are more common when the infant has low birthweight. The five most frequently reported complications of labor in 2003 were meconium (5 percent), breech/malpresentation (4 percent), fetal distress (4 percent), dysfunctional labor (3 percent), and premature rupture of membrane (2 percent). Some of these complications had above-average occurences in mothers under 20 years of age, but some complication rates increased substantially after age 35. These were breech/malpresentation, dysfunctional labor, fetal distress, and premature rupture of membrane. The highest percentage (6 percent) applied to breech/malpresentation for mothers over 40 years old. Complication rates vary between White and Black mothers, with meconium and fetal distress occurring somewhat more frequently in Blacks and breech/malpresentation and cephalopelvic disproportion occurring more commonly in Whites.

Cord and placental complications are quite infrequent, but they are among the top 10 causes of infant death.

Table I-37. Live Births to Mothers with Selected Complications of Labor and/or Delivery and Rates, by Age and Race of Mother, 2003

(Number, rate of live births with specified complication per 1,000 live births in specified group.)

Complication and race of mother	All births [1]	Complication reported	Rate by age of mother							Not stated [2]
			All ages	Under 20 years	20–24 years	25–29 years	30–34 years	35–39 years	40–54 years	
All Races [3]										
Febrile [4]	3 863 502	59 787	15.5	20.5	16.2	15.6	14.7	12.3	10.6	15 296
Meconium, moderate/heavy	4 089 950	197 865	48.6	55.2	49.7	47.7	46.3	46.9	47.4	15 320
Premature rupture of membrane [4]	3 863 502	83 103	21.6	22.3	20.5	20.6	22.1	23.2	27.0	15 296
Abruptio placenta [4]	3 863 502	20 386	5.3	5.2	5.1	4.8	5.4	6.2	8.0	15 296
Placenta previa [4]	3 863 502	12 953	3.4	1.1	1.8	2.8	4.5	6.5	9.2	15 296
Other excessive bleeding [4]	3 863 502	22 787	5.9	5.8	5.6	5.7	6.0	6.6	8.4	15 296
Seizures during labor [4]	3 863 502	1 304	0.3	0.8	0.4	0.3	0.2	0.3	0.2	15 296
Precipitous labor	4 089 950	74 807	18.4	12.8	17.5	18.3	19.9	21.5	21.3	15 471
Prolonged labor [4]	3 863 502	26 130	6.8	7.8	6.7	6.7	6.7	6.3	7.1	15 296
Dysfunctional labor [4]	3 863 502	109 836	28.5	29.8	27.3	27.9	28.8	30.2	32.8	15 296
Breech/malpresentation	4 089 950	156 804	38.5	27.8	30.7	37.5	44.5	51.0	58.8	15 296
Cephalopelvic disproportion [4]	3 863 502	56 111	14.6	15.9	13.8	14.5	15.0	14.3	15.0	19 563
Cord prolapse [4]	3 863 502	6 385	1.7	1.3	1.6	1.6	1.7	2.0	2.2	15 296
Anesthetic complication [4,5]	3 486 026	2 415	0.7	0.5	0.6	0.7	0.8	0.9	1.0	15 253
Fetal distress [4,5]	3 486 026	132 377	38.1	44.1	37.8	36.2	36.8	39.0	45.8	15 253
White										
Febrile [4]	3 040 873	45 331	15.0	20.1	16.1	15.1	13.8	11.7	10.0	12 584
Meconium, moderate/heavy	3 225 848	146 301	45.5	51.2	46.6	44.7	43.7	44.4	45.2	11 842
Premature rupture of membrane [4]	3 040 873	62 759	20.7	20.9	19.4	20.0	21.4	22.4	26.5	12 584
Abruptio placenta [4]	3 040 873	15 392	5.1	4.9	4.8	4.6	5.2	5.9	8.0	12 584
Placenta previa [4]	3 040 873	10 072	3.3	1.1	1.7	2.8	4.4	6.1	8.6	12 584
Other excessive bleeding [4]	3 040 873	17 939	5.9	6.1	5.7	5.7	5.9	6.4	8.1	12 584
Seizures during labor [4]	3 040 873	938	0.3	0.7	0.3	0.2	0.2	0.3	0.3	12 584
Precipitous labor	3 225 848	57 757	18.0	11.8	16.6	17.8	19.8	21.6	21.7	11 960
Prolonged labor [4]	3 040 873	20 972	6.9	8.1	7.0	6.8	6.7	6.3	7.4	12 584
Dysfunctional labor [4]	3 040 873	85 039	28.1	29.6	27.2	27.4	28.0	29.5	32.2	12 584
Breech/malpresentation	3 225 848	127 933	39.8	29.3	31.7	38.5	45.7	51.8	59.4	15 418
Cephalopelvic disproportion [4]	3 040 873	45 314	15.0	16.6	14.6	14.9	15.0	14.3	15.1	12 584
Cord prolapse [4]	3 040 873	4 881	1.6	1.2	1.5	1.6	1.7	2.0	2.2	12 584
Anesthetic complication [4,5]	2 719 331	1 937	0.7	0.5	0.6	0.7	0.8	1.0	0.9	12 553
Fetal distress [4,5]	2 719 331	98 501	36.4	42.0	36.1	34.6	35.3	37.3	44.4	12 553
Black										
Febrile [4]	573 776	8 666	15.1	21.6	15.4	13.2	13.0	11.8	8.7	1 669
Meconium, moderate/heavy	599 847	38 349	64.1	67.5	61.7	63.1	66.2	65.7	63.7	1 803
Premature rupture of membrane [4]	573 776	14 401	25.2	25.1	24.0	23.5	27.1	29.8	30.3	1 669
Abruptio placenta [4]	573 776	3 892	6.8	6.3	6.3	6.3	7.7	9.8	9.7	1 669
Placenta previa [4]	573 776	1 680	2.9	1.1	1.7	2.9	4.4	7.4	9.0	1 669
Other excessive bleeding [4]	573 776	2 657	4.6	3.9	4.0	4.6	5.4	6.5	8.0	1 669
Seizures during labor [4]	573 776	288	0.5	0.9	0.5	0.3	0.3	0.5	*	1 669
Precipitous labor [4]	599 847	11 818	19.8	14.6	20.0	21.5	21.7	20.8	20.2	1 815
Prolonged labor [4]	573 776	3 006	5.3	6.2	5.1	4.8	5.5	4.9	5.1	1 669
Dysfunctional labor	573 776	16 027	28.0	29.5	26.4	27.0	29.3	31.4	29.8	1 669
Breech/malpresentation	599 847	19 075	31.9	23.2	26.7	32.6	39.4	48.0	54.3	1 987
Cephalopelvic disproportion [4]	573 776	6 074	10.6	13.7	10.2	9.4	10.4	9.4	11.2	1 669
Cord prolapse [4]	573 776	1 119	2.0	1.7	1.7	2.0	2.3	2.5	2.4	1 669
Anesthetic complication [4,5]	531 891	312	0.6	0.5	0.5	0.6	0.7	0.6	*	1 660
Fetal distress [4,5]	531 891	25 049	47.2	50.8	45.0	44.6	48.1	51.5	58.7	1 660

[1] Total number of births to residents of areas reporting specified complication.
[2] No response reported for the complications item.
[3] Includes races other than White and Black.
[4] Excludes data for Pennsylvania and Washington State, which implemented the 2003 Revision to the U.S. Standard Certificate of Live Birth for data year 2003.
[5] Texas does not report this complication.
* = Figure does not meet standards of reliability or precision; based on fewer than 20 births in numerator.

TABLE I-38. LIVE BIRTHS, BY ATTENDANT, PLACE OF DELIVERY, AND RACE AND HISPANIC ORIGIN OF MOTHER, 2003

The share of births delivered by physicians in hospitals declined from 98.7 percent in 1975 to 91.2 percent in 2003. This reflected an increase in births attended by midwives, the number of which increased from 1.0 percent to 8.0 percent over the same period. (Midwife-attended births are in fact underreported, so these are considered low estimates.) The vast majority of midwives were certified nurse midwives who generally used a hos-

pital as the place of delivery. Less than 1 percent of all births took place outside a hospital and occurred either in the mother's residence (23,000) or in a freestanding birthing center (almost 10,000).

Hispanic women were more likely to have a midwife-attended hospital birth in 2003 (9.1 percent) than non-Hispanic White and Black women (6.8 and 7.0 percent, respectively). Among Hispanic subgroups, the lowest rate of midwife attendance was among Cuban women (4 percent, data not shown).

Table I-38. Live Births, by Attendant, Place of Delivery, and Race and Hispanic Origin of Mother, 2003

(Number.)

Place of delivery and race and Hispanic origin of mother	All births	Physician			Midwife			Other	Unspecified
		Total	Doctor of medicine	Doctor of osteopathy	Total	Certified nurse midwife	Other midwife		
All Races [1]									
Total	4 089 950	3 733 750	3 554 819	178 931	328 153	310 342	17 811	20 599	7 448
In hospital [2]	4 053 987	3 730 008	3 551 650	178 358	305 513	300 931	4 582	11 535	6 931
Not in hospital	35 723	3 622	3 049	573	22 588	9 362	13 226	9 015	498
Freestanding birthing center	9 779	923	611	312	8 664	5 828	2 836	185	7
Clinic or doctor's office	397	225	196	29	108	57	51	62	2
Residence	23 221	1 813	1 613	200	13 403	3 272	10 131	7 631	374
Other	2 326	661	629	32	413	205	208	1 137	115
Not specified	240	120	120	-	52	49	3	49	19
White Total [3]									
Total	3 225 848	2 940 517	2 787 768	152 749	262 462	246 108	16 354	16 513	6 356
In hospital [2]	3 193 825	2 937 737	2 785 519	152 218	241 079	237 436	3 643	9 034	5 975
Not in hospital	31 829	2 681	2 150	531	21 335	8 626	12 709	7 445	368
Freestanding birthing center	9 096	908	597	311	8 021	5 337	2 684	160	7
Clinic or doctor's office	334	191	167	24	96	51	45	46	1
Residence	20 698	1 193	1 018	175	12 860	3 082	9 778	6 356	289
Other	1 701	389	368	21	358	156	202	883	71
Not specified	194	99	99	-	48	46	2	34	13
Non-Hispanic White									
Total	2 321 904	2 126 099	2 005 392	120 707	177 765	163 709	14 056	12 336	5 704
In hospital [2]	2 293 934	2 123 733	2 003 534	120 199	158 723	156 009	2 714	6 013	5 465
Not in hospital	27 836	2 294	1 786	508	19 008	7 668	11 340	6 299	235
Freestanding birthing center	7 723	880	572	308	6 697	4 607	2 090	139	7
Clinic or doctor's office	289	168	145	23	82	44	38	38	1
Residence	18 556	981	817	164	11 917	2 897	9 020	5 455	203
Other	1 268	265	252	13	312	120	192	667	24
Not specified	134	72	72	-	34	32	2	24	4
Black Total [3]									
Total	599 847	552 884	534 344	18 540	43 433	42 539	894	2 726	804
In hospital [2]	597 024	552 099	533 587	18 512	42 708	42 063	645	1 502	715
Not in hospital	2 788	769	741	28	723	474	249	1 212	84
Freestanding birthing center	430	6	5	1	406	316	90	18	-
Clinic or doctor's office	18	11	10	1	5	3	2	2	-
Residence	1 883	533	515	18	280	125	155	1 016	54
Other	457	219	211	8	32	30	2	176	30
Not specified	35	16	16	-	2	2	-	12	5
Non-Hispanic Black									
Total	576 033	531 655	513 916	17 739	41 055	40 226	829	2 609	714
In hospital [2]	573 941	530 913	513 201	17 712	40 376	39 783	593	1 427	631
Not in hospital	2 661	729	702	27	678	442	236	1 175	79
Freestanding birthing center	408	5	4	1	386	299	87	17	-
Clinic or doctor's office	17	10	10	-	5	3	2	2	-
Residence	1 803	503	485	18	257	112	145	993	50
Other	433	211	203	8	30	28	2	163	29
Not specified	25	13	13	-	1	1	-	7	4
Hispanic [4]									
Total	912 329	822 611	790 349	32 262	85 070	82 968	2 102	3 975	673
In hospital [2]	908 745	822 205	789 967	32 238	82 940	82 078	862	3 032	568
Not in hospital	3 549	390	366	24	2 116	876	1 240	939	104
Freestanding birthing center	1 341	29	26	3	1 291	692	599	21	-
Clinic or doctor's office	40	19	17	2	12	4	8	9	-
Residence	1 753	216	205	11	771	143	628	696	70
Other	415	126	118	8	42	37	5	213	34
Not specified	35	16	16	-	14	14	-	4	1

[1]Includes races other than White and Black and origin not stated.
[2]Includes births occurring en route to or on arrival at hospital.
[3]Race and Hispanic origin are reported separately on the birth certificate. Data for persons of Hispanic origin are included in the data for each race group according to the mother's reported race.
[4]May be of any race.
- = Quantity zero.

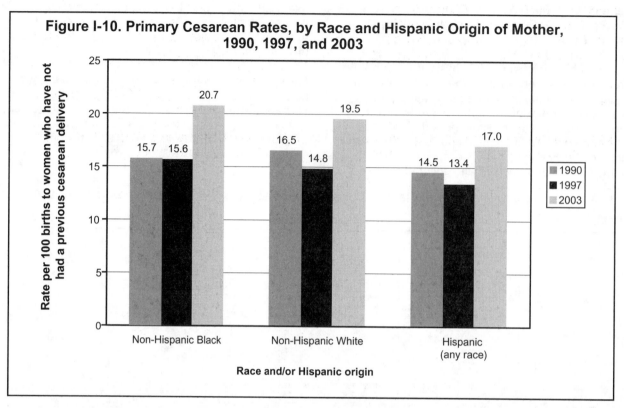

Figure I-10. Primary Cesarean Rates, by Race and Hispanic Origin of Mother, 1990, 1997, and 2003

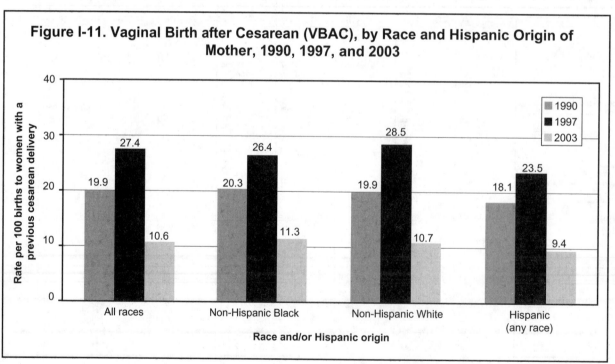

Figure I-11. Vaginal Birth after Cesarean (VBAC), by Race and Hispanic Origin of Mother, 1990, 1997, and 2003

TABLE I-39. LIVE BIRTHS BY METHOD OF DELIVERY AND RATES OF CESAREAN DELIVERY AND VAGINAL BIRTH AFTER PREVIOUS CESAREAN DELIVERY, BY RACE AND HISPANIC ORIGIN OF MOTHER, 1989–2003

The rate of cesarean delivery has risen every year since 1996, reaching a new high of 27.5 percent of all births in 2003. The continuing increases in the cesarean rate may be associated with nonclinical factors, such as physician practice patterns and maternal choice. (See: Minkoff, H., et al. 2004. Ethical dimensions of elective primary cesarean delivery. *Obstet Gynecol* 103(2): 387-92. 2004. See also: Zinberg, S. 2001. Vaginal delivery after previous cesarean delivery: A continuing controversy. *Clin Obstet Gynecol* 44(3): 561-9.)

Table I-39. Live Births by Method of Delivery and Rates of Cesarean Delivery and Vaginal Birth after Previous Cesarean Delivery, by Race and Hispanic Origin of Mother, 1989–2003

(Number, percent.)

| Year and race and Hispanic origin of mother | Births by method of delivery | | | | | | | Cesarean delivery rate | | Rate of vaginal birth after previous cesarean [5] |
| | All births | Vaginal | | Cesarean | | | Not stated | Total [3] | Primary [4] | |
		Total [1]	After previous cesarean	Total [2]	Primary	Repeat				
All Races[6]										
2003	4 089 950	2 949 853	51 602	1 119 388	684 484	434 699	20 709	27.5	19.1	10.6
2002	4 021 726	2 958 423	59 248	1 043 846	634 426	409 420	19 457	26.1	18.0	12.6
2001	4 025 933	3 027 993	74 048	978 411	601 383	377 028	19 529	24.4	16.9	16.4
2000	4 058 814	3 108 188	89 978	923 991	577 638	346 353	26 635	22.9	16.1	20.6
1999	3 959 417	3 063 870	97 680	862 086	542 080	320 006	33 461	22.0	15.5	23.4
1998	3 941 553	3 078 537	108 903	825 870	519 975	305 895	37 146	21.2	14.9	26.3
1997	3 880 894	3 046 621	112 145	799 033	502 526	296 507	35 240	20.8	14.6	27.4
1996	3 891 494	3 061 092	116 045	797 119	503 724	293 395	33 283	20.7	14.6	28.3
1995	3 899 589	3 063 724	112 439	806 722	510 104	296 618	29 143	20.8	14.7	27.5
1994	3 952 767	3 087 576	110 341	830 517	520 647	309 870	34 674	21.2	14.9	26.3
1993	4 000 240	3 098 796	103 581	861 987	539 251	322 736	39 457	21.8	15.3	24.3
1992	4 065 014	3 100 710	97 549	888 622	554 662	333 960	75 682	22.3	15.6	22.6
1991	4 110 907	3 100 891	90 690	905 077	569 195	335 882	104 939	22.6	15.9	21.3
1990 [7]	4 110 563	3 111 421	84 299	914 096	575 066	339 030	85 046	22.7	16.0	19.9
1989 [8]	3 798 734	2 793 463	71 019	826 955	521 873	305 082	178 316	22.8	16.1	18.9
White Total [9]										
2003	3 225 848	2 332 605	39 696	876 595	531 486	344 954	16 648	27.3	18.8	10.3
2002	3 174 760	2 340 512	46 004	818 347	493 002	325 345	15 901	25.9	17.7	12.4
2001	3 177 626	2 394 930	58 053	766 771	467 285	299 486	15 925	24.3	16.7	16.2
2000	3 194 005	2 449 264	70 414	723 209	449 161	274 048	21 532	22.8	15.9	20.4
1999	3 132 501	2 426 092	77 158	678 952	424 148	254 804	27 457	21.9	15.3	23.2
1998	3 118 727	2 440 113	86 495	649 987	406 439	243 548	28 627	21.0	14.7	26.2
1997	3 072 640	2 415 236	89 522	630 613	393 603	237 010	26 791	20.7	14.5	27.4
1996	3 093 057	2 434 079	93 783	631 409	395 851	235 558	27 569	20.6	14.5	28.5
1995	3 098 885	2 435 191	90 940	639 818	401 098	238 720	23 876	20.8	14.6	27.6
1994	3 121 004	2 435 965	88 471	656 400	407 946	248 454	28 639	21.2	14.8	26.3
1993	3 149 833	2 435 229	82 995	682 355	423 540	258 815	32 249	21.9	15.3	24.3
1992	3 201 678	2 434 959	77 977	705 841	437 398	268 443	60 878	22.5	15.7	22.5
1991	3 241 273	2 434 900	72 564	723 088	452 534	270 554	83 285	22.9	16.1	21.1
1990 [7]	3 252 473	2 453 857	67 191	732 713	458 656	274 057	65 903	23.0	16.1	19.7
1989 [8]	3 022 537	2 212 843	56 851	667 114	418 177	248 937	142 580	23.2	16.2	18.6
Non-Hispanic White										
2003	2 321 904	1 671 414	28 751	637 482	398 368	238 990	13 008	27.6	19.5	10.7
2002	2 298 156	1 687 144	33 440	598 682	370 339	228 343	12 330	26.2	18.3	12.8
2001	2 326 578	1 746 551	43 215	567 488	353 977	213 511	12 539	24.5	17.2	16.8
2000	2 362 968	1 804 550	52 912	540 794	342 732	198 062	17 624	23.1	16.4	21.1
1999	2 346 450	1 810 682	59 480	514 051	327 106	186 945	21 717	22.1	15.7	24.1
1998	2 361 462	1 842 420	67 787	495 550	315 138	180 412	23 492	21.2	15.1	27.3
1997	2 333 363	1 829 213	70 284	481 982	305 605	176 377	22 168	20.9	14.8	28.5
1996	2 358 989	1 851 058	73 973	485 530	308 482	177 048	22 401	20.8	14.8	29.5
1995	2 382 638	1 867 024	72 124	496 103	313 933	182 170	19 511	21.0	14.9	28.4
1994	2 438 855	1 896 609	71 597	518 021	324 236	193 785	24 225	21.5	15.1	27.0
1993	2 472 031	1 902 433	67 536	542 013	338 236	203 777	27 585	22.2	15.6	24.9
1992 [10]	2 527 207	1 916 414	63 828	566 788	352 470	214 318	44 005	22.8	16.0	22.9
1991 [10]	2 589 878	1 941 726	60 174	587 802	368 721	219 081	60 350	23.2	16.4	21.5
1990 [7,11]	2 626 500	1 972 754	55 952	603 467	378 508	224 959	50 279	23.4	16.5	19.9
1989 [8,11]	2 526 367	1 806 753	47 559	556 585	349 858	206 727	163 029	23.6	16.6	18.7

[1] For 2003, includes unknown type of vaginal delivery.
[2] For 2003, includes unknown type of cesarean delivery.
[3] Percent of all live births by cesarean delivery.
[4] Number of primary cesareans per 100 live births to women who have not had a previous cesarean.
[5] Number of vaginal births after previous cesarean delivery per 100 live births to women with a previous cesarean delivery.
[6] Includes races other than White and Black and origin not stated.
[7] Excludes data for Oklahoma, which did not report method of delivery on the birth certificate.
[8] Excludes data for Louisiana, Maryland, Nebraska, Nevada, and Oklahoma, which did not report method of delivery on the birth certificate.
[9] Race and Hispanic origin are reported separately on the birth certificate. Data for persons of Hispanic origin are included in the data for each race group according to the mother's reported race.
[10] Excludes data for New Hampshire, which did not report Hispanic origin.
[11] Excludes data for New Hampshire and Oklahoma, which did not report Hispanic origin.

The primary cesarean rate (the rate for mothers who did not have a previous cesarean) increased to 19.1 percent in 2003, 31 percent higher than in 1997. The rate of vaginal birth after previous cesarean delivery fell to 10.6 percent in 2003; it had reached a temporary high of 28.3 percent in 1996. The steep decline of vaginal births after a previous cesarean delivery implies a corresponding rise in the rate of repeat cesarean deliveries: the data indicate that once a woman has had a cesarean delivery, there is an almost 90 percent likelihood that subsequent deliveries will be through a cesarean section. These recent trends were shared by the major racial and ethnic groups.

Table I-39. Live Births by Method of Delivery and Rates of Cesarean Delivery and Vaginal Birth after Previous Cesarean Delivery, by Race and Hispanic Origin of Mother, 1989–2003—*Continued*

(Number, percent.)

Year and race and Hispanic origin of mother	All births	Births by method of delivery					Not stated	Cesarean delivery rate		Rate of vaginal birth after previous cesarean [5]
		Vaginal		Cesarean				Total [3]	Primary [4]	
		Total [1]	After previous cesarean	Total [2]	Primary	Repeat				
Black Total [9]										
2003	599 847	423 033	8 484	173 834	107 603	66 217	2 980	29.1	20.6	11.4
2002	593 691	427 801	9 567	163 295	100 621	62 674	2 595	27.6	19.4	13.2
2001	606 156	447 458	11 747	156 071	97 429	58 642	2 627	25.9	18.3	16.7
2000	622 598	468 497	14 382	150 401	94 767	55 634	3 700	24.3	17.3	20.5
1999	605 970	462 401	15 438	139 471	88 269	51 202	4 098	23.2	16.5	23.2
1998	609 902	470 088	17 062	135 727	86 438	49 289	4 087	22.4	16.0	25.7
1997	599 913	466 001	16 986	130 142	83 025	47 117	3 770	21.8	15.6	26.5
1996	594 781	462 378	16 866	128 357	82 646	45 711	4 046	21.7	15.6	27.0
1995	603 139	468 984	16 224	130 482	84 441	46 041	3 673	21.8	15.7	26.1
1994	636 391	493 879	16 970	138 067	88 636	49 431	4 445	21.8	15.7	25.6
1993	658 875	509 816	16 179	143 452	91 677	51 775	5 607	22.0	15.7	23.8
1992	673 633	514 929	15 382	146 480	93 165	53 315	12 224	22.1	15.7	22.4
1991	682 602	519 047	14 213	145 583	92 645	52 938	17 972	21.9	15.5	21.2
1990 [7]	679 236	516 581	13 496	146 472	93 476	52 996	16 183	22.1	15.7	20.3
1989 [8]	611 147	452 921	11 104	127 907	82 695	45 212	30 319	22.0	15.8	19.7
Non-Hispanic Black										
2003	576 033	405 671	8 109	167 506	103 694	63 802	2 856	29.2	20.7	11.3
2002	578 335	416 516	9 317	159 297	98 245	61 052	2 522	27.7	19.4	13.2
2001	589 917	435 455	11 417	151 908	94 912	56 996	2 554	25.9	18.3	16.7
2000	604 346	454 736	13 910	146 042	92 044	53 998	3 568	24.3	17.3	20.5
1999	588 981	449 580	14 999	135 508	85 898	49 610	3 893	23.2	16.5	23.2
1998	593 127	457 186	16 510	131 999	84 169	47 830	3 942	22.4	16.0	25.7
1997	581 431	451 744	16 353	126 138	80 599	45 539	3 549	21.8	15.6	26.4
1996	578 099	449 544	16 322	124 836	80 457	44 379	3 719	21.7	15.7	26.9
1995	587 781	457 104	15 721	127 171	82 395	44 776	3 506	21.8	15.7	26.0
1994	619 198	480 551	16 478	134 526	86 411	48 115	4 121	21.9	15.7	25.5
1993	641 273	496 333	15 675	139 702	89 315	50 387	5 238	22.0	15.7	23.7
1992 [10]	657 450	502 669	14 950	143 153	91 086	52 067	11 628	22.2	15.7	22.3
1991 [10]	666 758	507 522	13 847	142 417	90 664	51 753	16 819	21.9	15.5	21.1
1990 [7,11]	661 701	503 720	13 157	142 838	91 175	51 663	15 143	22.1	15.7	20.3
1989 [8,12]	611 269	440 310	10 726	125 290	81 177	44 113	45 669	22.2	15.9	19.6
Hispanic [13]										
2003	912 329	667 656	11 153	241 159	134 231	106 912	3 514	26.5	17.0	9.4
2002	876 642	653 516	12 610	219 777	122 603	97 174	3 349	25.2	16.1	11.5
2001	851 851	648 821	14 846	199 874	113 529	86 345	3 156	23.6	15.2	14.7
2000	815 868	633 220	17 062	179 583	104 597	74 986	3 065	22.1	14.5	18.5
1999	764 339	599 118	16 915	161 035	94 433	66 602	4 186	21.2	14.0	20.3
1998	734 661	580 143	17 803	150 317	88 763	61 554	4 201	20.6	13.6	22.4
1997	709 767	563 114	17 942	142 907	84 410	58 497	3 746	20.2	13.4	23.5
1996	701 339	558 105	18 491	139 554	83 392	56 162	3 680	20.0	13.4	24.8
1995	679 768	539 731	17 396	136 640	82 662	53 978	3 397	20.2	13.7	24.4
1994	665 026	525 928	16 206	135 569	81 961	53 608	3 529	20.5	13.9	23.2
1993	654 418	514 493	14 586	136 279	82 576	53 703	3 646	20.9	14.2	21.4
1992 [10]	643 271	494 338	13 111	133 369	81 211	52 158	15 564	21.2	14.4	20.1
1991 [10]	623 085	472 126	11 615	129 752	80 228	49 524	21 207	21.6	14.8	19.0
1990 [7,11]	595 073	458 242	10 395	122 969	76 027	46 942	13 862	21.2	14.5	18.1
1989 [8,12]	532 249	385 462	8 549	105 268	64 905	40 363	41 519	21.5	14.7	17.5

[1]For 2003, includes unknown type of vaginal delivery.
[2]For 2003, includes unknown type of cesarean delivery.
[3]Percent of all live births by cesarean delivery.
[4]Number of primary cesareans per 100 live births to women who have not had a previous cesarean.
[5]Number of vaginal births after previous cesarean delivery per 100 live births to women with a previous cesarean delivery.
[7]Excludes data for Oklahoma, which did not report method of delivery on the birth certificate.
[8]Excludes data for Louisiana, Maryland, Nebraska, Nevada, and Oklahoma, which did not report method of delivery on the birth certificate.
[9]Race and Hispanic origin are reported separately on the birth certificate. Data for persons of Hispanic origin are included in the data for each race group according to the mother's reported race.
[10]Excludes data for New Hampshire, which did not report Hispanic origin.
[11]Excludes data for New Hampshire and Oklahoma, which did not report Hispanic origin.
[12]Excludes data for Louisiana, New Hampshire, and Oklahoma, which did not report Hispanic origin.
[13]May be of any race.

TABLE I-40. LIVE BIRTHS BY METHOD OF DELIVERY AND RATES OF CESAREAN DELIVERY AND VAGINAL BIRTH AFTER PREVIOUS CESAREAN DELIVERY, BY AGE, RACE, AND HISPANIC ORIGIN OF MOTHER, 2003

As in past years, the rate of primary cesareans rose with advancing maternal age. The rate for women age 35–39 years was 24.2 percent in 2003, compared to an average of 19.1 percent for all ages. The primary cesarean rate for all mothers age 40 years and over was 30.4 percent (34.3 percent for non-Hispanic Blacks). The increased likelihood of cesareans for middle-aged mothers may be related to their high rate of multiple births, to increased concerns by patients or practitioners, and to biological factors.

The frequency of vaginal births after previous cesareans (VBAC) was not as strongly related to the age of the mother as primary cesareans. (This frequency compares vaginal births after previous cesareans to all births with previous cesarean deliveries.) Somewhat higher than average rates for VBAC were observed among mothers age 25–29 years. For Hispanics and non-Hispanic Blacks, mothers above 35 years of age had lower than average rates of VBAC, but non-Hispanic Whites had rates that were marginally higher than average.

Table I-40. Live Births by Method of Delivery and Rates of Cesarean Delivery and Vaginal Birth after Previous Cesarean Delivery, by Age, Race, and Hispanic Origin of Mother, 2003

(Number, percent.)

Age and race and Hispanic origin of mother	Births by method of delivery						Not stated	Cesarean delivery rate		Rate of vaginal birth after previous cesarean [3]
	All births	Vaginal		Cesarean				Total [1]	Primary [2]	
		Total	After previous cesarean	Total	Primary	Repeat				
All Races [4]	4 089 950	2 949 853	51 602	1 119 388	684 484	434 699	20 709	27.5	19.1	10.6
Under 20 years	421 241	339 393	1 171	80 182	70 150	10 030	1 666	19.1	17.2	10.5
20–24 years	1 032 305	795 078	9 003	232 579	154 407	78 157	4 648	22.6	16.4	10.3
25–29 years	1 086 366	795 736	14 123	285 231	172 845	112 353	5 399	26.4	18.1	11.2
30–34 years	975 546	665 025	16 004	305 102	170 728	134 296	5 419	31.4	20.8	10.6
35–39 years	467 642	293 643	9 194	171 142	90 685	80 403	2 857	36.8	24.2	10.3
40–54 years	106 850	60 978	2 107	45 152	25 669	19 460	720	42.5	30.4	9.8
White Total [5]	3 225 848	2 332 605	39 696	876 595	531 486	344 954	16 648	27.3	18.8	10.3
Under 20 years	302 024	244 706	708	56 101	49 264	6 835	1 217	18.7	16.8	9.4
20–24 years	790 910	612 917	6 360	174 405	116 293	58 102	3 588	22.2	16.1	9.9
25–29 years	871 496	640 765	10 764	226 343	136 887	89 434	4 388	26.1	17.8	10.7
30–34 years	795 902	544 355	12 646	247 011	136 885	110 068	4 536	31.2	20.5	10.3
35–39 years	379 773	240 412	7 495	137 017	71 959	65 015	2 344	36.3	23.6	10.3
40–54 years	85 743	49 450	1 723	35 718	20 198	15 500	575	41.9	29.7	10.0
Non-Hispanic White	2 321 904	1 671 414	28 751	637 482	398 368	238 990	13 008	27.6	19.5	10.7
Under 20 years	174 019	140 063	326	33 137	29 808	3 327	819	19.1	17.6	8.9
20–24 years	522 275	403 708	3 719	115 906	80 222	35 680	2 661	22.3	16.7	9.4
25–29 years	627 437	462 787	7 202	161 278	103 308	57 952	3 372	25.8	18.5	11.1
30–34 years	626 315	431 212	9 848	191 321	110 359	80 912	3 782	30.7	20.8	10.9
35–39 years	303 354	193 777	6 212	107 661	58 334	49 293	1 916	35.7	23.7	11.2
40–54 years	68 504	39 867	1 444	28 179	16 337	11 826	458	41.4	29.8	10.9
Black Total [5]	599 847	423 033	8 484	173 834	107 603	66 217	2 980	29.1	20.6	11.4
Under 20 years	103 677	81 467	430	21 813	18 862	2 951	397	21.1	18.9	12.7
20–24 years	196 268	145 662	2 217	49 712	31 975	17 733	894	25.4	18.2	11.1
25–29 years	139 947	98 252	2 502	40 995	23 174	17 817	700	29.4	19.5	12.3
30–34 years	97 529	62 270	2 077	34 694	19 106	15 583	565	35.8	24.1	11.8
35–39 years	49 889	28 710	1 019	20 839	11 154	9 684	340	42.1	28.7	9.5
40–54 years	12 537	6 672	239	5 781	3 332	2 449	84	46.4	34.1	8.9
Non-Hispanic Black	576 033	405 671	8 109	167 506	103 694	63 802	2 856	29.2	20.7	11.3
Under 20 years	100 151	78 599	414	21 165	18 288	2 877	387	21.2	19.0	12.6
20–24 years	189 020	140 017	2 129	48 132	30 843	17 287	871	25.6	18.3	11.0
25–29 years	133 821	93 804	2 383	39 351	22 249	17 098	666	29.6	19.6	12.2
30–34 years	93 346	59 483	1 987	33 324	18 381	14 940	539	35.9	24.2	11.7
35–39 years	47 661	27 374	966	19 972	10 716	9 255	315	42.2	28.9	9.5
40–54 years	12 034	6 394	230	5 562	3 217	2 345	78	46.5	34.3	8.9
Hispanic [6]	912 329	667 656	11 153	241 159	134 231	106 912	3 514	26.5	17.0	9.4
Under 20 years	130 880	106 994	394	23 487	19 916	3 571	399	18.0	15.7	9.9
20–24 years	273 311	212 886	2 728	59 513	36 802	22 707	912	21.8	14.9	10.7
25–29 years	246 361	179 603	3 650	65 781	33 872	31 907	977	26.8	16.1	10.3
30–34 years	169 054	112 629	2 835	55 702	26 397	29 300	723	33.1	19.4	8.8
35–39 years	75 801	46 157	1 272	29 246	13 467	15 775	398	38.8	23.1	7.5
40–54 years	16 922	9 387	274	7 430	3 777	3 652	105	44.2	29.3	7.0

[1]Percent of all live births by cesarean delivery.
[2]Number of primary cesareans per 100 live births to women who have not had a previous cesarean.
[3]Number of vaginal births after previous cesarean delivery per 100 live births to women with a previous cesarean delivery.
[4]Includes races other than White and Black and origin not stated.
[5]Race and Hispanic origin are reported separately on the birth certificate. Data for persons of Hispanic origin are included in the data for each race group according to the mother's reported race.
[6]May be of any race.

TABLE I-41. RATES OF CESAREAN DELIVERY AND VAGINAL BIRTH AFTER PREVIOUS CESAREAN DELIVERY, BY RACE AND HISPANIC ORIGIN OF MOTHER, FOR EACH STATE AND TERRITORY, 2003

Cesarean rates increased in all states from 2002 to 2003, as they had in the two previous years. Rates varied considerably by state in 2003, ranging from under 22 percent in New Mexico, Utah, Idaho, Alaska, and Wisconsin to over 30 percent in New Jersey, Mississippi, Louisiana, West Virginia, Florida, Texas, and Kentucky. Puerto Rico had an astounding cesarean delivery rate of 46.1 percent.

In contrast to the national average rate of 10.6 percent of vaginal births after previous cesarean delivery, Vermont, Utah, and Pennsylvania had frequencies above 20 percent in this category. Louisiana, Florida, and Mississippi reported rates of less than 6 percent for such vaginal births. Puerto Rico was an outlier again, with a rate of only 3.2 percent for vaginal births after previous cesarean.

Table I-41. Rates of Cesarean Delivery and Vaginal Birth after Previous Cesarean Delivery, by Race and Hispanic Origin of Mother, for Each State and Territory, 2003

(Percent.)

State	Cesarean delivery rate [1]						Rate of vaginal births after previous cesarean [2]					
	All races [3]	White		Black		Hispanic [5]	All races [3]	White		Black		Hispanic [5]
		Total [4]	Non-Hispanic	Total [4]	Non-Hispanic			Total [4]	Non-Hispanic	Total [4]	Non-Hispanic	
UNITED STATES [6]	27.5	27.3	27.6	29.1	29.2	26.5	10.6	10.3	10.7	11.4	11.3	9.4
Alabama	29.6	29.4	29.9	30.3	30.3	22.9	6.9	6.9	6.5	7.0	6.9	12.1
Alaska	21.4	24.3	23.9	27.0	29.2	22.0	16.5	11.1	10.5	*	*	*
Arizona	22.2	22.2	23.7	24.7	25.5	20.8	7.8	7.1	8.1	8.2	8.1	6.0
Arkansas	29.5	29.1	29.7	31.3	31.3	24.3	8.7	8.8	7.7	7.9	7.8	16.7
California	27.9	27.8	28.5	31.3	31.4	27.2	6.6	6.3	6.8	7.1	7.1	6.1
Colorado	22.2	22.1	22.9	24.4	24.4	20.6	14.9	14.3	13.6	25.6	25.5	15.5
Connecticut	27.2	27.3	28.1	27.9	28.2	24.0	11.2	10.7	10.6	13.0	13.5	10.5
Delaware	29.1	28.5	28.5	31.4	31.6	27.5	10.9	10.5	9.6	11.0	11.0	14.9
District of Columbia	27.4	28.9	29.2	26.8	28.2	20.2	10.3	12.1	*	10.1	9.5	*
Florida	30.8	31.0	29.8	30.2	30.1	33.3	5.7	5.4	6.2	6.4	6.5	4.1
Georgia	27.2	26.9	28.4	28.1	28.1	21.0	9.2	9.1	8.2	8.9	8.7	13.3
Hawaii	22.0	21.1	21.1	20.2	21.1	22.3	16.7	12.9	13.3	*	*	13.2
Idaho	21.1	21.1	21.0	*	*	21.6	14.1	14.3	13.6	*	*	17.6
Illinois	25.7	25.5	26.5	26.2	26.2	23.1	13.5	13.5	12.7	13.1	13.1	15.3
Indiana	25.6	25.5	25.5	26.2	26.3	25.3	10.2	10.1	9.9	11.0	10.9	12.8
Iowa	25.4	25.5	25.4	26.9	27.0	26.6	10.4	10.3	10.5	11.8	12.0	7.9
Kansas	26.5	26.6	26.9	27.2	27.2	25.1	9.0	8.7	8.6	8.9	9.1	9.3
Kentucky	30.1	30.2	30.3	29.4	29.4	27.7	6.6	6.4	6.0	8.6	8.6	14.5
Louisiana	31.7	32.8	32.8	30.3	30.3	33.0	5.1	3.9	3.9	6.8	6.8	*
Maine	26.3	26.3	26.3	25.1	26.1	30.7	8.2	7.9	8.1	*	*	*
Maryland	28.5	27.4	27.7	30.7	31.2	24.2	15.4	15.6	15.2	14.7	14.5	18.4
Massachusetts	29.2	29.4	30.0	29.6	30.4	25.8	12.6	12.3	12.1	14.0	15.8	12.7
Michigan	26.4	26.5	26.7	25.8	25.9	25.1	11.4	11.5	11.3	10.9	10.9	13.3
Minnesota	23.3	23.6	23.8	23.9	23.9	22.2	13.9	12.8	11.9	22.8	23.4	20.2
Mississippi	32.5	33.0	33.2	31.9	31.9	24.6	5.8	4.8	4.8	6.9	6.9	*
Missouri	27.3	27.4	27.6	26.5	26.5	23.9	11.2	10.7	10.5	14.2	14.4	13.7
Montana	23.6	23.2	23.1	*	*	24.3	15.8	17.2	17.2	*	*	*
Nebraska	27.7	27.9	28.2	25.4	25.2	26.6	8.6	8.3	7.8	13.0	12.7	11.7
Nevada	27.5	26.8	29.4	31.6	31.8	23.6	8.0	8.0	7.0	10.1	10.1	9.4
New Hampshire	26.5	26.2	26.4	33.3	35.3	25.5	11.2	11.2	11.1	*	*	*
New Jersey	33.1	33.0	33.6	34.4	34.2	31.8	14.3	13.7	13.7	16.5	17.9	12.9
New Mexico	20.3	20.9	21.8	21.1	21.0	20.4	18.7	17.1	17.8	*	*	16.5
New York	28.4	28.5	29.1	29.1	29.3	27.1	16.2	15.9	16.1	17.3	17.5	15.4
North Carolina	27.4	26.9	28.1	29.2	29.2	22.0	10.7	10.8	9.8	10.1	10.1	15.5
North Dakota	24.3	24.3	24.1	21.1	21.7	30.4	13.7	13.7	13.7	*	*	*
Ohio	25.1	24.9	25.0	25.7	25.7	23.1	14.6	13.9	13.9	17.7	17.8	15.8
Oklahoma	29.4	29.1	29.8	32.5	32.6	24.9	7.6	7.5	7.2	5.7	5.8	9.8
Oregon	24.9	24.6	25.1	30.3	30.1	22.8	13.6	13.7	12.1	*	*	19.6
Pennsylvania	26.1	26.2	26.3	25.9	26.4	24.6	20.4	19.3	19.4	26.4	26.2	18.3
Rhode Island	28.3	29.0	30.3	25.7	25.4	26.1	11.2	10.3	10.2	15.3	*	11.5
South Carolina	29.9	29.7	30.3	30.3	30.3	25.3	8.3	8.2	7.4	8.2	8.2	15.4
South Dakota	25.4	25.6	25.8	23.0	24.1	20.2	14.6	13.8	13.5	*	*	*
Tennessee	28.6	28.9	29.3	27.7	27.7	24.2	9.6	8.3	8.1	14.2	14.2	11.2
Texas	30.2	29.8	31.0	33.2	33.3	28.9	6.6	6.6	5.7	5.9	5.9	7.3
Utah	19.2	19.0	18.5	27.3	28.9	21.9	21.8	21.7	22.1	*	*	20.4
Vermont	22.6	22.4	22.4	*	*	*	24.0	23.5	23.5	*	*	*
Virginia	28.3	28.0	28.4	28.3	28.5	25.0	10.7	10.0	9.5	12.3	12.1	13.5
Washington	25.5	25.3	25.5	28.2	28.7	23.8	17.7	17.3	16.5	20.9	20.0	21.6
West Virginia	31.6	31.5	31.5	34.0	34.3	28.8	8.8	8.8	8.8	*	*	*
Wisconsin	21.9	22.2	22.3	21.2	21.1	21.1	15.4	14.7	14.6	18.3	18.3	15.7
Wyoming	23.8	23.9	23.9	...	...	24.4	13.4	13.4	13.7	*	*	*
Puerto Rico	46.1	46.3	...	44.2	...	...	3.2	3.1	...	3.3	...	...
Virgin Islands	26.6	29.3	21.2	25.5	24.8	30.6	24.3	*	*	22.5	24.3	...
Guam	24.4	16.1	16.3	*	*	*	10.8	*	*	*	*	*
American Samoa	...	...	...	...	...	...	...	...	...	...	...	...
Northern Marianas	20.3	*	...	*	...	...	*	*	...	*	...	...

[1] Percent of all live births by cesarean delivery.
[2] Number of vaginal births after previous cesarean delivery per 100 live births to women with a previous cesarean delivery.
[3] Includes races other than White and Black and origin not stated.
[4] Race and Hispanic origin are reported separately on the birth certificate. Data for persons of Hispanic origin are included in the data for each race group according to the mother's reported race.
[5] May be of any race.
[6] Excludes data for the territories.
* = Figure does not meet standards of reliability or precision; based on fewer than 20 births in numerator.
. . . = Not available.

TABLE I-42. RATES OF CESAREAN DELIVERY AND VAGINAL BIRTH AFTER PREVIOUS CESAREAN DELIVERY, BY SELECTED MATERNAL MEDICAL RISK FACTORS AND COMPLICATIONS OF LABOR AND/OR DELIVERY, 2003

In the case of some medical risk factors, mothers are especially likely to have a cesarean delivery. High rates of cesareans (in the neighborhood of 40 to 50 percent) occurred for women with diabetes, chronic as well as pregnancy-associated hypertension, eclampsia, and other conditions. In the case of complications during labor and/or delivery, mothers received cesarean deliveries with the following frequencies: dysfunctional labor, 72 percent; breech/malpresentation, 87 percent; and cephalopelvic disproportion, 96 percent. However, the fairly frequent complication of meconium, moderate/heavy, was associated with a relatively low rate of cesarean delivery of 23.5 percent.

In cases of precipitous labor (less than 3 hours) the total cesarean rate was as low as 2.7 percent; the rate of vaginal birth after previous cesarean delivery surged to 73 percent.

Table I-42. Rates of Cesarean Delivery and Vaginal Birth after Previous Cesarean Delivery, by Selected Maternal Medical Risk Factors and Complications of Labor and/or Delivery, 2003

(Number, percent.)

Medical risk factor and complication	All births to mothers with specified condition and/or procedure	Cesarean delivery rate		Rate of vaginal birth after previous cesarean [3]
		Total [1]	Primary [2]	
Medical Risk Factors				
Anemia [4]	91 535	28.2	19.2	13.4
Cardiac disease [4]	18 639	32.2	23.0	11.3
Acute or chronic lung disease [4]	46 356	31.1	22.3	12.4
Diabetes	133 547	43.0	31.2	8.0
Genital herpes [4,5]	31 567	36.6	29.2	13.4
Hydramnios/oligohydramnios [4]	53 141	41.4	35.3	9.5
Hemoglobinopathy [4]	3 112	31.2	22.4	11.8
Hypertension, chronic	35 953	47.8	37.1	6.4
Hypertension, pregnancy-associated	152 268	43.1	37.1	6.9
Eclampsia	12 059	55.4	49.7	4.6
Incompetent cervix [4]	11 464	41.6	33.4	14.2
Renal disease [4]	11 668	29.3	20.9	12.7
Rh sensitization [4,6]	26 040	27.7	19.5	12.6
Uterine bleeding [4,5]	18 494	37.9	29.8	13.2
Complications of Labor and/or Delivery				
Febrile [4]	59 787	32.2	31.1	39.2
Meconium, moderate/heavy	197 865	23.5	20.5	30.8
Premature rupture of membrane [4]	83 103	30.8	26.8	21.9
Abruptio placenta [4]	20 386	64.3	59.7	8.0
Placenta previa [4]	12 953	81.7	77.5	2.3
Other excessive bleeding [4]	22 787	33.7	26.5	15.1
Seizures during labor [4]	1 304	58.6	55.3	*
Precipitous labor (less than 3 hours)	74 807	2.7	1.8	73.0
Prolonged labor (more than 20 hours) [4]	26 130	38.2	37.6	41.4
Dysfunctional labor [4]	109 836	72.3	71.2	10.9
Breech/malpresentation	156 804	87.2	85.7	2.9
Cephalopelvic disproportion [4]	56 111	96.0	95.9	1.9
Cord prolapse [4]	6 385	68.4	66.6	8.0
Anesthetic complication [4,5]	2 415	45.2	37.1	8.0
Fetal distress [4,5]	132 377	63.2	61.6	14.0

[1] Percent of all live births by cesarean delivery.
[2] Number of primary cesareans per 100 live births to women who have not had a previous cesarean.
[3] Number of vaginal births after previous cesarean delivery per 100 live births to women with a previous cesarean delivery.
[4] Excludes data for Pennsylvania and Washington State, which implemented the 2003 Revision to the U.S. Standard Certificate of Live Birth for data year 2003.
[5] Texas does not report this risk factor or complication.
[6] Kansas does not report this risk factor.
* = Figure does not meet standards of reliability or precision; based on fewer than 20 births in numerator.

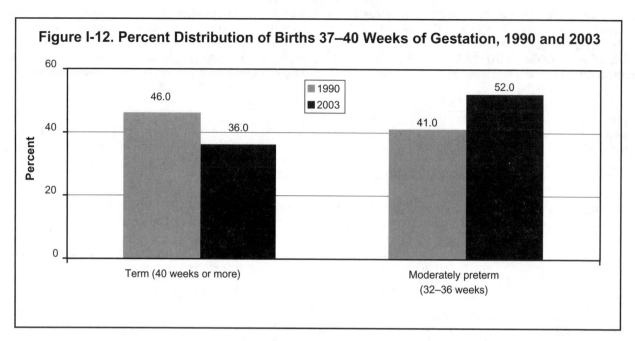

Figure I-12. Percent Distribution of Births 37–40 Weeks of Gestation, 1990 and 2003

TABLE I-43. LIVE BIRTHS BY BIRTHWEIGHT AND PERCENT VERY LOW AND LOW BIRTHWEIGHT, BY PERIOD OF GESTATION, RACE, AND HISPANIC ORIGIN OF MOTHER, 2003

Very low birthweight (under 3.25 pounds) occurred in 1.4 percent of all births, and 7.9 percent of all births resulted in low birthweight (under 5.5 pounds), the highest level reported in more than three decades. When the period of gestation becomes very short, these percentages increase dramatically. For all preterm deliveries, or deliveries with a period of gestation of less than 37 weeks, the incidence of very low birthweight was 11.3 percent and the low birthweight rate was 43.1 percent. For periods of gestation of 37–41 weeks, the frequency of very low birth-

weight dropped to 0.1 percent, while low birthweight declined to 3.0 percent. For deliveries after 41 weeks of gestation, the low birthweight percentage dropped even further to 2.4 percent.

When comparing the same gestation periods between Black mothers and non-Hispanic White mothers, Blacks showed a greater incidence of infants with very low birthweight and low birthweight, especially among near-full-term and full-term births. The results for Hispanic mothers were similar to those for non-Hispanic Whites, except in the case of preterm babies; for these, Hispanics reported somewhat smaller percentages of underweight newborns.

Table I-43. Live Births by Birthweight and Percent Very Low and Low Birthweight, by Period of Gestation, Race, and Hispanic Origin of Mother, 2003

(Number, percent.)

Birthweight, race, and Hispanic origin of mother	All births	Period of gestation [1]										Not stated
		Preterm					Term				Postterm	
		Total under 37 weeks	Under 28 weeks	28–31 weeks	32–35 weeks	36 weeks	Total 37–41 weeks	37–39 weeks	40 weeks	41 weeks	42 weeks and over	
ALL RACES [2]												
Total Number	4 089 950	499 008	30 061	49 545	234 074	185 328	3 288 548	2 097 771	807 157	383 620	258 552	43 842
Less than 500 grams	6 307	6 132	5 857	247	23	5	6	2	3	1	1	168
500–999 grams	22 980	22 319	16 587	5 172	528	32	183	133	35	15	19	459
1,000–1,499 grams	29 930	27 759	3 905	16 085	7 179	590	1 508	1 080	297	131	213	450
1,500–1,999 grams	63 791	53 171	957	12 259	34 790	5 165	8 984	7 419	1 095	470	794	842
2,000–2,499 grams	201 056	105 163	612	4 193	68 175	32 183	88 377	73 882	9 883	4 612	5 175	2 341
2,500–2,999 grams	711 003	133 242	908	4 162	60 025	68 147	537 339	412 555	87 702	37 082	32 922	7 500
3,000–3,499 grams	1 557 864	100 835	-	4 827	41 100	54 908	1 340 828	888 504	314 513	137 811	99 990	16 211
3,500–3,999 grams	1 131 577	39 471	-	2 461	17 514	19 496	993 872	559 499	290 910	143 463	86 878	11 356
4,000–4,499 grams	309 721	7 721	-	-	3 805	3 916	271 493	132 782	88 291	50 420	27 172	3 335
4,500–4,999 grams	46 690	1 243	-	-	577	666	40 228	18 893	12 804	8 531	4 720	499
5,000 grams or more	5 431	211	-	-	98	113	4 577	2 324	1 306	947	566	77
Not stated	3 600	1 741	1 235	139	260	107	1 153	698	318	137	102	604
Percent												
Very low birthweight [3]	1.4	11.3	91.4	43.5	3.3	0.3	0.1	0.1	0.0	0.0	0.1	2.5
Low birthweight [4]	7.9	43.1	96.9	76.8	47.3	20.5	3.0	3.9	1.4	1.4	2.4	9.9
WHITE TOTAL [5]												
Total Number	3 225 848	365 358	17 967	34 155	172 141	141 095	2 618 961	1 659 139	648 700	311 122	206 544	34 985
Less than 500 grams	3 593	3 475	3 299	159	14	3	4	1	2	1	-	114
500–999 grams	14 096	13 618	9 947	3 292	356	23	138	102	28	8	12	328
1,000–1,499 grams	20 173	18 698	2 460	10 984	4 847	407	1 012	733	202	77	155	308
1,500–1,999 grams	44 419	37 217	575	8 780	24 316	3 546	6 035	5 014	699	322	548	619
2,000–2,499 grams	141 331	75 862	378	2 804	49 885	22 795	60 221	50 388	6 660	3 173	3 568	1 680
2,500–2,999 grams	511 317	99 112	564	2 735	44 617	51 196	383 324	295 407	61 647	26 270	23 389	5 492
3,000–3,499 grams	1 220 632	77 218	-	3 400	30 561	43 257	1 052 594	699 863	244 945	107 786	77 864	12 956
3,500–3,999 grams	951 782	31 556	-	1 909	13 722	15 925	837 969	472 654	244 546	120 769	72 640	9 617
4,000–4,499 grams	270 180	6 300	-	-	3 087	3 213	237 343	115 942	77 176	44 225	23 626	2 911
4,500–4,999 grams	41 156	1 020	-	-	467	553	35 514	16 540	11 415	7 559	4 174	448
5,000 grams or more	4 664	171	-	-	78	93	3 930	1 969	1 132	829	495	68
Not stated	2 505	1 111	744	92	191	84	877	526	248	103	73	444
Percent												
Very low birthweight [3]	1.2	9.8	91.2	42.4	3.0	0.3	0.0	0.1	0.0	0.0	0.1	2.2
Low birthweight [4]	6.9	40.9	96.7	76.4	46.2	19.0	2.6	3.4	1.2	1.2	2.1	8.8
NON-HISPANIC WHITE												
Total Number	2 321 904	260 947	12 639	24 251	121 222	102 835	1 904 575	1 211 016	469 198	224 361	144 119	12 263
Less than 500 grams	2 529	2 485	2 352	117	13	3	2	1	1	-	-	42
500–999 grams	9 998	9 785	7 048	2 475	245	17	94	70	18	6	6	113
1,000–1,499 grams	14 882	13 981	1 751	8 240	3 680	310	661	490	121	50	111	129
1,500–1,999 grams	32 915	27 963	354	6 567	18 396	2 646	4 302	3 611	483	208	377	273
2,000–2,499 grams	103 007	57 100	245	1 891	37 837	17 127	42 794	36 111	4 558	2 125	2 493	620
2,500–2,999 grams	356 232	72 108	362	1 635	31 901	38 210	266 678	207 843	41 369	17 466	15 627	1 819
3,000–3,499 grams	858 305	51 795	-	2 047	18 736	31 012	749 648	503 605	171 317	74 726	52 630	4 232
3,500–3,999 grams	700 819	20 131	-	1 206	8 064	10 861	625 749	355 104	181 568	89 077	51 528	3 411
4,000–4,499 grams	206 407	4 033	-	-	1 879	2 154	183 514	89 671	59 815	34 028	17 709	1 151
4,500–4,999 grams	31 570	654	-	-	282	372	27 533	12 691	8 892	5 950	3 201	182
5,000 grams or more	3 415	110	-	-	48	62	2 901	1 401	862	638	380	24
Not stated	1 825	802	527	73	141	61	699	418	194	87	57	267
Percent												
Very low birthweight [3]	1.2	10.1	92.1	44.8	3.3	0.3	0.0	0.0	0.0	0.0	0.1	2.4
Low birthweight [4]	7.0	42.8	97.0	79.8	49.7	19.6	2.5	3.3	1.1	1.1	2.1	9.8

[1] Expressed in completed weeks.
[2] Includes races other than White and Black and origin not stated.
[3] Birthweight of less than 1,500 grams (3 lb 4 oz).
[4] Birthweight of less than 2,500 grams (5 lb 8 oz).
[5] Race and Hispanic origin are reported separately on the birth certificate. Data for persons of Hispanic origin are included in the data for each race group according to the mother's reported race.
- = Quantity zero.

Table I-43. Live Births by Birthweight and Percent Very Low and Low Birthweight, by Period of Gestation, Race, and Hispanic Origin of Mother, 2003—*Continued*

(Number, percent.)

Birthweight, race, and Hispanic origin of mother	All births	Period of gestation [1]										Not stated
		Preterm					Term				Postterm	
		Total under 37 weeks	Under 28 weeks	28–31 weeks	32–35 weeks	36 weeks	Total 37–41 weeks	37–39 weeks	40 weeks	41 weeks	42 weeks and over	
BLACK TOTAL [5]												
Total Number	599 847	105 101	10 675	12 789	48 486	33 151	454 209	299 385	106 021	48 803	36 234	4 303
Less than 500 grams	2 427	2 382	2 300	72	8	2	2	1	1	-	1	42
500–999 grams	7 765	7 630	5 865	1 625	133	7	37	27	6	4	7	91
1,000–1,499 grams	8 204	7 656	1 248	4 329	1 923	156	406	290	69	47	49	93
1,500–1,999 grams	15 654	12 919	331	2 902	8 436	1 250	2 383	1 934	326	123	203	149
2,000–2,499 grams	46 038	23 077	192	1 161	14 472	7 252	21 283	17 656	2 499	1 128	1 278	400
2,500–2,999 grams	143 176	26 071	303	1 160	11 945	12 663	108 977	82 712	18 483	7 782	7 132	996
3,000–3,499 grams	228 356	17 831	-	1 097	8 137	8 597	193 652	126 959	46 445	20 248	15 460	1 413
3,500–3,999 grams	117 889	5 795	-	405	2 802	2 588	101 871	56 971	30 108	14 792	9 457	766
4,000–4,499 grams	25 428	1 026	-	-	501	525	21 955	10 967	7 020	3 968	2 246	201
4,500–4,999 grams	3 546	151	-	-	73	78	3 040	1 529	901	610	333	22
5,000 grams or more	504	30	-	-	13	17	426	236	115	75	46	2
Not stated	860	533	436	38	43	16	177	103	48	26	22	128
Percent												
Very low birthweight [3]	3.1	16.9	91.9	47.3	4.3	0.5	0.1	0.1	0.1	0.1	0.2	5.4
Low birthweight [4]	13.4	51.3	97.0	79.1	51.5	26.2	5.3	6.7	2.7	2.7	4.2	18.6
NON-HISPANIC BLACK												
Total Number	576 033	101 984	10 386	12 452	47 067	32 079	435 340	287 620	101 268	46 452	34 669	4 040
Less than 500 grams	2 350	2 310	2 229	71	8	2	2	1	1	-	1	37
500–999 grams	7 575	7 444	5 715	1 593	129	7	37	27	6	4	7	87
1,000–1,499 grams	7 998	7 466	1 215	4 216	1 885	150	391	279	66	46	48	93
1,500–1,999 grams	15 211	12 553	320	2 819	8 202	1 212	2 320	1 884	316	120	196	142
2,000–2,499 grams	44 813	22 477	187	1 133	14 098	7 059	20 717	17 189	2 425	1 103	1 239	380
2,500–2,999 grams	138 440	25 295	298	1 131	11 596	12 270	105 299	79 977	17 817	7 505	6 894	952
3,000–3,499 grams	218 901	17 220	-	1 064	7 873	8 283	185 532	121 808	44 413	19 311	14 824	1 325
3,500–3,999 grams	112 139	5 555	-	391	2 678	2 486	96 862	54 274	28 606	13 982	8 998	724
4,000–4,499 grams	23 992	975	-	-	473	502	20 738	10 406	6 618	3 714	2 094	185
4,500–4,999 grams	3 340	147	-	-	71	76	2 869	1 453	844	572	305	19
5,000 grams or more	484	29	-	-	13	16	408	227	111	70	45	2
Not stated	790	513	422	34	41	16	165	95	45	25	18	94
Percent												
Very low birthweight [3]	3.1	17.0	91.9	47.4	4.3	0.5	0.1	0.1	0.1	0.1	0.2	5.5
Low birthweight [4]	13.6	51.5	97.0	79.2	51.7	26.3	5.4	6.7	2.8	2.7	4.3	18.7
HISPANIC [6]												
Total Number	912 329	105 688	5 378	10 026	51 536	38 748	721 266	452 575	181 123	87 568	63 292	22 083
Less than 500 grams	1 037	965	922	42	1	-	2	-	1	1	-	70
500–999 grams	4 140	3 884	2 948	821	109	6	41	31	8	2	6	209
1,000–1,499 grams	5 366	4 778	736	2 766	1 174	102	363	252	83	28	44	181
1,500–1,999 grams	11 655	9 383	231	2 237	5 996	919	1 767	1 425	227	115	171	334
2,000–2,499 grams	38 775	18 963	140	930	12 163	5 730	17 685	14 491	2 142	1 052	1 102	1 025
2,500–2,999 grams	157 583	27 359	202	1 118	12 859	13 180	118 701	89 047	20 682	8 972	7 944	3 579
3,000–3,499 grams	366 508	25 760	-	1 382	11 982	12 396	306 547	198 452	74 561	33 534	25 679	8 522
3,500–3,999 grams	252 230	11 569	-	710	5 755	5 104	213 311	118 177	63 258	31 876	21 274	6 076
4,000–4,499 grams	63 688	2 310	-	-	1 236	1 074	53 687	26 170	17 352	10 165	5 958	1 733
4,500–4,999 grams	9 619	368	-	-	184	184	8 002	3 870	2 516	1 616	984	265
5,000 grams or more	1 246	62	-	-	30	32	1 029	573	266	190	114	41
Not stated	482	287	199	20	47	21	131	87	27	17	16	48
Percent												
Very low birthweight [3]	1.2	9.1	88.9	36.3	2.5	0.3	0.1	0.1	0.1	0.0	0.1	2.1
Low birthweight [4]	6.7	36.0	96.1	67.9	37.8	17.4	2.8	3.6	1.4	1.4	2.1	8.3

[1]Expressed in completed weeks.
[3]Birthweight of less than 1,500 grams (3 lb 4 oz).
[4]Birthweight of less than 2,500 grams (5 lb 8 oz).
[5]Race and Hispanic origin are reported separately on the birth certificate. Data for persons of Hispanic origin are included in the data for each race group according to the mother's reported race.
[6]May be of any race.
- = Quantity zero.

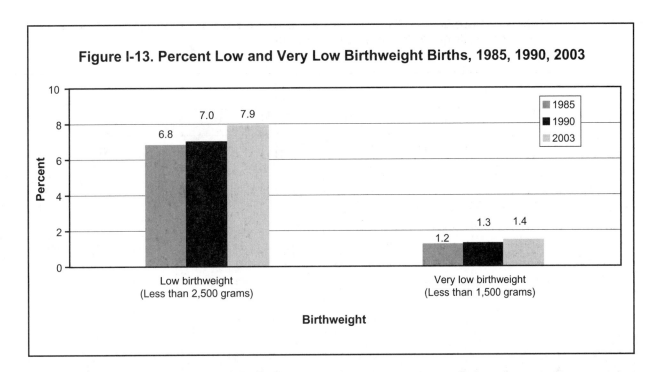

Figure I-13. Percent Low and Very Low Birthweight Births, 1985, 1990, 2003

TABLE I-44. PERCENT OF LIVE BIRTHS THAT ARE VERY PRETERM, PRETERM, VERY LOW BIRTHWEIGHT, AND LOW BIRTHWEIGHT, BY RACE AND HISPANIC ORIGIN OF MOTHER, 1981–2003

The preterm birth rate (including births at less than 37 completed weeks of gestation) rose to 12.3 percent of all births for 2003, the highest level recorded in two decades. The "very preterm birth rate" (defined as less than 32 completed weeks of gestation) was 1.97 percent in 2003, up approximately 9 percent from the 1981 level of 1.81 percent. Preterm birth is among the leading causes of infant death. It is associated with nearly half of all congenital neurological defects, such as cerebral palsy. In 2001, 41 percent of all infants born earlier than 28 weeks of gestation did not survive their first year of life, as compared with 0.3 percent of those that had gestation periods of 37–41 weeks. The rise of multiple births over the past two decades has had an important influence on the preterm birth rate, as these births are much more likely to occur early.

Preterm rates increased between 2002 and 2003 for non-Hispanic Whites, non-Hispanic Blacks, and Hispanics. The long-term trend of increasing preterm births, however, has been concentrated among non-Hispanic Whites—a 33 percent increase from 1990 (8.5 percent) to 2003 (11.3 percent). Rates for non-Hispanic Blacks declined from 19 percent in the early 1990s, plateaued around 17.5 percent in the late 1990s, and gradually rose to 17.8 percent in the early 2000s. Risk levels for Blacks remain considerably greater than those for Hispanics and non-Hispanic Whites. Preterm rates for Hispanics have risen by 8 percent (from 11.0 to 11.9 percent of live births) since 1990.

Trends in the rates of low birthweight correspond to developments in preterm births. Thus, for all births since 1981, the frequency of low-birthweight infants has increased to 7.9 percent. On the basis of detailed data available since 1989, the frequency of low-birthweight infants has increased for non-Hispanic Whites and, to a small extent, for Hispanics. For non-Hispanic Blacks, the incidence of low birthweight declined slightly from 1989 to the mid-1990s, but had climbed back to the 1989 level of 13.6 percent by 2003. The risk of low birthweight remains relatively high for non-Hispanic Blacks: singleton infants born to Black mothers continue to be more than twice as likely as non-Hispanic White or Hispanic infants to weigh less than 5.5 pounds at birth.

Among non-Hispanic Whites, there was a steep rise in multiple births. Infants born in multiple deliveries are approximately 10 times as likely to have low birthweight than singletons. Also, according to a recent study, singletons conceived with assisted-reproductive technology are at greater risk of low birthweight than those conceived without such intervention.

Table I-44. Percent of Live Births That Are Very Preterm, Preterm, Very Low Birthweight, and Low Birthweight, by Race and Hispanic Origin of Mother, 1981–2003

(Percent.)

Year	Very preterm [1]						Preterm [2]					
	All races [3]	White		Black		Hispanic [5]	All races [3]	White		Black		Hispanic [5]
		Total [4]	Non-Hispanic	Total [4]	Non-Hispanic			Total [4]	Non-Hispanic	Total [4]	Non-Hispanic	
2003	1.97	1.63	1.60	3.94	3.99	1.73	12.3	11.5	11.3	17.6	17.8	11.9
2002	1.96	1.60	1.56	4.01	4.04	1.72	12.1	11.1	11.0	17.5	17.7	11.6
2001	1.95	1.59	1.55	4.02	4.05	1.69	11.9	11.0	10.8	17.5	17.6	11.4
2000	1.93	1.55	1.51	4.04	4.09	1.69	11.6	10.6	10.4	17.3	17.4	11.2
1999	1.96	1.57	1.54	4.13	4.18	1.68	11.8	10.7	10.5	17.5	17.6	11.4
1998	1.96	1.57	1.52	4.11	4.15	1.72	11.6	10.5	10.2	17.5	17.6	11.4
1997	1.94	1.53	1.49	4.17	4.19	1.68	11.4	10.2	9.9	17.5	17.6	11.2
1996	1.89	1.48	1.43	4.13	4.17	1.66	11.0	9.8	9.5	17.4	17.5	10.9
1995	1.89	1.46	1.41	4.25	4.29	1.66	11.0	9.7	9.4	17.7	17.8	10.9
1994	1.91	1.45	1.39	4.32	4.36	1.67	11.0	9.6	9.3	18.1	18.2	10.9
1993	1.93	1.45	1.39	4.41	4.45	1.67	11.0	9.5	9.1	18.5	18.6	11.0
1992 [8]	1.91	1.40	1.33	4.47	4.50	1.64	10.7	9.1	8.7	18.4	18.5	10.7
1991 [8]	1.94	1.41	1.35	4.62	4.65	1.65	10.8	9.1	8.7	18.9	19.0	11.0
1990 [9]	1.92	1.39	1.33	4.61	4.63	1.69	10.6	8.9	8.5	18.8	18.9	11.0
1989 [10]	1.95	1.41	1.34	4.64	4.68	1.76	10.6	8.8	8.4	18.9	19.0	11.1
1988	1.96	1.42	...	4.72	...	...	10.2	8.5	...	18.7	...	...
1987	1.96	1.44	...	4.61	...	...	10.2	8.5	...	18.4	...	...
1986	1.90	1.41	...	4.47	...	...	10.0	8.4	...	18.0	...	...
1985	1.88	1.42	...	4.37	...	...	9.8	8.2	...	17.8	...	...
1984	1.83	1.38	...	4.22	...	...	9.4	7.9	...	17.1	...	...
1983	1.86	1.40	...	4.34	...	...	9.6	8.0	...	17.7	...	...
1982	1.84	1.40	...	4.22	...	...	9.5	8.0	...	17.4	...	...
1981	1.81	1.37	...	4.13	...	...	9.4	7.9	...	17.3	...	...

Year	Very low birthweight [6]						Low birthweight [7]					
	All races [3]	White		Black		Hispanic [5]	All races [3]	White		Black		Hispanic [5]
		Total [4]	Non-Hispanic	Total [4]	Non-Hispanic			Total [4]	Non-Hispanic	Total [4]	Non-Hispanic	
2003	1.45	1.17	1.18	3.07	3.12	1.16	7.9	6.9	7.0	13.4	13.6	6.7
2002	1.46	1.17	1.17	3.13	3.15	1.17	7.8	6.8	6.9	13.3	13.4	6.5
2001	1.44	1.16	1.17	3.04	3.08	1.14	7.7	6.7	6.8	13.0	13.1	6.5
2000	1.43	1.14	1.14	3.07	3.10	1.14	7.6	6.5	6.6	13.0	13.1	6.4
1999	1.45	1.15	1.15	3.14	3.18	1.14	7.6	6.6	6.6	13.1	13.2	6.4
1998	1.45	1.15	1.15	3.08	3.11	1.15	7.6	6.5	6.6	13.0	13.2	6.4
1997	1.42	1.13	1.12	3.04	3.05	1.13	7.5	6.5	6.5	13.0	13.1	6.4
1996	1.37	1.09	1.08	2.99	3.02	1.12	7.4	6.3	6.4	13.0	13.1	6.3
1995	1.35	1.06	1.04	2.97	2.98	1.11	7.3	6.2	6.2	13.1	13.2	6.3
1994	1.33	1.02	1.01	2.96	2.99	1.08	7.3	6.1	6.1	13.2	13.3	6.2
1993	1.33	1.01	1.00	2.96	2.99	1.06	7.2	6.0	5.9	13.3	13.4	6.2
1992 [8]	1.29	0.96	0.94	2.96	2.97	1.04	7.1	5.8	5.7	13.3	13.4	6.1
1991 [8]	1.29	0.96	0.94	2.96	2.97	1.02	7.1	5.8	5.7	13.6	13.6	6.1
1990 [9]	1.27	0.95	0.93	2.92	2.93	1.03	7.0	5.7	5.6	13.3	13.3	6.1
1989 [10]	1.28	0.95	0.93	2.95	2.97	1.05	7.0	5.7	5.6	13.5	13.6	6.2
1988	1.24	0.93	...	2.86	...	...	6.9	5.7	...	13.3	...	...
1987	1.24	0.94	...	2.79	...	...	6.9	5.7	...	13.0	...	...
1986	1.21	0.93	...	2.73	...	...	6.8	5.7	...	12.8	...	...
1985	1.21	0.93	...	2.71	...	...	6.8	5.7	...	12.6	...	...
1984	1.19	0.93	...	2.60	...	...	6.7	5.6	...	12.6	...	...
1983	1.19	0.92	...	2.60	...	...	6.8	5.7	...	12.8	...	...
1982	1.18	0.91	...	2.56	...	...	6.8	5.6	...	12.6	...	...
1981	1.16	0.91	...	2.52	...	...	6.8	5.7	...	12.7	...	...

[1]Births of less than 32 completed weeks of gestation.
[2]Births of less than 37 completed weeks of gestation.
[3]Includes races other than White and Black and origin not stated.
[4]Race and Hispanic origin are reported separately on the birth certificate. Data for persons of Hispanic origin are included in the data for each race group according to the mother's reported race.
[5]May be of any race.
[6]Less than 1,500 grams (3 lb 4 oz).
[7]Less than 2,500 grams (5 lb 8 oz).
[8]Data by Hispanic origin exclude New Hampshire, which did not report Hispanic origin.
[9]Data by Hispanic origin exclude New Hampshire and Oklahoma, which did not report Hispanic origin.
[10]Data by Hispanic origin exclude New Hampshire, Oklahoma, and Louisiana, which did not report Hispanic origin.
. . . = Not available.

TABLE I-44A. LOW-BIRTHWEIGHT LIVE BIRTHS, ACCORDING TO MOTHER'S DETAILED RACE, HISPANIC ORIGIN, AND SMOKING STATUS, SELECTED YEARS, 1970–2003

Low birthweight is associated with an elevated risk of death and disability in infants. In 2003, the rate of low birthweight (infants weighing less than 5.5 pounds at birth) increased to 7.8 percent overall, up from 7.0 percent in 1990 and 6.75 percent in 1985. Throughout these years, non-Hispanic Blacks have had particularly high rates of low and of very low birthweight babies. Mothers who smoke cigarettes also show higher rates of low birthweight than nonsmokers.

Birthweight is sensitive to the length of gestation. Preterm infants (less than 37 weeks of gestation) have a 43 percent chance of being of low birthweight (see Table I–45), and the frequency of preterm deliveries has increased over the last two decades. In addition, the rise in multiple births has increased the incidence of low birthweight babies.

Table I-44A. Low-Birthweight Live Births, According to Mother's Detailed Race, Hispanic Origin, and Smoking Status, Selected Years, 1970–2003

(Percent.)

Birthweight, race, Hispanic origin of mother, and smoking status of mother	2003	2002	2001	2000	1999	1998	1995	1990	1985	1980	1975	1970
PERCENT OF LIVE BIRTHS [1]												
Low Birthweight, (Less Than 2,500 Grams)												
All Races	7.93	7.82	7.68	7.57	7.62	7.57	7.32	6.97	6.75	6.84	7.38	7.93
White	6.94	6.80	6.68	6.55	6.57	6.52	6.22	5.70	5.65	5.72	6.27	6.85
Black or African American	13.37	13.29	12.95	12.99	13.11	13.05	13.13	13.25	12.65	12.69	13.19	13.90
American Indian or Alaska Native	7.37	7.23	7.33	6.76	7.15	6.81	6.61	6.11	5.86	6.44	6.41	7.97
Asian or Pacific Islander	7.78	7.78	7.51	7.31	7.45	7.42	6.90	6.45	6.16	6.68	. . .	. . .
Chinese	. . .	5.52	5.33	5.10	5.19	5.34	5.29	4.69	4.98	5.21	5.29	6.67
Japanese	. . .	7.57	7.28	7.14	7.95	7.50	7.26	6.16	6.21	6.60	7.47	9.03
Filipino	. . .	8.61	8.66	8.46	8.30	8.23	7.83	7.30	6.95	7.40	8.08	10.02
Hawaiian	. . .	8.14	7.91	6.76	7.69	7.15	6.84	7.24	6.49	7.23	. . .	. . .
Other Asian or Pacific Islander	. . .	8.16	7.76	7.67	7.76	7.76	7.05	6.65	6.19	6.83	. . .	. . .
Hispanic or Latino [2]	6.69	6.55	6.47	6.41	6.38	6.44	6.29	6.06	6.16	6.12	. . .	. . .
Mexican	6.28	6.16	6.08	6.01	5.94	5.97	5.81	5.55	5.77	5.62	. . .	. . .
Puerto Rican	10.01	9.68	9.34	9.30	9.30	9.68	9.41	8.99	8.69	8.95	. . .	. . .
Cuban	7.04	6.50	6.49	6.49	6.80	6.50	6.50	5.67	6.02	5.62	. . .	. . .
Central and South American	6.70	6.53	6.49	6.34	6.38	6.47	6.20	5.84	5.68	5.76	. . .	. . .
Other and unknown Hispanic or Latino	8.01	7.87	7.96	7.84	7.63	7.59	7.55	6.87	6.83	6.96	. . .	. . .
Not Hispanic or Latino [2]												
White	7.04	6.91	6.76	6.60	6.64	6.55	6.20	5.61	5.61	5.69	. . .	. . .
Black or African American	13.55	13.39	13.07	13.13	13.23	13.17	13.21	13.32	12.62	12.71	. . .	. . .
Cigarette smoker [3]	12.40	12.15	11.90	11.88	12.06	12.01	12.18	11.25	. . .	. . .	. . .	. . .
Nonsmoker [3]	7.66	7.48	7.32	7.19	7.21	7.18	6.79	6.14	. . .	. . .	. . .	. . .
Very Low Birthweight, (Less Than 1,500 Grams)												
All Races	1.45	1.46	1.44	1.43	1.45	1.45	1.35	1.27	1.21	1.15	1.16	1.17
White	1.17	1.17	1.16	1.14	1.15	1.15	1.06	0.95	0.94	0.90	0.92	0.95
Black or African American	3.07	3.13	3.04	3.07	3.14	3.08	2.97	2.92	2.71	2.48	2.40	2.40
American Indian or Alaska Native	1.30	1.28	1.26	1.16	1.26	1.24	1.10	1.01	1.01	0.92	0.95	0.98
Asian or Pacific Islander	1.09	1.12	1.03	1.05	1.08	1.10	0.91	0.87	0.85	0.92	. . .	. . .
Chinese	. . .	0.74	0.69	0.77	0.68	0.75	0.67	0.51	0.57	0.66	0.52	0.80
Japanese	. . .	0.97	0.71	0.75	0.86	0.84	0.87	0.73	0.84	0.94	0.89	1.48
Filipino	. . .	1.31	1.23	1.38	1.41	1.35	1.13	1.05	0.86	0.99	0.93	1.08
Hawaiian	. . .	1.55	1.50	1.39	1.41	1.53	0.94	0.97	1.03	1.05	. . .	. . .
Other Asian or Pacific Islander	. . .	1.17	1.06	1.04	1.09	1.12	0.91	0.92	0.91	0.96	. . .	. . .
Hispanic or Latino [2]	1.16	1.17	1.14	1.14	1.14	1.15	1.11	1.03	1.01	0.98	. . .	. . .
Mexican	1.06	1.06	1.05	1.03	1.04	1.02	1.01	0.92	0.97	0.92	. . .	. . .
Puerto Rican	2.01	1.96	1.85	1.93	1.86	1.86	1.79	1.62	1.30	1.29	. . .	. . .
Cuban	1.37	1.15	1.27	1.21	1.49	1.33	1.19	1.20	1.18	1.02	. . .	. . .
Central and South American	1.17	1.20	1.19	1.20	1.15	1.23	1.13	1.05	1.01	0.99	. . .	. . .
Other and unknown Hispanic or Latino	1.28	1.44	1.27	1.42	1.32	1.38	1.28	1.09	0.96	1.01	. . .	. . .
Not Hispanic or Latino [2]												
White	1.18	1.17	1.17	1.14	1.15	1.15	1.04	0.93	0.91	0.87	. . .	. . .
Black or African American	3.12	3.15	3.08	3.10	3.18	3.11	2.98	2.93	2.67	2.47	. . .	. . .
Cigarette smoker [3]	1.92	1.88	1.88	1.91	1.91	1.87	1.85	1.73	. . .	. . .	. . .	. . .
Nonsmoker [3]	1.44	1.45	1.42	1.40	1.43	1.44	1.31	1.18	. . .	. . .	. . .	. . .

Note: Data are based on birth certificates.

[1] Excludes live births with unknown birthweight. Percent based on live births with known birthweight.
[2] Prior to 1993, data from states lacking an Hispanic-origin item on the birth certificate were excluded.
[3] Percent based on live births with known smoking status of mother and known birthweight. Data from states that did not require the reporting of mother's tobacco use during pregnancy on the birth certificate are not included.
. . . =Not available.

TABLE I-44B. PRETERM BIRTH RATES, BY STATE, 1990 AND 2003

The proportion of births delivered at gestational ages of less than 37 weeks increased between 1990 and 2003 for all states (the District of Columbia was the sole exception). Preterm rates in 2003 ranged from more than 15 percent in Alabama and Louisiana to less than 10 percent in Connecticut, New Hampshire, and Vermont.

TABLE I-44C. RATE OF VERY LOW BIRTHWEIGHT AND LOW BIRTHWEIGHT AND MEAN BIRTHWEIGHT AMONG SINGLETONS, BY RACE AND HISPANIC ORIGIN OF MOTHER, SELECTED YEARS, 1990–2003

Examining singleton births reveals trends without the influence of the increase in multiple births. Low birthweight in singletons rose for all age groups between 2002 and 2003. Since 1990, low birthweight rates for singletons have risen 6 and 12 percent for Hispanic and non-Hispanic White infants, respectively, but have declined 3 percent for non-Hispanic Black newborns.

In 2003, the average birthweight for infants delivered in single deliveries was 3,325 grams (7 lb 5 oz). Since 1990, the average birthweight has declined by about 1 percent for U.S. births overall and for non-Hispanic White and Hispanic births. The mean birthweight for non-Hispanic Black infants has been essentially stable over this period.

Table I-44B. Preterm Birth Rates, by State, 1990 and 2003

(Percent.)

State	2003	1990	Percent change, 1990–2003
UNITED STATES	12.3	10.6	16
Alabama	15.7	13.1	20
Alaska	11.1	9.0	23
Arizona	13.1	10.2	28
Arkansas	13.0	12.5	4
California	10.5	9.8	7
Colorado	12.1	9.6	26
Connecticut	9.7	8.9	9
Delaware	13.7	11.1	24
District of Columbia	14.8	20.7	-28
Florida	13.0	11.6	13
Georgia	13.1	12.8	2
Hawaii	12.6	10.0	26
Idaho	10.7	8.7	24
Illinois	12.8	11.4	13
Indiana	12.9	9.9	30
Iowa	11.4	8.7	31
Kansas	11.6	9.5	22
Kentucky	14.0	10.5	34
Louisiana	15.6	13.9	12
Maine	10.1	7.6	32
Maryland	13.1	11.2	16
Massachusetts	10.7	7.7	39
Michigan	11.9	10.7	11
Minnesota	10.2	8.2	25
Mississippi	17.9	15.1	19
Missouri	13.1	10.7	22
Montana	11.1	8.5	31
Nebraska	12.4	8.5	45
Nevada	13.6	11.1	22
New Hampshire	9.2	6.8	36
New Jersey	12.1	10.7	13
New Mexico	12.7	11.0	15
New York	11.4	10.7	7
North Carolina	13.6	12.5	9
North Dakota	12.0	8.3	45
Ohio	12.5	10.6	18
Oklahoma	12.7	10.1	26
Oregon	10.1	8.0	25
Pennsylvania	11.6	10.3	12
Rhode Island	11.6	9.6	21
South Carolina	14.5	12.3	18
South Dakota	11.2	8.9	25
Tennessee	14.1	12.6	12
Texas	13.9	11.2	23
Utah	10.4	8.7	20
Vermont	9.5	7.1	34
Virginia	12.1	11.0	9
Washington	10.3	8.4	22
West Virginia	13.3	9.9	34
Wisconsin	11.3	9.2	23
Wyoming	11.8	10.3	15

Note: Preterm is defined as less than 37 completed weeks of gestation.

Table I-44C. Rate of Very Low Birthweight and Low Birthweight and Mean Birthweight Among Singletons, by Race and Hispanic Origin of Mother, Selected Years, 1990–2003

(Percent, number.)

Mean birthweight and rate of low birthweight by race and Hispanic origin	2003	2002	2000	1995	1990 [1]
Total, All Races [2]					
Percent very low birthweight	1.11	1.11	1.11	1.08	1.05
Percent low birthweight	6.20	6.12	6.00	6.05	5.90
Mean birthweight in grams	3 325	3 332	3 348	3 353	3 365
Non-Hispanic White					
Percent very low birthweight	0.82	0.81	0.80	0.78	0.73
Percent low birthweight	5.11	5.02	4.88	4.87	4.56
Mean birthweight in grams	3 384	3 392	3 410	3 416	3 433
Non-Hispanic Black					
Percent very low birthweight	2.61	2.63	2.62	2.55	2.54
Percent low birthweight	11.58	11.44	11.28	11.66	11.92
Mean birthweight in grams	3 122	3 128	3 141	3 132	3 128
Hispanic [3]					
Percent very low birthweight	0.94	0.96	0.94	0.93	0.87
Percent low birthweight	5.55	5.44	5.36	5.36	5.23
Mean birthweight in grams	3 324	3 332	3 344	3 343	3 351

[1] Data for 1990 by race and Hispanic origin exclude data for New Hampshire and Oklahoma, which did not require reporting of Hispanic origin of mother.
[2] Includes births to races not shown separately.
[3] May be of any race.

TABLE I-45. NUMBER AND PERCENT WITH LOW BIRTHWEIGHT AND NUMBER OF LIVE BIRTHS BY BIRTHWEIGHT, BY AGE, RACE, AND HISPANIC ORIGIN OF MOTHER, 2003

For mothers between 25 and 29 years of age, the risk of low birthweight (newborns less than 5.5 pounds) is smallest (7.1 percent). For younger mothers, the risk increases (peaking at 9.7 percent for women 15–19 years of age). The risk increases rapidly to 10.6 percent for women 40–44 years of age and to 20.5 percent for mothers 45–54 years of age. These patterns also apply to Hispanics and non-Hispanic Blacks, although the level of low birthweight risk is substantially greater for Blacks in each age group. Non-Hispanic Blacks also have a higher than average proportion of teenage mothers, and teenagers in turn have a greater risk of low birthweight than the average risk for all ages.

Much of the increase in risk among older mothers can be attributed to their higher rates of multiple births. In 2003, multiples accounted for almost two-thirds of all low birthweight infants delivered to mothers 45 years old and over. For these mothers, singleton births had roughly half the rate of low birthweight compared to all births (10 percent versus 20 percent) and about half the rate of very low birthweight (2 percent versus 4 percent, data not shown).

Table I-45. Number and Percent with Low Birthweight and Number of Live Births by Birthweight, by Age, Race, and Hispanic Origin of Mother, 2003

(Number.)

Age and race and Hispanic origin of mother	Low birthweight [1] Number	Low birthweight [1] Percent	Birthweight Total	Less than 500 grams	500–999 grams	1,000–1,499 grams	1,500–1,999 grams	2,000–2,499 grams	2,500–2,999 grams	3,000–3,499 grams	3,500–3,999 grams	4,000–4,499 grams	4,500–4,999 grams	5,000 grams or more	Not stated
All Races [2]															
All ages	324 064	7.9	4 089 950	6 307	22 980	29 930	63 791	201 056	711 003	1 557 864	1 131 577	309 721	46 690	5 431	3 600
Under 15 years	848	12.7	6 661	32	85	87	149	495	1 698	2 694	1 220	179	14	1	7
15–19 years	40 211	9.7	414 580	804	3 152	3 637	7 462	25 156	92 531	169 390	91 699	18 154	2 014	178	403
15 years	2 103	11.5	18 238	50	191	210	412	1 240	4 423	7 548	3 524	553	59	2	26
16 years	4 402	10.7	41 344	77	381	414	825	2 705	9 843	16 996	8 390	1 502	146	19	46
17 years	7 549	10.1	74 802	161	622	670	1 383	4 713	16 990	30 720	16 087	3 053	295	32	76
18 years	11 268	9.6	117 750	234	858	981	2 066	7 129	26 522	48 060	26 044	5 127	574	43	112
19 years	14 889	9.2	162 446	282	1 100	1 362	2 776	9 369	34 753	66 066	37 654	7 919	940	82	143
20–24 years	82 494	8.0	1 032 305	1 604	5 732	7 084	15 167	52 907	199 835	412 228	264 313	63 142	8 526	878	889
25–29 years	76 631	7.1	1 086 366	1 522	5 399	6 943	14 862	47 905	178 150	415 463	314 316	86 511	12 886	1 477	932
30–34 years	71 477	7.3	975 546	1 454	4 944	6 822	14 636	43 621	148 022	357 144	293 569	88 696	14 155	1 701	782
35–39 years	40 550	8.7	467 642	685	2 863	4 059	8 797	24 146	72 708	164 600	137 185	43 764	7 397	991	447
40–44 years	10 655	10.6	101 005	194	730	1 151	2 403	6 177	16 858	34 639	27 995	8 908	1 626	198	126
45–54 years	1 198	20.5	5 845	12	75	147	315	649	1 201	1 706	1 280	367	72	7	14
White Total [3]															
All ages	223 612	6.9	3 225 848	3 593	14 096	20 173	44 419	141 331	511 317	1 220 632	951 782	270 180	41 156	4 664	2 505
Under 15 years	378	10.3	3 677	8	41	42	68	219	838	1 573	752	124	10	1	1
15–19 years	24 774	8.3	298 347	409	1 771	2 193	4 604	15 797	61 144	123 409	72 095	14 884	1 666	138	237
15 years	1 107	9.6	11 484	26	93	107	221	660	2 503	4 899	2 522	396	45	2	10
16 years	2 536	9.0	28 151	30	199	247	482	1 578	6 120	11 844	6 301	1 197	119	12	22
17 years	4 669	8.8	52 941	78	357	418	849	2 967	11 026	21 981	12 452	2 487	249	27	50
18 years	7 054	8.2	85 734	127	496	596	1 281	4 554	17 756	35 474	20 627	4 246	467	33	77
19 years	9 408	7.8	120 037	148	626	825	1 771	6 038	23 739	49 211	30 193	6 558	786	64	78
20–24 years	53 600	6.8	790 910	824	3 323	4 447	9 751	35 255	140 299	316 971	217 687	53 701	7 340	717	595
25–29 years	54 143	6.2	871 496	901	3 401	4 750	10 617	34 474	130 541	330 559	267 011	75 912	11 397	1 267	666
30–34 years	52 407	6.6	795 902	882	3 209	4 927	10 888	32 501	110 515	287 041	252 401	78 817	12 650	1 503	568
35–39 years	29 593	7.8	379 773	435	1 791	2 878	6 520	17 969	54 448	132 207	117 123	38 636	6 593	854	319
40–44 years	7 751	9.6	81 031	125	500	824	1 718	4 584	12 592	27 513	23 658	7 799	1 436	177	105
45–54 years	966	20.6	4 712	9	60	112	253	532	940	1 359	1 055	307	64	7	14
Non-Hispanic White															
All ages	163 331	7.0	2 321 904	2 529	9 998	14 882	32 915	103 007	356 232	858 305	700 819	206 407	31 570	3 415	1 825
Under 15 years	144	10.3	1 399	3	19	18	30	74	309	551	323	67	5	-	5
15–19 years	14 904	8.6	172 620	258	1 122	1 369	2 811	9 344	33 960	69 160	43 514	9 726	1 120	75	161
15 years	525	10.8	4 878	10	46	53	113	303	994	1 973	1 152	208	21	-	5
16 years	1 266	9.5	13 375	16	111	119	232	788	2 703	5 432	3 208	684	68	4	10
17 years	2 666	9.3	28 550	49	218	253	509	1 637	5 654	11 474	6 991	1 556	159	16	34
18 years	4 316	8.6	50 484	88	321	380	789	2 738	10 061	20 199	12 708	2 795	323	21	61
19 years	6 131	8.1	75 333	95	426	564	1 168	3 878	14 548	30 082	19 455	4 483	549	34	51
20–24 years	36 764	7.0	522 275	571	2 273	3 141	6 777	24 002	91 307	204 117	146 151	37 745	5 273	497	421
25–29 years	39 730	6.3	627 437	615	2 438	3 503	7 900	25 274	92 116	233 898	194 930	56 873	8 508	904	478
30–34 years	41 263	6.6	626 315	661	2 383	3 849	8 613	25 757	85 088	223 247	201 188	63 791	10 175	1 132	431
35–39 years	23 634	7.8	303 354	319	1 334	2 282	5 231	14 468	42 777	104 440	94 704	31 608	5 284	665	242
40–44 years	6 083	9.4	64 600	95	380	628	1 340	3 640	9 895	21 760	19 149	6 344	1 152	137	80
45–54 years	809	20.8	3 904	7	49	92	213	448	780	1 132	860	253	53	5	12
Black Total [3]															
All ages	80 088	13.4	599 847	2 427	7 765	8 204	15 654	46 038	143 176	228 356	117 889	25 428	3 546	504	860
Under 15 years	437	16.1	2 726	20	42	41	76	258	807	1 016	416	41	3	-	6
15–19 years	14 092	14.0	100 951	359	1 281	1 328	2 620	8 504	27 963	39 811	16 167	2 493	246	33	146
15 years	913	15.1	6 056	21	92	93	178	529	1 777	2 361	852	125	13	-	15
16 years	1 686	14.5	11 654	41	172	154	312	1 007	3 374	4 565	1 739	243	20	6	21
17 years	2 648	13.8	19 145	74	249	238	483	1 604	5 349	7 643	3 020	436	22	4	23
18 years	3 861	13.9	27 817	100	329	348	729	2 355	7 808	10 877	4 474	678	81	8	30
19 years	4 984	13.8	36 279	123	439	495	918	3 009	9 655	14 365	6 082	1 011	110	15	57
20–24 years	25 500	13.0	196 268	730	2 228	2 386	4 856	15 300	49 599	76 813	36 184	6 970	838	114	250
25–29 years	17 182	12.3	139 947	557	1 733	1 816	3 341	9 735	31 287	53 465	29 962	6 744	958	146	203
30–34 years	13 021	13.4	97 529	495	1 431	1 471	2 601	7 023	20 197	35 739	21 850	5 546	907	120	149
35–39 years	7 712	15.5	49 889	200	865	904	1 652	4 091	10 553	17 226	10 784	2 965	476	76	97
40–44 years	2 007	16.9	11 895	64	171	237	470	1 065	2 632	4 086	2 400	632	114	15	9
45–54 years	137	21.3	642	2	14	21	38	62	138	200	126	37	4	-	-

[1]Less than 2,500 grams (5 lb 8 oz).
[2]Includes races other than White and Black and origin not stated.
[3]Race and Hispanic origin are reported separately on the birth certificate. Data for persons of Hispanic origin are included in the data for each race group according to the mother's reported race.
- = Quantity zero.

Table I-45. Number and Percent with Low Birthweight and Number of Live Births by Birthweight, by Age, Race, and Hispanic Origin of Mother, 2003—*Continued*

(Number.)

Age and race and Hispanic origin of mother	Low birthweight [1] Number	Low birthweight [1] Percent	Total	Less than 500 grams	500–999 grams	1,000–1,499 grams	1,500–1,999 grams	2,000–2,499 grams	2,500–2,999 grams	3,000–3,499 grams	3,500–3,999 grams	4,000–4,499 grams	4,500–4,999 grams	5,000 grams or more	Not stated
Non-Hispanic Black															
All ages	77 947	13.6	576 033	2 350	7 575	7 998	15 211	44 813	138 440	218 901	112 139	23 992	3 340	484	790
Under 15 years	423	16.0	2 642	20	40	40	75	248	784	986	402	38	3	-	6
15–19 years	13 738	14.1	97 509	342	1 250	1 296	2 562	8 288	27 154	38 392	15 462	2 364	229	32	138
15 years	884	15.1	5 852	21	90	88	175	510	1 726	2 279	818	120	13	-	12
16 years	1 637	14.6	11 247	37	165	151	307	977	3 277	4 396	1 660	234	17	6	20
17 years	2 575	14.0	18 431	70	238	230	472	1 565	5 169	7 352	2 884	406	20	3	22
18 years	3 779	14.1	26 915	98	323	343	710	2 305	7 601	10 502	4 282	639	76	8	28
19 years	4 863	13.9	35 064	116	434	484	898	2 931	9 381	13 863	5 818	965	103	15	56
20–24 years	24 899	13.2	189 020	707	2 179	2 333	4 735	14 945	48 011	73 795	34 567	6 620	786	103	56
25–29 years	16 668	12.5	133 821	544	1 694	1 772	3 228	9 430	30 194	51 072	28 330	6 332	895	109	233
30–34 years	12 667	13.6	93 346	480	1 396	1 432	2 523	6 836	19 462	34 164	20 738	5 202	865	142	188
35–39 years	7 484	15.7	47 661	195	837	872	1 606	3 974	10 166	16 383	10 230	2 798	446	112	136
40–44 years	1 933	16.9	11 419	60	165	232	445	1 031	2 532	3 923	2 290	605	112	74	80
45–54 years	135	22.0	615	2	14	21	37	61	137	186	120	33	4	15	9
Hispanic [4]															
All ages	60 973	6.7	912 329	1 037	4 140	5 366	11 655	38 775	157 583	366 508	252 230	63 688	9 619	1 246	482
Under 15 years	244	10.4	2 356	5	24	24	36	155	556	1 045	444	61	5	-	1
15–19 years	10 120	7.9	128 524	160	669	853	1 834	6 604	27 891	55 455	29 109	5 255	565	60	69
15 years	610	9.0	6 818	16	50	60	110	374	1 552	3 021	1 409	194	25	2	5
16 years	1 303	8.6	15 151	15	91	129	256	812	3 520	6 566	3 163	524	57	8	10
17 years	2 054	8.2	24 986	28	147	171	348	1 360	5 533	10 756	5 573	952	93	11	14
18 years	2 791	7.8	35 927	40	174	226	503	1 848	7 866	15 574	8 050	1 472	146	12	16
19 years	3 362	7.4	45 642	61	207	267	617	2 210	9 420	19 538	10 914	2 113	244	27	24
20–24 years	17 173	6.3	273 311	254	1 075	1 339	3 052	11 453	50 176	114 882	72 521	16 079	2 105	225	150
25–29 years	14 624	5.9	246 361	274	975	1 266	2 780	9 329	38 964	97 748	72 557	19 065	2 921	364	118
30–34 years	11 122	6.6	169 054	209	813	1 075	2 277	6 748	25 497	63 815	50 866	14 839	2 460	370	85
35–39 years	5 914	7.8	75 801	104	455	601	1 272	3 482	11 665	27 649	22 118	6 939	1 281	190	45
40–44 years	1 641	10.2	16 172	29	119	190	374	929	2 692	5 689	4 432	1 399	272	35	12
45–54 years	135	18.0	750	2	10	18	30	75	142	225	183	51	10	2	2

[1]Less than 2,500 grams (5 lb 8 oz).
[4]May be of any race.
- = Quantity zero.

TABLE I-46. NUMBER AND PERCENT OF BIRTHS OF LOW BIRTHWEIGHT, BY RACE AND HISPANIC ORIGIN OF MOTHER, FOR EACH STATE AND TERRITORY, 2003

Low birthweight (newborns less than 5.5 pounds) was encountered least frequently in Alaska, Oregon, and Washington; these states had rates between 6.0 and 6.1 percent. Rates of 10 percent or more were reported for Mississippi (11.4 percent), the District of Columbia (10.9 percent), Louisiana (10.7 percent), South Carolina (10.1 percent), and Alabama (10.0 percent), as well as for Puerto Rico and the Virgin Islands.

For every state in which non-Hispanic Blacks could be separately identified, infants of this groups were found to have low birthweights more frequently than infants born to non-Hispanic Whites and Hispanics. Among states with at least 1,000 non-Hispanic Black births, the non-Hispanic Black low birthweight rate had lows in Minnesota (10.3 percent) and Washington State (11.1 percent), and highs in Colorado (15.7 percent) and Mississippi (15.2 percent). The low birthweight rate for Hispanics (in states with at least 1,000 Hispanic births) had lows in Minnesota (5.1 percent) and Oregon (5.3 percent) and highs in Pennsylvania (8.9 percent), Rhode Island (8.9 percent), and New Mexico (8.7 percent).

Table I-46. Number and Percent of Births of Low Birthweight, by Race and Hispanic Origin of Mother, for Each State and Territory, 2003

(Number, percent.)

State	Number						Percent					
	All races[1]	White		Black		Hispanic[3]	All races[1]	White		Black		Hispanic[3]
		Total[2]	Non-Hispanic	Total[2]	Non-Hispanic			Total[2]	Non-Hispanic	Total[2]	Non-Hispanic	
UNITED STATES[4]	324 064	223 612	163 331	80 088	77 947	60 973	7.9	6.9	7.0	13.4	13.6	6.7
Alabama	5 923	3 271	3 084	2 588	2 583	194	10.0	8.0	8.1	14.4	14.5	6.7
Alaska	600	369	255	39	24	39	6.0	5.7	5.2	9.7	9.1	5.1
Arizona	6 414	5 410	2 696	368	320	2 727	7.1	6.9	6.9	11.3	12.1	6.9
Arkansas	3 348	2 247	2 044	1 053	1 048	205	8.9	7.6	7.7	14.6	14.6	6.3
California	35 628	26 554	10 183	3 965	3 842	16 172	6.6	6.1	6.1	12.3	12.4	6.0
Colorado	6 224	5 432	3 720	457	439	1 783	9.0	8.6	8.8	15.6	15.7	8.3
Connecticut	3 218	2 435	1 791	617	600	651	7.5	6.9	6.4	11.9	12.5	8.6
Delaware	1 068	616	511	411	407	106	9.4	7.8	7.8	14.2	14.3	7.7
District of Columbia	833	136	113	677	627	73	10.9	6.5	6.1	12.9	13.7	7.6
Florida	18 007	11 231	7 532	6 206	6 103	3 791	8.5	7.1	7.2	13.1	13.2	6.9
Georgia	12 205	6 223	5 104	5 606	5 480	1 047	9.0	7.1	7.4	13.0	13.0	5.7
Hawaii	1 554	339	277	71	64	219	8.6	6.7	6.5	12.2	13.3	8.4
Idaho	1 413	1 363	1 163	8	8	191	6.5	6.5	6.5	*	*	6.5
Illinois	15 081	9 780	7 098	4 546	4 518	2 709	8.3	6.9	7.1	14.4	14.4	6.4
Indiana	6 767	5 404	4 993	1 239	1 236	400	7.9	7.2	7.3	13.1	13.3	5.9
Iowa	2 512	2 242	2 087	168	168	155	6.6	6.3	6.3	13.1	13.3	6.2
Kansas	2 908	2 406	2 068	354	349	334	7.4	6.9	7.1	12.8	12.8	6.1
Kentucky	4 809	4 071	3 949	660	659	121	8.7	8.2	8.3	13.6	13.7	6.2
Louisiana	6 944	2 885	2 760	3 910	3 901	133	10.7	7.7	7.7	14.9	14.9	7.9
Maine	904	874	863	13	13	10	6.5	6.5	6.6	*	*	*
Maryland	6 782	3 148	2 766	3 250	3 145	490	9.1	7.0	7.1	12.7	13.0	7.0
Massachusetts	6 095	4 745	4 024	903	773	812	7.6	7.2	7.0	10.5	11.8	8.3
Michigan	10 706	7 134	6 473	3 171	3 149	504	8.2	6.9	6.9	14.1	14.1	6.6
Minnesota	4 374	3 430	3 152	550	539	252	6.2	5.8	5.8	10.3	10.3	5.1
Mississippi	4 846	1 988	1 948	2 825	2 825	39	11.4	8.6	8.6	15.2	15.2	7.2
Missouri	6 169	4 538	4 340	1 492	1 473	214	8.0	7.1	7.2	13.4	13.4	6.1
Montana	776	650	606	7	7	35	6.8	6.6	6.5	*	*	9.2
Nebraska	1 792	1 547	1 318	168	166	212	6.9	6.6	6.8	11.5	11.5	6.1
Nevada	2 716	2 053	1 204	381	366	855	8.1	7.4	7.7	13.1	13.3	7.0
New Hampshire	895	832	772	26	21	31	6.2	6.1	6.1	10.7	12.2	5.9
New Jersey	9 498	6 095	4 350	2 543	2 345	1 935	8.1	7.1	7.0	12.6	13.3	7.3
New Mexico	2 346	1 984	707	82	75	1 288	8.5	8.5	8.2	15.6	16.0	8.7
New York	19 985	12 534	8 745	5 748	5 347	4 124	7.9	6.8	6.6	12.0	12.2	7.5
North Carolina	10 631	6 348	5 368	3 852	3 837	990	9.0	7.3	7.6	14.2	14.2	6.2
North Dakota	517	436	417	10	9	8	6.5	6.3	6.4	*	*	*
Ohio	12 477	9 124	8 727	3 060	3 021	387	8.3	7.4	7.4	13.5	13.6	7.2
Oklahoma	3 951	2 913	2 579	632	621	347	7.8	7.3	7.5	13.7	13.6	6.1
Oregon	2 822	2 470	2 018	119	113	449	6.1	5.9	6.1	11.7	11.6	5.3
Pennsylvania	11 718	8 278	7 464	2 985	2 629	960	8.1	7.0	6.9	13.7	14.0	8.9
Rhode Island	1 127	891	566	149	137	221	8.5	8.0	7.8	11.9	12.3	8.9
South Carolina	5 595	2 758	2 533	2 750	2 740	235	10.1	7.6	7.8	15.0	15.0	6.4
South Dakota	732	581	552	9	9	32	6.6	6.5	6.4	*	*	9.4
Tennessee	7 380	4 858	4 565	2 404	2 391	302	9.4	8.0	8.1	14.8	14.8	6.1
Texas	29 745	22 937	10 054	5 692	5 631	12 886	7.9	7.1	7.3	13.6	13.7	7.0
Utah	3 260	3 054	2 556	58	52	496	6.5	6.5	6.4	15.2	15.3	7.0
Vermont	460	451	445	2	2	4	7.0	7.1	7.1	*	*	*
Virginia	8 297	4 890	4 287	2 887	2 835	652	8.2	6.8	6.9	12.8	13.0	6.3
Washington	4 843	3 756	3 001	404	338	744	6.0	5.7	5.6	10.1	11.1	5.6
West Virginia	1 808	1 705	1 686	86	86	10	8.6	8.5	8.5	12.0	12.1	*
Wisconsin	4 764	3 638	3 314	884	873	341	6.8	6.0	6.0	13.6	13.6	6.2
Wyoming	597	558	503	3	3	58	8.9	8.9	8.9	*	*	8.7
Puerto Rico	5 815	5 266	. . .	545	. . .	. . .	11.5	11.4	. . .	11.9	. . .	. . .
Virgin Islands	164	28	6	134	103	32	10.8	8.0	*	11.7	11.3	9.4
Guam	301	13	11	2	2	2	9.2	*	*	*	. . .	. . .
American Samoa	67	-	. . .	-	. . .	. . .	4.2	*	. . .	*	. . .	. . .
Northern Marianas	103	-	. . .	-	. . .	. . .	7.6	. . .	. . .	. . .	. . .	. . .

Note: Low birthweight is birthweight of less than 2,500 grams (5 lb 8 oz).

[1]Includes races other than White and Black and origin not stated.
[2]Race and Hispanic origin are reported separately on the birth certificate. Data for persons of Hispanic origin are included in the data for each race group according to the mother's reported race.
[3]May be of any race.
[4]Excludes data for the territories.
* = Figure does not meet standards of reliability or precision; based on fewer than 20 births in numerator.
- = Quantity zero.
. . . = Not available.

TABLE I-47. NUMBER AND PERCENT OF BIRTHS OF VERY LOW BIRTHWEIGHT, BY RACE AND HISPANIC ORIGIN OF MOTHER, FOR EACH STATE AND TERRITORY, 2003

For non-Hispanic White and Hispanic mothers, the rate of very low birthweight (less than 3.25 pounds) averaged 1.2 percent nationally in 2003; for non-Hispanic Blacks, this rate was 3.1 percent. The highest rates across all races in the United States (not including territories) were 2.2 percent in the District of Columbia and Mississippi and 2.1 percent in South Carolina. The lowest rates were recorded in Alaska, at 0.9 percent, and Idaho, Utah, Oregon, and Washington, all at 1.0 percent.

Table I-47. Number and Percent of Births of Very Low Birthweight, by Race and Hispanic Origin of Mother, for Each State and Territory, 2003

(Number, percent.)

| State | Number | | | | | | Percent | | | | | |
| | All races [1] | White | | Black | | Hispanic [3] | All races [1] | White | | Black | | Hispanic [3] |
		Total [2]	Non-Hispanic	Total [2]	Non-Hispanic			Total [2]	Non-Hispanic	Total [2]	Non-Hispanic	
UNITED STATES [4]	59 217	37 862	27 409	18 396	17 923	10 543	1.4	1.2	1.2	3.1	3.1	1.2
Alabama	1 197	568	530	622	620	39	2.0	1.4	1.4	3.5	3.5	1.3
Alaska	95	57	31	4	2	5	0.9	0.9	0.6	*	*	*
Arizona	994	837	429	66	63	415	1.1	1.1	1.1	2.0	2.4	1.0
Arkansas	610	373	346	229	229	27	1.6	1.3	1.3	3.2	3.2	0.8
California	6 293	4 694	1 726	842	810	2 929	1.2	1.1	1.0	2.6	2.6	1.1
Colorado	890	757	499	98	93	267	1.3	1.2	1.2	3.4	3.3	1.2
Connecticut	626	441	323	161	160	118	1.5	1.2	1.2	3.1	3.3	1.6
Delaware	231	121	101	102	102	20	2.0	1.5	1.5	3.5	3.6	1.4
District of Columbia	169	21	14	144	140	12	2.2	1.0	*	2.7	3.1	*
Florida	3 292	1 847	1 185	1 355	1 331	678	1.6	1.2	1.1	2.9	2.9	1.2
Georgia	2 373	1 030	839	1 290	1 251	184	1.7	1.2	1.2	3.0	3.0	1.0
Hawaii	252	51	40	19	19	46	1.4	1.0	0.9	*	*	1.8
Idaho	224	214	180	1	1	32	1.0	1.0	1.0	*	*	1.1
Illinois	2 914	1 741	1 265	1 062	1 056	479	1.6	1.2	1.3	3.4	3.4	1.1
Indiana	1 211	895	834	301	301	59	1.4	1.2	1.2	3.2	3.2	0.9
Iowa	436	395	361	34	34	34	1.1	1.1	1.1	2.6	2.7	1.4
Kansas	441	356	303	71	71	55	1.1	1.0	1.0	2.6	2.6	1.0
Kentucky	847	688	670	148	148	18	1.5	1.4	1.4	3.1	3.1	*
Louisiana	1 398	455	438	919	915	20	2.2	1.2	1.2	3.5	3.5	1.2
Maine	159	157	152	2	2	5	1.1	1.2	1.2	*	*	*
Maryland	1 386	536	462	812	794	90	1.9	1.2	1.2	3.2	3.3	1.3
Massachusetts	1 093	815	690	216	189	130	1.4	1.2	1.2	2.5	2.9	1.3
Michigan	2 155	1 332	1 210	771	764	99	1.6	1.3	1.3	3.4	3.4	1.3
Minnesota	742	563	508	118	115	46	1.1	0.9	0.9	2.2	2.2	0.9
Mississippi	952	314	305	633	633	9	2.2	1.4	1.3	3.4	3.4	*
Missouri	1 215	811	770	380	375	45	1.6	1.3	1.3	3.4	3.4	1.3
Montana	120	100	90	1	1	6	1.1	1.0	1.0	*	*	*
Nebraska	310	261	223	37	36	37	1.2	1.1	1.1	2.5	2.5	1.1
Nevada	431	314	194	74	72	117	1.3	1.1	1.2	2.6	2.6	1.0
New Hampshire	165	150	138	9	8	7	1.1	1.1	1.1	*	*	*
New Jersey	1 840	1 101	751	629	586	390	1.6	1.3	1.2	3.1	3.3	1.5
New Mexico	318	263	119	14	12	146	1.1	1.1	1.4	*	*	1.0
New York	3 846	2 207	1 468	1 385	1 299	792	1.5	1.2	1.1	2.9	3.0	1.4
North Carolina	2 099	1 111	927	924	922	185	1.8	1.3	1.3	3.4	3.4	1.2
North Dakota	86	74	70	4	4	1	1.1	1.1	1.1	*	*	*
Ohio	2 325	1 545	1 462	729	717	77	1.6	1.3	1.2	3.2	3.2	1.4
Oklahoma	608	433	378	117	114	58	1.2	1.1	1.1	2.5	2.5	1.0
Oregon	465	417	339	24	23	76	1.0	1.0	1.0	2.4	2.4	0.9
Pennsylvania	2 252	1 524	1 336	671	583	201	1.5	1.3	1.2	3.1	3.1	1.9
Rhode Island	227	179	115	30	27	42	1.7	1.6	1.6	2.4	2.4	1.7
South Carolina	1 149	507	470	628	625	40	2.1	1.4	1.4	3.4	3.4	1.1
South Dakota	120	92	85	1	1	7	1.1	1.0	1.0	*	*	*
Tennessee	1 316	778	738	521	517	44	1.7	1.3	1.3	3.2	3.2	0.9
Texas	5 121	3 734	1 680	1 237	1 231	2 053	1.4	1.2	1.2	3.0	3.0	1.1
Utah	516	479	395	14	13	84	1.0	1.0	1.0	*	*	1.2
Vermont	75	74	73	1	1	1	1.1	1.2	1.2	*	*	*
Virginia	1 590	869	773	643	635	104	1.6	1.2	1.2	2.8	2.9	1.0
Washington	790	613	485	73	52	128	1.0	0.9	0.9	1.8	1.7	1.0
West Virginia	282	264	261	14	14	1	1.3	1.3	1.3	*	*	*
Wisconsin	897	639	572	215	211	76	1.3	1.1	1.0	3.3	3.3	1.4
Wyoming	74	65	56	1	1	9	1.1	1.0	1.0	*	*	*
Puerto Rico	706	618	. . .	88	. . .	. . .	1.4	1.3	. . .	1.9	. . .	. . .
Virgin Islands	37	6	-	30	19	5	2.4	*	*	2.6	. . .	. . .
Guam	45	2	2	-	-	-	1.4	*	*	*	*	*
American Samoa	10	-	. . .	-	. . .	. . .	*	*	*	*	. . .	. . .
Northern Marianas	9	-	. . .	-	. . .	. . .	*	*	. . .	*	. . .	. . .

Note: Very low birthweight is birthweight of less than 1,500 grams (3lb 4oz).

[1]Includes races other than White and Black and origin not stated.
[2]Race and Hispanic origin are reported separately on the birth certificate. Data for persons of Hispanic origin are included in the data for each race group according to the mother's reported race.
[3]May be of any race.
[4]Excludes data for the territories.
* = Figure does not meet standards of reliability or precision; based on fewer than 20 births in numerator.
- = Quantity zero.
. . . = Not available.

For non-Hispanic Whites, the smallest rate of very low birthweight was in Alaska (0.6 percent), and the highest rates were in Rhode Island (1.6 percent) and Delaware (1.5 percent). For non-Hispanic Blacks, the lowest rates were in Washington (1.7 percent), Oregon (2.4 percent), and Rhode Island (2.4 percent); while the highest rates were in Delaware (3.6 percent), Louisiana (3.5 percent), and Alabama (3.5 percent). For Hispanics, the lowest rate was recorded in Arkansas (0.8 percent), and the highest rates were in Pennsylvania (1.9 percent), Hawaii (1.8 percent), and Rhode Island (1.7 percent). Hispanics residing in the Northeast, including in New Jersey, New York, and Pennsylvania, generally had relatively high rates of very low birthweight, possibly associated with the sizable presence of residents of Puerto Rican origin.

TABLE I-48. LIVE BIRTHS WITH SELECTED ABNORMAL CONDITIONS OF THE NEWBORN AND RATES, BY AGE AND RACE OF MOTHER: UNITED STATES EXCLUDING PENNSYLVANIA AND WASHINGTON STATE, 2003

Eight abnormal conditions are reported on the birth cer-

tificate. Every year (since the beginning of data collection in 1989), the three most frequently reported conditions have been assisted ventilation less than 30 minutes, assisted ventilation 30 minutes or longer, and hyaline membrane disease/respiratory distress syndrome. There may be underreporting of abnormal conditions on the birth certificate, especially for conditions difficult to identify at birth, such as fetal alcohol syndrome. In 2003, the rate for assisted ventilation of less than 30 minutes was 21.4 per 1,000 births, nearly twice the rate in 1989. The rate of assisted ventilation 30 minutes or longer was 9.3 per 1,000 births, which was not significantly different from the 2002 rate, although this rate has increased gradually since 1989. The rate for hyaline membrane disease/respiratory distress syndrome (a frequent cause of morbidity in preterm infants) was 6.0 per 1,000 births in 2003; this rate has been declining since the mid-1990s. Since 1989, the rate for meconium aspiration syndrome has slowly decreased and the rate for anemia has decreased by 50 percent. Both conditions were more common in Blacks than Whites, while birth injury was reported more frequently in Whites.

Table I-48. Live Births with Selected Abnormal Conditions of the Newborn and Rates, by Age and Race of Mother: United States Excluding Pennsylvania and Washington State, 2003

(Number, rate of live births with specified abnormal condition per 1,000 live births in specified group.)

Abnormal condition and race of mother	All births [1]	Abnormal condition reported	Rate by age of mother							Not stated [2]
			All ages	Under 20 years	20–24 years	25–29 years	30–34 years	35–39 years	40–54 years	
All Races [3]										
Anemia	3 863 502	3 604	0.9	1.0	0.9	0.9	0.9	1.0	1.2	22 046
Birth injury [4]	3 460 109	9 774	2.8	3.1	3.0	2.8	2.9	2.4	2.5	21 979
Fetal alcohol syndrome [5]	3 793 462	132	0.0	*	0.0	0.0	0.0	0.0	*	21 963
Hyaline membrane disease/RDS	3 863 502	23 214	6.0	6.6	6.3	5.8	5.7	6.1	6.9	22 046
Meconium aspiration syndrome	3 863 502	4 788	1.2	1.5	1.4	1.2	1.1	1.2	1.5	22 046
Assisted ventilation less than 30 minutes [6]	3 743 733	79 727	21.4	21.6	20.3	20.8	22.2	23.1	24.1	21 364
Assisted ventilation 30 minutes or longer [6]	3 743 733	34 699	9.3	10.8	9.2	8.6	8.9	10.1	12.0	21 364
Seizures	3 863 502	1 755	0.5	0.5	0.5	0.4	0.4	0.4	0.6	22 046
White										
Anemia	3 040 873	2 668	0.9	0.9	0.8	0.9	0.9	1.0	1.1	18 133
Birth injury [4]	2 695 955	8 043	3.0	3.4	3.2	3.0	3.0	2.5	2.5	18 081
Fetal alcohol syndrome [5]	2 980 629	90	0.0	*	*	*	0.0	*	*	18 053
Hyaline membrane disease/RDS	3 040 873	18 626	6.2	6.5	6.3	6.0	5.9	6.3	7.1	18 133
Meconium aspiration syndrome	3 040 873	3 583	1.2	1.5	1.4	1.1	1.1	1.0	1.5	18 133
Assisted ventilation less than 30 minutes [6]	2 971 066	64 570	21.9	21.6	20.4	21.2	22.9	23.9	24.8	17 639
Assisted ventilation 30 minutes or longer [6]	2 971 066	26 782	9.1	10.3	8.9	8.5	8.8	9.8	12.1	17 639
Seizures	3 040 873	1 415	0.5	0.5	0.5	0.5	0.4	0.4	0.6	18 133
Black										
Anemia	573 776	724	1.3	1.0	1.1	1.3	1.5	1.5	1.8	2 356
Birth injury [4]	530 423	897	1.7	1.8	1.8	1.6	1.6	1.7	*	2 345
Fetal alcohol syndrome [5]	567 282	28	0.0	*	*	*	*	*	*	2 355
Hyaline membrane disease/RDS	573 776	3 702	6.5	6.9	6.6	5.9	6.4	7.0	6.7	2 356
Meconium aspiration syndrome	573 776	909	1.6	1.5	1.4	1.7	1.6	2.1	1.8	2 356
Assisted ventilation less than 30 minutes [6]	540 060	11 323	21.1	22.1	20.4	20.5	20.9	22.7	23.5	2 274
Assisted ventilation 30 minutes or longer [6]	540 060	6 309	11.7	12.0	11.1	10.9	12.5	14.2	13.0	2 274
Seizures	573 776	247	0.4	0.4	0.4	0.4	0.4	0.5	*	2 356

Note: Excludes data for Pennsylvania and Washington State, which implemented a forthcoming revision in the standard birth certificate and thus impaired comparability with the data from other states.

[1]Total number of births to residents of areas reporting specified abnormal condition.
[2]No response reported for the abnormal condition item.
[3]Includes races other than White and Black.
[4]Nebraska and Texas do not report this condition.
[5]Wisconsin does not report this condition.
[6]New York City does not report this condition.
0.0 = Quantity more than zero but less than 0.05.
* = Figure does not meet standards of reliability or precision; based on fewer than 20 births in numerator.

TABLE I-49. LIVE BIRTHS WITH SELECTED CONGENITAL ANOMALIES AND RATES, BY AGE AND RACE OF MOTHER: UNITED STATES EXCLUDING NEW MEXICO, 2003

Twenty-one types of malformations are reported on the birth certificate. Some of these are underreported due to difficulties of detection at birth. These anomalies are rare, but together they remain the leading causes of infant death. The most frequent among them are heart malformations (128.9 per 100,000 births), other circulatory/respiratory anomalies (126.1 per 100,000 births), and other musculoskeletal/integumental anomalies (208.2 per 100,000 births).

Table I-49. Live Births with Selected Congenital Anomalies and Rates, by Age and Race of Mother: United States Excluding New Mexico, 2003

(Number, rate of live births with specified congenital anomaly per 100,000 live births in specified group.)

Congenital anomaly and race of mother	All births [1]	Congenital anomaly reported	Rate by age of mother							Not stated [2]
			All ages	Under 20 years	20–24 years	25–29 years	30–34 years	35–39 years	40–54 years	
All Races [3]										
Anencephalus	4 062 129	460	11.4	14.0	12.7	10.1	12.5	8.0	*	20 877
Spina bifida/meningocele	4 062 129	755	18.7	18.3	20.6	19.7	16.2	15.8	26.5	20 877
Hydrocephalus	3 835 681	847	22.2	28.4	23.5	20.5	20.9	20.1	24.2	22 705
Microcephalus	3 835 681	214	5.6	6.6	5.7	4.6	4.7	7.6	*	22 705
Other central nervous system anomalies	3 835 681	803	21.1	21.5	21.2	19.6	18.7	27.7	25.2	22 705
Heart malformation	3 835 681	4 916	128.9	107.6	118.9	123.1	131.9	150.9	247.4	22 705
Other circulatory/respiratory anomalies	3 835 681	4 807	126.1	113.5	121.1	115.4	123.2	158.1	220.1	22 705
Rectal atresia/stenosis	3 835 681	298	7.8	6.1	8.6	6.7	7.6	9.5	*	22 705
Tracheoesophageal fistula/esophageal atresia	3 835 681	411	10.8	11.6	10.7	10.9	8.1	13.8	*	22 705
Omphalocele/gastroschisis	4 062 129	1 313	32.5	84.4	47.8	20.9	15.3	16.9	24.6	20 877
Other gastrointestinal anomalies	3 835 681	1 259	33.0	40.8	33.4	31.2	28.0	35.3	52.5	22 705
Malformed genitalia	3 835 681	3 038	79.7	72.9	76.5	84.4	78.8	82.4	84.8	22 705
Renal agenesis	3 835 681	533	14.0	14.2	13.8	13.3	15.7	12.5	*	22 705
Other urogenital anomalies	3 835 681	3 438	90.2	79.5	84.3	87.2	95.9	104.8	104.0	22 705
Cleft lip/palate	4 062 129	3 066	75.9	73.8	86.4	76.4	64.4	73.3	92.9	22 705
Polydactyly/syndactyly/adactyly	3 835 681	2 915	76.4	102.1	87.8	72.5	63.8	60.9	87.8	20 877
Clubfoot	3 835 681	2 198	57.6	64.6	65.3	58.4	49.0	51.2	55.5	22 705
Diaphragmatic hernia	3 835 681	436	11.4	9.1	10.8	12.0	11.0	14.1	*	22 705
Other musculoskeletal/integumental anomalies	3 835 681	7 937	208.2	248.4	222.5	202.6	190.0	186.9	223.1	22 705
Down's syndrome	4 062 129	1 881	46.5	25.1	26.0	26.1	37.4	111.6	336.5	20 877
Other chromosomal anomalies	3 835 681	1 147	30.1	21.5	22.7	24.1	26.8	54.2	122.2	22 705
White										
Anencephalus	3 202 564	364	11.4	13.8	12.3	11.0	12.1	8.5	*	16 132
Spina bifida/meningocele	3 202 564	630	19.8	20.5	20.5	21.0	17.5	17.8	27.2	16 132
Hydrocephalus	3 017 589	660	22.0	29.3	23.8	19.9	20.5	20.0	*	18 140
Microcephalus	3 017 589	148	4.9	*	5.0	4.1	3.8	7.1	*	18 140
Other central nervous system anomalies	3 017 589	642	21.4	20.5	21.9	20.0	19.3	27.1	29.0	18 140
Heart malformation	3 017 589	3 688	123.0	102.5	113.1	117.8	125.2	142.1	234.8	18 140
Other circulatory/respiratory anomalies	3 017 589	3 759	125.3	115.6	124.5	112.5	119.5	155.2	220.9	18 140
Rectal atresia/stenosis	3 017 589	251	8.4	*	8.5	7.3	8.3	10.8	*	18 140
Tracheoesophageal fistula/esophageal atresia	3 017 589	350	11.7	14.1	10.8	12.3	8.3	14.5	*	18 140
Omphalocele/gastroschisis	3 202 564	1 039	32.6	96.3	48.7	20.7	15.2	15.7	*	16 132
Other gastrointestinal anomalies	3 017 589	1 002	33.4	41.0	35.4	30.8	29.0	34.8	48.0	18 140
Malformed genitalia	3 017 589	2 543	84.8	76.7	81.4	89.8	83.4	89.9	83.3	18 140
Renal agenesis	3 017 589	438	14.6	16.6	14.1	13.1	16.6	13.7	*	18 140
Other urogenital anomalies	3 017 589	2 855	95.2	85.6	89.2	90.4	99.9	115.0	103.5	18 140
Cleft lip/palate	3 202 564	2 617	82.1	85.8	97.2	83.0	67.7	74.6	89.8	16 132
Polydactyly/syndactyly/adactyly	3 017 589	1 620	54.0	64.0	59.7	51.4	50.3	44.8	66.9	18 140
Clubfoot	3 017 589	1 872	62.4	72.1	71.7	61.9	53.6	57.1	51.7	18 140
Diaphragmatic hernia	3 017 589	366	12.2	9.9	12.0	12.8	11.7	14.3	*	18 140
Other musculoskeletal/integumental anomalies	3 017 589	5 152	171.8	206.1	180.7	168.1	157.4	158.6	194.4	18 140
Down's syndrome	3 202 564	1 631	51.2	30.0	27.3	28.7	41.0	120.9	360.3	16 132
Other chromosomal anomalies	3 017 589	916	30.5	22.6	24.4	21.3	27.1	57.3	123.7	18 140
Black										
Anencephalus	599 315	61	10.2	*	12.3	*	*	*	*	2 532
Spina bifida/meningocele	599 315	95	15.9	*	21.0	16.5	*	*	*	2 532
Hydrocephalus	573 244	144	25.2	24.4	24.6	25.5	26.9	*	*	2 613
Microcephalus	573 244	51	8.9	*	*	*	*	*	*	2 613
Other central nervous system anomalies	573 244	112	19.6	24.4	14.4	19.5	*	*	*	2 613
Heart malformation	573 244	915	160.3	119.9	135.8	168.3	195.0	208.9	327.8	2 613
Other circulatory/respiratory anomalies	573 244	677	118.6	104.6	98.4	120.9	137.9	162.5	201.7	2 613
Rectal atresia/stenosis	573 244	33	5.8	*	*	*	*	*	*	2 613
Tracheoesophageal fistula/esophageal atresia	573 244	43	7.5	*	*	*	*	*	*	2 613
Omphalocele/gastroschisis	599 315	224	37.5	54.2	42.5	26.6	23.7	*	*	2 532
Other gastrointestinal anomalies	573 244	189	33.1	36.6	27.3	36.8	23.7	46.4	*	2 613
Malformed genitalia	573 244	323	56.6	59.9	56.2	57.1	51.7	54.9	*	2 613
Renal agenesis	573 244	67	11.7	*	11.8	16.5	*	*	*	2 613
Other urogenital anomalies	573 244	358	62.7	54.9	56.2	69.9	73.3	57.0	*	2 613
Cleft lip/palate	599 315	244	40.9	28.1	36.9	43.1	45.4	48.4	*	2 532
Polydactyly/syndactyly/adactyly	573 244	1 181	207.0	211.3	209.1	212.6	195.0	189.9	235.3	2 613
Clubfoot	573 244	238	41.7	43.7	44.9	45.1	31.2	*	*	2 613
Diaphragmatic hernia	573 244	52	9.1	*	*	*	*	*	*	2 613
Other musculoskeletal/integumental anomalies	573 244	2 291	401.5	375.9	386.7	421.4	417.0	405.1	487.5	2 613
Down's syndrome	599 315	168	28.2	*	21.0	15.8	22.7	76.6	265.0	2 532
Other chromosomal anomalies	573 244	163	28.6	*	17.6	38.3	32.3	*	*	2 613

Note: Excludes data for New Mexico, which did not report congenital anomalies.

[1] Total number of births to residents of areas reporting specified congenital anomaly.
[2] No response reported for the congenital anomalies item.
[3] Includes races other than White and Black.
* = Figure does not meet standards of reliability or precision; based on fewer than 20 births in numerator.

Studies have found a positive association between maternal smoking and certain birth defects, including cleft lip/palate and clubfoot. Since 1998, there has been mandatory fortification of cereal and grain products with folic acid in a successful effort to reduce spina bifida and anencephalus. By 2002, the rate for anencephalus had decreased to 9.9 per 100,000 births; this rate increased to 11.4 per 100,000 births in 2003. The spina bifida/meningocele rate was 18.7 per 100,000 births in 2003, compared with a rate of 20.0 for 2002. This rate also declined between 1997 and 2003.

Rates for Down's syndrome, heart malformations, and other circulatory/respiratory anomalies increase significantly for infants of mothers over 34 years of age.

Maternal age-specific rates for Down's syndrome are lower among Blacks than Whites. By contrast, rates for polydactyly/syndactyly/adactyly (digit abnormalities) and other musculoskeletal/integumental anomalies are markedly higher among Blacks.

TABLE I-50. NUMBER AND RATE OF LIVE BIRTHS, BY PLURALITY OF BIRTH, AGE, RACE, AND HISPANIC ORIGIN OF MOTHER, 2003

There has been an upsurge in multiple births over the last two decades. This is associated with two related trends: greater access to fertility therapies and an increase in childbearing among women in their thirties and forties (who are more likely to have multiple births

Table I-50. Number and Rate of Live Births, by Plurality of Birth, Age, Race, and Hispanic Origin of Mother, 2003

(Number, rate.)

Plurality and race and Hispanic origin of mother	All ages	Under 15 years	15–19 years Total	15–17 years	18–19 years	20–24 years	25–29 years	30–34 years	35–39 years	40–44 years	45–54 years
NUMBER											
All Live Births											
All races [1]	4 089 950	6 661	414 580	134 384	280 196	1 032 305	1 086 366	975 546	467 642	101 005	5 845
White total [2]	3 225 848	3 677	298 347	92 576	205 771	790 910	871 496	795 902	379 773	81 031	4 712
Non-Hispanic White	2 321 904	1 399	172 620	46 803	125 817	522 275	627 437	626 315	303 354	64 600	3 904
Black total [2]	599 847	2 726	100 951	36 855	64 096	196 268	139 947	97 529	49 889	11 895	642
Non-Hispanic Black	576 033	2 642	97 509	35 530	61 979	189 020	133 821	93 346	47 661	11 419	615
Hispanic [3]	912 329	2 356	128 524	46 955	81 569	273 311	246 361	169 054	75 801	16 172	750
Live Births in Single Deliveries											
All races [1]	3 953 622	6 588	408 155	132 574	275 581	1 008 698	1 052 490	934 283	443 355	95 493	4 560
White total [2]	3 117 818	3 646	294 172	91 462	202 710	774 749	844 743	761 360	359 261	76 293	3 594
Non-Hispanic White	2 234 291	1 389	170 035	46 168	123 867	510 878	606 336	596 838	285 449	60 464	2 902
Black total [2]	578 564	2 684	98 908	36 224	62 684	189 610	134 532	93 244	47 536	11 492	558
Non-Hispanic Black	555 392	2 605	95 521	34 923	60 598	182 516	128 575	89 208	45 399	11 037	531
Hispanic [3]	892 073	2 332	126 892	46 454	80 438	268 472	240 679	164 105	73 291	15 631	671
Live Births in Twin Deliveries											
All races [1]	128 665	73	6 371	1 794	4 577	23 107	32 150	38 248	22 372	5 178	1 166
White total [2]	101 297	31	4 134	1 101	3 033	15 801	25 270	31 812	18 773	4 463	1 013
Non-Hispanic White	81 691	10	2 565	628	1 937	11 115	19 805	27 041	16 356	3 890	909
Black total [2]	20 633	42	2 032	628	1 404	6 538	5 231	4 114	2 234	369	73
Non-Hispanic Black	20 010	37	1 977	604	1 373	6 390	5 067	3 975	2 143	348	73
Hispanic [3]	19 472	24	1 611	495	1 116	4 761	5 492	4 673	2 326	515	70
Live Births in Higher Order Multiple Deliveries [4]											
All races [1]	7 663	-	54	16	38	500	1 726	3 015	1 915	334	119
White total [2]	6 733	-	41	13	28	360	1 483	2 730	1 739	275	105
Non-Hispanic White	5 922	-	20	7	13	282	1 296	2 436	1 549	246	93
Black total [2]	650	-	11	3	8	120	184	171	119	34	11
Non-Hispanic Black	631	-	11	3	8	114	179	163	119	34	11
Hispanic [3]	784	-	21	6	15	78	190	276	184	26	9
RATE PER 1,000 LIVE BIRTHS											
All Multiple Births											
All races [1]	33.3	11.0	15.5	13.5	16.5	22.9	31.2	42.3	51.9	54.6	219.8
White total [2]	33.5	8.4	14.0	12.0	14.9	20.4	30.7	43.4	54.0	58.5	237.3
Non-Hispanic White	37.7	*	15.0	13.6	15.5	21.8	33.6	47.1	59.0	64.0	256.7
Black total [2]	35.5	15.4	20.2	17.1	22.0	33.9	38.7	43.9	47.2	33.9	130.8
Non-Hispanic Black	35.8	14.0	20.4	17.1	22.3	34.4	39.2	44.3	47.5	33.5	136.6
Hispanic [3]	22.2	10.2	12.7	10.7	13.9	17.7	23.1	29.3	33.1	33.5	105.3
Twin Births											
All races [1]	31.5	11.0	15.4	13.3	13.3	22.4	29.6	39.2	47.8	51.3	199.5
White total [2]	31.4	8.4	13.9	11.9	11.9	20.0	29.0	40.0	49.4	55.1	215.0
Non-Hispanic White	35.2	*	14.9	13.4	13.4	21.3	31.6	43.2	53.9	60.2	232.8
Black total [2]	34.4	15.4	20.1	17.0	17.0	33.3	37.4	42.2	44.8	31.0	113.7
Non-Hispanic Black	34.7	14.0	20.3	17.0	17.0	33.8	37.9	42.6	45.0	30.5	118.7
Hispanic [3]	21.3	10.2	12.5	10.5	10.5	17.4	22.3	27.6	30.7	31.8	93.3
RATE PER 100,000 LIVE BIRTHS											
Higher Order Multiple Births [4]											
All races [1]	187.4	*	13.0	*	13.6	48.4	158.9	309.1	409.5	330.7	2 035.9
White total [2]	208.7	*	13.7	*	13.6	45.5	170.2	343.0	457.9	339.4	2 228.4
Non-Hispanic White	255.0	*	11.6	*	*	54.0	206.6	388.9	510.6	380.8	2 382.2
Black total [2]	108.4	*	*	*	*	61.1	131.5	175.3	238.5	285.8	*
Non-Hispanic Black	109.5	*	*	*	*	60.3	133.8	174.6	249.7	297.7	*
Hispanic [3]	85.9	*	16.3	*	*	28.5	77.1	163.3	242.7	160.8	*

[1] Includes races other than White and Black and origin not stated.
[2] Race and Hispanic origin are reported separately on the birth certificate. Data for persons of Hispanic origin are included in the data for each race group according to the mother's reported race.
[3] May be of any race.
[4] Births in greater than twin deliveries.
* = Figure does not meet standards of reliability or precision; based on fewer than 20 births in numerator.
- = Quantity zero.

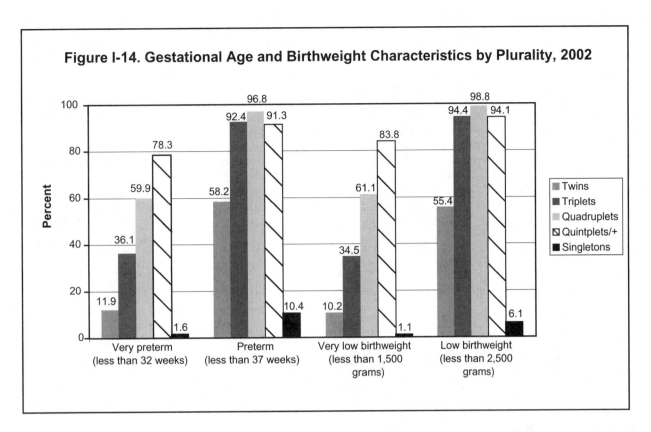

Figure I-14. Gestational Age and Birthweight Characteristics by Plurality, 2002

even without the use of fertility therapies). In 2003, there were over 128,000 births in twin deliveries, which accounted for a record 3.15 percent of total births. This rate was 67 percent higher than the rate in 1980. The most rapid increases in twin deliveries have been for mothers over 40 years old. Twinning rates have increased among the three largest racial and ethnic groups. Since 1990, the likelihood of giving births to twins has risen by more than 50 percent among non-Hispanic Whites, 30 percent among non-Hispanic Blacks, and 15 percent among Hispanics.

In contrast to the continued rise in twin birth rates, the remarkable growth of triplet and higher-order multiples of the past two decades has at least temporarily ended. Such births numbered 7,663 in 2003, which represents a rate of 187 per 100,000 live births. The rate in 2003 was roughly 4 percent less than the 1998 high. Despite the stability in the rate since 1999, the number of triplet or greater multiple births was 7,663, in 2003 the highest ever reported. Refinements and less aggressive techniques in assisted reproductive technologies may be contributing to the current abatement of higher-order multiple births. Obstetric and reproductive medicine organizations have recommended limiting the number of embryos transferred to the mother to prevent higher-order multiple pregnancies. The higher the plurality of a pregnancy, the greater the likelihood of a shorter gestational period, low birthweight, and other adverse conditions.

TABLE I-50A. GESTATIONAL AGE AND BIRTHWEIGHT CHARACTERISTICS, BY PLURALITY, 2002

The higher the plurality of a pregnancy, the greater the risk of a poor perinatal outcome. The average twin in 2002 was delivered more than three weeks earlier than the average singleton (35.3 compared with 38.8 weeks) and weighed about 2 pounds less. The typical triplet weighed about half of its singleton counterpart (4 pounds) at birth; the average quintuplet less than one-third (only 3 pounds). As a result, twins are nearly 5 times as likely to die by their first birthday; for triplets or higher plurality, the risk was 12 times higher than that for singletons. Updates of this information were not available for 2003.

TABLE I-50B. NUMBER AND RATES OF MULTIPLE BIRTHS, SELECTED YEARS, 1980–2003

The twin birth rate rose to another record high of 31.5 per 1,000 live births in 2003. This was a 1 percent increase from the 2002 level, which was 31.1 per 1,000. Since 1980, the twinning rate has climbed by two-thirds (from 18.9 per 1,000 live births) and the number of births in twin deliveries has increased by more than three-fourths, from 68,339 to 128,665.

The birth rate for triplets and higher-order multiples held relatively steady for 2003. Between 1980 and 1998, this birth rate surged by more than 500 percent, rising from 37.0 to 193.5 per 100,000 live births. In 1999, however, it fell slightly and has remained fairly stable since. Despite the stability in the rate, the number of triplets and higher-order births in 2003 was 7,663—the highest ever reported. The rising incidence of multiple births over the last two decades has been associated with two related trends: older age at childbearing (older mothers are more likely to spontaneously conceive multiples) and the increased use of fertility therapies. A study of multiples born in 2000 estimated that natural conception accounted for 67 percent of the twins and only 18

percent of the triplets and higher-order births that year. The highest rates and fastest growth in multiples are reported for non-Hispanic White mothers, who are also more likely to receive infertility services. Between 1990 and 2003, the twin birth rate rose by more than 50 percent among non-Hispanic White women, and the triplet and higher-order rate rose by 184 percent. In comparison, twinning rates rose 30 percent among non-Hispanic Black mothers and 18 percent among Hispanic mothers; triplet and higher order birth rates rose by 137 and 117 percent, respectively.

Table I-50A. Gestational Age and Birthweight Characteristics, by Plurality, 2002

(Number, percent.)

Characteristic	Twins	Triplets	Quadruplets	Quintuplets/+	Singletons
Number	125 134	6 898	434	69	3 889 191
Percent very preterm [1]	11.9	36.1	59.9	78.3	1.6
Percent preterm [2]	58.2	92.4	96.8	91.3	10.4
Mean gestational age (standard deviation) in weeks	35.3 (3.7)	32.2 (3.8)	29.9 (4.0)	28.5 (4.7)	38.8 (2.5)
Percent very low birthweight [3]	10.2	34.5	61.1	83.8	1.1
Percent low birthweight [4]	55.4	94.4	98.8	94.1	6.1
Mean birthweight (standard deviation) in grams	2 347 (645)	1 687 (561)	1 309 (522)	1 105 (777)	3 332 (573)

[1]Very preterm is less than 32 completed weeks of gestation.
[2]Preterm is less than 37 completed weeks of gestation.
[3]Very low birthweight is less than 1,500 grams.
[4]Low birthweight is less than 2,500 grams.

Table I-50B. Number and Rates of Multiple Births, Selected Years, 1980–2003

(Number, percent.)

Year	Twins	Triplets [1]	Quadruplets [1]	Quintuplets and higher order multiples [2]	Triplet/+	Twin birth rate [3]	Triplet/+ birth rate [4]
2003	128 665	7 110	468	85	7 663	31.5	187.4
2002	125 134	6 898	434	69	7 401	31.1	184.0
2001	121 246	6 885	501	85	7 471	30.1	185.6
2000	118 916	6 742	506	77	7 325	29.3	180.5
1995	96 736	4 551	365	57	4 973	24.8	127.5
1990	93 865	2 830	185	13	3 028	22.6	72.8
1985	77 102	[5]1 925	. . .	. . .	1 925	20.5	51.2
1980	68 339	[5]1 337	. . .	. . .	1 337	18.9	37.0

[1]Triplets, quadruplets, and quintuplets and other higher order multiple births were not differentiated in the national data set until 1989.
[2]Quintuplets, sextuplets, and higher order multiple births are not differentiated in the national data set.
[3]Births in twin deliveries per 1,000 live births.
[4]Births in triplet and higher order multiple deliveries per 100,000 live births.
[5]Includes quadruplets and higher order multiple births.
. . . = Not available.

TABLE I-51. LEGAL ABORTIONS AND LEGAL ABORTION RATIOS, ACCORDING TO SELECTED PATIENT CHARACTERISTICS, SELECTED YEARS, 1973–2001

The Alan Guttmacher Institute estimated that 1,300,000 abortions were performed in 2001. CDC estimates were considerably smaller, partly because four reporting areas, including California, have not been reporting abortions to the CDC. Even without complete coverage, the ratios obtained in the CDC sample are informative.

Pregnant unmarried women were about 10 times more likely to have an abortion than those who were married. Abortions were concentrated among teenagers, especially those under 15 years of age. For every two live births, Black women tended to have one abortion. For White women, the number of abortions was equivalent to 17 percent of live births; and for Hispanics, the ratio was 23 percent.

In total, the ratio of abortions to live births has moderated since its high points in the 1980s.

Table I-51. Legal Abortions and Legal Abortion Ratios, According to Selected Patient Characterisitics, Selected Years, 1973–2001

(Number, percent.)

Characteristic	2001 [1]	2000 [1]	1999 [2]	1998 [2]	1997	1995	1990	1985	1980	1975	1973
NUMBER OF LEGAL ABORTIONS IN THOUSANDS											
Centers for Disease Control and Prevention	853	857	862	884	1 186	1 211	1 429	1 329	1 298	855	616
Alan Guttmacher Institute [3]	1 303	1 313	1 315	1 319	1 335	1 359	1 609	1 589	1 554	1 034	745
ABORTIONS PER 100 LIVE BIRTHS [4]											
Total	24.6	24.5	25.6	26.4	30.6	31.1	34.4	35.4	35.9	27.2	19.6
Age											
Under 15 years	74.4	70.8	70.9	75.0	72.9	66.4	81.8	137.6	139.7	119.3	123.7
15–19 years	36.6	36.1	37.5	39.1	40.7	39.9	51.1	68.8	71.4	54.2	53.9
20–24 years	30.4	30.0	31.6	32.9	34.5	34.8	37.8	38.6	39.5	28.9	29.4
25–29 years	20.0	19.8	20.8	21.6	22.4	22.0	21.8	21.7	23.7	19.2	20.7
30–34 years	14.7	14.5	15.2	15.7	16.1	16.1	16.4	19.0	19.9	25.0	28.0
35–39 years	18.0	18.1	19.3	20.0	20.9	22.3	27.3	33.6	41.0	42.2	45.1
40 years and over	30.4	30.1	32.9	33.8	35.2	38.5	50.6	62.3	80.7	66.8	68.4
Race											
White [5]	16.5	16.7	17.7	18.9	19.4	20.3	25.8	27.7	33.2	27.7	32.6
Black or African American [6]	49.1	50.3	52.9	51.2	54.3	53.1	53.7	47.2	54.3	47.6	42.0
Hispanic Origin [7]											
Hispanic or Latino	23.0	22.5	26.1	27.3	26.8	27.1	. . .	. . .	. . .	. . .	. . .
Not Hispanic or Latino	23.2	23.3	25.2	27.1	27.2	27.9	. . .	. . .	. . .	. . .	. . .
Marital Status											
Married	6.5	6.5	7.0	7.1	7.4	7.6	8.7	8.0	10.5	9.6	7.6
Unmarried	57.2	57.0	60.4	62.7	65.9	64.5	86.3	117.4	147.6	161.0	139.8
Previous Live Births [8]											
0	26.4	22.6	24.3	25.5	26.4	28.6	36.0	45.1	45.7	38.4	43.7
1	18.0	19.4	20.6	21.4	22.3	22.0	22.7	21.6	20.2	22.0	23.5
2	25.5	27.4	29.0	30.0	31.0	30.6	31.5	29.9	29.5	36.8	36.8
3	26.4	28.5	29.8	30.5	31.1	30.7	30.1	18.2	29.8	47.7	46.9
4 or more [9]	21.9	23.7	24.2	24.3	24.5	23.7	26.6	21.5	24.3	43.5	44.7
Percent Distribution [10]											
Total	100.0	100.0	100.0	100.0	100.0	100.0	100.0	100.0	100.0	100.0	100.0
Period of Gestation											
Under 9 weeks	59.1	58.1	57.6	55.7	55.4	54.0	51.6	50.3	51.7	44.6	36.1
9–10 weeks	19.0	19.8	20.2	21.5	22.0	23.1	25.3	26.6	26.2	28.4	29.4
11–12 weeks	10.0	10.2	10.2	10.9	10.7	10.9	11.7	12.5	12.2	14.9	17.9
13–15 weeks	6.2	6.2	6.2	6.4	6.2	6.3	6.4	5.9	5.1	5.0	6.9
16–20 weeks	4.3	4.3	4.3	4.1	4.3	4.3	4.0	3.9	3.9	6.1	8.0
21 weeks and over	1.4	1.4	1.5	1.4	1.4	1.4	1.0	0.8	0.9	1.0	1.7
Previous Induced Abortions											
0	55.5	54.7	53.7	53.8	53.4	55.1	57.1	60.1	67.6	81.9	. . .
1	25.8	26.4	27.1	27.0	27.5	26.9	26.9	25.7	23.5	14.9	. . .
2	11.0	11.3	11.5	11.4	11.5	10.9	10.1	9.8	6.6	2.5	. . .
3 or more	7.7	7.6	7.7	7.8	7.6	7.1	5.9	4.4	2.3	0.7	. . .

[1] In 2000 and 2001, Alaska, California, and New Hampshire did not report abortion data to CDC.
[2] In 1998 and 1999, Alaska, California, New Hampshire, and Oklahoma did not report abortion data to CDC. For comparison, in 1997, the 48 corresponding reporting areas reported about 900,000 legal abortions.
[3] No surveys were conducted in 1983, 1986, 1989, 1990, 1993, 1994, 1997, or 1998. Data for these years were estimated by interpolation.
[4] For calculation of ratios by each characteristic, abortions with characteristic unknown were distributed in proportion to abortions with characteristic known.
[5] For 1989 and later years, White race includes women of Hispanic ethnicity.
[6] Before 1989, Black race includes races other than White.
[7] Reporting area increased from 20–22 states, the District of Columbia (DC), and New York City (NYC) in 1991–1995 to 31 states and NYC in 2001. California, Florida, Illinois, Arizona, and states with large Hispanic populations do not report Hispanic ethnicity.
[8] For 1973–1975, data indicate number of living children.
[9] For 1975, data refer to four previous live births, not four or more. For five or more previous live births, the ratio is 47.3.
[10] For calculation of percent distribution by each characteristic, abortions with characteristic unknown were excluded.
. . . = Not available.

TABLE I-52. CONTRACEPTIVE USE AMONG WOMEN 15–44 YEARS OF AGE, ACCORDING TO AGE, RACE, HISPANIC ORIGIN, AND METHOD OF CONTRACEPTION, SELECTED YEARS, 1982–2002

In 2002, some 62 percent of women age 15–44 years were using contraception. This was an increase from 1982, when 56 percent of women used contraception. The use of contraception in 2002 was only moderately different among the major race and ethnic groups: 65 percent of non-Hispanic Whites, 58 percent of non-Hispanic Blacks, and 59 percent of Hispanics used contraception.

Contraception use among teenage women was relatively low (about 32 percent).

Female sterilization represented a major method of contraception; it was particularly prevalent among women 35 to 44 years of age. Birth control pills were the most frequent method used (31 percent of contracepting women). This was followed by the use of condoms and by male sterilization. Diaphragms and intrauterine devices, which were used by 15 percent of contracepting women in 1982, were only used by about 3.0 percent of women by 2002.

Table I-52. Contraceptive Use Among Women 15–44 Years of Age, According to Age, Race, Hispanic Origin, and Method of Contraception, Selected Years, 1982–2002

(Number, percent.)

Characteristic	Age in years				
	15–44 years	15–19 years	20–24 years	25–34 years	35–44 years
NUMBER IN THOUSANDS					
All Women [1]					
2002	61 561	9 834	9 840	19 522	22 365
1995	60 201	8 961	9 041	20 758	21 440
1988	57 900	9 179	9 413	21 726	17 582
1982	54 099	9 521	10 629	19 644	14 305
Not Hispanic or Latino					
White					
2002	39 498	6 069	5 938	12 073	15 418
1995	42 154	5 865	6 020	14 471	15 798
1988	42 575	6 531	6 630	15 929	13 486
1982	41 279	7 010	8 081	14 945	11 243
Black or African American					
2002	8 250	1 409	1 396	2 587	2 857
1995	8 060	1 334	1 305	2 780	2 641
1988	7 408	1 362	1 322	2 760	1 965
1982	6 825	1 383	1 456	2 392	1 593
Hispanic or Latino [2]					
2002	9 107	1 521	1 632	3 249	2 705
1995	6 702	1 150	1 163	2 450	1 940
1988	4 393	886	811	1 677	1 018
1982	5 557	999	1 003	2 104	1 451
PERCENT OF WOMEN USING CONTRACEPTION					
All Women [1]					
2002	61.9	31.5	60.7	68.6	69.9
1995	64.2	29.8	63.5	71.1	72.3
1988	60.3	32.1	59.0	66.3	68.3
1982	55.7	24.2	55.8	66.7	61.6
Not Hispanic or Latino					
White					
2002	64.6	35.0	66.3	69.9	71.4
1995	66.2	30.5	65.4	72.9	73.6
1988	63.0	34.0	62.6	67.7	71.5
1982	57.3	23.6	58.7	67.8	63.5
Black or African American					
2002	57.6	32.9	50.8	67.9	63.8
1995	62.3	36.1	67.6	66.8	68.3
1988	56.8	35.7	61.8	63.5	58.7
1982	51.6	29.8	52.3	63.5	52.0
Hispanic or Latino [2]					
2002	59.0	20.4	57.4	66.2	72.9
1995	59.0	26.1	50.6	69.2	70.8
1988	50.4	*18.3	40.8	67.4	54.3
1982	50.6	*	*36.8	67.2	59.0

Note: Data are based on household interviews of samples of women in the childbearing ages.

[1] Includes women of other or unknown race not shown separately.
[2] May be of any race.
* = Figure does not meet standards of reliability or precision.

Table I-52. Contraceptive Use Among Women 15–44 Years of Age, According to Age, Race, Hispanic Origin, and Method of Contraception, Selected Years, 1982–2002—*Continued*

(Number, percent.)

Characteristic	Age in years				
	15–44 years	15–19 years	20–24 years	25–34 years	35–44 years
PERCENT OF CONTRACEPTING WOMEN					
Female Sterilization					
2002	27.0	-	3.6	21.7	45.8
1995	27.8	*	4.0	23.8	45.0
1988	27.6	*	*4.6	25.0	47.6
1982	23.2	-	*4.5	22.1	43.5
Male Sterilization					
2002	10.2	-	*	7.2	18.2
1995	10.9	-	*	7.8	19.5
1988	11.7	*	*	10.2	20.8
1982	10.9	*	*3.6	10.1	19.9
Implant [3]					
2002	1.2	*	*	*1.9	*
1995	1.3	*	3.7	*1.3	*
1988	. . .	. . .	. . .	. . .	. . .
1982	. . .	. . .	. . .	. . .	. . .
Injectable [3]					
2002	5.4	13.9	10.2	5.3	*1.8
1995	3.0	9.7	6.1	2.9	*0.8
1988	. . .	. . .	. . .	. . .	. . .
1982	. . .	. . .	. . .	. . .	. . .
Birth Control Pill					
2002	31.0	53.8	52.5	34.8	15.0
1995	27.0	43.8	52.1	33.4	8.7
1988	30.8	58.8	68.2	32.6	4.3
1982	28.0	63.9	55.1	25.7	*3.7
Intrauterine Device					
2002	2.2	*	1.8	3.7	*
1995	0.8	-	*	*0.8	1.1
1988	2.0	-	*	2.1	3.1
1982	7.1	*	*4.2	9.7	6.9
Diaphragm					
2002	0.6	-	*	*	*
1995	1.9	*	*	1.7	2.8
1988	5.7	*	*3.7	7.3	6.0
1982	8.1	*6.0	10.2	10.3	4.0
Condom					
2002	23.8	44.6	36.0	23.1	15.6
1995	23.4	45.8	33.7	23.7	15.3
1988	14.6	32.8	14.5	13.7	11.2
1982	12.0	20.8	10.7	11.4	11.3
Periodic Abstinence-Calendar Rhythm					
2002	2.0	*	*2.3	*1.7	*2.4
1995	3.3	*	*1.5	3.7	3.9
1988	1.7	*	1.1	1.8	2.0
1982	3.3	2.0	3.1	3.3	3.7
Periodic Abstinence-Natural Family Planning					
2002	*0.4	-	-	*	*
1995	*0.5	-	*	*0.7	*
1988	0.6	-	*	0.7	0.7
1982	0.6	-	*	0.9	*
Withdrawal					
2002	8.8	15.0	11.9	10.7	4.7
1995	6.1	13.2	7.1	6.0	4.5
1988	2.2	3.0	3.4	2.8	0.8
1982	2.0	2.9	3.0	1.8	1.3
Other Methods [4]					
2002	1.7	*	*	*1.5	*1.8
1995	3.2	*	3.2	3.1	3.4
1988	3.2	*	1.8	3.8	3.5
1982	4.9	2.6	5.4	4.8	5.3

Note: Data are based on household interviews of samples of women in the childbearing ages.

[3]Data collected starting with the 1995 survey only.
[4]In 2002, includes female condom, foam, cervical cap, sponge, suppository or insert, jelly or cream, and other methods.
* = Figure does not meet standards of reliability or precision.
- = Quantity zero.
. . . = Not available.

Table I-52. Contraceptive Use Among Women 15–44 Years of Age, According to Age, Race, Hispanic Origin, and Method of Contraception, Selected Years, 1982–2002—Continued

(Number, percent.)

Characteristic	Not Hispanic or Latino		Hispanic or Latino
	White	Black or African American	
PERCENT OF CONTRACEPTING WOMEN			
Female Sterilization			
2002	23.9	39.2	33.8
1995	24.5	39.9	36.6
1988	25.6	37.8	31.7
1982	22.0	30.0	23.0
Male Sterilization			
2002	12.9	*	4.7
1995	13.7	*1.8	*4.0
1988	14.3	*0.9	-
1982	13.0	*1.5	-
Implant [3]			
2002	*0.8	*	*1.3
1995	*1.0	*2.4	*2.0
1988	. . .	. . .	. . .
1982	. . .	. . .	. . .
Injectable [3]			
2002	4.2	9.4	7.3
1995	2.4	5.4	4.7
1988	. . .	. . .	. . .
1982	. . .	. . .	. . .
Birth Control Pill			
2002	34.9	23.1	22.1
1995	28.7	23.7	23.0
1988	29.5	38.2	33.4
1982	26.4	37.9	30.2
Intrauterine Device			
2002	1.7	*	5.3
1995	0.7	*	*
1988	1.5	3.2	*5.0
1982	5.8	9.3	19.2
Diaphragm			
2002	*	*	-
1995	2.3	*	*
1988	6.6	*2.0	*
1982	9.2	*3.2	*
Condom			
2002	21.7	29.6	24.1
1995	22.5	24.9	21.2
1988	15.2	10.1	13.7
1982	13.1	6.3	*6.9
Periodic Abstinence-Calendar Rhythm			
2002	2.3	*	*
1995	3.3	*1.7	3.2
1988	1.6	1.9	*
1982	3.2	2.9	3.9
Periodic Abstinence-Natural Family Planning			
2002	*	*	*
1995	0.7	*	*
1988	0.7	*	*
1982	0.7	0.3	-
Withdrawal			
2002	9.5	4.9	6.3
1995	6.4	3.3	5.7
1988	2.0	1.4	4.5
1982	2.1	1.3	2.6
Other Methods [4]			
2002	*1.7	*1.9	*1.2
1995	3.3	3.8	*2.2
1988	3.0	4.4	2.6
1982	4.6	7.3	5.0

Note: Data are based on household interviews of samples of women in the childbearing ages.

[3]Data collected starting with the 1995 survey only.
[4]In 2002, includes female condom, foam, cervical cap, sponge, suppository or insert, jelly or cream, and other methods.
* = Figure does not meet standards of reliability or precision.
- = Quantity zero.
. . . = Not available.

TABLE I-53. BREASTFEEDING BY MOTHERS 15–44 YEARS OF AGE BY YEAR OF BABY'S BIRTH, ACCORDING TO SELECTED CHARACTERISTICS OF MOTHER: ANNUAL AVERAGES, 1986–2001

In 1999–2001, about 67 percent of babies were breastfed, and 48 percent were breastfed for 3 months or more.

Breastfeeding increased strongly with educational attainment, with the age of the mother, and with geographic location in the West. Non-Hispanic Black mothers used breastfeeding much less frequently than their White and Hispanic counterparts.

Table 1-53. Breastfeeding by Mothers 15–44 Years of Age by Year of Baby's Birth, According to Selected Characteristics of Mother: Annual Averages, 1986–2001

(Percent.)

Selected characteristics of mother	1999–2001	1995–1998	1992–1994	1989–1991	1986–1988
PERCENT OF BABIES BREASTFED					
Total	66.5	64.4	57.6	53.3	54.1
Age at Baby's Birth					
Under 20 years	47.3	49.5	41.0	34.7	28.4
20-24 years	59.3	55.9	50.0	44.3	48.2
25-29 years	63.5	68.1	57.4	56.4	58.2
30-44 years	80.0	72.8	70.2	66.0	68.6
Race and Hispanic Origin [1]					
Non-Hispanic White	68.7	66.5	61.7	58.4	59.1
Non-Hispanic Black	45.3	47.9	26.1	22.4	22.3
Hispanic or Latino	76.0	71.2	63.8	57.0	55.6
Education [2]					
No high school diploma or GED [3]	46.6	50.6	44.6	36.5	31.8
High school diploma or GED [3]	61.6	55.9	51.1	45.5	47.4
Some college, no bachelor's degree	75.6	70.1	64.3	61.4	62.2
Bachelor's degree or higher	81.3	82.0	82.5	80.6	78.4
Geographic Region					
Northeast	66.9	61.6	56.5	53.5	51.3
Midwest	61.9	61.7	51.7	49.6	52.3
South	60.9	58.1	48.6	43.6	44.6
West	78.9	78.1	77.3	69.5	71.4
PERCENT BREASTFED 3 MONTHS OR MORE					
Total	48.4	45.8	33.6	31.8	34.6
Age at Baby's Birth					
Under 20 years	30.0	30.0	*11.7	*10.5	18.5
20–24 years	41.8	36.6	25.1	24.1	26.1
25–29 years	43.7	46.3	35.6	32.3	36.9
30–44 years	62.4	57.5	46.7	46.8	50.1
Race and Hispanic Origin [1]					
Non-Hispanic White	49.7	47.8	36.6	35.2	37.7
Non-Hispanic Black	33.7	29.6	13.3	11.5	11.6
Hispanic or Latino	54.3	49.7	35.0	33.9	38.2
Education [2]					
No high school diploma or GED [3]	37.0	33.9	25.2	17.6	21.8
High school diploma or GED [3]	43.1	36.9	27.4	28.0	28.2
Some college, no bachelor's degree	52.8	49.6	38.7	33.1	38.7
Bachelor's degree or higher	64.1	64.5	59.3	56.1	55.0
Geographic Region					
Northeast	48.8	48.2	36.4	37.2	29.9
Midwest	42.8	42.0	30.1	31.5	30.3
South	44.4	38.9	26.2	20.1	27.7
West	59.2	58.2	45.3	42.9	52.4

Note: Low birthweight is defined as weight of less than 2,500 grams (5lb 8oz).

[1] May be of any race.
[2] For women 22–44 years of age. Education is as of year of interview.
[3] General equivalency diploma.
* = Figure does not meet standards of reliability or precision.

CHAPTER II: MORTALITY

Most of this chapter is based on three releases from the National Center for Health Statistics (NCHS), a component of the Centers for Disease Control and Prevention (CDC). They are "Deaths: Final Data for 2002," "Deaths: Preliminary Data for 2003," and "Deaths: Final Data for 2003." Thus, some tables cover data for 2003, but many end with 2002. The bulk of this information has been derived by NCHS through an examination of the death certificates collected by individual states and the District of Columbia. Following the overview presented in Table II-1, data are shown for the number of deaths and for death rates by sex, age, race, and Hispanic origin. Subsequent tables show life expectancy and its derivation. A major part of this chapter classifies deaths according to groups of causes, including 113 selected causes with detail by sex, age, race, and Hispanic origin. Certain additional groupings, such as death through injury by firearms and alcohol-induced deaths, are shown separately. Statistics on infant mortality are presented the end of the chapter.

TABLE II-1. OVERVIEW OF DEATHS, DEATH RATES, AND LIFE EXPECTANCY AT BIRTH, BY SEX AND RACE, 2002 AND 2003

The number of deaths increased slightly in 2003, reflecting the United States' growing population. The age-adjusted death rate decreased in 2003 for both Whites and Blacks, and reached 832.7 per 100,000 of the overall U.S. population.

Life expectancy at birth reached a record high of 77.5 years, compared to 77.3 years in 2002. Both males and females, as well Blacks and Whites, experienced increased life expectancies.

The number of maternal deaths—deaths from physical conditions aggravated during pregnancy—increased to 495 cases in 2003, up from 357 fatalities in 2002. This jump was at least partly due to the fact that an increasing number of states introduced a separate item for pregnancy status on the death certificate, which focused attention on the possibility of maternal death.

The rate of infant deaths declined to 6.85 per 1,000 live births in 2003, after rising to nearly 7.0 per 1,000 live births in 2002, contrary to its downward trend over previous years. The record low for this rate was 6.8 per 1,000 birth rates in 2001.

Table II-1. Overview of Deaths, Death Rates, and Life Expectancy at Birth, by Sex and Race, 2002 and 2003

(Number, rate.)

Measure and sex	All races [1,2]		White [2]		Black [2]	
	2003	2002	2003	2002	2003	2002
ALL DEATHS	2 448 288	2 443 387	2 103 714	2 102 589	291 300	290 051
Age-adjusted death rate [3]	832.7	845.3	817.0	829.0	1 065.9	1 083.3
Male	994.3	1 013.7	973.9	992.9	1 319.1	1 341.4
Female	706.2	715.2	693.1	701.3	885.6	901.8
Life expectancy at birth [4]	77.5	77.3	78.0	77.7	72.7	72.3
Male	74.8	74.5	75.3	75.1	69.0	68.8
Female	80.1	79.9	80.5	80.3	76.1	75.6
All maternal deaths	495	357	280	190	183	148
Maternal mortality rate [5]	12.1	8.9	8.7	6.0	30.5	24.9
All infant deaths	28 025	28 034	18 440	18 369	8 402	8 524
Infant mortality rate [6]	6.8	7.0	5.7	5.8	14.0	14.4

[1] Includes races other than White and Black.
[2] Race categories are consistent with the 1977 Office of Management and Budget (OMB) standards. California, Hawaii, Idaho, Maine, Montana, New York, and Wisconsin reported multiple-race data in 2003. The multiple-race data for these states were bridged to the single race categories established by the 1977 OMB standards for comparability with other states.
[3] Age-adjusted death rates are per 100,000 U.S. standard population, based on the year 2000 standard.
[4] Life expectancy at birth stated in years.
[5] Maternal deaths per 100,000 live births.
[6] Infant mortality rates are deaths under 1 year of age per 1,000 live births in specified group.

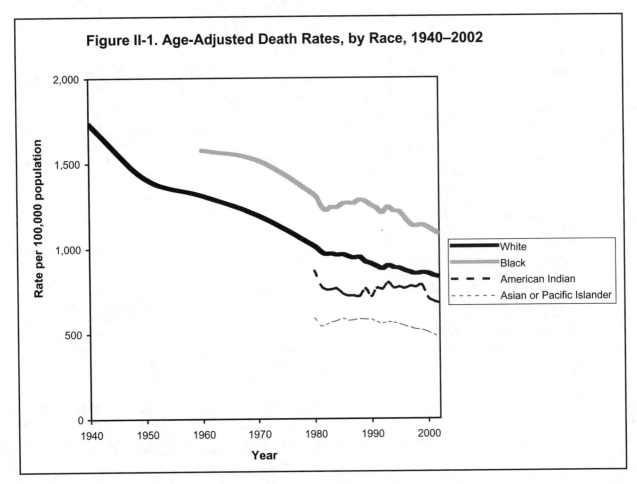

Figure II-1. Age-Adjusted Death Rates, by Race, 1940–2002

TABLE II-1A. NUMBER OF DEATHS, DEATH RATES, AND AGE-ADJUSTED DEATH RATES, BY RACE AND SEX, SELECTED YEARS, 1940–2002

In 2002, a total of 2.443 million resident deaths were registered in the United States, compared to 4.022 million births. The number of deaths in the United States has increased considerably over the years as the country's population grew. The crude death rate was 847.3 per 100,000 persons in 2002. This death rate indicated the health status of the population and its age distribution. The younger the age, the lower the crude death rate would tend to be.

An age-adjusted death rate is also shown in this table. This rate attempts to eliminate the effects of changes in the age distribution on mortality. Age-adjusted rates are calculated to show what mortality would be if the age distribution of the population did not change from year to year, and if it was the same for all of the various subgroups. These rates are constructed by measuring the age-specific death rates in a given population; a standard age distribution is substituted for the actual observed age distribution when the specific death rates are combined. The standard age distribution currently in use is that of the total U.S. population from the year 2000. Age-adjusted rates are better suited than crude rates for examining trends over time, and for comparing relative risk rates across geographic areas or subgroups for gender and race.

Age adjustment has tended to increase the death rate for populations with shorter than average life spans, such as White males and Blacks. However, the death rate decreased for White females, who tended to live longer. Asians and Pacific Islanders and American Indians had surprisingly low crude and age-adjusted death rates. It was estimated that these races were underreported on death certificates. Funeral directors generally supplied this information for the deceased, and their knowledge may have been less accurate than that of the family members who had previously reported race to the Census Bureau. The Census Bureau data provided the population estimates to which the death statistics are compared. Estimates of this bias have been made in research papers, and deaths were found to have been undercounted by approximately 21 percent for American Indians and 11 percent for Asians and Pacific Islanders. (Rosenberg, H.M., J.D. Maurer, et al. 1999. Quality of death rates by race and Hispanic origin: A summary of current research. *Vital Health Statistics* 2 (128). Hyattsville, MD: National Center for Health Statistics.)

In 2002, the age-adjusted death rate for the Black population was 1.3 times the rate for Whites. In other words, the average risk of death for Blacks was about 33 percent higher than that for Whites. For the total population, the age-adjusted death rate in the United States declined 18.7 percent between 1980 and 2002.

Table II-1A. Number of Deaths, Death Rates, and Age-Adjusted Death Rates, by Race and Sex, Selected Years, 1940–2002

(Number, rate per 100,000 population.)

Year	All races [1]			White			Black			American Indian [2]			Asian or Pacific Islander [3]		
	Both sexes	Male	Female	Both sexes	Male	Female	Both sexes	Male	Female	Both sexes	Male	Female	Both sexes	Male	Female
Number of Deaths															
2002	2 443 387	1 199 264	1 244 123	2 102 589	1 025 196	1 077 393	290 051	146 835	143 216	12 415	6 750	5 665	38 332	20 483	17 849
2001	2 416 425	1 183 421	1 233 004	2 079 691	1 011 218	1 068 473	287 709	145 908	141 801	11 977	6 466	5 511	37 048	19 829	17 219
2000	2 403 351	1 177 578	1 225 773	2 071 287	1 007 191	1 064 096	285 826	145 184	140 642	11 363	6 185	5 178	34 875	19 018	15 857
1999	2 391 399	1 175 460	1 215 939	2 061 348	1 005 335	1 056 013	285 064	145 703	139 361	11 312	6 092	5 220	33 675	18 330	15 345
1998	2 337 256	1 157 260	1 179 996	2 015 984	990 190	1 025 794	278 440	143 417	135 023	10 845	5 994	4 851	31 987	17 659	14 328
1997	2 314 245	1 154 039	1 160 206	1 996 393	986 884	1 009 509	276 520	144 110	132 410	10 576	5 985	4 591	30 756	17 060	13 696
1996	2 314 690	1 163 569	1 151 121	1 992 966	991 984	1 000 982	282 089	149 472	132 617	10 127	5 563	4 564	29 508	16 550	12 958
1995	2 312 132	1 172 959	1 139 173	1 987 437	997 277	990 160	286 401	154 175	132 226	9 997	5 574	4 423	28 297	15 933	12 364
1994	2 278 994	1 162 747	1 116 247	1 959 875	988 823	971 052	282 379	153 019	129 360	9 637	5 497	4 140	27 103	15 408	11 695
1993	2 268 553	1 161 797	1 106 756	1 951 437	988 329	963 108	282 151	153 502	128 649	9 579	5 434	4 145	25 386	14 532	10 854
1992	2 175 613	1 122 336	1 053 277	1 873 781	956 957	916 824	269 219	146 630	122 589	8 953	5 181	3 772	23 660	13 568	10 092
1991	2 169 518	1 121 665	1 047 853	1 868 904	956 497	912 407	269 525	147 331	122 194	8 621	4 948	3 673	22 173	12 727	9 446
1990	2 148 463	1 113 417	1 035 046	1 853 254	950 812	902 442	265 498	145 359	120 139	8 316	4 877	3 439	21 127	12 211	8 916
1989	2 150 466	1 114 190	1 036 276	1 853 841	950 852	902 989	267 642	146 393	121 249	8 614	5 066	3 548	20 042	11 688	8 354
1988	2 167 999	1 125 540	1 042 459	1 876 906	965 419	911 487	264 019	144 228	119 791	7 917	4 617	3 300	18 963	11 155	7 808
1987	2 123 323	1 107 958	1 015 365	1 843 067	953 382	889 685	254 814	139 551	115 263	7 602	4 432	3 170	17 689	10 496	7 193
1986	2 105 361	1 104 005	1 001 356	1 831 083	952 554	878 529	250 326	137 214	113 112	7 301	4 365	2 936	16 514	9 795	6 719
1985	2 086 440	1 097 758	988 682	1 819 054	950 455	868 599	244 207	133 610	110 597	7 154	4 181	2 973	15 887	9 441	6 446
1984	2 039 369	1 076 514	962 855	1 781 897	934 529	847 368	235 884	129 147	106 737	6 949	4 117	2 832	14 483	8 627	5 856
1983	2 019 201	1 071 923	947 278	1 765 582	931 779	833 803	233 124	127 911	105 213	6 839	4 064	2 775	13 554	8 126	5 428
1982	1 974 797	1 056 440	918 357	1 729 085	919 239	809 846	226 513	125 610	100 903	6 679	3 974	2 705	12 430	7 564	4 866
1981	1 977 981	1 063 772	914 209	1 731 233	925 490	805 743	228 560	127 296	101 264	6 608	4 016	2 592	11 475	6 908	4 567
1980	1 989 841	1 075 078	914 763	1 738 607	933 878	804 729	233 135	130 138	102 997	6 923	4 193	2 730	11 071	6 809	4 262
1970	1 921 031	1 078 478	842 553	1 682 096	942 437	739 659	225 647	127 540	98 107	5 675	3 391	2 284	. . .	. . .	. . .
1960	1 711 982	975 648	736 334	1 505 335	860 857	644 478	196 010	107 701	88 309	4 528	2 658	1 870	. . .	. . .	. . .
1950	1 452 454	827 749	624 705	1 276 085	731 366	544 719	169 606	92 004	77 602	4 440	2 497	1 943	. . .	. . .	. . .
1940	1 417 269	791 003	626 266	1 231 223	690 901	540 322	178 743	95 517	83 226	4 791	2 527	2 264	. . .	. . .	. . .
Death Rate															
2002	847.3	846.6	848.0	895.7	884.0	907.0	768.4	816.7	724.4	403.6	439.6	367.7	299.5	331.4	269.7
2001	848.5	846.4	850.4	895.1	881.9	907.9	773.5	823.9	727.7	392.1	424.2	360.2	303.8	335.0	274.4
2000	854.0	853.0	855.0	900.2	887.8	912.3	781.1	834.1	733.0	380.8	415.6	346.1	296.6	332.9	262.3
1999	857.0	859.2	854.9	901.4	892.1	910.4	788.1	847.4	734.3	399.3	431.8	367.1	296.8	333.2	262.5
1998	847.3	856.4	838.5	889.5	887.3	891.6	782.3	848.2	722.6	397.8	441.9	354.2	293.8	335.4	254.9
1997	848.8	864.6	833.6	889.1	893.3	885.0	789.9	867.1	720.1	402.7	458.2	347.7	294.1	336.8	253.9
1996	859.2	882.8	836.7	896.0	907.1	885.3	819.7	915.3	733.3	399.5	441.5	358.0	294.4	340.2	251.1
1995	868.3	900.8	837.2	901.8	921.0	883.2	846.2	960.2	743.2	409.4	459.4	360.1	294.6	341.4	250.4
1994	866.1	904.2	829.7	897.8	922.6	873.8	849.0	970.2	739.7	408.2	468.8	348.3	294.6	344.0	247.7
1993	872.8	915.0	832.5	902.7	931.8	874.6	864.6	992.2	749.6	419.8	479.6	360.7	288.0	338.1	240.3
1992	848.1	896.1	802.4	875.8	912.2	840.8	841.8	967.6	728.6	406.6	474.1	340.0	282.1	331.1	235.3
1991	857.6	908.8	808.7	883.2	922.7	845.2	861.4	994.8	741.4	405.3	468.9	342.7	278.7	326.9	232.4
1990	863.8	918.4	812.0	888.0	930.9	846.9	871.0	1 008.0	747.9	402.8	476.4	330.4	283.3	334.3	234.3
1989	871.3	926.3	818.9	893.2	936.5	851.8	887.9	1 026.7	763.2	430.5	510.7	351.3	280.9	334.5	229.4
1988	886.7	945.1	831.2	910.5	957.9	865.3	888.3	1 026.1	764.6	411.7	485.0	339.9	282.0	339.0	227.4
1987	876.4	939.3	816.7	900.1	952.7	849.8	868.9	1 006.2	745.7	410.7	483.8	339.0	278.9	338.3	222.0
1986	876.7	944.7	812.3	900.1	958.6	844.3	864.9	1 002.6	741.5	409.5	494.9	325.9	276.2	335.1	219.9
1985	876.9	948.6	809.1	900.4	963.6	840.1	854.8	989.3	734.2	416.4	492.5	342.5	283.4	344.6	224.9
1984	864.8	938.8	794.7	887.8	954.1	824.6	836.1	968.5	717.4	419.6	502.7	338.4	275.9	336.5	218.1
1983	863.7	943.2	788.4	885.4	957.7	816.4	836.6	971.2	715.9	428.5	515.1	343.9	276.1	339.1	216.1
1982	852.4	938.4	771.2	873.1	951.8	798.2	823.4	966.2	695.5	434.5	522.9	348.1	271.3	338.3	207.4
1981	862.0	954.0	775.0	880.4	965.2	799.8	842.4	992.6	707.7	445.6	547.9	345.6	272.3	336.2	211.5
1980	878.3	976.9	785.3	892.5	983.3	806.1	875.4	1 034.1	733.3	487.4	597.1	380.1	296.9	375.3	222.5
1970	945.3	1 090.3	807.8	946.3	1 086.7	812.6	999.3	1 186.6	829.2	. . .	. . .	. . .	. . .	. . .	. . .
1960	954.7	1 104.5	809.2	947.8	1 098.5	800.9	1 038.6	1 181.7	905.0	. . .	. . .	. . .	. . .	. . .	. . .
1950	963.8	1 106.1	823.5	945.7	1 089.5	803.3	. . .	. . .	. . .	. . .	. . .	. . .	. . .	. . .	. . .
1940	1 076.4	1 197.4	954.6	1 041.5	1 162.2	919.4	. . .	. . .	. . .	. . .	. . .	. . .	. . .	. . .	. . .
Age-Adjusted Death Rate															
2002	845.3	1 013.7	715.2	829.0	992.9	701.3	1 083.3	1 341.4	901.8	677.4	794.2	581.1	474.4	578.4	395.9
2001	854.5	1 029.1	721.8	836.5	1 006.1	706.7	1 101.2	1 375.0	912.5	686.7	798.9	594.0	492.1	597.4	412.0
2000	869.0	1 053.8	731.4	849.8	1 029.4	715.3	1 121.4	1 403.5	927.6	709.3	841.5	604.5	506.4	624.2	416.8
1999	875.6	1 067.0	734.0	854.6	1 040.0	716.6	1 135.7	1 432.6	933.6	780.9	925.9	668.2	519.7	641.2	427.5
1998	870.6	1 069.4	724.7	849.3	1 042.0	707.3	1 127.8	1 430.5	921.6	770.4	943.9	640.5	522.4	646.9	426.7
1997	878.1	1 088.1	725.6	855.7	1 059.1	707.8	1 139.8	1 458.8	922.1	774.0	974.8	625.3	531.8	660.2	432.6
1996	894.1	1 115.7	733.0	869.0	1 082.9	713.6	1 178.4	1 524.2	940.3	763.6	924.8	641.7	543.2	676.1	439.6
1995	909.8	1 143.9	739.4	882.3	1 107.5	718.7	1 213.9	1 585.7	955.9	771.2	932.0	643.9	554.8	693.4	446.7
1994	913.5	1 155.5	738.6	885.6	1 118.7	717.5	1 216.9	1 592.8	954.6	764.8	953.3	618.8	562.7	702.5	452.1
1993	926.1	1 177.3	745.9	897.0	1 138.9	724.1	1 241.2	1 632.2	969.5	796.4	1 006.3	641.6	565.8	709.9	450.4
1992	905.6	1 158.3	725.5	877.7	1 122.4	704.1	1 206.7	1 587.8	942.5	759.0	970.4	599.4	558.5	697.3	445.8
1991	922.3	1 180.5	738.2	893.2	1 143.1	716.1	1 235.4	1 626.1	963.3	763.9	970.6	608.3	566.2	703.4	453.2
1990	938.7	1 202.8	750.9	909.8	1 165.9	728.8	1 250.3	1 644.5	975.1	716.3	916.2	561.8	582.0	716.4	469.3
1989	950.5	1 215.0	761.8	920.2	1 176.6	738.8	1 275.5	1 670.1	998.1	761.6	999.8	586.3	581.3	729.6	458.4
1988	975.7	1 250.7	781.0	947.6	1 215.9	759.1	1 284.3	1 677.6	1 006.8	718.6	917.4	563.6	584.2	732.0	451.0
1987	970.0	1 246.1	774.2	943.4	1 213.4	753.3	1 263.1	1 650.3	989.7	719.8	899.3	583.7	577.3	732.4	448.1
1986	978.6	1 261.7	778.7	952.8	1 230.5	758.1	1 266.7	1 650.1	994.4	720.8	926.7	549.3	576.4	730.5	445.4
1985	988.1	1 278.1	784.5	963.6	1 249.8	764.3	1 261.2	1 634.5	994.4	731.7	926.1	577.2	586.5	755.4	456.7
1984	982.5	1 271.4	779.8	959.7	1 245.9	760.7	1 236.7	1 600.8	976.9	761.7	946.0	567.9	574.4	724.7	443.1
1983	990.0	1 284.5	783.3	967.3	1 259.4	763.9	1 240.5	1 600.7	980.7	757.3	945.0	605.5	565.1	718.8	428.8
1982	985.0	1 279.9	776.6	963.6	1 255.9	758.7	1 221.3	1 580.4	960.1	757.0	940.1	604.4	550.4	738.2	410.3
1981	1 007.1	1 308.2	792.7	984.0	1 282.2	773.6	1 258.4	1 626.6	986.6	784.6	1 030.2	588.0	544.7	710.3	405.3
1980	1 039.1	1 348.1	817.9	1 012.7	1 317.6	796.1	1 314.8	1 697.8	1 033.3	867.0	1 111.5	662.4	589.9	786.5	425.9
1970	1 222.6	1 542.1	971.4	1 193.3	1 513.7	944.0	1 518.1	1 873.9	1 228.7	. . .	. . .	. . .	. . .	. . .	. . .
1960	1 339.2	1 609.0	1 105.3	1 311.3	1 586.0	1 074.4	1 577.5	1 811.1	1 369.7	. . .	. . .	. . .	. . .	. . .	. . .
1950	1 446.0	1 674.2	1 236.0	1 410.8	1 642.5	1 198.0	. . .	. . .	. . .	. . .	. . .	. . .	. . .	. . .	. . .
1940	1 785.0	1 976.0	1 599.4	1 735.3	1 925.2	1 550.4	. . .	. . .	. . .	. . .	. . .	. . .	. . .	. . .	. . .

[1] For 1940–1991, includes deaths among races not shown separately; beginning in 1992, records coded as "other races" and records for which race was unknown, not stated, or not classifiable were assigned to the race of the previous record.
[2] Includes Aleuts and Eskimos.
[3] Includes Chinese, Filipino, Hawaiian, Japanese, and Other Asian or Pacific Islander.
. . . = Not available.

TABLE II-1B. DEATHS, DEATH RATES, AND AGE-ADJUSTED DEATH RATES, BY AGE, SEX, RACE, AND HISPANIC ORIGIN, 2002 AND PRELIMINARY 2003

While four tables with final data for 2003 have been released (such as Table II-1), other statistics for 2003 have been issued in a preliminary form. The preliminary data are based on 90 to 93 percent of the complete records. According to these preliminary data, age-adjusted death rates for all racial and ethnic groups declined in 2003, except for a small increase for American Indians.

Death rates for specific age brackets also tended to decline, with some exceptions. Among male Hispanics, the death rate for persons 85 years old and over increased somewhat. Among American Indians, there were increases in the death rates for those age 75 years and over.

Death rates for infants under 1 year of age were shown to have generally increased in the preliminary 2003 report, but the nation's infant mortality rate was edged

Table II-1B. Deaths, Death Rates, and Age-Adjusted Death Rates, by Age, Sex, Race, and Hispanic Origin, 2002 and Preliminary 2003

(Number, rate per 100,000 population.)

Age, race, and sex	2003 Number	2003 Rate	2002 Number	2002 Rate
ALL RACES, BOTH SEXES				
All Ages	2 443 908	840.4	2 443 387	847.3
Under 1 year [1]	28 428	710.1	28 034	695.0
1–4 years	4 905	31.1	4 858	31.2
5–14 years	6 903	16.8	7 150	17.4
15–24 years	33 050	80.2	33 046	81.4
25–34 years	40 731	102.2	41 355	103.6
35–44 years	88 433	199.3	91 140	202.9
45–54 years	175 591	430.3	172 385	430.1
55–64 years	261 505	937.3	253 342	952.4
65–74 years	413 227	2 253.5	422 990	2 314.7
75–84 years	702 641	5 460.1	707 654	5 556.9
85 years and over	687 959	14 595.6	681 076	14 828.3
Not stated	533	X	357	X
Age-adjusted rate	X	831.2	X	845.3
ALL RACES, MALE				
All Ages	1 198 454	837.9	1 199 264	846.6
Under 1 year [1]	16 131	788.6	15 717	761.5
1–4 years	2 807	34.8	2 806	35.2
5–14 years	4 116	19.6	4 198	20.0
15–24 years	24 232	114.4	24 416	117.3
25–34 years	28 216	139.5	28 736	142.2
35–44 years	55 839	252.3	57 593	257.5
45–54 years	109 830	548.0	107 722	547.5
55–64 years	155 748	1 160.2	151 363	1 184.0
65–74 years	231 375	2 771.2	237 021	2 855.3
75–84 years	341 875	6 632.9	343 504	6 760.5
85 years and over	227 932	15 774.7	225 906	16 254.5
Not stated	354	X	282	X
Age-adjusted rate	X	991.7	X	1 013.7
ALL RACES, FEMALE				
All Ages	1 245 454	842.8	1 244 123	848.0
Under 1 year [1]	12 297	628.0	12 317	625.3
1–4 years	2 098	27.2	2 052	27.0
5–14 years	2 787	13.9	2 952	14.7
15–24 years	8 818	44.0	8 630	43.7
25–34 years	12 516	63.7	12 619	64.0
35–44 years	32 594	146.6	33 547	148.8
45–54 years	65 762	316.8	64 663	316.9
55–64 years	105 757	730.6	101 979	738.0
65–74 years	181 852	1 820.8	185 969	1 864.7
75–84 years	360 766	4 676.5	364 150	4 757.9
85 years and over	460 027	14 074.4	455 170	14 209.6
Not stated	179	X	75	X
Age-adjusted rate	X	705.4	X	715.2
WHITE, [2] BOTH SEXES				
All Ages	2 101 860	889.3	2 102 589	895.7
Under 1 year [1]	18 768	601.8	18 369	586.7
1–4 years	3 458	28.1	3 406	28.1
5–14 years	4 975	15.6	5 138	16.1
15–24 years	24 590	75.9	24 641	77.1
25–34 years	29 293	93.1	29 571	93.5
35–44 years	65 948	183.5	68 093	186.6
45–54 years	133 702	395.1	131 816	395.3
55–64 years	212 254	889.8	205 414	902.5
65–74 years	350 587	2 207.2	360 047	2 267.6
75–84 years	627 597	5 459.1	632 353	5 544.2
85 years and over	630 297	14 806.5	623 455	15 015.9
Not stated	391	X	286	X
Age-adjusted rate	X	816.2	X	829.0

[1]Death rates for "Under 1 year" (based on population estimates) differ from infant mortality rates (based on live births).
[2]Race and Hispanic origin are reported separately on the death certificate. Data for persons of Hispanic origin are included in the data for each race group according to the decedent's reported race.
X = Not applicable.

lower in the final report. (See Table II-1.) One reason for this difference may have been the receipt of more complete final data, and another reason may have been the different denominators used in the two tallies. The infant death rates in Table II-1B were calculated by dividing the number of infant deaths in 2003 by the estimated population of infants under 1 year of age as of July 1, 2003. However, the infant mortality rates were calculated by dividing the number of infant deaths in 2003 by the number of live births during that year.

Table II-1B. Deaths, Death Rates, and Age-Adjusted Death Rates, by Age, Sex, Race, and Hispanic Origin, 2002 and Preliminary 2003—*Continued*

(Number, rate per 100,000 population.)

Age, race, and sex	2003		2002	
	Number	Rate	Number	Rate
WHITE, [2] MALE				
All Ages	1 023 610	875.8	1 025 196	884.0
Under 1 year [1]	10 670	669.4	10 433	650.9
1–4 years	1 967	31.2	1 958	31.5
5–14 years	2 989	18.3	3 005	18.4
15–24 years	17 905	107.0	18 082	109.7
25–34 years	20 531	127.1	20 798	128.3
35–44 years	42 616	235.1	43 955	239.3
45–54 years	85 031	505.9	83 651	505.4
55–64 years	127 302	1 098.4	123 551	1 118.6
65–74 years	197 937	2 708.5	203 735	2 795.4
75–84 years	306 964	6 618.7	308 654	6 738.8
85 years and over	209 425	16 026.4	207 144	16 473.2
Not stated	273	X	230	X
Age-adjusted rate	X	972.2	X	992.9
WHITE, [2] FEMALE				
All Ages	1 078 250	902.5	1 077 393	907.0
Under 1 year [1]	8 098	531.1	7 936	519.4
1–4 years	1 491	24.9	1 448	24.5
5–14 years	1 986	12.8	2 133	13.7
15–24 years	6 685	42.7	6 559	42.4
25–34 years	8 762	57.2	8 773	56.9
35–44 years	23 332	131.0	24 138	133.2
45–54 years	48 671	285.7	48 165	286.8
55–64 years	84 951	692.7	81 863	698.7
65–74 years	152 650	1 780.1	156 312	1 819.7
75–84 years	320 633	4 674.9	323 699	4 742.5
85 years and over	420 872	14 266.1	416 311	14 382.8
Not stated	119	X	56	X
Age-adjusted rate	X	692.9	X	701.3
NON-HISPANIC WHITE, BOTH SEXES				
All Ages	1 979 602	993.7	1 981 973	997.5
Under 1 year [1]	13 450	586.4	13 463	575.9
1–4 years	2 535	27.5	2 502	27.1
5–14 years	3 860	15.5	4 031	16.0
15–24 years	19 433	75.0	19 458	75.8
25–34 years	23 384	95.1	23 758	95.9
35–44 years	57 550	189.1	59 529	191.6
45–54 years	121 317	400.6	119 812	400.1
55–64 years	197 149	900.4	190 843	912.8
65–74 years	329 901	2 239.5	338 961	2 296.1
75–84 years	601 002	5 519.4	606 431	5 596.0
85 years and over	609 812	14 968.6	603 063	15 149.1
Not stated	211	X	122	X
Age-adjusted rate	X	826.0	X	837.5
NON-HISPANIC WHITE, MALE				
All Ages	955 463	978.4	957 645	983.9
Under 1 year [1]	7 706	657.0	7 706	643.5
1–4 years	1 433	30.4	1 431	30.3
5–14 years	2 305	18.0	2 365	18.3
15–24 years	13 881	104.9	13 957	106.7
25–34 years	15 983	129.0	16 339	130.9
35–44 years	36 843	242.0	38 049	244.9
45–54 years	76 789	511.1	75 724	509.9
55–64 years	118 022	1 107.1	114 535	1 126.5
65–74 years	186 357	2 742.1	191 844	2 824.1
75–84 years	293 885	6 694.8	295 763	6 801.7
85 years and over	202 122	16 232.3	199 834	16 641.9
Not stated	138	X	98	X
Age-adjusted rate	X	983.3	X	1 002.2

[1]Death rates for "Under 1 year" (based on population estimates) differ from infant mortality rates (based on live births).
[2]Race and Hispanic origin are reported separately on the death certificate. Data for persons of Hispanic origin are included in the data for each race group according to the decedent's reported race.
X = Not applicable.

Table II-1B. Deaths, Death Rates, and Age-Adjusted Death Rates, by Age, Sex, Race, and Hispanic Origin, 2002 and Preliminary 2003—Continued

(Number, rate per 100,000 population.)

Age, race, and sex	2003		2002	
	Number	Rate	Number	Rate
NON-HISPANIC WHITE, FEMALE				
All Ages	1 024 140	1 008.5	1 024 328	1 010.6
Under 1 year [1]	5 745	512.6	5 757	504.8
1–4 years	1 102	24.6	1 071	23.8
5–14 years	1 555	12.8	1 666	13.6
15–24 years	5 552	43.8	5 501	43.8
25–34 years	7 401	60.7	7 419	60.3
35–44 years	20 707	136.2	21 480	138.3
45–54 years	44 528	291.8	44 088	292.1
55–64 years	79 127	704.2	76 308	710.5
65–74 years	143 544	1 809.0	147 117	1 846.0
75–84 years	307 118	4 725.5	310 668	4 787.9
85 years and over	407 690	14 412.3	403 229	14 504.3
Not stated	73	X	24	X
Age-adjusted rate	X	702.4	X	709.9
BLACK, [2] BOTH SEXES				
All Ages	289 202	758.1	290 051	768.4
Under 1 year [1]	8 437	1 279.1	8 524	1 263.6
1–4 years	1 185	46.3	1 196	47.1
5–14 years	1 551	22.9	1 666	24.5
15–24 years	7 064	111.8	7 045	113.7
25–34 years	9 793	178.9	10 171	186.8
35–44 years	19 583	340.1	20 235	348.6
45–54 years	36 698	765.0	35 623	765.8
55–64 years	42 493	1 537.9	41 336	1 565.2
65–74 years	52 797	3 089.0	53 314	3 159.3
75–84 years	61 928	6 308.7	62 862	6 518.9
85 years and over	47 547	13 871.4	48 022	14 260.8
Not stated	125	X	57	X
Age-adjusted rate	X	1 058.0	X	1 083.3
BLACK, [2] MALE				
All Ages	146 818	807.1	146 835	816.7
Under 1 year [1]	4 772	1 419.5	4 652	1 351.5
1–4 years	691	53.1	702	54.4
5–14 years	907	26.3	998	28.9
15–24 years	5 351	168.3	5 364	172.6
25–34 years	6 604	252.7	6 848	264.5
35–44 years	11 424	422.3	11 849	434.7
45–54 years	21 745	980.5	21 122	983.0
55–64 years	24 605	1 997.8	24 000	2 039.2
65–74 years	28 151	3 961.6	28 198	4 024.5
75–84 years	28 278	7 976.1	28 478	8 169.6
85 years and over	14 219	14 825.2	14 584	15 635.5
Not stated	71	X	40	X
Age-adjusted rate	X	1 308.3	X	1 341.4
BLACK, [2] FEMALE				
All Ages	142 384	713.4	143 216	724.4
Under 1 year [1]	3 665	1 133.1	3 872	1 172.0
1–4 years	494	39.2	494	39.5
5–14 years	644	19.3	668	19.9
15–24 years	1 712	54.5	1 681	54.4
25–34 years	3 189	111.4	3 323	116.4
35–44 years	8 160	267.3	8 386	272.3
45–54 years	14 953	579.7	14 501	579.4
55–64 years	17 888	1 168.1	17 336	1 184.2
65–74 years	24 646	2 468.1	25 116	2 545.0
75–84 years	33 650	5 366.0	34 384	5 584.4
85 years and over	33 328	13 500.8	33 438	13 734.2
Not stated	55	X	17	X
Age-adjusted rate	X	879.8	X	901.8

[1]Death rates for "Under 1 year" (based on population estimates) differ from infant mortality rates (based on live births).
[2]Race and Hispanic origin are reported separately on the death certificate. Data for persons of Hispanic origin are included in the data for each race group according to the decedent's reported race.
X = Not applicable.

Table II-1B. Deaths, Death Rates, and Age-Adjusted Death Rates, by Age, Sex, Race, and Hispanic Origin, 2002 and Preliminary 2003—*Continued*

(Number, rate per 100,000 population.)

Age, race, and sex	2003		2002	
	Number	Rate	Number	Rate
NON-HISPANIC BLACK, BOTH SEXES				
All Ages	285 777	782.8	286 573	792.8
Under 1 year [1]	8 185	1 294.1	8 284	1 280.3
1–4 years	1 157	47.5	1 163	48.4
5–14 years	1 533	23.9	1 634	25.3
15–24 years	6 947	115.3	6 904	116.9
25–34 years	9 645	186.0	10 009	193.9
35–44 years	19 354	350.5	19 955	357.8
45–54 years	36 274	781.6	35 211	782.0
55–64 years	42 000	1 565.3	40 878	1 592.9
65–74 years	52 234	3 137.8	52 748	3 204.8
75–84 years	61 321	6 386.3	62 183	6 584.8
85 years and over	47 069	14 001.5	47 565	14 386.7
Not stated	56	X	39	X
Age-adjusted rate	X	1 074.9	X	1 099.2
NON-HISPANIC BLACK, MALE				
All Ages	144 881	833.4	144 802	842.3
Under 1 year [1]	4 626	1 435.5	4 520	1 369.3
1–4 years	676	54.7	681	55.8
5–14 years	896	27.5	977	29.8
15–24 years	5 253	173.5	5 248	177.4
25–34 years	6 498	262.8	6 723	274.3
35–44 years	11 282	435.2	11 661	445.7
45–54 years	21 465	1 001.4	20 839	1 002.9
55–64 years	24 281	2 032.0	23 706	2 074.5
65–74 years	27 810	4 019.9	27 859	4 078.9
75–84 years	27 980	8 074.2	28 137	8 246.2
85 years and over	14 086	15 007.6	14 422	15 776.9
Not stated	30	X	29	X
Age-adjusted rate	X	1 329.9	X	1 360.6
NON-HISPANIC BLACK, FEMALE				
All Ages	140 895	736.7	141 771	748.0
Under 1 year [1]	3 559	1 147.2	3 764	1 187.5
1–4 years	482	40.2	482	40.8
5–14 years	637	20.1	657	20.7
15–24 years	1 694	56.5	1 656	56.1
25–34 years	3 148	116.0	3 286	121.3
35–44 years	8 072	275.5	8 294	280.1
45–54 years	14 809	593.0	14 372	592.7
55–64 years	17 719	1 190.6	17 172	1 206.3
65–74 years	24 424	2 510.5	24 889	2 584.8
75–84 years	33 341	5 433.1	34 046	5 644.9
85 years and over	32 983	13 611.8	33 143	13 855.4
Not stated	27	X	10	X
Age-adjusted rate	X	893.7	X	915.3
AMERICAN INDIAN, [2, 3] BOTH SEXES				
All Ages	13 112	421.5	12 415	403.6
Under 1 year [1]	336	798.1	343	822.1
1–4 years	93	49.2	90	45.2
5–14 years	133	23.0	126	21.6
15–24 years	615	107.5	583	104.6
25–34 years	635	136.8	652	141.9
35–44 years	1 230	263.6	1 169	248.5
45–54 years	1 797	466.8	1 602	428.9
55–64 years	2 045	918.1	1 886	898.0
65–74 years	2 263	1 959.5	2 291	2 076.1
75–84 years	2 373	4 188.0	2 215	4 110.1
85 years and over	1 583	8 393.9	1 451	8 299.5
Not stated	9	X	7	X
Age-adjusted rate	X	683.8	X	677.4

[1]Death rates for "Under 1 year" (based on population estimates) differ from infant mortality rates (based on live births).
[2]Race and Hispanic origin are reported separately on the death certificate. Data for persons of Hispanic origin are included in the data for each race group according to the decedent's reported race.
[3]Includes deaths among Aleuts and Eskimos.
X = Not applicable.

Table II-1B. Deaths, Death Rates, and Age-Adjusted Death Rates, by Age, Sex, Race, and Hispanic Origin, 2002 and Preliminary 2003—*Continued*

(Number, rate per 100,000 population.)

Age, race, and sex	2003 Number	2003 Rate	2002 Number	2002 Rate
AMERICAN INDIAN, [2,3] MALE				
All Ages	7 075	455.6	6 750	439.6
Under 1 year [1]	199	930.2	191	896.8
1–4 years	52	54.2	49	48.3
5–14 years	83	28.3	65	22.0
15–24 years	445	151.4	416	145.1
25–34 years	438	182.8	457	193.1
35–44 years	782	337.2	749	321.5
45–54 years	1 076	576.1	978	539.4
55–64 years	1 136	1 058.3	1 074	1 059.2
65–74 years	1 191	2 237.3	1 201	2 366.5
75–84 years	1 090	4 635.5	1 048	4 748.3
85 years and over	577	9 567.2	516	9 219.2
Not stated	6	X	6	X
Age-adjusted rate	X	794.6	X	794.2
AMERICAN INDIAN, [2,3] FEMALE				
All Ages	6 037	387.5	5 665	367.7
Under 1 year [1]	137	661.7	152	744.1
1–4 years	41	44.1	41	42.0
5–14 years	50	17.5	61	21.2
15–24 years	170	61.1	167	61.7
25–34 years	197	87.8	195	87.5
35–44 years	448	190.9	420	176.8
45–54 years	721	363.8	624	324.7
55–64 years	909	787.6	812	747.5
65–74 years	1 072	1 721.9	1 090	1 828.9
75–84 years	1 283	3 870.5	1 167	3 667.4
85 years and over	1 006	7 842.2	935	7 866.4
Not stated	3	X	1	X
Age-adjusted rate	X	592.2	X	581.1
ASIAN OR PACIFIC ISLANDER, [2] BOTH SEXES				
All Ages	39 734	301.0	38 332	299.5
Under 1 year [1]	887	484.4	798	427.4
1–4 years	169	23.4	166	23.4
5–14 years	243	13.5	220	12.4
15–24 years	781	40.5	777	41.3
25–34 years	1 010	41.0	961	40.1
35–44 years	1 672	75.9	1 643	76.1
45–54 years	3 394	190.5	3 344	195.3
55–64 years	4 714	444.4	4 706	475.5
65–74 years	7 581	1 205.7	7 338	1 226.7
75–84 years	10 743	3 216.6	10 224	3 290.4
85 years and over	8 532	8 986.7	8 148	9 378.6
Not stated	8	X	7	X
Age-adjusted rate	X	461.2	X	474.4
ASIAN OR PACIFIC ISLANDER, [2] MALE				
All Ages	20 951	326.4	20 483	331.4
Under 1 year [1]	490	521.4	441	461.9
1–4 years	96	26.1	97	27.1
5–14 years	137	14.9	130	14.4
15–24 years	531	54.0	554	58.6
25–34 years	642	53.0	633	54.5
35–44 years	1 018	95.4	1 040	100.0
45–54 years	1 977	237.5	1 971	248.4
55–64 years	2 705	545.7	2 738	594.5
65–74 years	4 096	1 476.4	3 887	1 487.1
75–84 years	5 544	4 007.7	5 324	4 090.8
85 years and over	3 711	10 242.6	3 662	10 938.5
Not stated	5	X	6	X
Age-adjusted rate	X	556.7	X	578.4

[1]Death rates for "Under 1 year" (based on population estimates) differ from infant mortality rates (based on live births).
[2]Race and Hispanic origin are reported separately on the death certificate. Data for persons of Hispanic origin are included in the data for each race group according to the decedent's reported race.
[3]Includes deaths among Aleuts and Eskimos.
X = Not applicable.

TABLE II-2. NUMBER OF DEATHS, DEATH RATES, AND AGE-ADJUSTED DEATH RATES, BY RACE, HISPANIC ORIGIN, AND SEX, 1997–2002

The age-adjusted death rate for Hispanics was 25 percent lower in 2002 than the rate for non-Hispanic Whites. The Hispanic population had lower age-specific death rates at older ages. (See Table II-4.) The underreporting of deaths for certain races and ethnicities, mentioned in the discussion of Table II-1, applied to Hispanics, but its magnitude was estimated to have only affected 2 percent of all reported Hispanic deaths. The lower death rate for Hispanics could have been due to health reasons, such as low rates of smoking and drinking by Hispanic women. There was also a hypothesis that elderly immigrants tended to return to their country of origin before their death (the so-called "salmon bias effect").

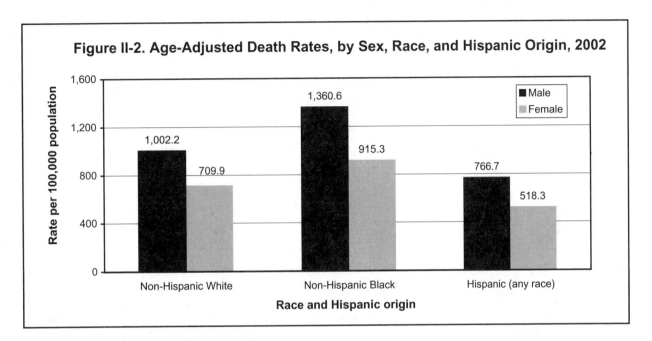

Figure II-2. Age-Adjusted Death Rates, by Sex, Race, and Hispanic Origin, 2002

Table II-2. Number of Deaths, Death Rates, and Age-Adjusted Death Rates, by Race, Hispanic Origin, and Sex, 1997–2002

(Number, rate per 100,000 population.)

Year	All origins [1]			Hispanic [2]			Non-Hispanic [3]			Non-Hispanic White			Non-Hispanic Black		
	Both sexes	Male	Female	Both sexes	Male	Female	Both sexes	Male	Female	Both sexes	Male	Female	Both sexes	Male	Female
Number of Deaths															
2002	2 443 387	1 199 264	1 244 123	117 135	65 703	51 432	2 318 269	1 129 090	1 189 179	1 981 973	957 645	1 024 328	286 573	144 802	141 771
2001	2 416 425	1 183 421	1 233 004	113 413	63 317	50 096	2 295 244	1 115 683	1 179 561	1 962 810	945 967	1 016 843	284 343	143 971	140 372
2000	2 403 351	1 177 578	1 225 773	107 254	60 172	47 082	2 287 846	1 112 704	1 175 142	1 959 919	944 781	1 015 138	282 676	143 297	139 379
1999	2 391 399	1 175 460	1 215 939	103 740	57 991	45 749	2 279 325	1 112 718	1 166 607	1 953 197	944 913	1 008 284	281 979	143 883	138 096
1998	2 337 256	1 157 260	1 179 996	98 406	55 821	42 585	2 230 127	1 096 677	1 133 450	1 912 802	931 844	980 958	275 264	141 627	133 637
1997	2 314 245	1 154 039	1 160 206	95 460	54 348	41 112	2 209 450	1 094 541	1 114 909	1 895 461	929 703	965 758	273 381	142 241	131 140
Death Rate															
2002	847.3	846.6	848.0	302.2	328.7	274.0	928.8	928.0	929.5	997.5	983.9	1 010.6	792.8	842.3	748.0
2001	848.5	846.4	850.4	306.8	332.9	279.0	926.2	923.6	928.6	991.1	975.6	1 006.1	798.1	849.7	751.2
2000	854.0	853.0	855.0	303.8	331.3	274.6	929.6	928.1	931.0	993.2	978.5	1 007.3	805.5	859.5	756.7
1999	857.0	859.2	854.9	305.7	332.6	277.2	929.9	932.2	927.8	990.7	979.6	1 001.3	812.1	872.8	757.3
1998	847.3	856.4	838.5	303.9	336.0	270.0	916.0	925.3	907.1	972.9	969.2	976.5	805.6	873.7	744.1
1997	848.8	864.6	833.6	309.0	343.2	272.9	913.9	930.4	898.3	967.4	970.6	964.3	813.5	892.9	741.9
Age-Adjusted Death Rate															
2002	845.3	1 013.7	715.2	629.3	766.7	518.3	856.5	1 026.5	725.8	837.5	1 002.2	709.9	1 099.2	1 360.6	915.3
2001	854.5	1 029.1	721.8	658.7	802.5	544.2	864.0	1 039.8	730.9	842.9	1 012.8	713.5	1 116.5	1 393.7	925.5
2000	869.0	1 053.8	731.4	665.7	818.1	546.0	877.9	1 063.8	740.0	855.5	1 035.4	721.5	1 137.0	1 422.0	941.2
1999	875.6	1 067.0	734.0	676.4	830.5	555.9	883.9	1 076.4	741.9	859.8	1 045.5	722.3	1 150.1	1 449.4	946.0
1998	870.6	1 069.4	724.7	665.4	833.6	536.9	878.4	1 078.2	732.4	854.1	1 046.7	712.8	1 141.8	1 448.2	932.9
1997	878.1	1 088.1	725.6	669.3	840.5	538.8	885.3	1 096.4	732.6	859.7	1 063.2	712.5	1 154.3	1 476.7	934.2

[1]Figures for origin not stated are included in "All origins" but are not distributed among specified origins.
[2]May be of any race.
[3]Includes races other than White and Black.

TABLE II-3. NUMBER OF DEATHS AND DEATH RATES, BY AGE, RACE, AND SEX, 2002

The death rate by age began at a high of 695 per 100,000 persons for infant deaths (under 1 year of age) in 2002. The rate dropped as age increased, reaching a low of 15 deaths per 100,000 persons in the 5- to 9-year-old age group. This indicated that a child who survived its first year of life had excellent subsequent survival chances. However, mortality rates increased for every successive age group, climbing slowly at first, then more rapidly. The death rate per 100,000 persons neared 1,200 by age 60–64 years and reached almost 15,000 by age 85 years and over.

The low death rates for Asians and Pacific Islanders, already noted in the discussion of Table II-1, were confirmed by their low age-specific death rates in this table. Table II-4 shows that Hispanics also had relatively low age-specific death rates, but the rates for Asians and Pacific Islanders were even lower. Bias would have occurred if the coverage of Asians and Pacific Islanders in the census had differed from the number of times the race was reported on death certificates. The funeral director, who often filled out the death certificate, could have marked the deceased as White instead of Asian. A study indicated an 11 percent net underreporting of deaths of Asians and Pacific Islanders. (For reference, see notes for Table II-1A.)

Table II-3. Number of Deaths and Death Rates, by Age, Race, and Sex, 2002

(Number, rate per 100,000 population.)

Age	All races			White			Black			American Indian [1]			Asian or Pacific Islander [2]		
	Both sexes	Male	Female	Both sexes	Male	Female	Both sexes	Male	Female	Both sexes	Male	Female	Both sexes	Male	Female
Number of Deaths															
All ages	2 443 387	1 199 264	1 244 123	2 102 589	1 025 196	1 077 393	290 051	146 835	143 216	12 415	6 750	5 665	38 332	20 483	17 849
Under 1 year	28 034	15 717	12 317	18 369	10 433	7 936	8 524	4 652	3 872	343	191	152	798	441	357
1–4 years	4 858	2 806	2 052	3 406	1 958	1 448	1 196	702	494	90	49	41	166	97	69
5–9 years	3 018	1 702	1 316	2 168	1 219	949	701	402	299	48	21	27	101	60	41
10–14 years	4 132	2 496	1 636	2 970	1 786	1 184	965	596	369	78	44	34	119	70	49
15–19 years	13 812	9 844	3 968	10 613	7 474	3 139	2 602	1 963	639	267	178	89	330	229	101
20–24 years	19 234	14 572	4 662	14 028	10 608	3 420	4 443	3 401	1 042	316	238	78	447	325	122
25–29 years	17 959	12 954	5 005	12 703	9 219	3 484	4 550	3 229	1 321	290	218	72	416	288	128
30–34 years	23 396	15 782	7 614	16 868	11 579	5 289	5 621	3 619	2 002	362	239	123	545	345	200
35–39 years	35 347	22 626	12 721	25 912	16 840	9 072	8 227	4 996	3 231	512	335	177	696	455	241
40–44 years	55 793	34 967	20 826	42 181	27 115	15 066	12 008	6 853	5 155	657	414	243	947	585	362
45–49 years	76 065	47 701	28 364	57 690	36 894	20 796	16 184	9 501	6 683	751	455	296	1 440	851	589
50–54 years	96 320	60 021	36 299	74 126	46 757	27 369	19 439	11 621	7 818	851	523	328	1 904	1 120	784
55–59 years	115 441	69 830	45 611	92 712	56 535	36 177	19 693	11 550	8 143	894	514	380	2 142	1 231	911
60–64 years	137 901	81 533	56 368	112 702	67 016	45 686	21 643	12 450	9 193	992	560	432	2 564	1 507	1 057
65–69 years	175 591	100 590	75 001	146 491	84 741	61 750	24 783	13 465	11 318	1 095	590	505	3 222	1 794	1 428
70–74 years	247 399	136 431	110 968	213 556	118 994	94 562	28 531	14 733	13 798	1 196	611	585	4 116	2 093	2 023
75–79 years	330 140	169 625	160 515	291 430	150 862	140 568	32 431	15 434	16 997	1 160	586	574	5 119	2 743	2 376
80–84 years	377 514	173 879	203 635	340 923	157 792	183 131	30 431	13 044	17 387	1 055	462	593	5 105	2 581	2 524
85 years and over	681 076	225 906	455 170	623 455	207 144	416 311	48 022	14 584	33 438	1 451	516	935	8 148	3 662	4 486
Not stated	357	282	75	286	230	56	57	40	17	7	6	1	7	6	1
Death Rate															
All ages [3]	847.3	846.6	848.0	895.7	884.0	907.0	768.4	816.7	724.4	403.6	439.6	367.7	299.5	331.4	269.7
Under 1 year [4]	695.0	761.5	625.3	586.7	650.9	519.4	1 263.6	1 351.5	1 172.0	822.1	896.8	744.1	427.4	461.9	391.4
1–4 years	31.2	35.2	27.0	28.1	31.5	24.5	47.1	54.4	39.5	45.2	48.3	42.0	23.4	27.1	19.6
5–9 years	15.2	16.7	13.5	14.0	15.4	12.6	21.3	24.1	18.5	17.3	15.0	19.8	11.5	13.5	9.5
10–14 years	19.5	23.1	15.9	18.1	21.2	14.8	27.5	33.4	21.3	25.5	28.4	22.5	13.4	15.3	11.3
15–19 years	67.8	94.0	40.1	66.3	90.5	40.4	82.0	121.7	41.0	91.2	119.1	62.1	37.0	50.5	23.1
20–24 years	95.2	140.8	47.3	88.0	128.9	44.4	146.8	227.6	68.0	119.5	173.6	61.2	45.2	66.1	24.5
25–29 years	94.7	134.4	53.6	85.0	119.7	48.1	172.1	255.7	95.7	126.2	182.7	65.2	36.2	51.7	21.6
30–34 years	111.6	149.4	73.3	101.1	136.0	64.8	200.7	272.9	135.7	157.5	203.6	109.4	43.7	56.9	31.2
35–39 years	161.3	206.6	116.1	146.8	188.7	103.9	284.0	366.5	210.6	217.8	284.5	150.8	61.8	83.1	41.6
40–44 years	242.6	306.4	179.7	224.0	287.2	160.5	412.9	502.9	333.6	279.1	359.3	202.3	91.8	118.8	67.2
45–49 years	357.1	454.7	262.4	327.4	420.4	235.1	634.1	801.4	489.0	365.2	455.2	280.0	155.7	197.5	119.3
50–54 years	512.8	653.5	378.2	471.3	601.2	344.3	925.9	1 206.6	688.0	507.0	642.8	379.2	241.9	309.0	184.6
55–59 years	770.1	961.8	590.0	723.5	902.0	552.6	1 321.6	1 719.3	995.2	730.0	868.2	600.7	379.7	470.2	301.3
60–64 years	1 187.7	1 476.0	926.0	1 133.0	1 402.7	883.7	1 880.7	2 464.7	1 423.7	1 133.0	1 327.2	952.3	602.6	758.1	466.3
65–69 years	1 832.7	2 265.9	1 458.7	1 777.6	2 196.1	1 409.1	2 632.0	3 357.1	2 093.9	1 726.0	1 992.2	1 493.0	961.2	1 196.0	772.4
70–74 years	2 845.9	3 533.0	2 296.7	2 796.3	3 469.7	2 247.4	3 824.9	4 918.1	3 091.2	2 549.7	2 891.1	2 269.7	1 563.3	1 879.0	1 331.8
75–79 years	4 449.1	5 522.7	3 690.9	4 407.8	5 469.3	3 648.0	5 571.3	7 088.6	4 664.6	3 493.9	4 189.6	2 987.4	2 646.4	3 371.4	2 120.0
80–84 years	7 103.8	8 652.3	6 162.2	7 111.3	8 660.8	6 161.6	7 962.2	9 968.4	6 917.8	5 098.8	5 715.0	4 703.7	4 352.6	5 290.5	3 684.6
85 years and over	14 828.3	16 254.5	14 209.6	15 015.9	16 473.2	14 382.8	14 260.8	15 635.5	13 734.2	8 299.5	9 219.2	7 866.4	9 378.6	10 938.5	8 400.6

[1] Includes Aleuts and Eskimos.
[2] Includes Chinese, Filipino, Hawaiian, Japanese, and Other Asian or Pacific Islander.
[3] Figures for age not stated are included in "All ages" but not distributed among age groups.
[4] Death rates for "Under 1 year" (based on population estimates) differ from infant mortality rates (based on live births).

TABLE II-4. NUMBER OF DEATHS AND DEATH RATES, BY RACE, HISPANIC ORIGIN, AGE, AND SEX, 2002

Death rates for Hispanic men and women were considerably lower than those for non-Hispanic Whites and non-Hispanic Blacks in all age groups above 24 years old. The comments for Table II-2 present some hypotheses for this finding.

TABLE II-5. NUMBER OF DEATHS, DEATH RATES, AND AGE-ADJUSTED DEATH RATES, ACCORDING TO SPECIFIED HISPANIC ORIGIN, RACE, AND SEX, 2002

Age-adjusted death rates for Cubans and Mexicans were particularly low relative to the rates for non-Hispanics. Data for Puerto Ricans are shown separately in this table, but Central and South American and other Hispanic deaths were combined for the computations of death rates, due to the small numbers of these populations.

Table II-4. Number of Deaths and Death Rates, by Race, Hispanic Origin, Age, and Sex, 2002

(Number, rate per 100,000 population.)

Age	All origins [1] Both sexes	Male	Female	Hispanic [2] Both sexes	Male	Female	Non-Hispanic [3] Both sexes	Male	Female	Non-Hispanic White Both sexes	Male	Female	Non-Hispanic Black Both sexes	Male	Female
Number of Deaths															
All ages	2 443 387	1 199 264	1 244 123	117 135	65 703	51 432	2 318 269	1 129 090	1 189 179	1 981 973	957 645	1 024 328	286 573	144 802	141 771
Under 1 year	28 034	15 717	12 317	4 943	2 746	2 197	22 816	12 815	10 001	13 463	7 706	5 757	8 284	4 520	3 764
1–4 years	4 858	2 806	2 052	933	546	387	3 904	2 250	1 654	2 502	1 431	1 071	1 163	681	482
5–9 years	3 018	1 702	1 316	538	303	235	2 472	1 394	1 078	1 643	923	720	686	392	294
10–14 years	4 132	2 496	1 636	586	344	242	3 530	2 140	1 390	2 388	1 442	946	948	585	363
15–19 years	13 812	9 844	3 968	2 086	1 614	472	11 671	8 192	3 479	8 552	5 884	2 668	2 542	1 914	628
20–24 years	19 234	14 572	4 662	3 169	2 568	601	15 987	11 937	4 050	10 906	8 073	2 833	4 362	3 334	1 028
25–29 years	17 959	12 954	5 005	2 803	2 239	564	15 073	10 657	4 416	9 900	6 988	2 912	4 487	3 179	1 308
30–34 years	23 396	15 782	7 614	3 013	2 235	778	20 256	13 457	6 799	13 858	9 351	4 507	5 522	3 544	1 978
35–39 years	35 347	22 626	12 721	3 644	2 514	1 130	31 512	19 976	11 536	22 230	14 299	7 931	8 102	4 906	3 196
40–44 years	55 793	34 967	20 826	4 823	3 314	1 509	50 713	31 475	19 238	37 299	23 750	13 549	11 853	6 755	5 098
45–49 years	76 065	47 701	28 364	5 527	3 695	1 832	70 178	43 743	26 435	52 044	33 102	18 942	16 002	9 372	6 630
50–54 years	96 320	60 021	36 299	6 218	4 024	2 194	89 665	55 690	33 975	67 768	42 622	25 146	19 209	11 467	7 742
55–59 years	115 441	69 830	45 611	6 634	4 247	2 387	108 370	65 283	43 087	85 916	52 169	33 747	19 483	11 414	8 069
60–64 years	137 901	81 533	56 368	7 581	4 515	3 066	129 815	76 683	53 132	104 927	62 366	42 561	21 395	12 292	9 103
65–69 years	175 591	100 590	75 001	9 060	5 214	3 846	165 934	94 990	70 944	137 191	79 363	57 828	24 508	13 292	11 216
70–74 years	247 399	136 431	110 968	11 416	6 262	5 154	235 248	129 716	105 532	201 770	112 481	89 289	28 240	14 567	13 673
75–79 years	330 140	169 625	160 515	12 797	6 654	6 143	316 397	162 434	153 963	278 144	143 909	134 235	32 076	15 246	16 830
80–84 years	377 514	173 879	203 635	12 041	5 637	6 404	364 481	167 757	196 724	328 287	151 854	176 433	30 107	12 891	17 216
85 years and over	681 076	225 906	455 170	19 265	6 977	12 288	660 078	218 367	441 711	603 063	199 834	403 229	47 565	14 422	33 143
Not stated	357	282	75	58	55	3	169	134	35	122	98	24	39	29	10
Death Rate															
All ages [4]	847.3	846.6	848.0	302.2	328.7	274.0	928.8	928.0	929.5	997.5	983.9	1 010.6	792.8	842.3	748.0
Under 1 year [5]	695.0	761.5	625.3	592.7	644.0	539.1	713.0	782.6	640.1	575.9	643.5	504.8	1 280.3	1 369.3	1 187.5
1–4 years	31.2	35.2	27.0	29.8	34.2	25.3	31.4	35.4	27.2	27.1	30.3	23.8	48.4	55.8	40.8
5–9 years	15.2	16.7	13.5	14.4	15.9	12.9	15.3	16.8	13.7	13.7	14.9	12.3	22.0	24.8	19.2
10–14 years	19.5	23.1	15.9	16.6	19.0	14.0	20.1	23.7	16.2	18.1	21.3	14.8	28.3	34.4	22.0
15–19 years	67.8	94.0	40.1	65.2	97.0	30.8	67.9	93.0	41.6	65.5	87.6	42.0	83.8	124.1	42.1
20–24 years	95.2	140.8	47.3	87.9	128.9	37.2	96.3	142.8	49.1	86.6	126.7	45.6	151.7	235.3	70.5
25–29 years	94.7	134.4	53.6	74.7	108.7	33.3	99.1	140.6	57.8	86.5	121.2	51.3	179.6	266.6	100.1
30–34 years	111.6	149.4	73.3	84.2	116.5	46.9	116.6	155.7	77.8	103.9	139.3	68.1	207.4	281.5	141.0
35–39 years	161.3	206.6	116.1	115.5	151.4	75.6	168.0	215.0	121.9	151.1	194.0	108.0	292.2	376.4	217.4
40–44 years	242.6	306.4	179.7	181.8	242.6	117.3	249.2	313.3	186.7	228.1	290.9	165.4	422.8	514.5	342.0
45–49 years	357.1	454.7	262.4	266.6	353.7	178.1	365.0	463.0	270.3	331.7	424.3	240.1	648.6	818.5	501.4
50–54 years	512.8	653.5	378.2	393.2	516.8	273.2	521.3	662.5	386.3	475.5	604.5	349.1	943.7	1 229.3	702.1
55–59 years	770.1	961.8	590.0	583.0	779.4	402.6	782.3	972.1	603.7	731.3	906.2	563.3	1 346.7	1 751.3	1 014.9
60–64 years	1 187.7	1 476.0	926.0	905.8	1 158.2	685.7	1 204.9	1 493.6	942.0	1 145.4	1 413.9	896.1	1 911.2	2 503.4	1 448.4
65–69 years	1 832.7	2 265.9	1 458.7	1 378.9	1 765.5	1 063.3	1 859.4	2 292.2	1 484.2	1 800.0	2 216.9	1 430.8	2 670.7	3 402.3	2 128.3
70–74 years	2 845.9	3 533.0	2 296.7	2 179.7	2 747.9	1 742.1	2 879.6	3 569.8	2 326.6	2 825.5	3 500.6	2 273.2	3 877.8	4 983.1	3 136.6
75–79 years	4 449.1	5 522.7	3 690.9	3 411.7	4 258.0	2 807.4	4 490.9	5 572.1	3 727.8	4 446.2	5 514.6	3 681.6	5 630.1	7 157.7	4 718.0
80–84 years	7 103.8	8 652.3	6 162.2	5 365.5	6 447.7	4 674.8	7 161.0	8 727.3	6 210.5	7 166.0	8 733.5	6 207.1	8 036.6	10 054.7	6 986.6
85 years and over	14 828.3	16 254.5	14 209.6	10 679.0	11 674.1	10 186.0	14 958.7	16 418.0	14 329.1	15 149.1	16 641.9	14 504.3	14 386.7	15 776.9	13 855.4

[1] Figures for origin not stated are included in "All origins" but not distributed among specified origins.
[2] May be of any race.
[3] Includes races other than White and Black.
[4] Figures for age not stated are included in "All ages" but not distributed among age groups.
[5] Death rates for "Under 1 year" (based on population estimates) differ from infant mortality rates (based on live births).

Table II-5. Number of Deaths, Death Rates, and Age-Adjusted Death Rates, According to Specified Hispanic Origin, Race, and Sex, 2002

(Number, rate per 100,000 population.)

Hispanic origin, race, and sex	All ages	Under 1 year [1]	1–4 years	5–14 years	15–24 years	25–34 years	35–44 years	45–54 years	55–64 years	65–74 years	75–84 years	85 years and over	Age not stated	Age-adjusted rate
NUMBER OF DEATHS														
All Origins	2 443 387	28 034	4 858	7 150	33 046	41 355	91 140	172 385	253 342	422 990	707 654	681 076	357	X
Male	1 199 264	15 717	2 806	4 198	24 416	28 736	57 593	107 722	151 363	237 021	343 504	225 906	282	X
Female	1 244 123	12 317	2 052	2 952	8 630	12 619	33 547	64 663	101 979	185 969	364 150	455 170	75	X
Hispanic [2]	117 135	4 943	933	1 124	5 255	5 816	8 467	11 745	14 215	20 476	24 838	19 265	58	X
Male	65 703	2 746	546	647	4 182	4 474	5 828	7 719	8 762	11 476	12 291	6 977	55	X
Female	51 432	2 197	387	477	1 073	1 342	2 639	4 026	5 453	9 000	12 547	12 288	3	X
Mexican	65 968	3 540	705	801	3 754	3 884	4 883	6 746	7 794	11 298	13 299	9 239	25	X
Male	38 180	1 978	407	470	3 033	3 026	3 432	4 435	4 744	6 275	6 744	3 612	24	X
Female	27 788	1 562	298	331	721	858	1 451	2 311	3 050	5 023	6 555	5 627	1	X
Puerto Rican	15 068	462	72	96	392	599	1 293	1 877	2 407	2 869	2 919	2 078	4	X
Male	8 367	257	50	48	293	421	853	1 254	1 518	1 620	1 348	701	4	X
Female	6 701	205	22	48	99	178	440	623	889	1 249	1 571	1 377	-	X
Cuban	11 743	67	6	10	71	117	310	569	1 057	2 197	3 600	3 739	-	X
Male	6 002	35	5	6	59	95	220	390	719	1 360	1 879	1 234	-	X
Female	5 741	32	1	4	12	22	90	179	338	837	1 721	2 505	-	X
Central and South American ...	11 490	402	74	127	648	803	1 039	1 270	1 459	1 956	2 091	1 617	4	X
Male	6 070	217	40	72	516	628	688	788	798	1 005	843	471	4	X
Female	5 420	185	34	55	132	175	351	482	661	951	1 248	1 146	-	X
Other and unknown Hispanic ..	12 866	472	76	90	390	413	942	1 283	1 498	2 156	2 929	2 592	25	X
Male	7 084	259	44	51	281	304	635	852	983	1 216	1 477	959	23	X
Female	5 782	213	32	39	109	109	307	431	515	940	1 452	1 633	2	X
Non-Hispanic [3]	2 318 269	22 816	3 904	6 002	27 658	35 329	82 225	159 843	238 185	401 182	680 878	660 078	169	X
Male	1 129 090	12 815	2 250	3 534	20 129	24 114	51 451	99 433	141 966	224 706	330 191	218 367	134	X
Female	1 189 179	10 001	1 654	2 468	7 529	11 215	30 774	60 410	96 219	176 476	350 687	441 711	35	X
White	1 981 973	13 463	2 502	4 031	19 458	23 758	59 529	119 812	190 843	338 961	606 431	603 063	122	X
Male	957 645	7 706	1 431	2 365	13 957	16 339	38 049	75 724	114 535	191 844	295 763	199 834	98	X
Female	1 024 328	5 757	1 071	1 666	5 501	7 419	21 480	44 088	76 308	147 117	310 668	403 229	24	X
Black	286 573	8 284	1 163	1 634	6 904	10 009	19 955	35 211	40 878	52 748	62 183	47 565	39	X
Male	144 802	4 520	681	977	5 248	6 723	11 661	20 839	23 706	27 859	28 137	14 422	29	X
Female	141 771	3 764	482	657	1 656	3 286	8 294	14 372	17 172	24 889	34 046	33 143	10	X
Not stated [4]	7 983	275	21	24	133	210	448	797	942	1 332	1 938	1 733	130	X
Male	4 471	156	10	17	105	148	314	570	635	839	1 022	562	93	X
Female	3 512	119	11	7	28	62	134	227	307	493	916	1 171	37	X
DEATH RATE [5]														
All Origins [6]	847.3	695.0	31.2	17.4	81.4	103.6	202.9	430.1	952.4	2 314.7	5 556.9	14 828.3	X	845.3
Male	846.6	761.5	35.2	20.0	117.3	142.2	257.5	547.5	1 184.0	2 855.3	6 760.5	16 254.5	X	1 013.7
Female	848.0	625.3	27.0	14.7	43.7	64.0	148.8	316.9	738.0	1 864.7	4 757.9	14 209.6	X	715.2
Hispanic	302.2	592.7	29.8	15.5	77.2	79.3	145.8	321.3	719.8	1 734.1	4 143.1	10 679.0	X	629.3
Male	328.7	644.0	34.2	17.4	114.4	112.5	192.5	423.4	937.4	2 193.4	5 043.5	11 674.1	X	766.7
Female	274.0	539.1	25.3	13.5	34.1	40.0	94.9	219.8	524.3	1 368.7	3 526.4	10 186.0	X	518.3
Mexican	254.4	565.1	30.2	15.4	80.3	76.8	133.0	307.3	684.1	1 862.0	3 969.5	10 048.7	X	612.8
Male	280.8	617.3	34.3	17.6	120.0	108.3	173.5	393.6	867.2	2 298.7	4 923.5	*	X	744.2
Female	225.3	510.4	26.0	13.1	33.6	37.9	85.7	216.3	514.9	1 504.8	3 309.7	9 528.4	X	503.8
Puerto Rican	431.6	841.8	31.5	14.6	66.3	101.7	245.5	485.1	984.2	2 042.3	5 688.8	*	X	766.2
Male	500.9	*	45.3	15.1	100.7	148.7	335.5	656.4	1 397.1	2 933.9	*	*	X	956.2
Female	368.1	*	*	14.2	33.0	58.2	161.5	318.1	654.1	1 464.9	*	*	X	623.3
Cuban	828.0	*	*	*	52.5	71.7	138.7	351.1	602.1	1 190.5	3 785.6	*	X	524.1
Male	838.0	*	*	*	*	100.1	183.7	475.6	943.3	1 510.8	*	*	X	628.7
Female	817.8	*	*	*	*	*	86.7	223.6	340.3	885.4	*	*	X	432.6
Other Hispanic [7]	307.3	635.8	29.5	17.3	74.0	79.7	142.9	280.4	712.0	1 651.7	4 252.1	*	X	761.8
Male	328.1	681.2	31.2	19.2	103.4	115.4	196.2	387.3	878.2	2 115.2	*		X	
Female	286.1	588.8	27.7	15.4	38.2	39.6	92.4	187.5	553.4	1 313.7	3 362.6	*	X	633.9
Non-Hispanic [3]	928.8	713.0	31.4	17.8	81.9	108.4	210.3	438.8	967.2	2 347.0	5 610.8	14 958.7	X	856.5
Male	928.0	782.6	35.4	20.4	117.3	148.6	266.0	557.0	1 198.1	2 889.1	6 825.9	16 418.0	X	1 026.5
Female	929.5	640.1	27.2	15.0	45.3	68.5	155.7	325.2	753.0	1 894.4	4 805.4	14 329.1	X	725.8
White	997.5	575.9	27.1	16.0	75.8	95.9	191.6	400.1	912.8	2 296.1	5 596.0	15 149.1	X	837.5
Male	983.9	643.5	30.3	18.3	106.7	130.9	244.9	509.9	1 126.5	2 824.1	6 801.7	16 641.9	X	1 002.2
Female	1 010.6	504.8	23.8	13.6	43.8	60.3	138.3	292.1	710.5	1 846.0	4 787.9	14 504.3	X	709.9
Black	792.8	1 280.3	48.4	25.3	116.9	193.9	357.8	782.0	1 592.9	3 204.8	6 584.8	14 386.7	X	1 099.2
Male	842.3	1 369.3	55.8	29.8	177.4	274.3	445.7	1 002.9	2 074.5	4 078.9	8 246.2	15 776.9	X	1 360.6
Female	748.0	1 187.5	40.8	20.7	56.1	121.3	280.1	592.7	1 206.3	2 584.8	5 644.9	13 855.4	X	915.3

[1]Death rates for "Under 1 year" (based on population estimates) differ from infant mortality rates (based on live births).
[2]May be of any race.
[3]Includes races other than White and Black.
[4]Includes deaths for which Hispanic origin was not reported on the death certificate.
[5]Figures for age not stated are included in "All ages" but not distributed among age groups.
[6]Figures for origin not stated are included in "All origins" but not distributed among specified origins.
[7]Includes Central and South American and other and unknown Hispanic.
* = Figure does not meet standards of reliability or precision.
- = Quantity zero.
X = Not applicable.

TABLE II-6. ABRIDGED LIFE TABLE FOR THE TOTAL POPULATION, 2002

Life expectancy at a given age represents the average number of years a group of that age could expect to live, if they were to continually experience the age-specific death rates present in that year throughout the rest of life. It does not reflect the changes in mortality rates that may occur in the future. The U.S. life expectancy in 2002 was 77.3 years at birth, 58.2 years at age 20, and 14.7 years at age 70.

Column 2 ("Probability of dying") shows the likelihood of dying between the ages shown at left. For example, for a 20- to 25-year-old person in 2002, the probability of dying was 0.00475. These probabilities were derived from vital statistics death rates for the population up to 85 years old, as well as from modeling data by Medicare for persons over 85 years old. All subsequent columns were derived from the calculations of the probability of dying.

Column 3 shows the number of persons, from a theoretical cohort of 100,000 live births, who survived to the beginning of each age interval. For example, 98,672 members of this cohort survived to age 20.

Column 4 shows the number of persons dying during each successive age interval out of the initial 100,000 live births. Each figure represents the difference between the two successive figures in Column 3.

Column 5 details the total number of person-years lived between the beginning and the end of a given age bracket. Person-years represent the total number of persons multiplied by years lived within a bracket.

Column 6 shows all of the person-years from the previous column cumulated from the bottom up (from the top age up). Starting with the cohort of 100,000 persons, the column shows how many person-years of life were left at the beginning of each age bracket.

Column 7 is derived by taking the total person-years that remained to be lived above a certain age and dividing this sum by the number of persons who survived to that age interval. Thus, it was the average number of years remaining to be lived by those who survived to a given age.

Table II-6. Abridged Life Table for the Total Population, 2002

(Number.)

Age x to x + n	Probability of dying between ages x to x + n $_nq_x$	Number surviving to age x l_x	Number dying between ages x to x + n $_nd_x$	Person-years lived between ages x to x + n $_nL_x$	Total number of person-years lived above age x T_x	Expectancy of life at age x e_x
0–1 year	0.00697	100 000	697	99 389	7 725 787	77.3
1–5 years	0.00124	99 303	123	396 921	7 626 399	76.8
5–10 years	0.00076	99 180	75	495 706	7 229 477	72.9
10–15 years	0.00098	99 105	97	495 311	6 733 771	67.9
15–20 years	0.00339	99 008	335	494 345	6 238 460	63.0
20–25 years	0.00475	98 672	468	492 189	5 744 116	58.2
25–30 years	0.00472	98 204	464	489 871	5 251 927	53.5
30–35 years	0.00557	97 740	545	487 395	4 762 056	48.7
35–40 years	0.00800	97 196	777	484 164	4 274 661	44.0
40–45 years	0.01207	96 419	1 163	479 362	3 790 497	39.3
45–50 years	0.01777	95 255	1 692	472 292	3 311 135	34.8
50–55 years	0.02538	93 563	2 375	462 186	2 838 843	30.3
55–60 years	0.03814	91 188	3 478	447 838	2 376 658	26.1
60–65 years	0.05819	87 711	5 104	426 603	1 928 820	22.0
65–70 years	0.08803	82 607	7 272	395 866	1 502 217	18.2
70–75 years	0.13308	75 335	10 025	352 791	1 106 350	14.7
75–80 years	0.20107	65 310	13 132	294 954	753 560	11.5
80–85 years	0.30423	52 178	15 874	222 013	458 606	8.8
85–90 years	0.44767	36 304	16 252	140 041	236 593	6.5
90–95 years	0.59962	20 052	12 024	67 822	96 552	4.8
95–100 years	0.73902	8 028	5 933	23 056	28 730	3.6
100 years and over	1.00000	2 095	2 095	5 675	5 675	2.7

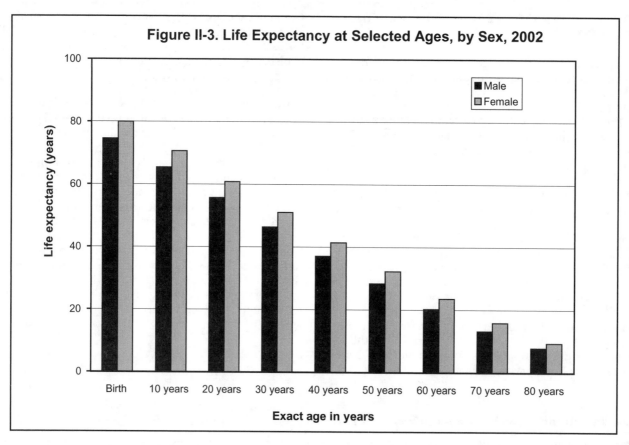

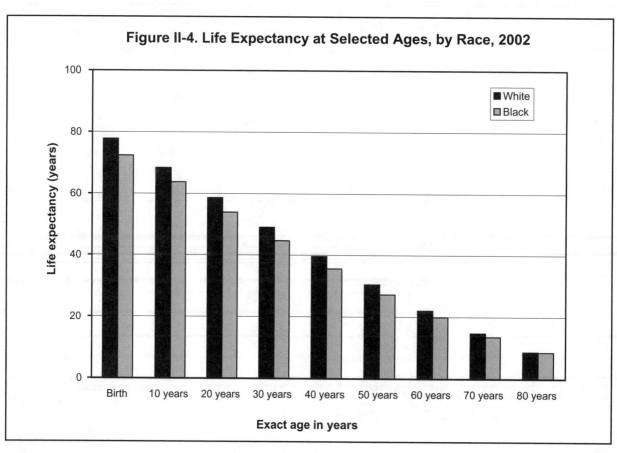

TABLE II-7. LIFE EXPECTANCY AT SELECTED AGES, BY RACE AND SEX, 2002

As expected, female life expectancy was longer than male life expectancy; the difference was 5.4 years at birth for all races and 6.8 years for Blacks. While life expectancy for young and mature Blacks was notably shorter than that for Whites, there was a reversal at about 85 years old, when surviving Blacks showed somewhat longer life expectancies than their White counterparts.

Table II-7. Life Expectancy at Selected Ages, by Race and Sex, 2002

(Years.)

Exact age in years	All races [1]			White			Black		
	Both sexes	Male	Female	Both sexes	Male	Female	Both sexes	Male	Female
0 years	77.3	74.5	79.9	77.7	75.1	80.3	72.3	68.8	75.6
1 year	76.8	74.1	79.4	77.2	74.6	79.7	72.4	68.8	75.6
5 years	72.9	70.2	75.4	73.3	70.7	75.8	68.5	65.0	71.7
10 years	67.9	65.3	70.5	68.3	65.7	70.8	63.6	60.1	66.8
15 years	63.0	60.3	65.5	63.4	60.8	65.9	58.7	55.2	61.8
20 years	58.2	55.6	60.7	58.6	56.1	61.0	53.9	50.5	57.0
25 years	53.5	51.0	55.8	53.8	51.4	56.1	49.3	46.0	52.1
30 years	48.7	46.3	51.0	49.0	46.7	51.2	44.7	41.6	47.4
35 years	44.0	41.6	46.1	44.3	42.0	46.4	40.1	37.1	47.4
40 years	39.3	37.0	41.4	39.6	37.4	41.6	35.6	32.8	42.7
45 years	34.8	32.6	36.7	35.0	32.9	36.9	31.3	28.5	38.1
50 years	30.3	28.3	32.2	30.5	28.5	32.4	27.3	24.6	33.7
55 years	26.1	24.1	27.7	26.2	24.3	27.9	23.4	21.0	29.5
60 years	22.0	20.2	23.5	22.1	20.3	23.6	19.9	17.6	25.4
65 years	18.2	16.6	19.5	18.2	16.6	19.5	16.6	14.6	21.6
70 years	14.7	13.2	15.8	14.7	13.3	15.8	13.5	11.8	18.0
75 years	11.5	10.3	12.4	11.5	10.3	12.3	10.9	9.5	14.7
80 years	8.8	7.8	9.4	8.7	7.7	9.3	8.6	7.5	11.7
85 years	6.5	5.7	6.9	6.4	5.7	6.8	6.6	5.8	9.2
90 years	4.8	4.2	5.0	4.7	4.1	4.9	5.1	4.5	7.0
95 years	3.6	3.2	3.7	3.4	3.0	3.5	3.9	3.6	5.3
100 years	2.7	2.5	2.8	2.4	2.3	2.5	3.0	2.9	4.0
									3.0

[1] Includes races other than White and Black.

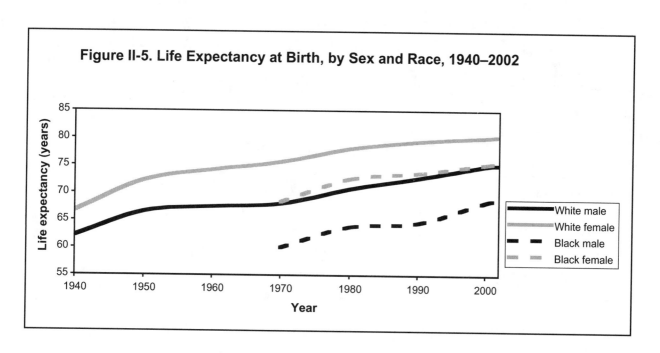

Figure II-5. Life Expectancy at Birth, by Sex and Race, 1940–2002

TABLE II-8. LIFE EXPECTANCY AT BIRTH, BY RACE AND SEX, SELECTED YEARS, 1940–2002

Life expectancy for the population as a whole has increased by 23 percent since 1940, a notable achievement. The life expectancy of 77.3 years at birth for the total population in 2002 was a record high, as were the life expectancies for all four race-sex groups. From 1900 (not shown in the table) through the late 1970s, the sex gap in life expectancy widened from 2.0 years to 7.8 years. However, this gap has been narrowing ever since,

dropping to 5.4 years in 2002. Summary data for 2003 are shown in Table II-1.

Since 1970, when separate data for Blacks became available, Black life expectancy has lengthened by 8.2 years, while the average life span of Whites has increased by 6.0 years. Nevertheless, there still remains an average difference of 5.4 years between the life spans of the two races. The increase in life expectancy did not occur evenly: between 1984 and 1989, Black life expectancy, especially male life expectancy, decreased.

Table II-8. Life Expectancy at Birth, by Race and Sex, Selected Years, 1940–2002

(Years.)

Year	All races [1]			White			Black		
	Both sexes	Male	Female	Both sexes	Male	Female	Both sexes	Male	Female
2002	77.3	74.5	79.9	77.7	75.1	80.3	72.3	68.8	75.6
2001	77.2	74.4	79.8	77.7	75.0	80.2	72.2	68.6	75.5
2000	77.0	74.3	79.7	77.6	74.9	80.1	71.9	68.3	75.2
1999	76.7	73.9	79.4	77.3	74.6	79.9	71.4	67.8	74.7
1998	76.7	73.8	79.5	77.3	74.5	80.0	71.3	67.6	74.8
1997	76.5	73.6	79.4	77.1	74.3	79.9	71.1	67.2	74.7
1996	76.1	73.1	79.1	76.8	73.9	79.7	70.2	66.1	74.2
1995	75.8	72.5	78.9	76.5	73.4	79.6	69.6	65.2	73.9
1994	75.7	72.4	79.0	76.5	73.3	79.6	69.5	64.9	73.9
1993	75.5	72.2	78.8	76.3	73.1	79.5	69.2	64.6	73.7
1992	75.8	72.3	79.1	76.5	73.2	79.8	69.6	65.0	73.9
1991	75.5	72.0	78.9	76.3	72.9	79.6	69.3	64.6	73.8
1990	75.4	71.8	78.8	76.1	72.7	79.4	69.1	64.5	73.6
1989	75.1	71.7	78.5	75.9	72.5	79.2	68.8	64.3	73.3
1988	74.9	71.4	78.3	75.6	72.2	78.9	68.9	64.4	73.2
1987	74.9	71.4	78.3	75.6	72.1	78.9	69.1	64.7	73.4
1986	74.7	71.2	78.2	75.4	71.9	78.8	69.1	64.8	73.4
1985	74.7	71.1	78.2	75.3	71.8	78.7	69.3	65.0	73.4
1984	74.7	71.1	78.2	75.3	71.8	78.7	69.5	65.3	73.6
1983	74.6	71.0	78.1	75.2	71.6	78.7	69.4	65.2	73.5
1982	74.5	70.8	78.1	75.1	71.5	78.7	69.4	65.1	73.6
1981	74.1	70.4	77.8	74.8	71.1	78.4	68.9	64.5	73.2
1980	73.7	70.0	77.4	74.4	70.7	78.1	68.1	63.8	72.5
1979	73.9	70.0	77.8	74.6	70.8	78.4	68.5	64.0	72.9
1978	73.5	69.6	77.3	74.1	70.4	78.0	68.1	63.7	72.4
1977	73.3	69.5	77.2	74.0	70.2	77.9	67.7	63.4	72.0
1976	72.9	69.1	76.8	73.6	69.9	77.5	67.2	62.9	71.6
1975	72.6	68.8	76.6	73.4	69.5	77.3	66.8	62.4	71.3
1970	70.8	67.1	74.7	71.7	68.0	75.6	64.1	60.0	68.3
1960	69.7	66.6	73.1	70.6	67.4	74.1	...	...	...
1950	68.2	65.6	71.1	69.1	66.5	72.2	...	...	...
1940	62.9	60.8	65.2	64.2	62.1	66.6	...	...	...

[1] Includes races other than White and Black.
... = Not available.

TABLE II-9. DEATH RATES, BY AGE AND AGE-ADJUSTED DEATH RATES FOR THE 15 LEADING CAUSES OF DEATH, 1999–2002

Between 2001 and 2002, the age-adjusted death rate for all causes decreased by 1.1 percent, reflecting decreases in deaths from heart disease, cancer, and stroke. However, these were largely offset by increases in deaths from other causes, such as influenza and pneumonia, Alzheimer's disease, and septicemia (blood poisoning). The number of deaths from accidents increased, but homicide deaths declined as the impact of the September 11, 2001, terror attacks moved into the past.

Diseases of the heart were the leading cause of death in the United States, accounting for 29 percent of the total. Cancer was the second leading cause, accounting for 22.8 percent of all deaths, and stroke was third with 6.7 percent. The death rates from each of the top three causes declined between 1999 and 2002, especially in the case of heart diseases. Of course, rankings of causes were not the same for each age group. Death rates from cancer exceeded those from heart diseases through the 65- to 74-year-old age bracket, but the incidence of heart diseases increased sharply thereafter, and jumped into first place for older age groups. Influenza and pneumonia and Alzheimer's disease, which ranked seventh and eighth in the general population, jumped to the fourth and fifth leading causes of death for those age 85 years and over.

The assault (homicide) rate ranked 14th overall and was somewhat lower than the rate for suicide, which ranked 11th. Deaths caused by HIV numbered 14,085, some 3,000 deaths short of being included in the top 15 causes. However, HIV still represented a major public health problem, although the age-adjusted death rate from this disease has declined for 7 consecutive years.

Table II-9. Death Rates, by Age and Age-Adjusted Death Rates for the 15 Leading Causes of Death, 1999–2002

(Rate per 100,000 population.)

Cause of death and year [1]	All ages [2]	Under 1 year [3]	1–4 years	5–14 years	15–24 years	25–34 years	35–44 years	45–54 years	55–64 years	65–74 years	75–84 years	85 years and over	Age-adjusted rate
All Causes													
2002	847.3	695.0	31.2	17.4	81.4	103.6	202.9	430.1	952.4	2 314.7	5 556.9	14 828.3	845.3
2001	848.5	683.4	33.3	17.3	80.7	105.2	203.6	428.9	964.6	2 353.3	5 582.4	15 112.8	854.5
2000	854.0	736.7	32.4	18.0	79.9	101.4	198.9	425.6	992.2	2 399.1	5 666.5	15 524.4	869.0
1999	857.0	736.0	34.2	18.6	79.3	102.2	198.0	418.2	1 005.0	2 457.3	5 714.5	15 554.6	875.6
Diseases of Heart (I00-I09, I11, I13, I20-I51)													
2002	241.7	12.4	1.1	0.6	2.5	7.9	30.5	93.7	241.5	615.9	1 677.2	5 466.8	240.8
2001	245.8	11.9	1.5	0.7	2.5	8.0	29.6	92.9	246.9	635.1	1 725.7	5 664.2	247.8
2000	252.6	13.0	1.2	0.7	2.6	7.4	29.2	94.2	261.2	665.6	1 780.3	5 926.1	257.6
1999	259.9	13.8	1.2	0.7	2.8	7.6	30.2	95.7	269.9	701.7	1 849.9	6 063.0	266.5
Malignant Neoplasms (C00-C97)													
2002	193.2	1.8	2.6	2.6	4.3	9.7	35.8	123.8	351.1	792.1	1 311.9	1 723.9	193.5
2001	194.4	1.6	2.7	2.5	4.3	10.1	36.8	126.5	356.5	802.8	1 315.8	1 765.6	196.0
2000	196.5	2.4	2.7	2.5	4.4	9.8	36.6	127.5	366.7	816.3	1 335.6	1 819.4	199.6
1999	197.0	1.8	2.7	2.5	4.5	10.0	37.1	127.6	374.6	827.1	1 331.5	1 805.8	200.8
Cerebrovascular Diseases (I60-I69)													
2002	56.4	2.9	0.3	0.2	0.4	1.4	5.4	15.1	37.2	120.3	431.0	1 445.9	56.2
2001	57.4	2.7	0.4	0.2	0.5	1.5	5.5	15.1	38.0	123.4	443.9	1 500.2	57.9
2000	59.6	3.3	0.3	0.2	0.5	1.5	5.8	16.0	41.0	128.6	461.3	1 589.2	60.9
1999	60.0	2.7	0.3	0.2	0.5	1.4	5.7	15.2	40.6	130.8	469.8	1 614.8	61.6
Chronic Lower Respiratory Diseases (J40-J47)													
2002	43.3	1.0	0.4	0.3	0.5	0.8	2.2	8.7	42.4	163.0	386.7	637.6	43.5
2001	43.2	1.0	0.3	0.3	0.4	0.7	2.2	8.5	44.1	167.9	379.8	644.7	43.7
2000	43.4	0.9	0.3	0.3	0.5	0.7	2.1	8.6	44.2	169.4	386.1	648.6	44.2
1999	44.5	0.9	0.4	0.3	0.5	0.8	2.0	8.5	47.5	177.2	397.8	646.0	45.4
Accidents (Unintentional Injuries) (V01-X59, Y85-Y86)													
2002	37.0	23.5	10.5	6.6	38.0	31.5	37.2	36.6	31.4	44.2	101.3	275.4	36.9
2001	35.7	24.2	11.2	6.9	36.1	29.9	35.4	34.1	30.3	42.8	100.9	276.4	35.7
2000	34.8	23.1	11.9	7.3	36.0	29.5	34.1	32.6	30.9	41.9	95.1	273.5	34.9
1999	35.1	22.3	12.4	7.6	35.3	29.6	33.8	31.8	30.6	44.6	100.5	282.4	35.3
Diabetes Mellitus (E10-E14)													
2002	25.4	*	*	0.1	0.4	1.6	4.8	13.7	37.7	91.4	182.8	320.6	25.4
2001	25.1	*	*	0.1	0.4	1.5	4.3	13.6	37.8	91.4	181.4	321.8	25.3
2000	24.6	*	*	0.1	0.4	1.6	4.3	13.1	37.8	90.7	179.5	319.7	25.0
1999	24.5	*	*	0.1	0.4	1.4	4.3	12.9	38.3	91.8	178.0	317.2	25.0
Influenza and Pneumonia (J10-J18)													
2002	22.8	6.5	0.7	0.2	0.4	0.9	2.2	4.8	11.2	37.5	156.9	696.6	22.6
2001	21.8	7.4	0.7	0.2	0.5	0.9	2.2	4.6	10.7	36.3	148.5	685.6	22.0
2000	23.2	7.6	0.7	0.2	0.5	0.9	2.4	4.7	11.9	39.1	160.3	744.1	23.7
1999	22.8	8.4	0.8	0.2	0.5	0.8	2.4	4.6	11.0	37.2	157.0	751.8	23.5

[1] Based on codes from the *International Classification of Diseases, Tenth Revision* (1992), except in cases where (*) precedes the cause of death code. Codes *U01-*U03 were added as of 2001 for deaths due to terrorism.
[2] Figures for age not stated are included in "All ages" but not distributed among age groups.
[3] Death rates for "Under 1 year" (based on population estimates) differ from infant mortality rates (based on live births).
* = Figure does not meet standards of reliability or precision.

Table II-9. Death Rates, by Age and Age-Adjusted Death Rates for the 15 Leading Causes of Death, 1999–2002—*Continued*

(Rate per 100,000 population.)

Cause of death and year [1]	All ages [2]	Under 1 year [3]	1–4 years	5–14 years	15–24 years	25–34 years	35–44 years	45–54 years	55–64 years	65–74 years	75–84 years	85 years and over	Age-adjusted rate
Alzheimer's Disease (G30)													
2002	20.4	*	*	*	*	*	*	0.1	1.9	19.7	158.1	752.3	20.2
2001	18.9	*	*	*	*	*	*	0.2	2.1	18.7	147.5	710.3	19.1
2000	17.6	*	*	*	*	*	*	0.2	2.0	18.7	139.6	667.7	18.1
1999	16.0	*	*	*	*	*	*	0.2	1.9	17.4	129.5	601.3	16.5
Nephritis, Nephrotic Syndrome, and Nephrosis (N00-N07, N17-N19, N25-N27)													
2002	14.2	4.3	*	0.1	0.2	0.7	1.7	4.7	13.0	39.2	109.1	288.6	14.2
2001	13.9	3.3	*	0.0	0.2	0.6	1.7	4.6	13.0	40.2	104.2	287.7	14.0
2000	13.2	4.3	*	0.1	0.2	0.6	1.6	4.4	12.8	38.0	100.8	277.8	13.5
1999	12.7	4.4	*	0.1	0.2	0.6	1.6	4.0	12.0	37.1	97.6	268.9	13.0
Septicemia (A40-A41)													
2002	11.7	7.3	0.5	0.2	0.3	0.8	1.9	5.2	12.6	34.7	86.5	203.0	11.7
2001	11.3	7.7	0.7	0.2	0.3	0.7	1.8	5.0	12.3	32.8	82.3	205.9	11.4
2000	11.1	7.2	0.6	0.2	0.3	0.7	1.9	4.9	11.9	31.0	80.4	215.7	11.3
1999	11.0	7.5	0.6	0.2	0.3	0.7	1.8	4.6	11.4	31.2	79.4	220.7	11.3
Intentional Self-Harm (Suicide) (*U03, X60-X84, Y87.0)													
2002	11.0	X	X	0.6	9.9	12.6	15.3	15.7	13.6	13.5	17.7	18.0	10.9
2001 [4]	10.8	X	X	0.7	9.9	12.8	14.7	15.2	13.1	13.3	17.4	17.5	10.7
2000	10.4	X	X	0.7	10.2	12.0	14.5	14.4	12.1	12.5	17.6	19.6	10.4
1999	10.5	X	X	0.6	10.1	12.7	14.3	13.9	12.2	13.4	18.1	19.3	10.5
Chronic Liver Disease and Cirrhosis (K70, K73-K74)													
2002	9.5	*	*	*	0.1	0.9	7.0	18.0	22.9	29.4	31.4	21.4	9.4
2001	9.5	*	*	*	0.1	1.0	7.4	18.5	22.7	30.0	30.2	22.2	9.5
2000	9.4	*	*	*	0.1	1.0	7.5	17.7	23.8	29.8	31.0	23.1	9.5
1999	9.4	*	*	*	0.1	1.0	7.3	17.4	23.7	30.6	31.9	23.2	9.6
Essential (Primary) Hypertension and Hypertensive Renal Disease (I10, I12)													
2002	7.0	*	*	*	0.1	0.2	0.8	2.3	5.7	16.0	48.2	180.4	7.0
2001	6.8	*	*	*	0.1	0.3	0.7	2.4	5.8	15.5	47.7	171.9	6.8
2000	6.4	*	*	*	*	0.2	0.8	2.3	5.9	15.1	45.5	162.9	6.5
1999	6.1	*	*	*	*	0.2	0.7	2.2	5.5	15.2	43.6	152.1	6.2
Assault (Homicide) (*U01-*U02, X85-Y09, Y87.1)													
2002	6.1	7.5	2.7	0.9	12.9	11.2	7.2	4.8	3.2	2.3	2.3	2.1	6.1
2001 [4]	7.1	8.2	2.7	0.8	13.3	13.1	9.5	6.3	4.0	2.9	2.5	2.4	7.1
2000	6.0	9.2	2.3	0.9	12.6	10.4	7.1	4.7	3.0	2.4	2.4	2.4	5.9
1999	6.1	8.7	2.5	1.1	12.9	10.5	7.1	4.6	3.0	2.6	2.5	2.4	6.0
Pneumonitis Due to Solids and Liquids (J69)													
2002	6.1	*	*	*	0.1	0.2	0.4	0.9	2.5	9.8	46.3	186.0	6.1
2001	6.1	*	*	*	0.1	0.2	0.4	1.0	2.6	10.0	45.8	189.4	6.1
2000	5.9	*	*	*	0.1	0.2	0.4	1.0	2.5	10.3	44.5	187.6	6.1
1999	5.5	*	*	*	0.1	0.2	0.4	0.8	2.5	9.5	41.1	175.6	5.6

[1]Based on codes from the *International Classification of Diseases, Tenth Revision* (1992), except in cases where (*) precedes the cause of death code. Codes *U01-*U03 were added as of 2001 for deaths due to terrorism.
[2]Figures for age not stated are included in "All ages" but not distributed among age groups.
[3]Death rates for "Under 1 year" (based on population estimates) differ from infant mortality rates (based on live births).
[4]Figures include September 11, 2001, related deaths for which death certificates were filed as of October 24, 2002.
* = Figure does not meet standards of reliability or precision.
X = Not applicable.

TABLE II-9A. THE 15 LEADING CAUSES OF DEATH AS PERCENT OF TOTAL DEATHS, AS DEATH RATES, AS AGE-ADJUSTED DEATH RATES, AS PERCENT CHANGE FROM 2001, AND AS RATIOS, BY SEX, RACE, AND ETHNICITY, 2002

The data shown here for 2002 are repeated in Table II-9B as part of the final data for 2003. During 2002, heart disease and cancer together accounted for over 51 percent of all deaths. Homicide fatalities declined 14 percent, reflecting the lessening of the influence of the September 11, 2001, terror attacks. Decreases of almost 3 percent each occurred for diseases of the heart and stroke. Death rates for heart disease have tended to decline since 1980, and those for stroke have been on a downward trend since 1958. Cancer mortality has also been declining since 1993. In 2002, the largest increases in mortality occurred for Alzheimer's disease (5.8 percent); accidents, or unintentional injuries (3.4 percent); hypertension and hypertensive renal disease (2.9 percent); and influenza and pneumonia (2.7 percent). The rapid rise in deaths from Alzheimer's disease over the last two decades partly reflected an increased awareness of this disease and a better diagnosis of it.

The relative risk of death in one population group compared to another can be expressed as a ratio. Ratios above the value of 1 indicate an increased risk for the first group, whereas ratios below 1 indicate an increased risk for the second group. Ratios of age-adjusted death rates showed that males had a higher risk than females for 12 of the 15 leading causes of death. The largest ratios were for suicide (4.4), homicide (3.4), and accidents (2.2). For the largest killers, heart disease and cancer, men had a 50 percent greater age-adjusted risk of death than women. The only leading cause of death with a lower risk for men was Alzheimer's disease (0.8).

Age-adjusted rates for the Black population were more than twice as great as those for Whites for 5 of the leading causes of death. The largest ratios were for homicide (5.7), hypertension (2.8), kidney disease (2.3), septicemia (blood poisoning—2.3), and diabetes (2.1). Rates were lower for Blacks for 3 leading causes of death. The lowest ratios for this group were for suicide (0.4), Alzheimer's diseases (0.7), and lower respiratory diseases (0.7).

Age-adjusted rates for Hispanics were lower than those for non-Hispanic Whites for 11 of the 15 leading causes of death. The lowest ratios were for suicide (0.4), Alzheimer's disease (0.5), and cancer (0.7). The highest ratios were for homicide (2.6), chronic liver disease and cirrhosis (1.7), and diabetes (1.6).

Table II-9A. The 15 Leading Causes of Death as Percent of Total Deaths, as Death Rates, as Age-Adjusted Death Rates, as Percent Change from 2001, and as Ratios, by Sex, Race, and Ethnicity, 2002

(Number, percent, rate per 100,000 population.)

Rank [1]	Cause of death [2]	Number	Percent of total deaths	2002 crude death rate	Age-adjusted death rate		Ratio		
					2002	Percent change, 2001–2002	Male to Female	Black to White	Hispanic to non-Hispanic White
	All Causes	2 443 387	100.0	847.3	845.3	-1.1	1.4	1.3	0.8
1	Diseases of heart (I00-I09, I11, I13, I20-I51)	696 947	28.5	241.7	240.8	-2.8	1.5	1.3	0.8
2	Malignant neoplasms (C00-C97)	557 271	22.8	193.2	193.5	-1.3	1.5	1.3	0.7
3	Cerebrovascular diseases (I60-I69)	162 672	6.7	56.4	56.2	-2.9	1.0	1.4	0.8
4	Chronic lower respiratory diseases (J40-J47)	124 816	5.1	43.3	43.5	-0.5	1.4	0.7	0.4
5	Accidents (unintentional injuries) (V01-X59, Y85-Y86)	106 742	4.4	37.0	36.9	3.4	2.2	1.0	0.8
6	Diabetes mellitus (E10-E14)	73 249	3.0	25.4	25.4	0.4	1.2	2.1	1.6
7	Influenza and pneumonia (J10-J18)	65 681	2.7	22.8	22.6	2.7	1.4	1.1	0.8
8	Alzheimer's disease (G30)	58 866	2.4	20.4	20.2	5.8	0.8	0.7	0.5
9	Nephritis, nephrotic syndrome, and nephrosis (N00-N07, N17-N19, N25-N27)	40 974	1.7	14.2	14.2	1.4	1.5	2.3	0.9
10	Septicemia (A40-A41)	33 865	1.4	11.7	11.7	2.6	1.2	2.3	0.8
11	Intentional self-harm (suicide) (*U03, X60-X84, Y87.0)	31 655	1.3	11.0	10.9	1.9	4.4	0.4	0.4
12	Chronic liver disease and cirrhosis (K70, K73-K74)	27 257	1.1	9.5	9.4	-1.1	2.0	0.9	1.7
13	Essential (primary) hypertension and hypertensive disease (I10, I12)	20 261	0.8	7.0	7.0	2.9	1.0	2.8	1.0
14	Assault (homicide) (*U01-*U02, X85-Y09, Y87.1)	17 638	0.7	6.1	6.1	-14.1	3.4	5.7	2.6
15	Pneumonitis due to solids and liquids (J69)	17 593	0.7	6.1	6.1	0.0	1.8	1.1	0.6
	All other causes (residual)	407 900	16.7	141.5	X	X	X	X	X

[1] Rank based on number of deaths.
[2] Based on codes from the *International Classification of Diseases, Tenth Revision* (1992), except in cases where (*) precedes the cause of death code. Codes *U01-*U03 were added as of 2001 for deaths due to terrorism.
X = Not applicable.

TABLE II-9B. THE 15 LEADING CAUSES OF DEATH AS PERCENT OF TOTAL DEATHS, AS DEATH RATES, AS AGE-ADJUSTED DEATH RATES, AS PERCENT CHANGE FROM 2002, AND AS RATIOS, BY SEX, RACE AND ETHNICITY, FINAL 2003

Overall, the age-adjusted death rate declined by 1.5 percent in 2003. Age-adjusted death rates from diseases of the heart, cancer, and stroke continued their downward trend, with each decreasing between 2 to 5 percent. However, these three causes of death still accounted for 57 percent of all deaths. In regard to cancer, 2003 was the first year in more than 70 years in which the absolute number of cancer deaths declined; fatalities in this category dropped from 557,271 to 556,902. Increases of 5 to 6 percent occurred in the age-adjusted death rates for Alzheimer's disease, hypertension and hypertensive renal disease, and Parkinson's disease.

As in 2002, males were more likely to suffer fatalities than females, especially from accidents, homicide, suicide, chronic liver disease and cirrhosis, and Parkinson's disease. Blacks had less than half the incidence rates of suicide and Parkinson's disease than Whites. On the other hand, Blacks suffered much more frequently from homicide, essential hypertension and hypertensive renal disease, septicemia (blood poisoning), nephritis, and diabetes. Hispanics generally had lower age-adjusted death rates from the 15 leading causes of death than non-Hispanic Whites. However, the reverse was true in the cases of homicide, diabetes, and chronic liver disease and cirrhosis.

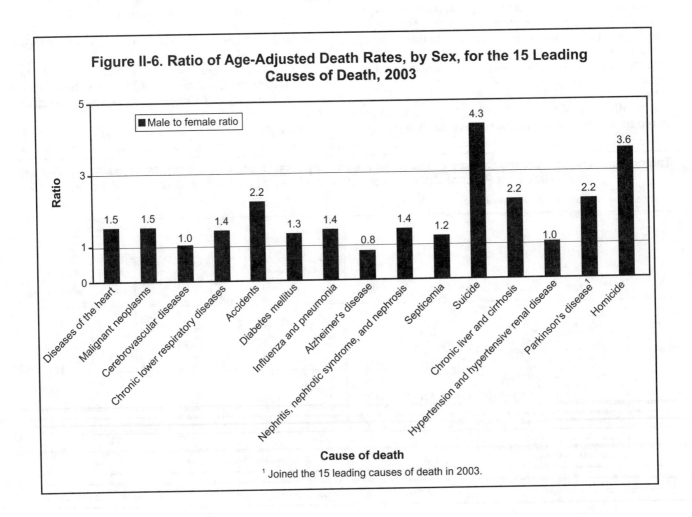

Figure II-6. Ratio of Age-Adjusted Death Rates, by Sex, for the 15 Leading Causes of Death, 2003

[1] Joined the 15 leading causes of death in 2003.

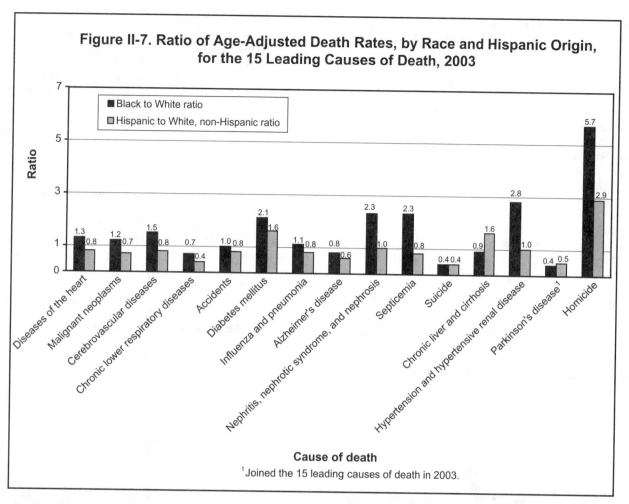

Figure II-7. Ratio of Age-Adjusted Death Rates, by Race and Hispanic Origin, for the 15 Leading Causes of Death, 2003

Cause of death

[1] Joined the 15 leading causes of death in 2003.

Table II-9B. The 15 Leading Causes of Death as Percent of Total Deaths, as Death Rates, as Age-Adjusted Death Rates, as Percent Change from 2002, and as Ratios, by Sex, Race, and Ethnicity, Final 2003

(Number, percent, rate per 100,000 population.)

Rank [1]	Cause of death [2]	Number	Percent of total deaths	2003 crude death rate	Age-adjusted death rate				
					2003	Percent change, 2002–2003	Ratio		
							Male to female	Black to White	Hispanic to non-Hispanic White
	All Causes	2 448 288	100.0	841.9	832.7	-1.5	1.4	1.3	0.8
1	Diseases of heart (I00-I09, I11, I13, I20-I51)	685 089	28.0	235.6	232.3	-3.5	1.5	1.3	0.8
2	Malignant neoplasms (C00-C97)	556 902	22.7	191.5	190.1	-1.8	1.5	1.2	0.7
3	Cerebrovascular diseases (I60-I69)	157 689	6.4	54.2	53.5	-4.8	1.0	1.5	0.8
4	Chronic lower respiratory diseases (J40-J47)	126 382	5.2	43.5	43.3	-0.5	1.4	0.7	0.4
5	Accidents (unintentional injuries) (V01-X59, Y85-Y86)	109 277	4.5	37.6	37.3	1.1	2.2	1.0	0.8
6	Diabetes mellitus (E10-E14)	74 219	3.0	25.5	25.3	-0.4	1.3	2.1	1.6
7	Influenza and pneumonia (J10-J18)	65 163	2.7	22.4	22.0	-2.7	1.4	1.1	0.8
8	Alzheimer's disease (G30)	63 457	2.6	21.8	21.4	5.9	0.8	0.8	0.6
9	Nephritis, nephrotic syndrome, and nephrosis (N00-N07, N17-N19, N25-N27)	42 453	1.7	14.6	14.4	1.4	1.4	2.3	1.0
10	Septicemia (A40-A41)	34 069	1.4	11.7	11.6	-0.9	1.2	2.3	0.8
11	Intentional self-harm (suicide) (*U03, X60-X84, Y87.0)	31 484	1.3	10.8	10.8	-0.9	4.3	0.4	0.4
12	Chronic liver disease and cirrhosis (K70, K73-K74)	27 503	1.1	9.5	9.3	-1.1	2.2	0.9	1.6
13	Essential (primary) hypertension and hypertensive disease (I10, I12)	21 940	0.9	7.5	7.4	5.7	1.0	2.8	1.0
14	Parkinson's disease (G20-G21)	17 997	0.7	6.2	6.2	5.1	2.2	0.4	0.5
15	Assault (homicide) (*U01-*U02, X85-Y09, Y87.1)	17 732	0.7	6.1	6.0	-1.6	3.6	5.7	2.9
	All other causes (residual)	416 932	17.0	143.4	X	X	X	X	X

[1] Rank based on number of deaths.

[2] Based on codes from the *International Classification of Diseases, Tenth Revision* (1992), except in cases where (*) precedes the cause of death code. Codes *U01-*U03 were added as of 2001 for deaths due to terrorism.

X = Not applicable.

TABLE II-9C. DEATHS AND DEATH RATES FOR 10 LEADING CAUSES OF DEATH IN SPECIFIED AGE GROUP, PRELIMINARY 2003

The preliminary count of deaths for 2003, which is used in this table, was 2.443 million. The final count, as shown by Table II-9B, was 2.448 million. These data provide a measure of comparison between the preliminary and the final data. Table II-9C shows the 10 leading causes of death, with detail for 6 age groups. The age groups start with 1- to 4-year-old age bracket and end with age 65 years and over. Detail for infants is provided in separate tables at the end of the chapter.

For the 1- to 4-year-old age group, accidents were the most frequent cause of death, compromising one-third of total fatalities. Congenital malformations were second,

accounting for one-tenth of fatalities for this age group. Accidents remained the leading cause of death for all age groups through the 25- to 44-year-old age bracket. In the 15- to 24-year-old age bracket, homicide and suicide followed accidents, becoming the second and third leading causes of death. But for those age 25 to 44 years, cancer and diseases of the heart increased in frequency and became the second and third leading causes of death. These causes moved up to the first and second most frequent causes of death for the 45- to 64-year-old age group.

For the oldest group, age 65 years and over, heart disease was the most frequent cause of death, and cancer was the second most frequent cause of death. Other high-ranking causes of death included stroke, chronic lower respiratory diseases, and Alzheimer's disease.

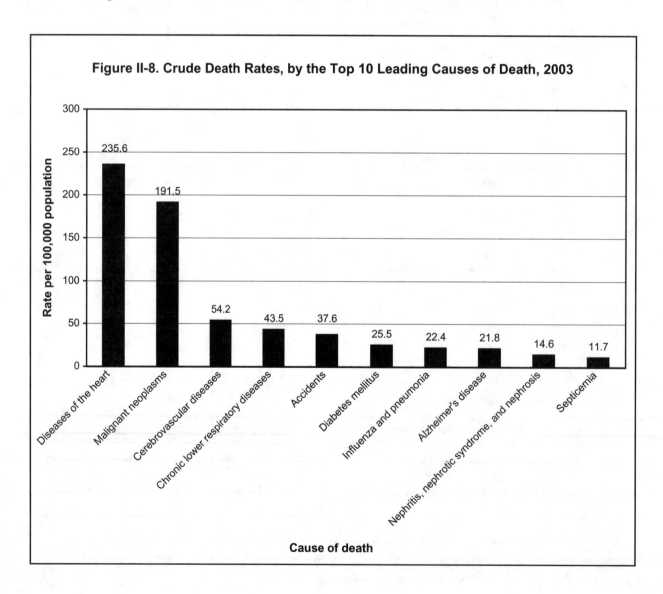

Figure II-8. Crude Death Rates, by the Top 10 Leading Causes of Death, 2003

Table II-9C. Deaths and Death Rates for the 10 Leading Causes of Death in Specified Age Group, Preliminary 2003

(Number, rate per 100,000 population.)

Rank[1] and age	Cause of death[2]	Number	Rate
All Ages[3]			
	All Causes	2 443 930	840.4
1	Diseases of heart (I00-I09, I11, I13, I20-I51)	684 462	235.4
2	Malignant neoplasms (C00-C97)	554 643	190.7
3	Cerebrovascular diseases (I60-I69)	157 803	54.3
4	Chronic lower respiratory diseases (J40-J47)	126 128	43.4
5	Accidents (unintentional injuries) (V01-X59, Y85-Y86)	105 695	36.3
	Motor vehicle accidents (V02-V04, V09.0, V09.2, V12-V14, V19.0-V19.2, V19.4-V19.6, V20-V79, V80.3-V80.5, V81.0-V81.1, V82.0-V82.1, V83-V86, V87.0-V87.8, V88.0-V88.8, V89.0, V89.2)	44 059	15.2
	All other accidents (V01, V05-V06, V09.1, V09.3-V09.9, V10-V12, V15-V18, V19.3, V19.8-V19.9, V80.0-V80.2, V80.6-V80.9, V81.2-V81.9, V82.2-V82.9, V87.9, V88.9, V89.1, V89.3, V89.9, V90-V99, W00-X59, Y85-Y86)	61 636	21.2
6	Diabetes mellitus (E10-E14)	73 965	25.4
7	Influenza and pneumonia (J10-J18)	64 847	22.3
8	Alzheimer's disease (G30)	63 343	21.8
9	Nephritis, nephrotic syndrome, and nephrosis (N00-N07, N17-N19, N25-N27)	42 536	14.6
10	Septicemia (A40-A41)	34 243	11.8
	All other causes (residual)	536 265	184.4
1–4 years			
	All Causes	4 911	31.1
1	Accidents (unintentional injuries) (V01-X59, Y85-Y86)	1 679	10.6
	Motor vehicle accidents (V02-V04, V09.0, V09.2, V12-V14, V19.0-V19.2, V19.4-V19.6, V20-V79, V80.3-V80.5, V81.0-V81.1, V82.0-V82.1, V83-V86, V87.0-V87.8, V88.0-V88.8, V89.0, V89.2)	591	3.7
	All other accidents (V01, V05-V06, V09.1, V09.3-V09.9, V10-V12, V15-V18, V19.3, V19.8-V19.9, V80.0-V80.2, V80.6-V80.9, V81.2-V81.9, V82.2-V82.9, V87.9, V88.9, V89.1, V89.3, V89.9, V90-V99, W00-X59, Y85-Y86)	1 088	6.9
2	Congenital malformations, deformations, and chromosomal abnormalities (Q00-Q99)	514	3.3
3	Malignant neoplasms (C00-C97)	383	2.4
4	Assault (homicide) (*U01-*U02, X85-Y09, Y87.1)	342	2.2
5	Diseases of heart (I00-I09, I11, I13, I20-I51)	186	1.2
6	Influenza and pneumonia (J10-J18)	151	1.0
7	Septicemia (A40-A41)	82	0.5
8	Certain conditions originating in the perinatal period (P00-P96)	76	0.5
9	In situ neoplasms, benign neoplasms, and neoplasms of uncertain or unknown behavior (D00-D48)	53	0.3
10	Chronic lower respiratory diseases (J40-J47)	47	0.3
	All other causes (residual)	1 398	8.9
5–14 years			
	All Causes	6 930	16.9
1	Accidents (unintentional injuries) (V01-X59, Y85-Y86)	2 561	6.3
	Motor vehicle accidents (V02-V04, V09.0, V09.2, V12-V14, V19.0-V19.2, V19.4-V19.6, V20-V79, V80.3-V80.5, V81.0-V81.1, V82.0-V82.1, V83-V86, V87.0-V87.8, V88.0-V88.8, V89.0, V89.2)	1 592	3.9
	All other accidents (V01, V05-V06, V09.1, V09.3-V09.9, V10-V12, V15-V18, V19.3, V19.8-V19.9, V80.0-V80.2, V80.6-V80.9, V81.2-V81.9, V82.2-V82.9, V87.9, V88.9, V89.1, V89.3, V89.9, V90-V99, W00-X59, Y85-Y86)	970	2.4
2	Malignant neoplasms (C00-C97)	1 060	2.6
3	Congenital malformations, deformations, and chromosomal abnormalities (Q00-Q99)	370	0.9
4	Assault (homicide) (*U01-*U02, X85-Y09, Y87.1)	310	0.8
5	Intentional self-harm (suicide) (*U03, X60-X84, Y87.0)	255	0.6
6	Diseases of heart (I00-I09, I11, I13, I20-I51)	252	0.6
7	Influenza and pneumonia (J10-J18)	134	0.3
8	Chronic lower respiratory diseases (J40-J47)	107	0.3
9	Septicemia (A40-A41)	77	0.2
10	In situ neoplasms, benign neoplasms, and neoplasms of uncertain or unknown behavior (D00-D48)	76	0.2
	All other causes (residual)	1 728	4.2
15–24 years			
	All Causes	33 022	80.1
1	Accidents (unintentional injuries) (V01-X59, Y85-Y86)	14 966	36.3
	Motor vehicle accidents (V02-V04, V09.0, V09.2, V12-V14, V19.0-V19.2, V19.4-V19.6, V20-V79, V80.3-V80.5, V81.0-V81.1, V82.0-V82.1, V83-V86, V87.0-V87.8, V88.0-V88.8, V89.0, V89.2)	10 857	26.3
	All other accidents (V01, V05-V06, V09.1, V09.3-V09.9, V10-V12, V15-V18, V19.3, V19.8-V19.9, V80.0-V80.2, V80.6-V80.9, V81.2-V81.9, V82.2-V82.9, V87.9, V88.9, V89.1, V89.3, V89.9, V90-V99, W00-X59, Y85-Y86)	4 109	10.0
2	Assault (homicide) (*U01-*U02, X85-Y09, Y87.1)	5 148	12.5
3	Intentional self-harm (suicide) (*U03, X60-X84, Y87.0)	3 921	9.5
4	Malignant neoplasms (C00-C97)	1 628	4.0
5	Diseases of heart (I00-I09, I11, I13, I20-I51)	1 083	2.6
6	Congenital malformations, deformations, and chromosomal abnormalities (Q00-Q99)	425	1.0
7	Influenza and pneumonia (J10-J18)	216	0.5
8	Cerebrovascular diseases (I60-I69)	204	0.5
9	Chronic lower respiratory diseases (J40-J47)	172	0.4
10	Human immunodeficiency virus (HIV) disease (B20-B24)	171	0.4
	All other causes (residual)	5 088	12.3

[1]Rank based on number of deaths.
[2]Based on codes from the *International Classification of Diseases, Tenth Revision* (1992), except in cases where (*) precedes the cause of death code. Codes *U01-*U03 were added as of 2001 for deaths due to terrorism.
[3]Includes deaths under 1 year of age.

Table II-9C. Deaths and Death Rates for the 10 Leading Causes of Death in Specified Age Group, Preliminary 2003—*Continued*

(Number, rate per 100,000 population.)

Rank[1] and age	Cause of death[2]	Number	Rate
25–44 years			
	All Causes	128 924	153.0
1	Accidents (unintentional injuries) (V01-X59, Y85-Y86)	27 844	33.1
	Motor vehicle accidents (V02-V04, V09.0, V09.2, V12-V14, V19.0-V19.2, V19.4-V19.6, V20-V79, V80.3-V80.5, V81.0-V81.1, V82.0-V82.1, V83-V86, V87.0-V87.8, V88.0-V88.8, V89.0, V89.2)	13 582	16.1
	All other accidents (V01, V05-V06, V09.1, V09.3-V09.9, V10-V12, V15-V18, V19.3, V19.8-V19.9, V80.0-V80.2, V80.6-V80.9, V81.2-V81.9, V82.2-V82.9, V87.9, V88.9, V89.1, V89.3, V89.9, V90-V99, W00-X59, Y85-Y86)	14 261	16.9
2	Malignant neoplasms (C00-C97)	19 041	22.6
3	Diseases of heart (I00-I09, I11, I13, I20-I51)	16 283	19.3
4	Intentional self-harm (suicide) (*U03, X60-X84, Y87.0)	11 251	13.4
5	Assault (homicide) (*U01-*U02, X85-Y09, Y87.1)	7 367	8.7
6	Human immunodeficiency virus (HIV) disease (B20-B24)	6 879	8.2
7	Chronic liver disease and cirrhosis (K70, K73-K74)	3 288	3.9
8	Cerebrovascular diseases (I60-I69)	3 004	3.6
9	Diabetes mellitus (E10-E14)	2 662	3.2
10	Influenza and pneumonia (J10-J18)	1 337	1.6
	All other causes (residual)	29 968	35.6
45–64 years			
	All Causes	437 058	636.1
1	Malignant neoplasms (C00-C97)	144 936	211.0
2	Diseases of heart (I00-I09, I11, I13, I20-I51)	101 713	148.0
3	Accidents (unintentional injuries) (V01-X59, Y85-Y86)	23 669	34.5
	Motor vehicle accidents (V02-V04, V09.0, V09.2, V12-V14, V19.0-V19.2, V19.4-V19.6, V20-V79, V80.3-V80.5, V81.0-V81.1, V82.0-V82.1, V83-V86, V87.0-V87.8, V88.0-V88.8, V89.0, V89.2)	9 891	14.4
	All other accidents (V01, V05-V06, V09.1, V09.3-V09.9, V10-V12, V15-V18, V19.3, V19.8-V19.9, V80.0-V80.2, V80.6-V80.9, V81.2-V81.9, V82.2-V82.9, V87.9, V88.9, V89.1, V89.3, V89.9, V90-V99, W00-X59, Y85-Y86)	13 778	20.1
4	Diabetes mellitus (E10-E14)	16 326	23.8
5	Cerebrovascular diseases (I60-I69)	15 971	23.2
6	Chronic lower respiratory diseases (J40-J47)	15 409	22.4
7	Chronic liver disease and cirrhosis (K70, K73-K74)	13 649	19.9
8	Intentional self-harm (suicide) (*U03, X60-X84, Y87.0)	10 057	14.6
9	Human immunodeficiency virus (HIV) disease (B20-B24)	5 917	8.6
10	Septicemia (A40-A41)	5 827	8.5
	All other causes (residual)	83 584	121.7
65 years and over			
	All Causes	1 804 131	5 022.8
1	Diseases of heart (I00-I09, I11, I13, I20-I51)	564 204	1 570.8
2	Malignant neoplasms (C00-C97)	387 475	1 078.7
3	Cerebrovascular diseases (I60-I69)	138 397	385.3
4	Chronic lower respiratory diseases (J40-J47)	109 199	304.0
5	Alzheimer's disease (G30)	62 707	174.6
6	Influenza and pneumonia (J10-J18)	57 507	160.1
7	Diabetes mellitus (E10-E14)	54 770	152.5
8	Nephritis, nephrotic syndrome, and nephrosis (N00-N07, N17-N19, N25-N27)	35 392	98.5
9	Accidents (unintentional injuries) (V01-X59, Y85-Y86)	33 976	94.6
	Motor vehicle accidents (V02-V04, V09.0, V09.2, V12-V14, V19.0-V19.2, V19.4-V19.6, V20-V79, V80.3-V80.5, V81.0-V81.1, V82.0-V82.1, V83-V86, V87.0-V87.8, V88.0-V88.8, V89.0, V89.2)	7 379	20.5
	All other accidents (V01, V05-V06, V09.1, V09.3-V09.9, V10-V12, V15-V18, V19.3, V19.8-V19.9, V80.0-V80.2, V80.6-V80.9, V81.2-V81.9, V82.2-V82.9, V87.9, V88.9, V89.1, V89.3, V89.9, V90-V99, W00-X59, Y85-Y86)	26 597	74.0
10	Septicemia (A40-A41)	26 609	74.1
	All other causes (residual)	333 895	929.6

[1]Rank based on number of deaths.
[2]Based on codes from the *International Classification of Diseases, Tenth Revision* (1992), except in cases where (*) precedes the cause of death code. Codes *U01-*U03 were added as of 2001 for deaths due to terrorism.

TABLE II-10. DEATHS, DEATH RATES, AND AGE-ADJUSTED DEATH RATES FOR 113 SELECTED CAUSES, WITH AN ADDENDUM FOR INJURIES AND DRUG- AND ALCOHOL-INDUCED DEATHS, FINAL 2002 AND PRELIMINARY 2003

This table shows causes of death in detail and provides a comparison between data for 2003 and 2002. However, the 2003 data are preliminary data. They are shown here because they encompassed 113 different causes of death, whereas the final figures available for 2003 (at the time this book went to press) showed only the 15 leading causes of death. Some caution must be used when interpreting the preliminary data; for instance, the preliminary age-adjusted cancer rate for 2003 is shown as 189.3 per 100,000 persons, but the final statistic was 190.1 per 100,000 persons.

In the preliminary 2003 report, the age-adjusted death rates for most major types of cancer (such as lung cancer and breast cancer) and major types of cardiovascular diseases showed decreases from 2002. Reductions in age-adjusted death rates were also reported for injury by firearms, drug-induced deaths, alcohol-induced deaths, and injuries at work.

Table II-10. Deaths, Death Rates, and Age-Adjusted Death Rates for 113 Selected Causes, with an Addendum for Injuries and Drug- and Alcohol-Induced Deaths, Final 2002 and Preliminary 2003

(Number, rate per 100,000 population.)

Cause of death[1]	2003			2002		
	Number	Rate	Age-adjusted rate	Number	Rate	Age-adjusted rate
ALL CAUSES	2 443 930	840.4	831.2	2 443 387	847.3	845.3
Salmonella infections (A01-A02)	42	0.0	0.0	21	0.0	0.0
Shigellosis and amebiasis (A03, A06)	11	*	*	8	*	*
Certain other intestinal infections (A04, A07-A09)	3 028	1.0	1.0	2 465	0.9	0.8
Tuberculosis (A16-A19)	704	0.2	0.2	784	0.3	0.3
Respiratory tuberculosis (A16)	564	0.2	0.2	626	0.2	0.2
Other tuberculosis (A17-A19)	140	0.0	0.0	158	0.1	0.0
Whooping cough (A37)	10	*	*	18	*	*
Scarlet fever and erysipelas (A38, A46)	1	*	*	2	*	*
Meningococcal infection (A39)	152	0.1	0.0	161	0.1	0.0
Septicemia (A40-A41)	34 243	11.8	11.7	33 865	11.7	11.7
Syphilis (A50-A53)	32	0.0	0.0	41	0.0	0.0
Acute poliomyelitis (A80)	5	*	*	-	*	*
Arthropod-borne viral encephalitis (A83-A84, A85.2)	12	*	*	9	*	*
Measles (B05)	1	*	*	-	*	*
Viral hepatitis (B15-B19)	5 345	1.8	1.8	5 793	2.0	2.0
Human immunodeficiency virus (HIV) disease (B20-B24)	13 544	4.7	4.7	14 095	4.9	4.9
Malaria (B50-B54)	5	*	*	12	*	*
Other and unspecified infectious and parasitic diseases and their sequelae (A00, A05, A20-A36, A42-A44, A48-A49, A54-A79, A81-A82, A85.0-A85.1, A85.8, A86-B04, B06-B09, B25-B49, B55-B99)	7 430	2.6	2.5	6 707	2.3	2.3
Malignant neoplasms (C00-C97)	554 643	190.7	189.3	557 271	193.2	193.5
Malignant neoplasms of lip, oral cavity, and pharynx (C00-C14)	7 712	2.7	2.6	7 737	2.7	2.7
Malignant neoplasm of esophagus (C15)	12 768	4.4	4.4	12 701	4.4	4.4
Malignant neoplasm of stomach (C16)	12 025	4.1	4.1	12 198	4.2	4.2
Malignant neoplasms of colon, rectum, and anus (C18-C21)	55 616	19.1	18.9	56 741	19.7	19.7
Malignant neoplasms of liver and intrahepatic bile ducts (C22)	14 572	5.0	5.0	14 047	4.9	4.9
Malignant neoplasm of pancreas (C25)	30 566	10.5	10.4	30 264	10.5	10.5
Malignant neoplasm of larynx (C32)	3 783	1.3	1.3	3 723	1.3	1.3
Malignant neoplasms of trachea, bronchus, and lung (C33-C34)	157 521	54.2	53.9	157 713	54.7	54.9
Malignant melanoma of skin (C43)	7 762	2.7	2.6	7 514	2.6	2.6
Malignant neoplasm of breast (C50)	41 941	14.4	14.2	41 883	14.5	14.5
Malignant neoplasm of cervix uteri (C53)	3 899	1.3	1.3	3 952	1.4	1.3
Malignant neoplasm of corpus uteri and uterus, part unspecified (C54-C55)	6 852	2.4	2.3	6 853	2.4	2.4
Malignant neoplasm of ovary (C56)	14 644	5.0	5.0	14 682	5.1	5.1
Malignant neoplasm of prostate (C61)	29 578	10.2	10.1	30 446	10.6	10.6
Malignant neoplasms of kidney and renal pelvis (C64-C65)	12 179	4.2	4.1	12 165	4.2	4.2
Malignant neoplasm of bladder (C67)	12 390	4.3	4.2	12 628	4.4	4.4
Malignant neoplasms of meninges, brain, and other parts of central nervous system (C70-C72)	12 804	4.4	4.4	12 830	4.4	4.4
Malignant neoplasms of lymphoid, hematopoietic, and related tissue (C81-C96)	55 571	19.1	19.0	56 225	19.5	19.5
Hodgkin's disease (C81)	1 340	0.5	0.5	1 352	0.5	0.5
Non-Hodgkin's lymphoma (C82-C85)	21 443	7.4	7.3	21 910	7.6	7.6
Leukemia (C91-C95)	21 446	7.4	7.3	21 498	7.5	7.5
Multiple myeloma and immunoproliferative neoplasms (C88, C90)	11 288	3.9	3.9	11 392	4.0	4.0
Other and unspecified malignant neoplasms of lymphoid, hematopoietic, and related tissue (C96)	54	0.0	0.0	73	0.0	0.0
All other and unspecified malignant neoplasms (C17, C23-C24, C26-C31, C37-C41, C44-C49, C51-C52, C57-C60, C62-C63, C66, C68-C69, C73-C80, C97)	62 458	21.5	21.3	62 969	21.8	21.8
In situ neoplasms, benign neoplasms, and neoplasms of uncertain or unknown behavior (D00-D48)	13 495	4.6	4.6	13 299	4.6	4.6
Anemias (D50-D64)	4 599	1.6	1.6	4 614	1.6	1.6
Diabetes mellitus (E10-E14)	73 965	25.4	25.2	73 249	25.4	25.4
Nutritional deficiencies (E40-E64)	3 358	1.2	1.1	3 779	1.3	1.3
Malnutrition (E40-E46)	3 170	1.1	1.1	3 510	1.2	1.2
Other nutritional deficiencies (E50-E64)	188	0.1	0.1	269	0.1	0.1
Meningitis (G00, G03)	708	0.2	0.2	700	0.2	0.2
Parkinson's disease (G20-G21)	17 898	6.2	6.1	16 959	5.9	5.9
Alzheimer's disease (G30)	63 343	21.8	21.4	58 866	20.4	20.2
Major cardiovascular diseases (I00-I78)	901 753	310.1	305.8	918 628	318.6	317.4
Diseases of heart (I00-I09, I11, I13, I20-I51)	684 462	235.4	232.1	696 947	241.7	240.8
Acute rheumatic fever and chronic rheumatic heart diseases (I00-I09)	3 554	1.2	1.2	3 579	1.2	1.2
Hypertensive heart disease (I11)	27 653	9.5	9.3	26 551	9.2	9.1
Hypertensive heart and renal disease (I13)	3 110	1.1	1.1	2 895	1.0	1.0
Ischemic heart diseases (I20-I25)	479 304	164.8	162.6	494 382	171.4	170.8
Acute myocardial infarction (I21-I22)	170 960	58.8	58.0	179 514	62.3	62.1
Other acute ischemic heart diseases (I24)	3 182	1.1	1.1	3 407	1.2	1.2
Other forms of chronic ischemic heart disease (I20, I25)	305 163	104.9	103.5	311 461	108.0	107.6
Atherosclerotic cardiovascular disease, so described (I25.0)	65 678	22.6	22.2	68 129	23.6	23.5
All other forms of chronic ischemic heart disease (I20, I25.1-I25.9)	239 485	82.4	81.2	243 332	84.4	84.1
Other heart diseases (I26-I51)	170 841	58.7	57.9	169 540	58.8	58.5
Acute and subacute endocarditis (I33)	1 214	0.4	0.4	1 154	0.4	0.4
Diseases of pericardium and acute myocarditis (I30-I31, I40)	826	0.3	0.3	848	0.3	0.3
Heart failure (I50)	57 218	19.7	19.3	56 494	19.6	19.5
All other forms of heart disease (I26-I28, I34-I38, I42-I49, I51)	111 583	38.4	37.9	111 044	38.5	38.4
Essential (primary) hypertension and hypertensive renal disease (I10, I12)	21 841	7.5	7.4	20 261	7.0	7.0
Cerebrovascular diseases (I60-I69)	157 803	54.3	53.6	162 672	56.4	56.2
Atherosclerosis (I70)	13 030	4.5	4.4	13 821	4.8	4.7
Other diseases of circulatory system (I71-I78)	24 617	8.5	8.4	24 927	8.6	8.7
Aortic aneurysm and dissection (I71)	14 751	5.1	5.1	14 818	5.1	5.2
Other diseases of arteries, arterioles, and capillaries (I72-I78)	9 867	3.4	3.4	10 109	3.5	3.5
Other disorders of circulatory system (I80-I99)	4 683	1.6	1.6	4 711	1.6	1.6

[1]Based on codes from the *International Classification of Diseases, Tenth Revision* (1992), except in cases where (*) precedes the cause of death code. Codes *U01-*U03 were added as of 2001 for deaths due to terrorism.
0.0 = Quantity more than zero but less than 0.05.
* = Figure does not meet standards of reliability or precision.
- = Quantity zero.

Table II-10. Deaths, Death Rates, and Age-Adjusted Death Rates for 113 Selected Causes, with an Addendum for Injuries and Drug- and Alcohol-Induced Deaths, Final 2002 and Preliminary 2003—*Continued*

(Number, rate per 100,000 population.)

Cause of death[1]	2003			2002		
	Number	Rate	Age-adjusted rate	Number	Rate	Age-adjusted rate
Influenza and pneumonia (J10-J18)	64 847	22.3	21.9	65 681	22.8	22.6
Influenza (J10-J11)	1 605	0.6	0.5	727	0.3	0.2
Pneumonia (J12-J18)	63 241	21.7	21.4	64 954	22.5	22.4
Other acute lower respiratory infections (J20-J22)	406	0.1	0.1	386	0.1	0.1
Acute bronchitis and bronchiolitis (J20-J21)	292	0.1	0.1	279	0.1	0.1
Unspecified acute lower respiratory infection (J22)	114	0.0	0.0	107	0.0	0.0
Chronic lower respiratory diseases (J40-J47)	126 128	43.4	43.2	124 816	43.3	43.5
Bronchitis, chronic and unspecified (J40-J42)	851	0.3	0.3	955	0.3	0.3
Emphysema (J43)	14 793	5.1	5.1	15 489	5.4	5.4
Asthma (J45-J46)	3 964	1.4	1.3	4 261	1.5	1.5
Other chronic lower respiratory diseases (J44, J47)	106 520	36.6	36.5	104 111	36.1	36.2
Pneumoconioses and chemical effects (J60-J66, J68)	1 107	0.4	0.4	1 114	0.4	0.4
Pneumonitis due to solids and liquids (J69)	17 457	6.0	5.9	17 593	6.1	6.1
Other diseases of respiratory system (J00-J06, J30-J39, J67, J70-J98)	25 304	8.7	8.6	25 039	8.7	8.7
Peptic ulcer (K25-K28)	3 888	1.3	1.3	4 079	1.4	1.4
Diseases of appendix (K35-K38)	432	0.1	0.1	480	0.2	0.2
Hernia (K40-K46)	1 617	0.6	0.6	1 595	0.6	0.5
Chronic liver disease and cirrhosis (K70, K73-K74)	27 201	9.4	9.2	27 257	9.5	9.4
Alcoholic liver disease (K70)	12 064	4.1	4.1	12 121	4.2	4.2
Other chronic liver disease and cirrhosis (K73-K74)	15 137	5.2	5.1	15 136	5.2	5.2
Cholelithiasis and other disorders of gallbladder (K80-K82)	2 934	1.0	1.0	2 979	1.0	1.0
Nephritis, nephrotic syndrome, and nephrosis (N00-N07, N17-N19, N25-N27)	42 536	14.6	14.5	40 974	14.2	14.2
Acute and rapidly progressive nephritic and nephrotic syndrome (N00-N01, N04)	149	0.1	0.1	166	0.1	0.0
Chronic glomerulonephritis, nephrosis, and nephropathy not specified as acute or chronic, and renal sclerosis unspecified (N02-N03, N05-N07, N26)	542	0.2	0.2	553	0.2	0.2
Renal failure (N17-N19)	41 818	14.4	14.2	40 222	13.9	13.9
Other disorders of kidney (N25, N27)	27	0.0	0.0	33	0.0	0.0
Infections of kidney (N10-N12, N13.6, N15.1)	821	0.3	0.3	788	0.3	0.3
Hyperplasia of prostate (N40)	487	0.2	0.2	437	0.2	0.1
Inflammatory diseases of female pelvic organs (N70-N76)	131	0.0	0.0	114	0.0	0.0
Pregnancy, childbirth, and the puerperium (O00-O99)	515	0.2	0.2	379	0.1	0.1
Pregnancy with abortive outcome (O00-O07)	42	0.0	0.0	22	0.0	0.0
Other complications of pregnancy, childbirth, and the puerperium (O10-O99)	473	0.2	0.2	357	0.1	0.1
Certain conditions originating in the perinatal period (P00-P96)	14 352	4.9	4.9	14 254	4.9	4.9
Congenital malformations, deformations, and chromosomal abnormalities (Q00-Q99)	10 430	3.6	3.6	10 687	3.7	3.7
Symptoms, signs, and abnormal clinical and laboratory findings, not elsewhere classified (R00-R99)	38 795	13.3	13.1	29 975	10.4	10.3
All other diseases (residual)	200 322	68.9	67.9	194 591	67.5	67.1
Accidents (unintentional injuries) (V01-X59, Y85-Y86)	105 695	36.3	36.1	106 742	37.0	36.9
Transport accidents (V01-V99, Y85)	47 325	16.3	16.1	48 366	16.8	16.7
Motor vehicle accidents (V02-V04, V09.0, V09.2, V12-V14, V19.0-V19.2, V19.4-V19.6, V20-V79, V80.3, V80.5, V81.1, V82.0, V82.1, V83, V86, V87.0, V87.8, V88.0, V88.8, V89.0, V89.2)	44 059	15.2	15.0	45 380	15.7	15.7
Other land transport accidents (V01, V05-V06, V09.1, V09.3-V09.9, V10-V11, V15-V18, V19.3, V19.8-V19.9, V80.0-V80.2, V80.6-V80.9, V81.2-V81.9, V82.2-V82.9, V87.9, V88.9, V89.1, V89.3, V89.9)	1 352	0.5	0.4	1 086	0.4	0.4
Water, air and space, and other and unspecified transport accidents and their sequelae (V90-V99, Y85)	1 913	0.7	0.7	1 900	0.7	0.6
Nontransport accidents (W00-X59, Y86)	58 371	20.1	19.9	58 376	20.2	20.2
Falls (W00-W19)	16 926	5.8	5.7	16 257	5.6	5.6
Accidental discharge of firearms (W32-W34)	752	0.3	0.2	762	0.3	0.3
Accidental drowning and submersion (W65-W74)	3 222	1.1	1.1	3 447	1.2	1.2
Accidental exposure to smoke, fire, and flames (X00-X09)	3 363	1.2	1.1	3 159	1.1	1.1
Accidental poisoning and exposure to noxious substances (X40-X49)	16 969	5.8	5.8	17 550	6.1	6.1
Other and unspecified nontransport accidents and their sequelae (W20-W31, W35-W64, W75-W99, X10-X39, X50-X59, Y86)	17 138	5.9	5.8	17 201	6.0	5.9
Intentional self-harm (suicide) (*U03, X60-X84, Y87.0)	30 642	10.5	10.5	31 655	11.0	10.9
Intentional self-harm (suicide) by discharge of firearms (X72-X74)	16 859	5.8	5.7	17 108	5.9	5.9
Intentional self-harm (suicide) by other and unspecified means and their sequelae (*U03, X60-X71, X75-X84, Y87.0)	13 782	4.7	4.7	14 547	5.0	5.0
Assault (homicide) (*U01-*U02, X85-Y09, Y87.1)	17 096	5.9	5.8	17 638	6.1	6.1
Assault (homicide) by discharge of firearms (*U01.4, X93-X95)	11 599	4.0	4.0	11 829	4.1	4.1
Assault (homicide) by other and unspecified means and their sequelae (*U01.0-*U01.3, *U01.5-*U01.9, *U02, X85-X92, X96-Y09, Y87.1)	5 498	1.9	1.9	5 809	2.0	2.0
Legal intervention (Y35, Y89.0)	394	0.1	0.1	384	0.1	0.1
Events of undetermined intent (Y10-Y34, Y87.2, Y89.9)	4 602	1.6	1.6	4 830	1.7	1.7
Discharge of firearms, undetermined intent (Y22-Y24)	197	0.1	0.1	243	0.1	0.1
Other and unspecified events of undetermined intent and their sequelae (Y10-Y21, Y25-Y34, Y87.2, Y89.9)	4 405	1.5	1.5	4 587	1.6	1.6
Operations of war and their sequelae (Y36, Y89.1)	16	*	*	20	0.0	0.0
Complications of medical and surgical care (Y40-Y84, Y88)	2 766	1.0	0.9	2 843	1.0	1.0
ADDENDUM						
Injury by firearms (*U01.4, W32-W34, X72-X74, X93-X95, Y22-Y24, Y35.0)[2]	29 730	10.2	10.1	30 242	10.5	10.4
Drug-induced deaths (F11.0, F11.5, F11.7, F11.9, F12.0, F12.5, F12.7, F12.9, F13.0, F13.5, F13.7 F13.9, F14.0-F14.5, F14.7-F14.9, F15.0-F15.5, F15.7-F15.9, F16.0-F16.5, F16.7-F16.9, F17.0, F17.3-F17.5, F17.7-F17.9, F18.0-F18.5, F18.7-F18.9, F19.0-F19.5, F19.7-F19.9, X40-X44, X60-X64, X85, Y10, Y14)[2]	25 162	8.7	8.7	26 018	9.0	9.0
Alcohol-induced deaths (F10, G31.2, G62.1, I42.6, K29.2, K70, R78.0, X45, X65, Y15)[2]	19 699	6.8	6.6	19 928	6.9	6.9
Injury at work	4 735	2.1	2.0	5 305	2.3	2.3

[1]Based on codes from the *International Classification of Diseases, Tenth Revision* (1992), except in cases where (*) precedes the cause of death code. Codes *U01-*U03 were added as of 2001 for deaths due to terrorism.
[2]Included in selected categories.
0.0 = Quantity more than zero but less than 0.05.
* = Figure does not meet standards of reliability or precision.

TABLE II-10A. NUMBER OF DEATHS FROM 113 SELECTED CAUSES, BY AGE, 2002

Of the 2.4 million deaths in 2002, 557,271 were caused by cancer. Lung cancer, with 158,000 deaths, was the leading type of fatal cancer. Major cardiovascular diseases caused 919,000 deaths in 2002; the principal component of this category was diseases of the heart, with 697,000 deaths. Stroke was the other major component of cardiovascular disease. Accidents accounted for about 100,000 deaths. This table contains a highly detailed listing of causes of death. For example, there are many different classifications for cancer and for heart diseases, as well as for different types of accidents. The classifications are based on the *International Classifications of Diseases, Tenth Revision* (1992).

TABLE II-11. DEATH RATES FOR 113 SELECTED CAUSES, BY AGE, 2002

The numbers of deaths shown in Table II-10 are converted in this table to rates per 100,000 persons. Data on deaths were obtained from death certificates, while population was based on updates of the population count from the 2000 census. Rates were not calculated for items with small numbers of deaths.

The typical pattern for many fatal diseases was to spike during infancy (representing low birthweight, congenital disorders, and susceptibility to infection), with a rapid drop in early childhood, followed by a steady increase with advancing age. Non-transportation accidents also followed this pattern. Some causes of death were extremely rare in infancy. For older persons, death rates from certain diseases, such as chronic liver disease, peaked before the highest age brackets were reached.

TABLE II-12. NUMBER OF DEATHS FROM 113 SELECTED CAUSES, BY RACE AND SEX, 2002

This table presents cause-specific death counts by sex for: 1) all races; 2) Whites, including non-Hispanic Whites; 3) total "all other," including Blacks; and 4) Blacks. The same format was used to calculate the crude rates in Table II-14 and the age-adjusted rates in Table II-16. In addition to their use in calculating death rates, the actual counts can help reveal the national burden of specific causes of death in the different race and sex groups.

Deaths from cardiovascular diseases were highly concentrated in the older age groups. Females (with their greater life expectancies) registered notably more fatalities from these diseases than males; this applied to both White and Black females. Male and female cancer fatalities were roughly equal, as cancer was less concentrated at the highest age levels.

Males were much more frequently the victims of accidents, whether motor vehicle or other types of accidents. For Black men, the number of fatalities from accidents in 2002 were twice as great as the number of fatalities for Black females. For Whites, the fatal accident rate was 80 percent higher for males than for females. In the case of suicide, fatalities for men were four times higher than those for women. For both sexes combined, the White rate of suicide was more than twice as high as the Black rate.

Table II-10A. Number of Deaths from 113 Selected Causes, by Age, 2002

(Number.)

Cause of death [1]	All ages	Under 1 year	1–4 years	5–14 years	15–24 years	25–34 years	35–44 years	45–54 years	55–64 years	65–74 years	75–84 years	85 years and over	Not stated
ALL CAUSES	2 443 387	28 034	4 858	7 150	33 046	41 355	91 140	172 385	253 342	422 990	707 654	681 076	357
Salmonella infections (A01-A02)	21	3	-	-	-	-	2	3	-	4	8	1	-
Shigellosis and amebiasis (A03, A06)	8	-	1	-	1	-	1	2	1	-	1	1	-
Certain other intestinal infections (A04, A07-A09)	2 465	13	8	3	6	4	18	56	142	362	889	964	-
Tuberculosis (A16-A19)	784	1	-	-	9	18	52	81	107	161	234	121	-
Respiratory tuberculosis (A16)	626	-	-	-	6	14	40	64	84	120	192	106	-
Other tuberculosis (A17-A19)	158	1	-	-	3	4	12	17	23	41	42	15	-
Whooping cough (A37)	18	18	-	-	-	-	-	-	-	-	-	-	-
Scarlet fever and erysipelas (A38, A46)	2	-	-	-	-	-	-	-	-	-	1	1	-
Meningococcal infection (A39)	161	17	12	20	33	16	9	19	13	7	10	5	-
Septicemia (A40-A41)	33 865	296	79	95	118	314	856	2 074	3 360	6 336	11 010	9 324	3
Syphilis (A50-A53)	41	1	1	-	-	-	2	5	5	6	12	9	-
Acute poliomyelitis (A80)	-	-	-	-	-	-	-	-	-	-	-	-	-
Arthropod-borne viral encephalitis (A83-A84, A85.2)	9	-	-	-	1	1	-	2	1	1	2	1	-
Measles (B05)	-	-	-	-	-	-	-	-	-	-	-	-	-
Viral hepatitis (B15-B19)	5 793	2	3	2	23	94	740	2 331	1 072	762	587	177	-
Human immunodeficiency virus (HIV) disease (B20-B24)	14 095	7	5	25	178	1 839	5 707	4 474	1 347	401	96	12	4
Malaria (B50-B54)	12	-	-	-	1	1	1	5	2	2	-	-	-
Other and unspecified infectious and parasitic diseases and their sequelae (A00, A05, A20-A36, A42-A44, A48-A49, A54-A79, A81-A82, A85.0-A85.1, A85.8, A86-B04, B06-B09, B25-B49, B55-B99)	6 707	224	61	84	97	169	453	916	889	1 223	1 594	997	-
Malignant neoplasms (C00-C97)	557 271	74	402	1 072	1 730	3 872	16 085	49 637	93 391	144 757	167 062	79 182	7
Malignant neoplasms of lip, oral cavity, and pharynx (C00-C14)	7 737	-	3	8	23	57	258	1 101	1 811	1 898	1 721	857	-
Malignant neoplasm of esophagus (C15)	12 701	-	-	1	6	19	311	1 390	2 763	3 691	3 389	1 130	1
Malignant neoplasm of stomach (C16)	12 198	-	1	-	29	138	436	1 106	1 831	2 816	3 656	2 185	-
Malignant neoplasms of colon, rectum, and anus (C18-C21)	56 741	1	-	1	50	290	1 425	4 573	8 421	13 392	17 498	11 089	1
Malignant neoplasms of liver and intrahepatic bile ducts (C22)	14 047	3	28	18	27	105	414	1 976	2 558	3 581	3 728	1 609	-
Malignant neoplasm of pancreas (C25)	30 264	1	-	-	7	39	596	2 433	5 105	8 187	9 555	4 340	1
Malignant neoplasm of larynx (C32)	3 723	-	-	-	-	11	76	425	904	1 084	969	253	1
Malignant neoplasms of trachea, bronchus, and lung (C33-C34)	157 713	-	1	4	21	165	2 698	12 150	30 684	50 256	48 082	13 652	-
Malignant melanoma of skin (C43)	7 514	-	3	1	41	194	604	1 135	1 351	1 616	1 748	820	1
Malignant neoplasm of breast (C50)	41 883	-	-	-	10	425	2 722	6 454	7 838	8 505	9 748	6 181	-
Malignant neoplasm of cervix uteri (C53)	3 952	-	-	-	17	208	666	894	725	630	528	284	-
Malignant neoplasms of corpus uteri and uterus, part unspecified (C54-C55)	6 853	-	-	-	-	23	146	565	1 199	1 835	1 957	1 128	-
Malignant neoplasm of ovary (C56)	14 682	1	1	2	37	97	469	1 717	2 748	3 601	4 259	1 750	-
Malignant neoplasm of prostate (C61)	30 446	-	-	-	1	1	32	382	2 020	6 300	12 753	8 957	-
Malignant neoplasms of kidney and renal pelvis (C64-C65)	12 165	4	8	30	20	48	306	1 322	2 340	3 239	3 355	1 493	-
Malignant neoplasm of bladder (C67)	12 628	-	-	3	1	14	123	503	1 310	2 907	4 707	3 059	1
Malignant neoplasms of meninges, brain, and other parts of central nervous system (C70-C72)	12 830	12	114	337	210	388	1 009	2 058	2 560	2 954	2 435	753	-
Malignant neoplasms of lymphoid, hematopoietic, and related tissue (C81-C96)	56 225	28	119	379	703	916	1 751	3 960	7 500	13 508	18 289	9 072	-
Hodgkin's disease (C81)	1 352	-	-	6	86	152	159	177	168	232	247	125	-
Non-Hodgkin's lymphoma (C82-C85)	21 910	2	15	57	142	281	687	1 581	3 049	5 264	7 283	3 549	-
Leukemia (C91-C95)	21 498	21	104	316	472	471	767	1 459	2 611	4 818	6 763	3 696	-
Multiple myeloma and immunoproliferative neoplasms (C88, C90)	11 392	2	-	-	2	12	138	736	1 669	3 176	3 971	1 686	-
Other and unspecified malignant neoplasms of lymphoid, hematopoietic, and related tissue (C96)	73	3	-	-	1	-	-	7	3	18	25	16	-
All other and unspecified malignant neoplasms (C17, C23-C24, C26-C31, C37-C41, C44-C49, C51-C52, C57-C60, C62-C63, C66, C68-C69, C73-C80, C97)	62 969	24	124	288	527	734	2 043	5 493	9 723	14 757	18 685	10 570	1
In situ neoplasms, benign neoplasms, and neoplasms of uncertain or unknown behavior (D00-D48)	13 299	69	60	89	87	163	366	714	1 193	2 348	4 597	3 613	-
Anemias (D50-D64)	4 614	18	21	53	111	180	196	250	264	508	1 161	1 852	-
Diabetes mellitus (E10-E14)	73 249	1	3	34	171	642	2 164	5 496	10 022	16 709	23 282	14 724	1
Nutritional deficiencies (E40-E64)	3 779	4	1	1	7	16	60	102	168	382	1 132	1 906	-
Malnutrition (E40-E46)	3 510	2	1	1	6	13	55	91	156	354	1 067	1 764	-
Other nutritional deficiencies (E50-E64)	269	2	-	-	1	3	5	11	12	28	65	142	-
Meningitis (G00, G03)	700	74	19	31	26	36	61	116	88	109	84	55	1
Parkinson's disease (G20-G21)	16 959	-	-	-	-	-	6	58	318	2 226	8 139	6 212	-
Alzheimer's disease (G30)	58 866	-	-	1	-	2	12	52	510	3 602	20 135	34 552	-

[1]Based on codes from the *International Classification of Diseases, Tenth Revision* (1992), except in cases where (*) precedes the cause of death code. Codes *U01-*U03 were added as of 2001 for deaths due to terrorism.
- = Quantity zero.

Table II-10A. Number of Deaths from 113 Selected Causes, by Age, 2002—*Continued*

(Number.)

Cause of death [1]	All ages	Under 1 year	1–4 years	5–14 years	15–24 years	25–34 years	35–44 years	45–54 years	55–64 years	65–74 years	75–84 years	85 years and over	Not stated
Major cardiovascular diseases (I00-I78)	918 628	640	223	358	1 283	3 986	16 962	45 800	78 430	144 071	287 415	339 409	51
Diseases of heart (I00-I09, I11, I13, I20-I51)	696 947	500	165	255	1 022	3 165	13 688	37 570	64 234	112 547	213 581	250 173	47
Acute rheumatic fever and chronic rheumatic heart diseases (I00-I09)	3 579	4	1	6	18	36	95	237	433	703	1 227	819	-
Hypertensive heart disease (I11)	26 551	-	-	2	30	297	1 213	2 882	3 320	3 895	6 321	8 587	4
Hypertensive heart and renal disease (I13)	2 895	-	-	-	5	28	77	165	273	402	866	1 079	-
Ischemic heart diseases (I20-I25)	494 382	23	7	20	133	996	7 683	25 575	47 262	83 867	155 391	173 388	37
Acute myocardial infarction (I21-I22)	179 514	11	5	7	62	400	3 161	10 619	19 933	34 003	56 590	54 718	5
Other acute ischemic heart diseases (I24)	3 407	2	-	1	4	18	77	345	460	631	898	971	-
Other forms of chronic ischemic heart disease (I20, I25)	311 461	10	2	12	67	578	4 445	14 611	26 869	49 233	97 903	117 699	32
Atherosclerotic cardiovascular disease, so described (I25.0)	68 129	2	-	1	17	181	1 515	5 366	8 793	11 817	18 618	21 796	23
All other forms of chronic ischemic heart disease (I20, I25.1-I25.9)	243 332	8	2	11	50	397	2 930	9 245	18 076	37 416	79 285	95 903	9
Other heart diseases (I26-I51)	169 540	473	157	227	836	1 808	4 620	8 711	12 946	23 680	49 776	66 300	6
Acute and subacute endocarditis (I33)	1 154	2	2	2	7	44	90	174	168	238	306	121	-
Diseases of pericardium and acute myocarditis (I30-I31, I40)	848	26	22	22	36	46	75	107	118	143	157	96	-
Heart failure (I50)	56 494	23	11	10	27	101	282	993	2 342	6 168	16 910	29 627	-
All other forms of heart disease (I26-I28, I34-I38, I42-I49, I51)	111 044	422	122	193	766	1 617	4 173	7 437	10 318	17 131	32 403	36 456	6
Essential (primary) hypertension and hypertensive renal disease (I10, I12)	20 261	5	1	1	21	85	354	923	1 526	2 922	6 138	8 285	-
Cerebrovascular diseases (I60-I69)	162 672	117	53	91	171	567	2 425	6 055	9 897	21 992	54 889	66 412	3
Atherosclerosis (I70)	13 821	4	-	-	3	9	50	182	487	1 300	4 062	7 723	1
Other diseases of circulatory system (I71-I78)	24 927	14	4	11	66	160	445	1 070	2 286	5 310	8 745	6 816	-
Aortic aneurysm and dissection (I71)	14 818	2	-	5	39	110	305	710	1 460	3 482	5 518	3 187	-
Other diseases of arteries, arterioles, and capillaries (I72-I78)	10 109	12	4	6	27	50	140	360	826	1 828	3 227	3 629	-
Other disorders of circulatory system (I80-I99)	4 711	27	4	2	35	139	305	531	595	697	1 253	1 123	-
Influenza and pneumonia (J10-J18)	65 681	263	110	91	167	345	971	1 918	2 987	6 847	19 984	31 995	3
Influenza (J10-J11) [2]	727	7	5	12	7	4	8	17	30	56	177	404	-
Pneumonia (J12-J18)	64 954	256	105	79	160	341	963	1 901	2 957	6 791	19 807	31 591	3
Other acute lower respiratory infections (J20-J22)	386	52	23	8	3	5	8	18	18	33	66	152	-
Acute bronchitis and bronchiolitis (J20-J21)	279	49	23	8	2	5	6	17	13	23	39	94	-
Unspecified acute lower respiratory infection (J22)	107	3	-	-	1	-	2	1	5	10	27	58	-
Chronic lower respiratory diseases (J40-J47)	124 816	39	65	136	192	301	1 008	3 475	11 280	29 788	49 241	29 284	7
Bronchitis, chronic and unspecified (J40-J42)	955	24	13	5	6	6	18	36	54	135	286	372	-
Emphysema (J43)	15 489	1	3	-	2	10	94	454	1 703	4 388	6 109	2 724	1
Asthma (J45-J46)	4 261	4	43	123	169	235	472	608	536	583	812	675	1
Other chronic lower respiratory diseases (J44, J47)	104 111	10	6	8	15	50	424	2 377	8 987	24 682	42 034	25 513	5
Pneumoconioses and chemical effects (J60-J66, J68)	1 114	2	-	-	-	-	5	17	75	223	480	312	-
Pneumonitis due to solids and liquids (J69)	17 593	2	7	16	44	74	192	351	671	1 793	5 900	8 543	-
Other diseases of respiratory system (J00-J06, J30-J39, J67, J70-J98)	25 039	278	85	84	126	185	528	1 288	2 440	5 237	8 658	6 130	-
Peptic ulcer (K25-K28)	4 079	1	1	1	-	22	113	272	411	665	1 291	1 302	-
Diseases of appendix (K35-K38)	480	3	-	7	12	10	27	54	64	89	120	94	-
Hernia (K40-K46)	1 595	29	3	7	5	11	35	77	126	225	489	588	-
Chronic liver disease and cirrhosis (K70, K73-K74)	27 257	6	3	6	31	374	3 154	7 216	6 097	5 381	4 000	985	4
Alcoholic liver disease (K70)	12 121	-	1	-	8	242	1 971	4 137	3 083	1 849	730	98	2
Other chronic liver disease and cirrhosis (K73-K74)	15 136	6	2	6	23	132	1 183	3 079	3 014	3 532	3 270	887	2
Cholelithiasis and other disorders of gallbladder (K80-K82)	2 979	-	-	-	9	21	54	129	216	504	992	1 054	-
Nephritis, nephrotic syndrome, and nephrosis (N00-N07, N17-N19, N25-N27)	40 974	173	14	21	84	269	749	1 893	3 455	7 164	13 896	13 256	-
Acute and rapidly progressive nephritic and nephrotic syndrome (N00-N01, N04)	166	6	5	2	3	1	4	9	16	27	51	42	-
Chronic glomerulonephritis, nephritis, and nephropathy, not specified as acute or chronic, and renal sclerosis, unspecified (N02-N03, N05-N07, N26)	553	2	-	3	4	23	26	53	52	85	178	127	-
Renal failure (N17-N19)	40 222	165	9	15	77	243	718	1 829	3 383	7 046	13 657	13 080	-
Other disorders of kidney (N25, N27)	33	-	-	1	-	2	1	2	4	6	10	7	-
Infections of kidney (N10-N12, N13.6, N15.1)	788	2	-	3	5	13	28	40	59	110	238	290	1
Hyperplasia of prostate (N40)	437	-	-	-	-	-	1	-	10	41	164	220	1
Inflammatory diseases of female pelvic organs (N70-N76)	114	1	-	-	2	4	17	11	6	8	29	36	-
Pregnancy, childbirth, and the puerperium (O00-O99)	379	X	X	1	89	175	105	8	-	-	-	1	-
Pregnancy with abortive outcome (O00-O07)	22	X	X	1	4	9	7	1	-	-	-	-	-
Other complications of pregnancy, childbirth, and the puerperium (O10-O99)	357	X	X	-	85	166	98	7	-	-	-	1	-
Certain conditions originating in the perinatal period (P00-P96)	14 254	14 106	65	31	21	10	10	2	1	3	2	1	2
Congenital malformations, deformations, and chromosomal abnormalities (Q00-Q99)	10 687	5 623	530	417	492	475	572	709	634	440	489	305	1
Symptoms, signs, and abnormal clinical and laboratory findings, not elsewhere classified (R00-R99)	29 975	3 456	248	139	740	1 319	2 402	2 672	2 002	2 398	4 936	9 554	109
All other diseases (residual)	194 591	1 144	661	868	1 853	3 136	8 506	15 151	17 378	25 689	51 618	68 574	13

[1]Based on codes from the *International Classification of Diseases, Tenth Revision* (1992), except in cases where (*) precedes the cause of death code. Codes *U01-*U03 were added as of 2001 for deaths due to terrorism.
[2]Cause of death coding changes may affect comparability with the previous year's data for this cause.
- = Quantity zero.
X = Not applicable.

Table II-10A. Number of Deaths from 113 Selected Causes, by Age, 2002—*Continued*

(Number.)

Cause of death [1]	All ages	Under 1 year	1–4 years	5–14 years	15–24 years	25–34 years	35–44 years	45–54 years	55–64 years	65–74 years	75–84 years	85 years and over	Not stated
Accidents (unintentional injuries) (V01-X59, Y85-Y86)	106 742	946	1 641	2 718	15 412	12 569	16 710	14 675	8 345	8 086	12 904	12 651	85
Transport accidents (V01-V99, Y85)	48 366	127	640	1 738	11 816	7 484	7 688	6 563	4 165	3 351	3 433	1 322	39
Motor vehicle accidents (V02-V04, V09.0, V09.2, V12-V14, V19.0-V19.2, V19.4-V19.6, V20-V79, V80.3-80.5, V81.0-V81.1, V82.0-V82.1, V83-V86, V87.0-V87.8, V88.0-V88.8, V89.0, V89.2)	45 380	123	610	1 614	11 459	7 092	7 077	5 937	3 764	3 113	3 271	1 285	35
Other land transport accidents (V01, V05-V06, V09.1, V09.3-V09.9, V10-V11, V15-V18, V19.3, V19.8-V19.9, V80.0-V80.2, V80.6-V80.9, V81.2-V81.9, V82.2-V82.9, V87.9, V88.9, V89.1, V89.3, V89.9)	1 086	2	17	70	159	138	223	211	109	70	66	17	4
Water, air and space, and other and unspecified transport accidents and their sequelae (V90-V99, Y85)	1 900	2	13	54	198	254	388	415	292	168	96	20	-
Nontransport accidents (W00-X59, Y86)	58 376	819	1 001	980	3 596	5 085	9 022	8 112	4 180	4 735	9 471	11 329	46
Falls (W00-W19)	16 257	16	37	42	247	307	664	1 017	1 089	1 967	4 880	5 990	1
Accidental discharge of firearms (W32-W34)	762	1	11	48	210	143	123	95	56	36	32	7	-
Accidental drowning and submersion (W65-W74) ...	3 447	63	454	321	629	433	526	374	212	169	167	79	20
Accidental exposure to smoke, fire, and flames (X00-X09)	3 159	36	221	253	193	266	361	448	340	385	432	221	3
Accidental poisoning and exposure to noxious substances (X40-X49)	17 550	26	31	43	1 679	3 116	6 007	4 682	1 098	383	295	181	9
Other and unspecified nontransport accidents and their sequelae (W20-W31, W35-W64, W75-W99, X10-X39, X50-X59, Y86)	17 201	677	247	273	638	820	1 341	1 496	1 385	1 795	3 665	4 851	13
Intentional self-harm (suicide) (*U03, X60-X84, Y87.0)	31 655	X	X	264	4 010	5 046	6 851	6 308	3 618	2 463	2 259	826	10
Intentional self-harm (suicide) by discharge of firearms (X72-X74)	17 108	X	X	86	2 088	2 399	3 157	3 136	2 234	1 776	1 680	550	2
Intentional self-harm (suicide) by other and unspecified means and their sequelae (*U03, X60-X71, X75-X84, Y87.0)	14 547	X	X	178	1 922	2 647	3 694	3 172	1 384	687	579	276	8
Assault (homicide) (*U01-*U02, X85-Y09, Y87.1)	17 638	303	423	356	5 219	4 489	3 239	1 915	841	421	296	95	41
Assault (homicide) by discharge of firearms (*U01.4, X93-X95)	11 829	9	49	205	4 317	3 465	2 042	1 025	409	161	115	19	13
Assault (homicide) by other and unspecified means and their sequelae (*U01.0-*U01.3, *U01.5-*U01.9, *U02, X85-X92, X96-Y09, Y87.1) ..	5 809	294	374	151	902	1 024	1 197	890	432	260	181	76	28
Legal intervention (Y35, Y89.0)	384	-	-	3	91	102	109	56	16	6	1	-	-
Events of undetermined intent (Y10-Y34, Y87.2, Y89.9)	4 830	101	57	68	487	828	1 516	1 140	320	139	95	65	14
Discharge of firearms, undetermined intent (Y22-Y24)	243	-	1	6	79	46	50	29	12	15	5	-	-
Other and unspecified events of undetermined intent and their sequelae (Y10-Y21, Y25-Y34, Y87.2, Y89.9)	4 587	101	56	62	408	782	1 466	1 111	308	124	90	65	14
Operations of war and their sequelae (Y36, Y89.1)	20	-	-	-	-	1	1	1	3	3	10	1	-
Complications of medical and surgical care (Y40-Y84, Y88)	2 843	15	19	35	35	79	171	265	351	560	792	521	-

[1]Based on codes from the *International Classification of Diseases, Tenth Revision* (1992), except in cases where (*) precedes the cause of death code. Codes *U01-*U03 were added as of 2001 for deaths due to terrorism.
- = Quantity zero.
X = Not applicable.

Table II-11. Death Rates for 113 Selected Causes, by Age, 2002

(Rate per 100,000 population.)

Cause of death [1]	All ages [2]	Under 1 year [3]	1–4 years	5–14 years	15–24 years	25–34 years	35–44 years	45–54 years	55–64 years	65–74 years	75–84 years	85 years and over
ALL CAUSES	847.3	695.0	31.2	17.4	81.4	103.6	202.9	430.1	952.4	2 314.7	5 556.9	14 828.3
Salmonella infections (A01-A02)	0.0	*	*	*	*	*	*	*	*	*	*	*
Shigellosis and amebiasis (A03, A06)	*	*	*	*	*	*	*	*	*	*	*	*
Certain other intestinal infections (A04, A07-A09)	0.9	*	*	*	*	*	*	0.1	0.5	2.0	7.0	21.0
Tuberculosis (A16-A19)	0.3	*	*	*	*	*	0.1	0.2	0.4	0.9	1.8	2.6
Respiratory tuberculosis (A16)	0.2	*	*	*	*	*	0.1	0.2	0.3	0.7	1.5	2.3
Other tuberculosis (A17-A19)	0.1	*	*	*	*	*	*	*	0.1	0.2	0.3	*
Whooping cough (A37)	*	*	*	*	*	*	*	*	*	*	*	*
Scarlet fever and erysipelas (A38, A46)	*	*	*	*	*	*	*	*	*	*	*	*
Meningococcal infection (A39)	0.1	*	*	0.0	0.1	*	*	*	*	*	*	*
Septicemia (A40-A41)	11.7	7.3	0.5	0.2	0.3	0.8	1.9	5.2	12.6	34.7	86.5	203.0
Syphilis (A50-A53)	0.0	*	*	*	*	*	*	*	*	*	*	*
Acute poliomyelitis (A80)	*	*	*	*	*	*	*	*	*	*	*	*
Arthropod-borne viral encephalitis (A83-A84, A85.2)	*	*	*	*	*	*	*	*	*	*	*	*
Measles (B05)	*	*	*	*	*	*	*	*	*	*	*	*
Viral hepatitis (B15-B19)	2.0	*	*	*	0.1	0.2	1.6	5.8	4.0	4.2	4.6	3.9
Human immunodeficiency virus (HIV) disease (B20-B24)	4.9	*	*	0.1	0.4	4.6	12.7	11.2	5.1	2.2	0.8	*
Malaria (B50-B54)	*	*	*	*	*	*	*	*	*	*	*	*
Other and unspecified infectious and parasitic diseases and their sequelae (A00, A05, A20-A36, A42-A44, A48-A49, A54-A79, A81-A82, A85.0-A85.1, A85.8, A86-B04, B06-B09, B25-B49, B55-B99)	2.3	5.6	0.4	0.2	0.2	0.4	1.0	2.3	3.3	6.7	12.5	21.7
Malignant neoplasms (C00-C97)	193.2	1.8	2.6	2.6	4.3	9.7	35.8	123.8	351.1	792.1	1 311.9	1 723.9
Malignant neoplasms of lip, oral cavity, and pharynx (C00-C14)	2.7	*	*	*	0.1	0.1	0.6	2.7	6.8	10.4	13.5	18.7
Malignant neoplasm of esophagus (C15)	4.4	*	*	*	*	*	0.7	3.5	10.4	20.2	26.6	24.6
Malignant neoplasm of stomach (C16)	4.2	*	*	*	0.1	0.3	1.0	2.8	6.9	15.4	28.7	47.6
Malignant neoplasms of colon, rectum, and anus (C18-C21)	19.7	*	*	*	0.1	0.7	3.2	11.4	31.7	73.3	137.4	241.4
Malignant neoplasms of liver and intrahepatic bile ducts (C22)	4.9	*	0.2	*	0.1	0.3	0.9	4.9	9.6	19.6	29.3	35.0
Malignant neoplasm of pancreas (C25)	10.5	*	*	*	*	0.1	1.3	6.1	19.2	44.8	75.0	94.5
Malignant neoplasm of larynx (C32)	1.3	*	*	*	*	*	0.2	1.1	3.4	5.9	7.6	5.5
Malignant neoplasms of trachea, bronchus, and lung (C33-C34)	54.7	*	*	*	0.1	0.4	6.0	30.3	115.3	275.0	377.6	297.2
Malignant melanoma of skin (C43)	2.6	*	*	*	0.1	0.5	1.3	2.8	5.1	8.8	13.7	17.9
Malignant neoplasm of breast (C50)	14.5	*	*	*	*	1.1	6.1	16.1	29.5	46.5	76.5	134.6
Malignant neoplasm of cervix uteri (C53)	1.4	*	*	*	*	0.5	1.5	2.2	2.7	3.4	4.1	6.2
Malignant neoplasms of corpus uteri and uterus, part unspecified (C54-C55)	2.4	*	*	*	*	0.1	0.3	1.4	4.5	10.0	15.4	24.6
Malignant neoplasm of ovary (C56)	5.1	*	*	*	0.1	0.2	1.0	4.3	10.3	19.7	33.4	38.1
Malignant neoplasm of prostate (C61)	10.6	*	*	*	*	*	0.1	1.0	7.6	34.5	100.1	195.0
Malignant neoplasms of kidney and renal pelvis (C64-C65)	4.2	*	*	0.1	0.0	0.1	0.7	3.3	8.8	17.7	26.3	32.5
Malignant neoplasm of bladder (C67)	4.4	*	*	*	*	*	0.3	1.3	4.9	15.9	37.0	66.6
Malignant neoplasms of meninges, brain, and other parts of central nervous system (C70-C72)	4.4	*	0.7	0.8	0.5	1.0	2.2	5.1	9.6	16.2	19.1	16.4
Malignant neoplasms of lymphoid, hematopoietic, and related tissue (C81-C96)	19.5	0.7	0.8	0.9	1.7	2.3	3.9	9.9	28.2	73.9	143.6	197.5
Hodgkin's disease (C81)	0.5	*	*	*	0.2	0.4	0.4	0.4	0.6	1.3	1.9	2.7
Non-Hodgkin's lymphoma (C82-C85)	7.6	*	*	0.1	0.3	0.7	1.5	3.9	11.5	28.8	57.2	77.3
Leukemia (C91-C95)	7.5	0.5	0.7	0.8	1.2	1.2	1.7	3.6	9.8	26.4	53.1	80.5
Multiple myeloma and immunoproliferative neoplasms (C88, C90)	4.0	*	*	*	*	*	0.3	1.8	6.3	17.4	31.2	36.7
Other and unspecified malignant neoplasms of lymphoid, hematopoietic, and related tissue (C96)	0.0	*	*	*	*	*	*	*	*	*	0.2	*
All other and unspecified malignant neoplasms (C17, C23-C24, C26-C31, C37-C41, C44-C49, C51-C52, C57-C60, C62-C63, C66, C68-C69, C73-C80, C97)	21.8	0.6	0.8	0.7	1.3	1.8	4.5	13.7	36.6	80.8	146.7	230.1
In situ neoplasms, benign neoplasms, and neoplasms of uncertain or unknown behavior (D00-D48)	4.6	1.7	0.4	0.2	0.2	0.4	0.8	1.8	4.5	12.8	36.1	78.7
Anemias (D50-D64)	1.6	*	0.1	0.1	0.3	0.5	0.4	0.6	1.0	2.8	9.1	40.3
Diabetes mellitus (E10-E14)	25.4	*	*	0.1	0.4	1.6	4.8	13.7	37.7	91.4	182.8	320.6
Nutritional deficiencies (E40-E64)	1.3	*	*	*	*	*	0.1	0.3	0.6	2.1	8.9	41.5
Malnutrition (E40-E46)	1.2	*	*	*	*	*	0.1	0.2	0.6	1.9	8.4	38.4
Other nutritional deficiencies (E50-E64)	0.1	*	*	*	*	*	*	*	*	0.2	0.5	3.1
Meningitis (G00, G03)	0.2	1.8	*	0.1	0.1	0.1	0.1	0.3	0.3	0.6	0.7	1.2
Parkinson's disease (G20-G21)	5.9	*	*	*	*	*	*	0.1	1.2	12.2	63.9	135.2
Alzheimer's disease (G30)	20.4	*	*	*	*	*	*	0.1	1.9	19.7	158.1	752.3

[1]Based on codes from the *International Classification of Diseases, Tenth Revision* (1992), except in cases where (*) precedes the cause of death code. Codes *U01-*U03 were added as of 2001 for deaths due to terrorism.

[2]Figures for age not stated are included in "All ages" but not distributed among age groups.

[3]Death rates for "Under 1 year" (based on population estimates) differ from infant mortality rates (based on live births).

0.0 = Quantity more than zero but less than 0.05.

* = Figure does not meet standards of reliability or precision.

Table II-11. Death Rates for 113 Selected Causes, by Age, 2002—*Continued*

(Rate per 100,000 population.)

Cause of death [1]	All ages [2]	Under 1 year [3]	1–4 years	5–14 years	15–24 years	25–34 years	35–44 years	45–54 years	55–64 years	65–74 years	75–84 years	85 years and over
Major cardiovascular diseases (I00-I78)	318.6	15.9	1.4	0.9	3.2	10.0	37.8	114.3	294.8	788.4	2 257.0	7 389.6
Diseases of heart (I00-I09, I11, I13, I20-I51)	241.7	12.4	1.1	0.6	2.5	7.9	30.5	93.7	241.5	615.9	1 677.2	5 446.8
Acute rheumatic fever and chronic rheumatic heart diseases (I00-I09)	1.2	*	*	*	*	0.1	0.2	0.6	1.6	3.8	9.6	17.8
Hypertensive heart disease (I11)	9.2	*	*	*	0.1	0.7	2.7	7.2	12.5	21.3	49.6	187.0
Hypertensive heart and renal disease (I13)	1.0	*	*	*	*	0.1	0.2	0.4	1.0	2.2	6.8	23.5
Ischemic heart diseases (I20-I25)	171.4	0.6	*	0.0	0.3	2.5	17.1	63.8	177.7	458.9	1 220.2	3 775.0
Acute myocardial infarction (I21-I22)	62.3	*	*	*	0.2	1.0	7.0	26.5	74.9	186.1	444.4	1 191.3
Other acute ischemic heart diseases (I24)	1.2	*	*	*	*	*	0.2	0.9	1.7	3.5	7.1	21.1
Other forms of chronic ischemic heart disease (I20, I25)	108.0	*	*	*	0.2	1.4	9.9	36.5	101.0	269.4	768.8	2 562.5
Atherosclerotic cardiovascular disease, so described (I25.0)	23.6	*	*	*	*	0.5	3.4	13.4	33.1	64.7	146.2	474.5
All other forms of chronic ischemic heart disease (I20, I25.1-I25.9)	84.4	*	*	*	0.1	1.0	6.5	23.1	68.0	204.7	622.6	2 088.0
Other heart diseases (I26-I51)	58.8	11.7	1.0	0.6	2.1	4.5	10.3	21.7	48.7	129.6	390.9	1 443.5
Acute and subacute endocarditis (I33)	0.4	*	*	*	*	0.1	0.2	0.4	0.6	1.3	2.4	2.6
Diseases of pericardium and acute myocarditis (I30-I31, I40)	0.3	0.6	0.1	0.1	0.1	0.1	0.2	0.3	0.4	0.8	1.2	2.1
Heart failure (I50)	19.6	0.6	*	*	0.1	0.3	0.6	2.5	8.8	33.8	132.8	645.0
All other forms of heart disease (I26-I28, I34-I38, I42-I49, I51)	38.5	10.5	0.8	0.5	1.9	4.0	9.3	18.6	38.8	93.7	254.4	793.7
Essential (primary) hypertension and hypertensive renal disease (I10, I12)	7.0	*	*	*	0.1	0.2	0.8	2.3	5.7	16.0	48.2	180.4
Cerebrovascular diseases (I60-I69)	56.4	2.9	0.3	0.2	0.4	1.4	5.4	15.1	37.2	120.3	431.0	1 445.9
Atherosclerosis (I70)	4.8	*	*	*	*	*	0.1	0.5	1.8	7.1	31.9	168.1
Other diseases of circulatory system (I71-I78)	8.6	*	*	*	0.2	0.4	1.0	2.7	8.6	29.1	68.7	148.4
Aortic aneurysm and dissection (I71)	5.1	*	*	*	0.1	0.3	0.7	1.8	5.5	19.1	43.3	69.4
Other diseases of arteries, arterioles, and capillaries (I72-I78)	3.5	*	*	*	0.1	0.1	0.3	0.9	3.1	10.0	25.3	79.0
Other disorders of circulatory system (I80-I99)	1.6	0.7	*	*	0.1	0.3	0.7	1.3	2.2	3.8	9.8	24.4
Influenza and pneumonia (J10-J18)	22.8	6.5	0.7	0.2	0.4	0.9	2.2	4.8	11.2	37.5	156.9	696.6
Influenza (J10-J11) [4]	0.3	*	*	*	*	*	*	*	0.1	0.3	1.4	8.8
Pneumonia (J12-J18)	22.5	6.3	0.7	0.2	0.4	0.9	2.1	4.7	11.1	37.2	155.5	687.8
Other acute lower respiratory infections (J20-J22)	0.1	1.3	0.1	*	*	*	*	*	*	0.2	0.5	3.3
Acute bronchitis and bronchiolitis (J20-J21)	0.1	1.2	0.1	*	*	*	*	*	*	0.1	0.3	2.0
Unspecified acute lower respiratory infection (J22)	0.0	*	*	*	*	*	*	*	*	*	0.2	1.3
Chronic lower respiratory diseases (J40-J47)	43.3	1.0	0.4	0.3	0.5	0.8	2.2	8.7	42.4	163.0	386.7	637.6
Bronchitis, chronic and unspecified (J40-J42)	0.3	0.6	*	*	*	*	*	0.1	0.2	0.7	2.2	8.1
Emphysema (J43)	5.4	*	*	*	*	*	0.2	1.1	6.4	24.0	48.0	59.3
Asthma (J45-J46)	1.5	*	0.3	0.3	0.4	0.6	1.1	1.5	2.0	3.2	6.4	14.7
Other chronic lower respiratory diseases (J44, J47)	36.1	*	*	*	*	*	0.1	0.9	5.9	33.8	135.1	330.1	555.5
Pneumoconioses and chemical effects (J60-J66, J68)	0.4	*	*	*	*	*	*	*	*	0.3	1.2	3.8	6.8
Pneumonitis due to solids and liquids (J69)	6.1	*	*	*	0.1	0.2	0.4	0.9	2.5	9.8	46.3	186.0
Other diseases of respiratory system (J00-J06, J30-J39, J67, J70-J98)	8.7	6.9	0.5	0.2	0.3	0.5	1.2	3.2	9.2	28.7	68.0	133.5
Peptic ulcer (K25-K28)	1.4	*	*	*	*	0.1	0.3	0.7	1.5	3.6	10.1	28.3
Diseases of appendix (K35-K38)	0.2	*	*	*	*	0.1	0.1	0.2	0.5	0.9	2.0
Hernia (K40-K46)	0.6	0.7	*	*	*	*	0.1	0.2	0.5	1.2	3.8	12.8
Chronic liver disease and cirrhosis (K70, K73-K74)	9.5	*	*	*	0.1	0.9	7.0	18.0	22.9	29.4	31.4	21.4
Alcoholic liver disease (K70)	4.2	*	*	*	*	0.6	4.4	10.3	11.6	10.1	5.7	2.1
Other chronic liver disease and cirrhosis (K73-K74)	5.2	*	*	*	0.1	0.3	2.6	7.7	11.3	19.3	25.7	19.3
Cholelithiasis and other disorders of gallbladder (K80-K82)	1.0	*	*	*	*	0.1	0.1	0.3	0.8	2.8	7.8	22.9
Nephritis, nephrotic syndrome, and nephrosis (N00-N07, N17-N19, N25-N27)	14.2	4.3	*	0.1	0.2	0.7	1.7	4.7	13.0	39.2	109.1	288.6
Acute and rapidly progressive nephritic and nephrotic syndrome (N00-N01, N04)	0.1	*	*	*	*	*	*	*	*	0.1	0.4	0.9
Chronic glomerulonephritis, nephritis, and nephropathy, not specified as acute or chronic, and renal sclerosis, unspecified (N02-N03, N05-N07, N26)	0.2	*	*	*	*	0.1	0.1	0.1	0.2	0.5	1.4	2.8
Renal failure (N17-N19)	13.9	4.1	*	*	0.2	0.6	1.6	4.6	12.7	38.6	107.2	284.8
Other disorders of kidney (N25, N27)	0.0	*	*	*	*	*	*	*	*	*	*	*
Infections of kidney (N10-N12, N13.6, N15.1)	0.3	*	*	*	*	*	0.1	0.1	0.2	0.6	1.9	6.3
Hyperplasia of prostate (N40)	0.2	*	*	*	*	*	*	*	*	0.2	1.3	4.8
Inflammatory diseases of female pelvic organs (N70-N76)	0.0	*	*	*	*	*	*	*	*	*	0.2	0.8
Pregnancy, childbirth, and the puerperium (O00-O99)	0.1	X	X	*	0.2	0.4	0.2	*	*	*	*	*
Pregnancy with abortive outcome (O00-O07)	0.0	X	X	*	*	*	*	*	*	*	*	*
Other complications of pregnancy, childbirth, and the puerperium (O10-O99)	0.1	X	X	0.0	0.2	0.4	0.2	*	*	*	*	*
Certain conditions originating in the perinatal period (P00-P96)	4.9	349.7	0.4	0.1	0.1	*	*	*	*	*	*	*
Congenital malformations, deformations, and chromosomal abnormalities (Q00-Q99)	3.7	139.4	3.4	1.0	1.2	1.2	1.3	1.8	2.4	2.4	3.8	6.6
Symptoms, signs, and abnormal clinical and laboratory findings, not elsewhere classified (R00-R99)	10.4	85.7	1.6	0.3	1.8	3.3	5.3	6.7	7.5	13.1	38.8	208.0
All other diseases (residual)	67.5	28.4	4.2	2.1	4.6	7.9	18.9	37.8	65.3	140.6	405.3	1 493.0

[1]Based on codes from the *International Classification of Diseases, Tenth Revision* (1992), except in cases where (*) precedes the cause of death code. Codes *U01-*U03 were added as of 2001 for deaths due to terrorism.
[2]Figures for age not stated are included in "All ages" but not distributed among age groups.
[3]Death rates for "Under 1 year" (based on population estimates) differ from infant mortality rates (based on live births).
[4]Cause of death coding changes may affect comparability with the previous year's data for this cause.
0.0 = Quantity more than zero but less than 0.05.
* = Figure does not meet standards of reliability or precision.
X = Not applicable.

Table II-11. Death Rates for 113 Selected Causes, by Age, 2002—*Continued*

(Rate per 100,000 population.)

Cause of death [1]	All ages [2]	Under 1 year [3]	1–4 years	5–14 years	15–24 years	25–34 years	35–44 years	45–54 years	55–64 years	65–74 years	75–84 years	85 years and over
Accidents (unintentional injuries) (V01-X59, Y85-Y86)	37.0	23.5	10.5	6.6	38.0	31.5	37.2	36.6	31.4	44.2	101.3	275.4
Transport accidents (V01-V99, Y85)	16.8	3.1	4.1	4.2	29.1	18.7	17.1	16.4	15.7	18.3	27.0	28.8
Motor vehicle accidents (V02-V04, V09.0, V09.2, V12-V14, V19.0-V19.2, V19.4-V19.6, V20-V79, V80.3-80.5, V81.0-V81.1, V82.0-V82.1, V83-V86, V87.0-V87.8, V88.0-V88.8, V89.0, V89.2)	15.7	3.0	3.9	3.9	28.2	17.8	15.8	14.8	14.1	17.0	25.7	28.0
Other land transport accidents (V01, V05-V06, V09.1, V09.3-V09.9, V10-V11, V15-V18, V19.3, V19.8-V19.9, V80.0-V80.2, V80.6-V80.9, V81.2-V81.9, V82.2-V82.9, V87.9, V88.9, V89.1, V89.3, V89.9)	0.4	*	*	0.2	0.4	0.3	0.5	0.5	0.4	0.4	0.5	*
Water, air and space, and other and unspecified transport accidents and their sequelae (V90-V99, Y85)	0.7	*	*	0.1	0.5	0.6	0.9	1.0	1.1	0.9	0.8	0.4
Nontransport accidents (W00-X59, Y86)	20.2	20.3	6.4	2.4	8.9	12.7	20.1	20.2	15.7	25.9	74.4	246.7
Falls (W00-W19)	5.6	*	0.2	0.1	0.6	0.8	1.5	2.5	4.1	10.8	38.3	130.4
Accidental discharge of firearms (W32-W34)	0.3	*	*	0.1	0.5	0.4	0.3	0.2	0.2	0.2	0.3	*
Accidental drowning and submersion (W65-W74) ...	1.2	1.6	2.9	0.8	1.5	1.1	1.2	0.9	0.8	0.9	1.3	1.7
Accidental exposure to smoke, fire, and flames (X00-X09)	1.1	0.9	1.4	0.6	0.5	0.7	0.8	1.1	1.3	2.1	3.4	4.8
Accidental poisoning and exposure to noxious substances (X40-X49)	6.1	0.6	0.2	0.1	4.1	7.8	13.4	11.7	4.1	2.1	2.3	3.9
Other and unspecified nontransport accidents and their sequelae (W20-W31, W35-W64, W75-W99, X10-X39, X50-X59, Y86)	6.0	16.8	1.6	0.7	1.6	2.1	3.0	3.7	5.2	9.8	28.8	105.6
Intentional self-harm (suicide) (*U03, X60-X84, Y87.0)	11.0	X	X	0.6	9.9	12.6	15.3	15.7	13.6	13.5	17.7	18.0
Intentional self-harm (suicide) by discharge of firearms (X72-X74)	5.9	X	X	0.2	5.1	6.0	7.0	7.8	8.4	9.7	13.2	12.0
Intentional self-harm (suicide) by other and unspecified means and their sequelae (*U03, X60-X71, X75-X84, Y87.0)	5.0	X	X	0.4	4.7	6.6	8.2	7.9	5.2	3.8	4.5	6.0
Assault (homicide) (*U01-*U02, X85-Y09, Y87.1)	6.1	7.5	2.7	0.9	12.9	11.2	7.2	4.8	3.2	2.3	2.3	2.1
Assault (homicide) by discharge of firearms (*U01.4, X93-X95)	4.1	*	0.3	0.5	10.6	8.7	4.5	2.6	1.5	0.9	0.9	*
Assault (homicide) by other and unspecified means and their sequelae (*U01.0-*U01.3, *U01.5-*U01.9, *U02, X85-X92, X96-Y09, Y87.1) ..	2.0	7.3	2.4	0.4	2.2	2.6	2.7	2.2	1.6	1.4	1.4	1.7
Legal intervention (Y35, Y89.0)	0.1	*	*	*	0.2	0.3	0.2	0.1	*	*	*	*
Events of undetermined intent (Y10-Y34, Y87.2, Y89.9) ..	1.7	2.5	0.4	0.2	1.2	2.1	3.4	2.8	1.2	0.8	0.7	1.4
Discharge of firearms, undetermined intent (Y22-Y24)	0.1	*	*	*	0.2	0.1	0.1	0.1	*	*	*	*
Other and unspecified events of undetermined intent and their sequelae (Y10-Y21, Y25-Y34, Y87.2, Y89.9)	1.6	2.5	0.4	0.2	1.0	2.0	3.3	2.8	1.2	0.7	0.7	1.4
Operations of war and their sequelae (Y36, Y89.1)	0.0	*	*	*	*	*	*	*	*	*	*	*
Complications of medical and surgical care (Y40-Y84, Y88)	1.0	*	*	0.1	0.1	0.2	0.4	0.7	1.3	3.1	6.2	11.3

[1]Based on codes from the *International Classification of Diseases, Tenth Revision* (1992), except in cases where (*) precedes the cause of death code. Codes *U01-*U03 were added as of 2001 for deaths due to terrorism.
[2]Figures for age not stated are included in "All ages" but not distributed among age groups.
[3]Death rates for "Under 1 year" (based on population estimates) differ from infant mortality rates (based on live births).
* = Figure does not meet standards of reliability or precision.
X = Not applicable.

Table II-12. Number of Deaths from 113 Selected Causes, by Race and Sex, 2002

(Number.)

Cause of death [1]	All races			White			All other Total			All other Black		
	Both sexes	Male	Female	Both sexes	Male	Female	Both sexes	Male	Female	Both sexes	Male	Female
ALL CAUSES	2 443 387	1 199 264	1 244 123	2 102 589	1 025 196	1 077 393	340 798	174 068	166 730	290 051	146 835	143 216
Salmonella infections (A01-A02)	21	10	11	18	9	9	3	1	2	3	1	2
Shigellosis and amebiasis (A03, A06)	8	4	4	7	4	3	1	-	1	-	-	-
Certain other intestinal infections (A04, A07-A09)	2 465	947	1 518	2 287	872	1 415	178	75	103	156	66	90
Tuberculosis (A16-A19)	784	462	322	461	272	189	323	190	133	204	127	77
Respiratory tuberculosis (A16)	626	372	254	374	223	151	252	149	103	164	104	60
Other tuberculosis (A17-A19)	158	90	68	87	49	38	71	41	30	40	23	17
Whooping cough (A37)	18	6	12	15	5	10	3	1	2	2	1	1
Scarlet fever and erysipelas (A38, A46)	2	-	2	2	-	2	-	-	-	-	-	-
Meningococcal infection (A39)	161	83	78	125	67	58	36	16	20	29	12	17
Septicemia (A40-A41)	33 865	14 947	18 918	27 110	11 919	15 191	6 755	3 028	3 727	6 137	2 703	3 434
Syphilis (A50-A53)	41	21	20	18	9	9	23	12	11	23	12	11
Acute poliomyelitis (A80)	-	-	-	-	-	-	-	-	-	-	-	-
Arthropod-borne viral encephalitis (A83-A84, A85.2)	9	4	5	6	2	4	3	2	1	3	2	1
Measles (B05)	-	-	-	-	-	-	-	-	-	-	-	-
Viral hepatitis (B15-B19)	5 793	3 770	2 023	4 620	3 049	1 571	1 173	721	452	865	541	324
Human immunodeficiency virus (HIV) disease (B20-B24)	14 095	10 468	3 627	6 089	5 028	1 061	8 006	5 440	2 566	7 835	5 301	2 534
Malaria (B50-B54)	12	8	4	7	7	-	5	1	4	4	1	3
Other and unspecified infectious and parasitic diseases and their sequelae (A00, A05, A20-A36, A42-A44, A48-A49, A54-A79, A81-A82, A85.0-A85.1, A85.8, A86-B04, B06-B09, B25-B49, B55-B99)	6 707	3 622	3 085	5 528	2 967	2 561	1 179	655	524	943	526	417
Malignant neoplasms (C00-C97)	557 271	288 768	268 503	482 481	249 867	232 614	74 790	38 901	35 889	62 617	32 627	29 990
Malignant neoplasms of lip, oral cavity, and pharynx (C00-C14)	7 737	5 184	2 553	6 432	4 256	2 176	1 305	928	377	1 044	766	278
Malignant neoplasm of esophagus (C15)	12 701	9 789	2 912	10 910	8 510	2 400	1 791	1 279	512	1 590	1 133	457
Malignant neoplasm of stomach (C16)	12 198	7 133	5 065	9 319	5 542	3 777	2 879	1 591	1 288	2 131	1 194	937
Malignant neoplasms of colon, rectum, and anus (C18-C21)	56 741	28 501	28 240	48 562	24 439	24 123	8 179	4 062	4 117	6 874	3 351	3 523
Malignant neoplasms of liver and intrahepatic bile ducts (C22)	14 047	9 011	5 036	11 250	7 114	4 136	2 797	1 897	900	1 734	1 165	569
Malignant neoplasm of pancreas (C25)	30 264	14 877	15 387	26 031	12 921	13 110	4 233	1 956	2 277	3 494	1 617	1 877
Malignant neoplasm of larynx (C32)	3 723	2 922	801	3 012	2 351	661	711	571	140	675	542	133
Malignant neoplasms of trachea, bronchus, and lung (C33-C34)	157 713	90 171	67 542	138 661	78 465	60 196	19 052	11 706	7 346	16 316	10 075	6 241
Malignant melanoma of skin (C43)	7 514	4 725	2 789	7 353	4 639	2 714	161	86	75	102	52	50
Malignant neoplasm of breast (C50)	41 883	369	41 514	35 382	300	35 082	6 501	69	6 432	5 636	64	5 572
Malignant neoplasm of cervix uteri (C53)	3 952	X	3 952	2 967	X	2 967	985	X	985	829	X	829
Malignant neoplasms of corpus uteri and uterus, part unspecified (C54-C55)	6 853	X	6 853	5 567	X	5 567	1 286	X	1 286	1 119	X	1 119
Malignant neoplasm of ovary (C56)	14 682	X	14 682	13 202	X	13 202	1 480	X	1 480	1 163	X	1 163
Malignant neoplasm of prostate (C61)	30 446	30 446	X	24 918	24 918	X	5 528	5 528	X	5 145	5 145	X
Malignant neoplasms of kidney and renal pelvis (C64-C65)	12 165	7 587	4 578	10 856	6 803	4 053	1 309	784	525	1 069	630	439
Malignant neoplasm of bladder (C67)	12 628	8 504	4 124	11 512	7 908	3 604	1 116	596	520	940	481	459
Malignant neoplasms of meninges, brain, and other parts of central nervous system (C70-C72)	12 830	7 125	5 705	11 794	6 554	5 240	1 036	571	465	781	409	372
Malignant neoplasms of lymphoid, hematopoietic, and related tissue (C81-C96)	56 225	30 302	25 923	49 943	27 087	22 856	6 282	3 215	3 067	5 151	2 622	2 529
Hodgkin's disease (C81)	1 352	751	601	1 193	655	538	159	96	63	130	82	48
Non-Hodgkin's lymphoma (C82-C85)	21 910	11 538	10 372	19 996	10 535	9 461	1 914	1 003	911	1 474	775	699
Leukemia (C91-C95)	21 498	12 016	9 482	19 273	10 835	8 438	2 225	1 181	1 044	1 770	923	847
Multiple myeloma and immunoproliferative neoplasms (C88, C90)	11 392	5 953	5 439	9 420	5 024	4 396	1 972	929	1 043	1 771	840	931
Other and unspecified malignant neoplasms of lymphoid, hematopoietic, and related tissue (C96)	73	44	29	61	38	23	12	6	6	6	2	4
All other and unspecified malignant neoplasms (C17, C23-C24, C26-C31, C37-C41, C44-C49, C51-C52, C57-C60, C62-C63, C66, C68-C69, C73-C80, C97)	62 969	32 122	30 847	54 810	28 060	26 750	8 159	4 062	4 097	6 824	3 381	3 443
In situ neoplasms, benign neoplasms, and neoplasms of uncertain or unknown behavior (D00-D48)	13 299	6 536	6 763	11 913	5 902	6 011	1 386	634	752	1 143	500	643
Anemias (D50-D64)	4 614	1 781	2 833	3 460	1 267	2 193	1 154	514	640	1 064	479	585
Diabetes mellitus (E10-E14)	73 249	34 301	38 948	58 459	28 110	30 349	14 790	6 191	8 599	12 687	5 207	7 480
Nutritional deficiencies (E40-E64)	3 779	1 321	2 458	3 213	1 102	2 111	566	219	347	502	188	314
Malnutrition (E40-E46)	3 510	1 233	2 277	2 979	1 029	1 950	531	204	327	472	175	297
Other nutritional deficiencies (E50-E64)	269	88	181	234	73	161	35	15	20	30	13	17
Meningitis (G00, G03)	700	389	311	498	270	228	202	119	83	178	107	71
Parkinson's disease (G20-G21)	16 959	9 593	7 366	16 135	9 130	7 005	824	463	361	557	313	244
Alzheimer's disease (G30)	58 866	16 989	41 877	55 058	15 874	39 184	3 808	1 115	2 693	3 341	959	2 382

[1]Based on codes from the *International Classification of Diseases, Tenth Revision* (1992), except in cases where (*) precedes the cause of death code. Codes *U01-*U03 were added as of 2001 for deaths due to terrorism.
- = Quantity zero.
X = Not applicable.

Table II-12. Number of Deaths from 113 Selected Causes, by Race and Sex, 2002—*Continued*

(Number.)

Cause of death [1]	All races			White			All other					
							Total			Black		
	Both sexes	Male	Female	Both sexes	Male	Female	Both sexes	Male	Female	Both sexes	Male	Female
Major cardiovascular diseases (I00-I78)	918 628	429 682	488 946	796 748	372 088	424 660	121 880	57 594	64 286	104 215	48 264	55 951
Diseases of heart (I00-I09, I11, I13, I20-I51)	696 947	340 933	356 014	606 876	296 904	309 972	90 071	44 029	46 042	77 621	37 094	40 527
Acute rheumatic fever and chronic rheumatic heart diseases (I00-I09)	3 579	1 078	2 501	3 204	950	2 254	375	128	247	252	93	159
Hypertensive heart disease (I11)	26 551	11 660	14 891	19 530	8 234	11 296	7 021	3 426	3 595	6 480	3 146	3 334
Hypertensive heart and renal disease (I13)	2 895	1 205	1 690	1 925	760	1 165	970	445	525	903	405	498
Ischemic heart diseases (I20-I25)	494 382	252 760	241 622	435 170	223 262	211 908	59 212	29 498	29 714	50 174	24 322	25 852
Acute myocardial infarction (I21-I22)	179 514	93 830	85 684	157 922	83 288	74 634	21 592	10 542	11 050	18 322	8 680	9 642
Other acute ischemic heart diseases (I24)	3 407	1 767	1 640	2 907	1 494	1 413	500	273	227	446	243	203
Other forms of chronic ischemic heart disease (I20, I25)	311 461	157 163	154 298	274 341	138 480	135 861	37 120	18 683	18 437	31 406	15 399	16 007
Atherosclerotic cardiovascular disease, so described (I25.0)	68 129	36 047	32 082	56 569	29 604	26 965	11 560	6 443	5 117	10 195	5 598	4 597
All other forms of chronic ischemic heart disease (I20, I25.1-I25.9)	243 332	121 116	122 216	217 772	108 876	108 896	25 560	12 240	13 320	21 211	9 801	11 410
Other heart diseases (I26-I51)	169 540	74 230	95 310	147 047	63 698	83 349	22 493	10 532	11 961	19 812	9 128	10 684
Acute and subacute endocarditis (I33)	1 154	643	511	930	524	406	224	119	105	199	106	93
Diseases of pericardium and acute myocarditis (I30-I31, I40)	848	434	414	666	344	322	182	90	92	154	75	79
Heart failure (I50)	56 494	21 698	34 796	50 672	19 335	31 337	5 822	2 363	3 459	5 186	2 069	3 117
All other forms of heart disease (I26-I28, I34-I38, I42-I49, I51)	111 044	51 455	59 589	94 779	43 495	51 284	16 265	7 960	8 305	14 273	6 878	7 395
Essential (primary) hypertension and hypertensive renal disease (I10, I12)	20 261	7 647	12 614	15 587	5 719	9 868	4 674	1 928	2 746	4 196	1 717	2 479
Cerebrovascular diseases (I60-I69)	162 672	62 622	100 050	139 719	52 959	86 760	22 953	9 663	13 290	18 856	7 828	11 028
Atherosclerosis (I70)	13 821	5 171	8 650	12 631	4 688	7 943	1 190	483	707	1 017	414	603
Other diseases of circulatory system (I71-I78)	24 927	13 309	11 618	21 935	11 818	10 117	2 992	1 491	1 501	2 525	1 211	1 314
Aortic aneurysm and dissection (I71)	14 818	9 013	5 805	13 285	8 132	5 153	1 533	881	652	1 218	677	541
Other diseases of arteries, arterioles, and capillaries (I72-I78)	10 109	4 296	5 813	8 650	3 686	4 964	1 459	610	849	1 307	534	773
Other disorders of circulatory system (I80-I99)	4 711	1 944	2 767	3 853	1 545	2 308	858	399	459	797	366	431
Influenza and pneumonia (J10-J18)	65 681	28 918	36 763	58 346	25 381	32 965	7 335	3 537	3 798	5 871	2 768	3 103
Influenza (J10-J11) [2]	727	289	438	686	270	416	41	19	22	30	15	15
Pneumonia (J12-J18)	64 954	28 629	36 325	57 660	25 111	32 549	7 294	3 518	3 776	5 841	2 753	3 088
Other acute lower respiratory infections (J20-J22)	386	154	232	334	130	204	52	24	28	45	23	22
Acute bronchitis and bronchiolitis (J20-J21)	279	122	157	237	100	137	42	22	20	36	21	15
Unspecified acute lower respiratory infection (J22)	107	32	75	97	30	67	10	2	8	9	2	7
Chronic lower respiratory diseases (J40-J47)	124 816	60 713	64 103	115 395	55 409	59 986	9 421	5 304	4 117	7 831	4 341	3 490
Bronchitis, chronic and unspecified (J40-J42)	955	420	535	876	376	500	79	44	35	66	35	31
Emphysema (J43)	15 489	8 084	7 405	14 476	7 426	7 050	1 013	658	355	850	541	309
Asthma (J45-J46)	4 261	1 580	2 681	3 014	1 017	1 997	1 247	563	684	1 096	497	599
Other chronic lower respiratory diseases (J44, J47)	104 111	50 629	53 482	97 029	46 590	50 439	7 082	4 039	3 043	5 819	3 268	2 551
Pneumoconioses and chemical effects (J60-J66, J68)	1 114	1 057	57	1 048	998	50	66	59	7	58	52	6
Pneumonitis due to solids and liquids (J69)	17 593	8 876	8 717	15 773	7 954	7 819	1 820	922	898	1 537	760	777
Other diseases of respiratory system (J00-J06, J30-J39, J67, J70-J98)	25 039	12 057	12 982	22 184	10 693	11 491	2 855	1 364	1 491	2 279	1 084	1 195
Peptic ulcer (K25-K28)	4 079	1 951	2 128	3 587	1 685	1 902	492	266	226	380	212	168
Diseases of appendix (K35-K38)	480	275	205	404	225	179	76	50	26	63	42	21
Hernia (K40-K46)	1 595	599	996	1 433	533	900	162	66	96	137	56	81
Chronic liver disease and cirrhosis (K70, K73-K74)	27 257	17 401	9 856	23 809	15 278	8 531	3 448	2 123	1 325	2 588	1 622	966
Alcoholic liver disease (K70)	12 121	8 814	3 307	10 423	7 688	2 735	1 698	1 126	572	1 191	797	394
Other chronic liver disease and cirrhosis (K73-K74)	15 136	8 587	6 549	13 386	7 590	5 796	1 750	997	753	1 397	825	572
Cholelithiasis and other disorders of gallbladder (K80-K82)	2 979	1 341	1 638	2 614	1 179	1 435	365	162	203	273	110	163
Nephritis, nephrotic syndrome, and nephrosis (N00-N07, N17-N19, N25-N27)	40 974	19 695	21 279	32 615	15 850	16 765	8 359	3 845	4 514	7 488	3 427	4 061
Acute and rapidly progressive nephritic and nephrotic syndrome (N00-N01, N04)	166	70	96	130	56	74	36	14	22	29	11	18
Chronic glomerulonephritis, nephritis, and nephropathy, not specified as acute or chronic, and renal sclerosis, unspecified (N02-N03, N05-N07, N26)	553	278	275	450	233	217	103	45	58	82	37	45
Renal failure (N17-N19)	40 222	19 341	20 881	32 008	15 558	16 450	8 214	3 783	4 431	7 373	3 377	3 996
Other disorders of kidney (N25, N27)	33	6	27	27	3	24	6	3	3	4	2	2
Infections of kidney (N10-N12, N13.6, N15.1)	788	251	537	692	219	473	96	32	64	73	22	51
Hyperplasia of prostate (N40)	437	437	X	389	389	X	48	48	X	39	39	X
Inflammatory diseases of female pelvic organs (N70-N76)	114	X	114	92	X	92	22	X	22	20	X	20
Pregnancy, childbirth, and the puerperium (O00-O99)	379	X	379	203	X	203	176	X	176	157	X	157
Pregnancy with abortive outcome (O00-O07)	22	X	22	7	X	7	15	X	15	12	X	12
Other complications of pregnancy, childbirth, and the puerperium (O10-O99)	357	X	357	196	X	196	161	X	161	145	X	145
Certain conditions originating in the perinatal period (P00-P96)	14 254	8 047	6 207	8 777	5 011	3 766	5 477	3 036	2 441	4 931	2 725	2 206
Congenital malformations, deformations, and chromosomal abnormalities (Q00-Q99)	10 687	5 515	5 172	8 556	4 416	4 140	2 131	1 099	1 032	1 758	909	849
Symptoms, signs, and abnormal clinical and laboratory findings, not elsewhere classified (R00-R99)	29 975	14 269	15 706	24 749	11 421	13 328	5 226	2 848	2 378	4 638	2 536	2 102
All other diseases (residual)	194 591	79 007	115 584	168 631	67 452	101 179	25 960	11 555	14 405	22 519	9 847	12 672

[1]Based on codes from the *International Classification of Diseases, Tenth Revision* (1992), except in cases where (*) precedes the cause of death code. Codes *U01-*U03 were added as of 2001 for deaths due to terrorism.
[2]Cause of death coding changes may affect comparability with the previous year's data for this cause.
X = Not applicable.

Table II-12. Number of Deaths from 113 Selected Causes, by Race and Sex, 2002—*Continued*

(Number.)

Cause of death [1]	All races			White			All other					
							Total			Black		
	Both sexes	Male	Female	Both sexes	Male	Female	Both sexes	Male	Female	Both sexes	Male	Female
Accidents (unintentional injuries) (V01-X59, Y85-Y86)	106 742	69 257	37 485	90 866	58 467	32 399	15 876	10 790	5 086	12 513	8 612	3 901
Transport accidents (V01-V99, Y85)	48 366	33 533	14 833	40 614	28 118	12 496	7 752	5 415	2 337	5 796	4 156	1 640
Motor vehicle accidents (V02-V04, V09.0, V09.2, V12-V14, V19.0-V19.2, V19.4-V19.6, V20-V79, V80.3-80.5, V81.0-V81.1, V82.0-V82.1, V83-V86, V87.0-V87.8, V88.0-V88.8, V89.0, V89.2)	45 380	31 064	14 316	38 054	26 000	12 054	7 326	5 064	2 262	5 462	3 874	1 588
Other land transport accidents (V01, V05-V06, V09.1, V09.3-V09.9, V10-V11, V15-V18, V19.3, V19.8-V19.9, V80.0-V80.2, V80.6-V80.9, V81.2-V81.9, V82.2-V82.9, V87.9, V88.9, V89.1, V89.3, V89.9)	1 086	882	204	870	708	162	216	174	42	172	145	27
Water, air and space, and other and unspecified transport accidents and their sequelae (V90-V99, Y85)	1 900	1 587	313	1 690	1 410	280	210	177	33	162	137	25
Nontransport accidents (W00-X59, Y86)	58 376	35 724	22 652	50 252	30 349	19 903	8 124	5 375	2 749	6 717	4 456	2 261
Falls (W00-W19)	16 257	8 463	7 794	15 027	7 699	7 328	1 230	764	466	838	532	306
Accidental discharge of firearms (W32-W34)	762	667	95	591	510	81	171	157	14	155	142	13
Accidental drowning and submersion (W65-W74)	3 447	2 761	686	2 624	2 093	531	823	668	155	613	509	104
Accidental exposure to smoke, fire, and flames (X00-X09)	3 159	1 935	1 224	2 287	1 419	868	872	516	356	774	461	313
Accidental poisoning and exposure to noxious substances (X40-X49)	17 550	12 059	5 491	14 868	10 213	4 655	2 682	1 846	836	2 365	1 631	734
Other and unspecified nontransport accidents and their sequelae (W20-W31, W35-W64, W75-W99, X10-X39, X50-X59, Y86)	17 201	9 839	7 362	14 855	8 415	6 440	2 346	1 424	922	1 972	1 181	791
Intentional self-harm (suicide) (*U03, X60-X84, Y87.0)	31 655	25 409	6 246	28 731	23 049	5 682	2 924	2 360	564	1 939	1 633	306
Intentional self-harm (suicide) by discharge of firearms (X72-X74)	17 108	15 045	2 063	15 733	13 809	1 924	1 375	1 236	139	1 059	962	97
Intentional self-harm (suicide) by other and unspecified means and their sequelae (*U03, X60-X71, X75-X84, Y87.0)	14 547	10 364	4 183	12 998	9 240	3 758	1 549	1 124	425	880	671	209
Assault (homicide) (*U01-*U02, X85-Y09, Y87.1)	17 638	13 640	3 998	8 685	6 282	2 403	8 953	7 358	1 595	8 287	6 896	1 391
Assault (homicide) by discharge of firearms (*U01.4, X93-X95)	11 829	9 899	1 930	5 185	4 050	1 135	6 644	5 849	795	6 285	5 575	710
Assault (homicide) by other and unspecified means and their sequelae (*U01.0-*U01.3, *U01.5-*U01.9, *U02, X85-X92, X96-Y09, Y87.1)	5 809	3 741	2 068	3 500	2 232	1 268	2 309	1 509	800	2 002	1 321	681
Legal intervention (Y35, Y89.0)	384	369	15	257	246	11	127	123	4	110	106	4
Events of undetermined intent (Y10-Y34, Y87.2, Y89.9)	4 830	3 114	1 716	3 962	2 524	1 438	868	590	278	759	521	238
Discharge of firearms, undetermined intent (Y22-Y24)	243	199	44	192	153	39	51	46	5	41	39	2
Other and unspecified events of undetermined intent and their sequelae (Y10-Y21, Y25-Y34, Y87.2, Y89.9)	4 587	2 915	1 672	3 770	2 371	1 399	817	544	273	718	482	236
Operations of war and their sequelae (Y36, Y89.1)	20	20	-	15	15	-	5	5	-	5	5	-
Complications of medical and surgical care (Y40-Y84, Y88)	2 843	1 236	1 607	2 331	1 025	1 306	512	211	301	448	184	264

[1]Based on codes from the *International Classification of Diseases, Tenth Revision* (1992), except in cases where (*) precedes the cause of death code. Codes *U01-*U03 were added as of 2001 for deaths due to terrorism.
- = Quantity zero.

TABLE II-13. NUMBER OF DEATHS FROM 113 SELECTED CAUSES, BY RACE, HISPANIC ORIGIN, AND SEX, 2002

This table presents cause-specific death counts by sex for 1) all ethnic origins; 2) all Hispanics; 3) all non-Hispanics (all races); 4) non-Hispanic Whites; 5) non-Hispanic Blacks; and 6) origin not stated. The same format (without "origin not stated") was used for the crude rates in Table II-15 and the age-adjusted rates in Table II-17.

As discussed in Table II-2, the Hispanic population had special qualities of good health. Overall, Hispanics accounted for 4.8 percent of deaths in the United States in 2002, although this ethnic group represented as much as 14 percent of the U.S. population. A large part of this difference was due to the younger average age of the Hispanic population. However, this was also caused by the underreporting of Hispanic ethnicity on death certificates. Hispanic cancer fatalities accounted for 4.2 percent of the national total, and their deaths from lung cancer made up 2.6 percent of such deaths. However, Hispanics represented 8.1 percent of the population that died from diabetes. Hispanics also accounted for a substantial share of accidental deaths (9.5 percent). When an adjustment was made for differences in the age distribution, the Hispanic mortality rate increased to 74 percent of the rate of the total population. (See Table II-17.)

Table II-13. Number of Deaths from 113 Selected Causes, by Race, Hispanic Origin, and Sex, 2002

(Number.)

Cause of death [1]	All origins			Hispanic [2]			Non-Hispanic [3]		
	Both sexes	Male	Female	Both sexes	Male	Female	Both sexes	Male	Female
ALL CAUSES	2 443 387	1 199 264	1 244 123	117 135	65 703	51 432	2 318 269	1 129 090	1 189 179
Salmonella infections (A01-A02)	21	10	11	3	1	2	18	9	9
Shigellosis and amebiasis (A03, A06)	8	4	4	1	1	-	7	3	4
Certain other intestinal infections (A04, A07-A09) ...	2 465	947	1 518	78	31	47	2 381	915	1 466
Tuberculosis (A16-A19)	784	462	322	95	52	43	682	404	278
Respiratory tuberculosis (A16)	626	372	254	78	44	34	543	323	220
Other tuberculosis (A17-A19)	158	90	68	17	8	9	139	81	58
Whooping cough (A37)	18	6	12	3	2	1	15	4	11
Scarlet fever and erysipelas (A38, A46)	2	-	2	-	-	-	2	-	2
Meningococcal infection (A39)	161	83	78	19	9	10	142	74	68
Septicemia (A40-A41)	33 865	14 947	18 918	1 521	744	777	32 225	14 136	18 089
Syphilis (A50-A53)	41	21	20	1	1	-	39	20	19
Acute poliomyelitis (A80)	-	-	-	-	-	-	-	-	-
Arthropod-borne viral encephalitis (A83-A84, A85.2)	9	4	5	-	-	-	9	4	5
Measles (B05)	-	-	-	-	-	-	-	-	-
Viral hepatitis (B15-B19)	5 793	3 770	2 023	758	491	267	5 004	3 256	1 748
Human immunodeficiency virus (HIV) disease (B20-B24) ...	14 095	10 468	3 627	1 855	1 440	415	12 094	8 911	3 183
Malaria (B50-B54)	12	8	4	-	-	-	12	8	4
Other and unspecified infectious and parasitic diseases and their sequelae (A00, A05, A20-A36, A42-A44, A48-A49, A54-A79, A81-A82, A85.0-A85.1, A85.8, A86-B04, B06-B09, B25-B49, B55-B99)	6 707	3 622	3 085	593	363	230	6 097	3 250	2 847
Malignant neoplasms (C00-C97)	557 271	288 768	268 503	23 141	12 235	10 906	532 712	275 770	256 942
Malignant neoplasms of lip, oral cavity, and pharynx (C00-C14)	7 737	5 184	2 553	284	215	69	7 431	4 950	2 481
Malignant neoplasm of esophagus (C15)	12 701	9 789	2 912	411	329	82	12 254	9 431	2 823
Malignant neoplasm of stomach (C16)	12 198	7 133	5 065	1 185	671	514	10 974	6 438	4 536
Malignant neoplasms of colon, rectum, and anus (C18-C21)	56 741	28 501	28 240	2 364	1 287	1 077	54 244	27 140	27 104
Malignant neoplasms of liver and intrahepatic bile ducts (C22)	14 047	9 011	5 036	1 363	891	472	12 638	8 085	4 553
Malignant neoplasm of pancreas (C25)	30 264	14 877	15 387	1 363	667	696	28 839	14 181	14 658
Malignant neoplasm of larynx (C32)	3 723	2 922	801	165	139	26	3 548	2 775	773
Malignant neoplasms of trachea, bronchus, and lung (C33-C34)	157 713	90 171	67 542	4 038	2 617	1 421	153 292	87 335	65 957
Malignant melanoma of skin (C43)	7 514	4 725	2 789	147	77	70	7 349	4 640	2 709
Malignant neoplasm of breast (C50)	41 883	369	41 514	1 736	12	1 724	40 037	355	39 682
Malignant neoplasm of cervix uteri (C53)	3 952	X	3 952	388	X	388	3 551	X	3 551
Malignant neoplasms of corpus uteri and uterus, part unspecified (C54-C55)	6 853	X	6 853	337	X	337	6 487	X	6 487
Malignant neoplasm of ovary (C56)	14 682	X	14 682	622	X	622	14 031	X	14 031
Malignant neoplasm of prostate (C61)	30 446	30 446	X	1 209	1 209	X	29 151	29 151	X
Malignant neoplasms of kidney and renal pelvis (C64-C65)	12 165	7 587	4 578	659	426	233	11 477	7 141	4 336
Malignant neoplasms of bladder (C67)	12 628	8 504	4 124	387	252	135	12 211	8 235	3 976
Malignant neoplasms of meninges, brain, and other parts of central nervous system (C70-C72)	12 830	7 125	5 705	649	359	290	12 152	6 752	5 400
Malignant neoplasms of lymphoid, hematopoietic, and related tissue (C81-C96)	56 225	30 302	25 923	2 829	1 518	1 311	53 249	28 698	24 551
Hodgkin's disease (C81)	1 352	751	601	99	53	46	1 248	693	555
Non-Hodgkin's lymphoma (C82-C85)	21 910	11 538	10 372	1 068	549	519	20 780	10 953	9 827
Leukemia (C91-C95)	21 498	12 016	9 482	1 088	601	487	20 363	11 386	8 977
Multiple myeloma and immunoproliferative neoplasms (C88, C90)	11 392	5 953	5 439	572	314	258	10 787	5 623	5 164
Other and unspecified malignant neoplasms of lymphoid, hematopoietic, and related tissue (C96)	73	44	29	2	1	1	71	43	28
All other and unspecified malignant neoplasms (C17, C23-C24, C26-C31, C37-C41, C44-C49, C51-C52, C57-C60, C62-C63, C66, C68-C69, C73-C80, C97)	62 969	32 122	30 847	3 005	1 566	1 439	59 797	30 463	29 334
In situ neoplasms, benign neoplasms, and neoplasms of uncertain or unknown behavior (D00-D48)	13 299	6 536	6 763	563	282	281	12 708	6 237	6 471
Anemias (D50-D64)	4 614	1 781	2 833	208	106	102	4 391	1 671	2 720
Diabetes mellitus (E10-E14)	73 249	34 301	38 948	5 912	2 779	3 133	67 112	31 399	35 713
Nutritional deficiencies (E40-E64)	3 779	1 321	2 458	141	61	80	3 621	1 255	2 366
Malnutrition (E40-E46)	3 510	1 233	2 277	136	58	78	3 358	1 171	2 187
Other nutritional deficiencies (E50-E64)	269	88	181	5	3	2	263	84	179
Meningitis (G00, G03)	700	389	311	70	42	28	625	344	281
Parkinson's disease (G20-G21)	16 959	9 593	7 366	491	281	210	16 435	9 290	7 145
Alzheimer's disease (G30)	58 866	16 989	41 877	1 474	464	1 010	57 246	16 491	40 755

[1] Based on codes from the *International Classification of Diseases, Tenth Revision* (1992), except in cases where (*) precedes the cause of death code. Codes *U01-*U03 were added as of 2001 for deaths due to terrorism.
[2] May be of any race.
[3] Includes races other than White and Black.
- = Quantity zero.
X = Not applicable.

Table II-13. Number of Deaths from 113 Selected Causes, by Race, Hispanic Origin, and Sex, 2002
—Continued

(Number.)

Cause of death [1]	Non-Hispanic White			Non-Hispanic Black			Origin not stated [4]		
	Both sexes	Male	Female	Both sexes	Male	Female	Both sexes	Male	Female
ALL CAUSES	1 981 973	957 645	1 024 328	286 573	144 802	141 771	7 983	4 471	3 512
Salmonella infections (A01-A02)	15	8	7	3	1	2	-	-	-
Shigellosis and amebiasis (A03, A06)	6	3	3	-	-	-	-	-	-
Certain other intestinal infections (A04, A07-A09)	2 205	840	1 365	155	66	89	6	1	5
Tuberculosis (A16-A19)	366	218	148	198	123	75	7	6	1
Respiratory tuberculosis (A16)	296	177	119	160	101	59	5	5	
Other tuberculosis (A17-A19)	70	41	29	38	22	16	2	1	1
Whooping cough (A37)	12	3	9	2	1	1	-	-	-
Scarlet fever and erysipelas (A38, A46)	2	-	2	-	-	-	-	-	-
Meningococcal infection (A39)	106	58	48	29	12	17	-	-	-
Septicemia (A40-A41)	25 545	11 148	14 397	6 074	2 668	3 406	119	67	52
Syphilis (A50-A53)	16	8	8	23	12	11	1	-	1
Acute poliomyelitis (A80)	-	-	-	-	-	-	-	-	-
Arthropod-borne viral encephalitis (A83-A84, A85.2)	6	2	4	3	2	1	-	-	-
Measles (B05)	-	-	-	-	-	-	-	-	-
Viral hepatitis (B15-B19)	3 857	2 551	1 306	849	532	317	31	23	8
Human immunodeficiency virus (HIV) disease (B20-B24) ...	4 224	3 582	642	7 714	5 203	2 511	146	117	29
Malaria (B50-B54)	7	7	-	4	1	3	-	-	-
Other and unspecified infectious and parasitic diseases and their sequelae (A00, A05, A20-A36, A42-A44, A48-A49, A54-A79, A81-A82, A85.0-A85.1, A85.8, A86-B04, B06-B09, B25-B49, B55-B99)	4 939	2 608	2 331	927	516	411	17	9	8
Malignant neoplasms (C00-C97)	458 754	237 323	221 431	61 996	32 287	29 709	1 418	763	655
Malignant neoplasms of lip, oral cavity, and pharynx (C00-C14)	6 141	4 035	2 106	1 034	757	277	22	19	3
Malignant neoplasm of esophagus (C15)	10 484	8 169	2 315	1 572	1 118	454	36	29	7
Malignant neoplasm of stomach (C16)	8 124	4 864	3 260	2 112	1 184	928	39	24	15
Malignant neoplasms of colon, rectum, and anus (C18-C21)	46 147	23 119	23 028	6 817	3 322	3 495	133	74	59
Malignant neoplasms of liver and intrahepatic bile ducts (C22)	9 878	6 215	3 663	1 708	1 143	565	46	35	11
Malignant neoplasm of pancreas (C25)	24 647	12 242	12 405	3 466	1 606	1 860	62	29	33
Malignant neoplasm of larynx (C32)	2 838	2 205	633	674	541	133	10	8	2
Malignant neoplasms of trachea, bronchus, and lung (C33-C34)	134 435	75 754	58 681	16 170	9 983	6 187	383	219	164
Malignant melanoma of skin (C43)	7 190	4 555	2 635	102	52	50	18	8	10
Malignant neoplasm of breast (C50)	33 611	288	33 323	5 579	62	5 517	110	2	108
Malignant neoplasm of cervix uteri (C53)	2 580	X	2 580	820	X	820	13	X	13
Malignant neoplasms of corpus uteri and uterus, part unspecified (C54-C55)	5 213	X	5 213	1 107	X	1 107	29	X	29
Malignant neoplasm of ovary (C56)	12 560	X	12 560	1 155	X	1 155	29	X	29
Malignant neoplasm of prostate (C61)	23 690	23 690	X	5 085	5 085	X	86	86	X
Malignant neoplasms of kidney and renal pelvis (C64-C65)	10 179	6 363	3 816	1 062	626	436	29	20	9
Malignant neoplasm of bladder (C67)	11 109	7 649	3 460	931	475	456	30	17	13
Malignant neoplasms of meninges, brain, and other parts of central nervous system (C70-C72)	11 139	6 195	4 944	766	400	366	29	14	15
Malignant neoplasms of lymphoid, hematopoietic, and related tissue (C81-C96)	47 058	25 523	21 535	5 080	2 593	2 487	147	86	61
Hodgkin's disease (C81)	1 093	599	494	126	80	46	5	5	-
Non-Hodgkin's lymphoma (C82-C85)	18 901	9 961	8 940	1 446	767	679	62	36	26
Leukemia (C91-C95)	18 162	10 218	7 944	1 752	914	838	47	29	18
Multiple myeloma and immunoproliferative neoplasms (C88, C90)	8 843	4 708	4 135	1 750	830	920	33	16	17
Other and unspecified malignant neoplasms of lymphoid, hematopoietic, and related tissue (C96)	59	37	22	6	2	4	-	-	-
All other and unspecified malignant neoplasms (C17, C23-C24, C26-C31, C37-C41, C44-C49, C51-C52, C57-C60, C62-C63, C66, C68-C69, C73-C80, C97)	51 731	26 457	25 274	6 756	3 340	3 416	167	93	74
In situ neoplasms, benign neoplasms, and neoplasms of uncertain or unknown behavior (D00-D48)	11 332	5 607	5 725	1 134	496	638	28	17	11
Anemias (D50-D64)	3 253	1 164	2 089	1 048	472	576	15	4	11
Diabetes mellitus (E10-E14)	52 463	25 273	27 190	12 583	5 158	7 425	225	123	102
Nutritional deficiencies (E40-E64)	3 064	1 039	2 025	495	185	310	17	5	12
Malnutrition (E40-E46)	2 836	970	1 866	465	172	293	16	4	12
Other nutritional deficiencies (E50-E64)	228	69	159	30	13	17	1	1	-
Meningitis (G00, G03)	427	227	200	175	105	70	5	3	2
Parkinson's disease (G20-G21)	15 626	8 838	6 788	547	306	241	33	22	11
Alzheimer's disease (G30)	53 486	15 399	38 087	3 303	940	2 363	146	34	112

[1]Based on codes from the *International Classification of Diseases, Tenth Revision* (1992), except in cases where (*) precedes the cause of death code. Codes *U01-*U03 were added as of 2001 for deaths due to terrorism.
[4]Includes deaths for which Hispanic origin was not reported on the death certificate.
- = Quantity zero.
X = Not applicable.

Table II-13. Number of Deaths from 113 Selected Causes, by Race, Hispanic Origin, and Sex, 2002
—*Continued*

(Number.)

Cause of death [1]	All origins			Hispanic [2]			Non-Hispanic [3]		
	Both sexes	Male	Female	Both sexes	Male	Female	Both sexes	Male	Female
Major cardiovascular diseases (I00-I78)	918 628	429 682	488 946	36 543	18 824	17 719	879 170	409 343	469 827
Diseases of heart (I00-I09, I11, I13, I20-I51)	696 947	340 933	356 014	27 887	14 798	13 089	666 690	324 848	341 842
Acute rheumatic fever and chronic rheumatic heart diseases (I00-I09)	3 579	1 078	2 501	198	55	143	3 375	1 021	2 354
Hypertensive heart disease (I11)	26 551	11 660	14 891	1 424	781	643	24 976	10 790	14 186
Hypertensive heart and renal disease (I13)	2 895	1 205	1 690	172	80	92	2 714	1 120	1 594
Ischemic heart diseases (I20-I25)	494 382	252 760	241 622	20 941	11 295	9 646	471 655	240 462	231 193
Acute myocardial infarction (I21-I22)	179 514	93 830	85 684	7 631	4 125	3 506	171 441	89 480	81 961
Other acute ischemic heart diseases (I24)	3 407	1 767	1 640	64	40	24	3 339	1 725	1 614
Other forms of chronic ischemic heart disease (I20, I25)	311 461	157 163	154 298	13 246	7 130	6 116	296 875	149 257	147 618
Atherosclerotic cardiovascular disease, so described (I25.0)	68 129	36 047	32 082	3 166	1 946	1 220	64 528	33 809	30 719
All other forms of chronic ischemic heart disease (I20, I25.1-I25.9)	243 332	121 116	122 216	10 080	5 184	4 896	232 347	115 448	116 899
Other heart diseases (I26-I51)	169 540	74 230	95 310	5 152	2 587	2 565	163 970	71 455	92 515
Acute and subacute endocarditis (I33)	1 154	643	511	69	45	24	1 082	596	486
Diseases of pericardium and acute myocarditis (I30-I31, I40)	848	434	414	64	35	29	783	398	385
Heart failure (I50)	56 494	21 698	34 796	1 412	593	819	54 932	21 050	33 882
All other forms of heart disease (I26-I28, I34-I38, I42-I49, I51)	111 044	51 455	59 589	3 607	1 914	1 693	107 173	49 411	57 762
Essential (primary) hypertension and hypertensive renal disease (I10, I12)	20 261	7 647	12 614	942	385	557	19 254	7 232	12 022
Cerebrovascular diseases (I60-I69)	162 672	62 622	100 050	6 451	3 003	3 448	155 852	59 470	96 382
Atherosclerosis (I70)	13 821	5 171	8 650	416	175	241	13 369	4 984	8 385
Other diseases of circulatory system (I71-I78)	24 927	13 309	11 618	847	463	384	24 005	12 809	11 196
Aortic aneurysm and dissection (I71)	14 818	9 013	5 805	431	284	147	14 341	8 701	5 640
Other diseases of arteries, arterioles, and capillaries (I72-I78)	10 109	4 296	5 813	416	179	237	9 664	4 108	5 556
Other disorders of circulatory system (I80-I99)	4 711	1 944	2 767	219	95	124	4 479	1 842	2 637
Influenza and pneumonia (J10-J18)	65 681	28 918	36 763	2 824	1 398	1 426	62 657	27 417	35 240
Influenza (J10-J11) [5]	727	289	438	19	10	9	704	277	427
Pneumonia (J12-J18)	64 954	28 629	36 325	2 805	1 388	1 417	61 953	27 140	34 813
Other acute lower respiratory infections (J20-J22)	386	154	232	21	9	12	365	145	220
Acute bronchitis and bronchiolitis (J20-J21)	279	122	157	19	9	10	260	113	147
Unspecified acute lower respiratory infection (J22)	107	32	75	2	-	2	105	32	73
Chronic lower respiratory diseases (J40-J47)	124 816	60 713	64 103	3 058	1 625	1 433	121 424	58 896	62 528
Bronchitis, chronic and unspecified (J40-J42)	955	420	535	51	20	31	900	398	502
Emphysema (J43)	15 489	8 084	7 405	295	168	127	15 161	7 895	7 266
Asthma (J45-J46)	4 261	1 580	2 681	287	114	173	3 950	1 448	2 502
Other chronic lower respiratory diseases (J44, J47)	104 111	50 629	53 482	2 425	1 323	1 102	101 413	49 155	52 258
Pneumoconioses and chemical effects (J60-J66, J68)	1 114	1 057	57	33	31	2	1 078	1 023	55
Pneumonitis due to solids and liquids (J69)	17 593	8 876	8 717	547	282	265	17 006	8 565	8 441
Other diseases of respiratory system (J00-J06, J30-J39, J67, J70-J98)	25 039	12 057	12 982	1 273	635	638	23 706	11 397	12 309
Peptic ulcer (K25-K28)	4 079	1 951	2 128	187	115	72	3 879	1 829	2 050
Diseases of appendix (K35-K38)	480	275	205	28	16	12	451	258	193
Hernia (K40-K46)	1 595	599	996	81	35	46	1 504	558	946
Chronic liver disease and cirrhosis (K70, K73-K74)	27 257	17 401	9 856	3 409	2 437	972	23 733	14 876	8 857
Alcoholic liver disease (K70)	12 121	8 814	3 307	1 679	1 418	261	10 377	7 342	3 035
Other chronic liver disease and cirrhosis (K73-K74)	15 136	8 587	6 549	1 730	1 019	711	13 356	7 534	5 822
Cholelithiasis and other disorders of gallbladder (K80-K82)	2 979	1 341	1 638	196	93	103	2 776	1 244	1 532
Nephritis, nephrotic syndrome, and nephrosis (N00-N07, N17-N19, N25-N27)	40 974	19 695	21 279	1 898	937	961	38 933	18 682	20 251
Acute and rapidly progressive nephritic and nephrotic syndrome (N00-N01, N04)	166	70	96	10	4	6	155	66	89
Chronic glomerulonephritis, nephritis, and nephropathy, not specified as acute or chronic, and renal sclerosis, unspecified (N02-N03, N05-N07, N26)	553	278	275	32	15	17	520	263	257
Renal failure (N17-N19)	40 222	19 341	20 881	1 856	918	938	38 225	18 347	19 878
Other disorders of kidney (N25, N27)	33	6	27	-	-	-	33	6	27
Infections of kidney (N10-N12, N13.6, N15.1)	788	251	537	47	19	28	740	232	508
Hyperplasia of prostate (N40)	437	437	X	14	14	X	417	417	X
Inflammatory diseases of female pelvic organs (N70-N76)	114	X	114	3	X	3	110	X	110
Pregnancy, childbirth, and the puerperium (O00-O99)	379	X	379	70	X	70	305	X	305
Pregnancy with abortive outcome (O00-O07)	22	X	22	1	X	1	20	X	20
Other complications of pregnancy, childbirth, and the puerperium (O10-O99)	357	X	357	69	X	69	285	X	285
Certain conditions originating in the perinatal period (P00-P96)	14 254	8 047	6 207	2 402	1 352	1 050	11 673	6 596	5 077
Congenital malformations, deformations, and chromosomal abnormalities (Q00-Q99)	10 687	5 515	5 172	1 715	903	812	8 904	4 577	4 327
Symptoms, signs, and abnormal clinical and laboratory findings, not elsewhere classified (R00-R99)	29 975	14 269	15 706	1 548	926	622	28 211	13 206	15 005
All other diseases (residual)	194 591	79 007	115 584	8 377	4 221	4 156	185 608	74 500	111 108

[1]Based on codes from the *International Classification of Diseases, Tenth Revision* (1992), except in cases where (*) precedes the cause of death code. Codes *U01-*U03 were added as of 2001 for deaths due to terrorism.
[2]May be of any race.
[3]Includes races other than White and Black.
[5]Cause of death coding changes may affect comparability with the previous year's data for this cause.
- = Quantity zero.
X = Not applicable.

Table II-13. Number of Deaths from 113 Selected Causes, by Race, Hispanic Origin, and Sex, 2002 —Continued

(Number.)

Cause of death [1]	Non-Hispanic White			Non-Hispanic Black			Origin not stated [4]		
	Both sexes	Male	Female	Both sexes	Male	Female	Both sexes	Male	Female
Major cardiovascular diseases (I00-I78)	758 738	352 520	406 218	103 054	47 656	55 398	2 915	1 515	1 400
Diseases of heart (I00-I09, I11, I13, I20-I51)	577 761	281 442	296 319	76 694	36 596	40 098	2 370	1 287	1 083
Acute rheumatic fever and chronic rheumatic heart diseases (I00-I09)	3 007	897	2 110	249	91	158	6	2	4
Hypertensive heart disease (I11)	18 060	7 427	10 633	6 385	3 089	3 296	151	89	62
Hypertensive heart and renal disease (I13)	1 752	679	1 073	897	402	495	9	5	4
Ischemic heart diseases (I20-I25)	413 230	211 391	201 839	49 522	23 976	25 546	1 786	1 003	783
Acute myocardial infarction (I21-I22)	150 051	79 037	71 014	18 162	8 607	9 555	442	225	217
Other acute ischemic heart diseases (I24)	2 843	1 454	1 389	443	242	201	4	2	2
Other forms of chronic ischemic heart disease (I20, I25)	260 336	130 900	129 436	30 917	15 127	15 790	1 340	776	564
Atherosclerotic cardiovascular disease, so described (I25.0)	53 161	27 493	25 668	10 024	5 483	4 541	435	292	143
All other forms of chronic ischemic heart disease (I20, I25.1-I25.9)	207 175	103 407	103 768	20 893	9 644	11 249	905	484	421
Other heart diseases (I26-I51)	141 712	61 048	80 664	19 641	9 038	10 603	418	188	230
Acute and subacute endocarditis (I33)	862	481	381	197	104	93	3	2	1
Diseases of pericardium and acute myocarditis (I30-I31, I40)	601	308	293	154	75	79	1	1	-
Heart failure (I50)	49 162	18 705	30 457	5 143	2 055	3 088	150	55	95
All other forms of heart disease (I26-I28, I34-I38, I42-I49, I51)	91 087	41 554	49 533	14 147	6 804	7 343	264	130	134
Essential (primary) hypertension and hypertensive renal disease (I10, I12)	14 617	5 325	9 292	4 165	1 701	2 464	65	30	35
Cerebrovascular diseases (I60-I69)	133 118	49 908	83 210	18 691	7 754	10 937	369	149	220
Atherosclerosis (I70)	12 191	4 508	7 683	1 009	409	600	36	12	24
Other diseases of circulatory system (I71-I78)	21 051	11 337	9 714	2 495	1 196	1 299	75	37	38
Aortic aneurysm and dissection (I71)	12 831	7 834	4 997	1 200	664	536	46	28	18
Other diseases of arteries, arterioles, and capillaries (I72-I78)	8 220	3 503	4 717	1 295	532	763	29	9	20
Other disorders of circulatory system (I80-I99)	3 630	1 450	2 180	789	359	430	13	7	6
Influenza and pneumonia (J10-J18)	55 419	23 934	31 485	5 803	2 734	3 069	200	103	97
Influenza (J10-J11) [5]	663	258	405	30	15	15	4	2	2
Pneumonia (J12-J18)	54 756	23 676	31 080	5 773	2 719	3 054	196	101	95
Other acute lower respiratory infections (J20-J22)	314	122	192	44	22	22	-	-	-
Acute bronchitis and bronchiolitis (J20-J21)	219	92	127	35	20	15	-	-	-
Unspecified acute lower respiratory infection (J22)	95	30	65	9	2	7	-	-	-
Chronic lower respiratory diseases (J40-J47)	112 128	53 662	58 466	7 730	4 282	3 448	334	192	142
Bronchitis, chronic and unspecified (J40-J42)	821	354	467	66	35	31	4	2	2
Emphysema (J43)	14 157	7 241	6 916	842	538	304	33	21	12
Asthma (J45-J46)	2 720	895	1 825	1 083	488	595	24	18	6
Other chronic lower respiratory diseases (J44, J47)	94 430	45 172	49 258	5 739	3 221	2 518	273	151	122
Pneumoconioses and chemical effects (J60-J66, J68)	1 014	966	48	56	50	6	3	3	-
Pneumonitis due to solids and liquids (J69)	15 203	7 654	7 549	1 528	755	773	40	29	11
Other diseases of respiratory system (J00-J06, J30-J39, J67, J70-J98)	20 879	10 043	10 836	2 257	1 076	1 181	60	25	35
Peptic ulcer (K25-K28)	3 394	1 569	1 825	376	209	167	13	7	6
Diseases of appendix (K35-K38)	377	210	167	61	40	21	1	1	-
Hernia (K40-K46)	1 343	493	850	137	56	81	10	6	4
Chronic liver disease and cirrhosis (K70, K73-K74)	20 353	12 800	7 553	2 545	1 592	953	115	88	27
Alcoholic liver disease (K70)	8 713	6 242	2 471	1 173	783	390	65	54	11
Other chronic liver disease and cirrhosis (K73-K74)	11 640	6 558	5 082	1 372	809	563	50	34	16
Cholelithiasis and other disorders of gallbladder (K80-K82)	2 420	1 087	1 333	266	106	160	7	4	3
Nephritis, nephrotic syndrome, and nephrosis (N00-N07, N17-N19, N25-N27)	30 669	14 883	15 786	7 410	3 389	4 021	143	76	67
Acute and rapidly progressive nephritic and nephrotic syndrome (N00-N01, N04)	119	52	67	29	11	18	1	-	1
Chronic glomerulonephritis, nephritis, and nephropathy, not specified as acute or chronic, and renal sclerosis, unspecified (N02-N03, N05-N07, N26)	419	218	201	80	37	43	1	-	1
Renal failure (N17-N19)	30 104	14 610	15 494	7 297	3 339	3 958	141	76	65
Other disorders of kidney (N25, N27)	27	3	24	4	2	2	-	-	-
Infections of kidney (N10-N12, N13.6, N15.1)	645	200	445	73	22	51	1	-	1
Hyperplasia of prostate (N40)	370	370	X	38	38	X	6	6	X
Inflammatory diseases of female pelvic organs (N70-N76)	88	X	88	20	X	20	1	X	1
Pregnancy, childbirth, and the puerperium (O00-O99)	133	X	133	153	X	153	4	X	4
Pregnancy with abortive outcome (O00-O07)	6	X	6	11	X	11	1	X	1
Other complications of pregnancy, childbirth, and the puerperium (O10-O99)	127	X	127	142	X	142	3	X	3
Certain conditions originating in the perinatal period (P00-P96)	6 384	3 663	2 721	4 777	2 640	2 137	179	99	80
Congenital malformations, deformations, and chromosomal abnormalities (Q00-Q99)	6 830	3 510	3 320	1 716	887	829	68	35	33
Symptoms, signs, and abnormal clinical and laboratory findings, not elsewhere classified (R00-R99)	23 099	10 432	12 667	4 556	2 482	2 074	216	137	79
All other diseases (residual)	159 945	63 109	96 836	22 297	9 722	12 575	606	286	320

[1] Based on codes from the *International Classification of Diseases, Tenth Revision* (1992), except in cases where (*) precedes the cause of death code. Codes *U01-*U03 were added as of 2001 for deaths due to terrorism.
[4] Includes deaths for which Hispanic origin was not reported on the death certificate.
[5] Cause of death coding changes may affect comparability with the previous year's data for this cause.
- = Quantity zero.
X = Not applicable.

Table II-13. Number of Deaths from 113 Selected Causes, by Race, Hispanic Origin, and Sex, 2002
—Continued

(Number.)

Cause of death [1]	All origins			Hispanic [2]			Non-Hispanic [3]		
	Both sexes	Male	Female	Both sexes	Male	Female	Both sexes	Male	Female
Accidents (unintentional injuries) (V01-X59, Y85-Y86)	106 742	69 257	37 485	10 106	7 698	2 408	96 175	61 201	34 974
Transport accidents (V01-V99, Y85)	48 366	33 533	14 833	5 921	4 481	1 440	42 268	28 906	13 362
Motor vehicle accidents (V02-V04, V09.0, V09.2, V12-V14, V19.0-V19.2, V19.4-V19.6, V20-V79, V80.3-80.5, V81.0-V81.1, V82.0-V82.1, V83-V86, V87.0-V87.8, V88.0-V88.8, V89.0, V89.2)	45 380	31 064	14 316	5 659	4 262	1 397	39 567	26 677	12 890
Other land transport accidents (V01, V05-V06, V09.1, V09.3-V09.9, V10-V11, V15-V18, V19.3, V19.8-V19.9, V80.0-V80.2, V80.6-V80.9, V81.2-V81.9, V82.2-V82.9, V87.9, V88.9, V89.1, V89.3, V89.9)	1 086	882	204	144	119	25	929	752	177
Water, air and space, and other and unspecified transport accidents and their sequelae (V90-V99, Y85)	1 900	1 587	313	118	100	18	1 772	1 477	295
Nontransport accidents (W00-X59, Y86)	58 376	35 724	22 652	4 185	3 217	968	53 907	32 295	21 612
Falls (W00-W19)	16 257	8 463	7 794	832	563	269	15 365	7 856	7 509
Accidental discharge of firearms (W32-W34)	762	667	95	60	51	9	700	614	86
Accidental drowning and submersion (W65-W74)	3 447	2 761	686	464	409	55	2 952	2 326	626
Accidental exposure to smoke, fire, and flames (X00-X09)	3 159	1 935	1 224	223	144	79	2 918	1 780	1 138
Accidental poisoning and exposure to noxious substances (X40-X49)	17 550	12 059	5 491	1 652	1 324	328	15 789	10 649	5 140
Other and unspecified nontransport accidents and their sequelae (W20-W31, W35-W64, W75-W99, X10-X39, X50-X59, Y86)	17 201	9 839	7 362	954	726	228	16 183	9 070	7 113
Intentional self-harm (suicide) (*U03, X60-X84, Y87.0)	31 655	25 409	6 246	1 954	1 651	303	29 543	23 623	5 920
Intentional self-harm (suicide) by discharge of firearms (X72-X74)	17 108	15 045	2 063	834	763	71	16 213	14 226	1 987
Intentional self-harm (suicide) by other and unspecified means and their sequelae (*U03, X60-X71, X75-X84, Y87.0)	14 547	10 364	4 183	1 120	888	232	13 330	9 397	3 933
Assault (homicide) (*U01-*U02, X85-Y09, Y87.1)	17 638	13 640	3 998	3 129	2 635	494	14 346	10 881	3 465
Assault (homicide) by discharge of firearms (*U01.4, X93-X95)	11 829	9 899	1 930	2 168	1 942	226	9 575	7 884	1 691
Assault (homicide) by other and unspecified means and their sequelae (*U01.0-*U01.3, *U01.5-*U01.9, *U02, X85-X92, X96-Y09, Y87.1)	5 809	3 741	2 068	961	693	268	4 771	2 997	1 774
Legal intervention (Y35, Y89.0)	384	369	15	68	67	1	315	301	14
Events of undetermined intent (Y10-Y34, Y87.2, Y89.9)	4 830	3 114	1 716	320	242	78	4 470	2 836	1 634
Discharge of firearms, undetermined intent (Y22-Y24)	243	199	44	23	21	2	215	173	42
Other and unspecified events of undetermined intent and their sequelae (Y10-Y21, Y25-Y34, Y87.2, Y89.9)	4 587	2 915	1 672	297	221	76	4 255	2 663	1 592
Operations of war and their sequelae (Y36, Y89.1)	20	20	-	1	1	-	19	19	-
Complications of medical and surgical care (Y40-Y84, Y88)	2 843	1 236	1 607	137	57	80	2 695	1 175	1 520

[1]Based on codes from the *International Classification of Diseases, Tenth Revision* (1992), except in cases where (*) precedes the cause of death code. Codes *U01-*U03 were added as of 2001 for deaths due to terrorism.
[2]May be of any race.
[3]Includes races other than White and Black.
- = Quantity zero.

Table II-13. Number of Deaths from 113 Selected Causes, by Race, Hispanic Origin, and Sex, 2002
　—Continued

(Number.)

Cause of death [1]	Non-Hispanic White			Non-Hispanic Black			Origin not stated [4]		
	Both sexes	Male	Female	Both sexes	Male	Female	Both sexes	Male	Female
Accidents (unintentional injuries) (V01-X59, Y85-Y86)	80 605	50 652	29 953	12 285	8 428	3 857	461	358	103
Transport accidents (V01-V99, Y85)	34 689	23 628	11 061	5 665	4 051	1 614	177	146	31
Motor vehicle accidents (V02-V04, V09.0, V09.2, V12-V14, V19.0-V19.2, V19.4-V19.6, V20-V79, V80.3-80.5, V81.0-V81.1, V82.0-V82.1, V83-V86, V87.0-V87.8, V88.0-V88.8, V89.0, V89.2)	32 405	21 743	10 662	5 338	3 774	1 564	154	125	29
Other land transport accidents (V01, V05-V06, V09.1, V09.3-V09.9, V10-V11, V15-V18, V19.3, V19.8-V19.9, V80.0-V80.2, V80.6-V80.9, V81.2-V81.9, V82.2-V82.9, V87.9, V88.9, V89.1, V89.3, V89.9)	719	582	137	168	143	25	13	11	2
Water, air and space, and other and unspecified transport accidents and their sequelae (V90-V99, Y85)	1 565	1 303	262	159	134	25	10	10	-
Nontransport accidents (W00-X59, Y86)	45 916	27 024	18 892	6 620	4 377	2 243	284	212	72
Falls (W00-W19)	14 157	7 107	7 050	821	518	303	60	44	16
Accidental discharge of firearms (W32-W34)	531	459	72	153	140	13	2	2	-
Accidental drowning and submersion (W65-W74)	2 143	1 669	474	604	502	102	31	26	5
Accidental exposure to smoke, fire, and flames (X00-X09)	2 055	1 271	784	765	454	311	18	11	7
Accidental poisoning and exposure to noxious substances (X40-X49)	13 165	8 849	4 316	2 326	1 601	725	109	86	23
Other and unspecified nontransport accidents and their sequelae (W20-W31, W35-W64, W75-W99, X10-X39, X50-X59, Y86)	13 865	7 669	6 196	1 951	1 162	789	64	43	21
Intentional self-harm (suicide) (*U03, X60-X84, Y87.0)	26 691	21 323	5 368	1 896	1 595	301	158	135	23
Intentional self-harm (suicide) by discharge of firearms (X72-X74)	14 865	13 014	1 851	1 041	945	96	61	56	5
Intentional self-harm (suicide) by other and unspecified means and their sequelae (*U03, X60-X71, X75-X84, Y87.0)	11 826	8 309	3 517	855	650	205	97	79	18
Assault (homicide) (*U01-*U02, X85-Y09, Y87.1)	5 571	3 661	1 910	8 147	6 780	1 367	163	124	39
Assault (homicide) by discharge of firearms (*U01.4, X93-X95)	3 052	2 139	913	6 181	5 482	699	86	73	13
Assault (homicide) by other and unspecified means and their sequelae (*U01.0-*U01.3, *U01.5-*U01.9, *U02, X85-X92, X96-Y09, Y87.1)	2 519	1 522	997	1 966	1 298	668	77	51	26
Legal intervention (Y35, Y89.0)	191	181	10	109	105	4	1	1	-
Events of undetermined intent (Y10-Y34, Y87.2, Y89.9)	3 627	2 265	1 362	738	504	234	40	36	4
Discharge of firearms, undetermined intent (Y22-Y24)	169	132	37	37	35	2	5	5	-
Other and unspecified events of undetermined intent and their sequelae (Y10-Y21, Y25-Y34, Y87.2, Y89.9)	3 458	2 133	1 325	701	469	232	35	31	4
Operations of war and their sequelae (Y36, Y89.1)	14	14	-	5	5	-	-	-	-
Complications of medical and surgical care (Y40-Y84, Y88)	2 188	966	1 222	445	182	263	11	4	7

[1]Based on codes from the *International Classification of Diseases, Tenth Revision* (1992), except in cases where (*) precedes the cause of death code. Codes *U01-*U03 were added as of 2001 for deaths due to terrorism.
[4]Includes deaths for which Hispanic origin was not reported on the death certificate.
- = Quantity zero.

TABLE II-14. DEATH RATES FOR 113 SELECTED CAUSES, BY RACE AND SEX, 2002

Crude death rates can be utilized to characterize actual measures of mortality risk. However, due to differences in age distribution between sexes and races, age-adjusted death rates (see Table II-16) should be used to compare relative risk among different groups. An example of the influence of age on crude rates is that the death rates from major cardiovascular diseases in 2002 were higher for women, even though the age-adjusted rates for the same diseases were considerably higher for men.

Table II-14. Death Rates for 113 Selected Causes, by Race and Sex, 2002

(Rate per 100,000 population.)

Cause of death [1]	All races			White			All other					
							Total			Black		
	Both sexes	Male	Female	Both sexes	Male	Female	Both sexes	Male	Female	Both sexes	Male	Female
ALL CAUSES	847.3	846.6	848.0	895.7	884.0	907.0	635.6	677.5	597.0	768.4	816.7	724.4
Salmonella infections (A01-A02)	0.0	*	*	*	*	*	*	*	*	*	*	*
Shigellosis and amebiasis (A03, A06)	*	*	*	*	*	*	*	*	*	*	*	*
Certain other intestinal infections (A04, A07-A09)	0.9	0.7	1.0	1.0	0.8	1.2	0.3	0.3	0.4	0.4	0.4	0.5
Tuberculosis (A16-A19)	0.3	0.3	0.2	0.2	0.2	0.2	0.6	0.7	0.5	0.5	0.7	0.4
Respiratory tuberculosis (A16)	0.2	0.3	0.2	0.2	0.2	0.1	0.5	0.6	0.4	0.4	0.6	0.3
Other tuberculosis (A17-A19)	0.1	0.1	0.0	0.0	0.0	0.0	0.1	0.2	0.1	0.1	0.1	*
Whooping cough (A37)	*	*	*	*	*	*	*	*	*	*	*	*
Scarlet fever and erysipelas (A38, A46)	*	*	*	*	*	*	*	*	*	*	*	*
Meningococcal infection (A39)	0.1	0.1	0.1	0.1	0.1	0.0	0.1	*	0.1	0.1	*	*
Septicemia (A40-A41)	11.7	10.6	12.9	11.5	10.3	12.8	12.6	11.8	13.3	16.3	15.0	17.4
Syphilis (A50-A53)	0.0	0.0	0.0	*	*	*	0.0	*	*	0.1	*	*
Acute poliomyelitis (A80)	*	*	*	*	*	*	*	*	*	*	*	*
Arthropod-borne viral encephalitis (A83-A84, A85.2)	*	*	*	*	*	*	*	*	*	*	*	*
Measles (B05)	*	*	*	*	*	*	*	*	*	*	*	*
Viral hepatitis (B15-B19)	2.0	2.7	1.4	2.0	2.6	1.3	2.2	2.8	1.6	2.3	3.0	1.6
Human immunodeficiency virus (HIV) disease (B20-B24)	4.9	7.4	2.5	2.6	4.3	0.9	14.9	21.2	9.2	20.8	29.5	12.8
Malaria (B50-B54)	*	*	*	*	*	*	*	*	*	*	*	*
Other and unspecified infectious and parasitic diseases and their sequelae (A00, A05, A20-A36, A42-A44, A48-A49, A54-A79, A81-A82, A85.0-A85.1, A85.8, A86-B04, B06-B09, B25-B49, B55-B99)	2.3	2.6	2.1	2.4	2.6	2.2	2.2	2.5	1.9	2.5	2.9	2.1
Malignant neoplasms (C00-C97)	193.2	203.8	183.0	205.5	215.5	195.8	139.5	151.4	128.5	165.9	181.5	151.7
Malignant neoplasms of lip, oral cavity, and pharynx (C00-C14)	2.7	3.7	1.7	2.7	3.7	1.8	2.4	3.6	1.3	2.8	4.3	1.4
Malignant neoplasm of esophagus (C15)	4.4	6.9	2.0	4.6	7.3	2.0	3.3	5.0	1.8	4.2	6.3	2.3
Malignant neoplasm of stomach (C16)	4.2	5.0	3.5	4.0	4.8	3.2	5.4	6.2	4.6	5.6	6.6	4.7
Malignant neoplasms of colon, rectum, and anus (C18-C21)	19.7	20.1	19.2	20.7	21.1	20.3	15.3	15.8	14.7	18.2	18.6	17.8
Malignant neoplasms of liver and intrahepatic bile ducts (C22)	4.9	6.4	3.4	4.8	6.1	3.5	5.2	7.4	3.2	4.6	6.5	2.9
Malignant neoplasm of pancreas (C25)	10.5	10.5	10.5	11.1	11.1	11.0	7.9	7.6	8.2	9.3	9.0	9.5
Malignant neoplasm of larynx (C32)	1.3	2.1	0.5	1.3	2.0	0.6	1.3	2.2	0.5	1.8	3.0	0.7
Malignant neoplasms of trachea, bronchus, and lung (C33-C34)	54.7	63.7	46.0	59.1	67.7	50.7	35.5	45.6	26.3	43.2	56.0	31.6
Malignant melanoma of skin (C43)	2.6	3.3	1.9	3.1	4.0	2.3	0.3	0.3	0.3	0.3	0.3	0.3
Malignant neoplasm of breast (C50)	14.5	0.3	28.3	15.1	0.3	29.5	12.1	0.3	23.0	14.9	0.4	28.2
Malignant neoplasm of cervix uteri (C53)	1.4	X	2.7	1.3	X	2.5	1.8	X	3.5	2.2	X	4.2
Malignant neoplasms of corpus uteri and uterus, part unspecified (C54-C55)	2.4	X	4.7	2.4	X	4.7	2.4	X	4.6	3.0	X	5.7
Malignant neoplasm of ovary (C56)	5.1	X	10.0	5.6	X	11.1	2.8	X	5.3	3.1	X	5.9
Malignant neoplasm of prostate (C61)	10.6	21.5	X	10.6	21.5	X	10.3	21.5	X	13.6	28.6	X
Malignant neoplasms of kidney and renal pelvis (C64-C65)	4.2	5.4	3.1	4.6	5.9	3.4	2.4	3.1	1.9	2.8	3.5	2.2
Malignant neoplasm of bladder (C67)	4.4	6.0	2.8	4.9	6.8	3.0	2.1	2.3	1.9	2.5	2.7	2.3
Malignant neoplasms of meninges, brain, and other parts of central nervous system (C70-C72)	4.4	5.0	3.9	5.0	5.7	4.4	1.9	2.2	1.7	2.1	2.3	1.9
Malignant neoplasms of lymphoid, hematopoietic, and related tissue (C81-C96)	19.5	21.4	17.7	21.3	23.4	19.2	11.7	12.5	11.0	13.6	14.6	12.8
Hodgkin's disease (C81)	0.5	0.5	0.4	0.5	0.6	0.5	0.3	0.4	0.2	0.3	0.5	0.2
Non-Hodgkin's lymphoma (C82-C85)	7.6	8.1	7.1	8.5	9.1	8.0	3.6	3.9	3.3	3.9	4.3	3.5
Leukemia (C91-C95)	7.5	8.5	6.5	8.2	9.3	7.1	4.1	4.6	3.7	4.7	5.1	4.3
Multiple myeloma and immunoproliferative neoplasms (C88, C90)	4.0	4.2	3.7	4.0	4.3	3.7	3.7	3.6	3.7	4.7	4.7	4.7
Other and unspecified malignant neoplasms of lymphoid, hematopoietic, and related tissue (C96)	0.0	0.0	0.0	0.0	0.0	0.0	*	*	*	*	*	*
All other and unspecified malignant neoplasms (C17, C23-C24, C26-C31, C37-C41, C44-C49, C51-C52, C57-C60, C62-C63, C66, C68-C69, C73-C80, C97)	21.8	22.7	21.0	23.3	24.2	22.5	15.2	15.8	14.7	18.1	18.8	17.4
In situ neoplasms, benign neoplasms, and neoplasms of uncertain or unknown behavior (D00-D48)	4.6	4.6	4.6	5.1	5.1	5.1	2.6	2.5	2.7	3.0	2.8	3.3
Anemias (D50-D64)	1.6	1.3	1.9	1.5	1.1	1.8	2.2	2.0	2.3	2.8	2.7	3.0
Diabetes mellitus (E10-E14)	25.4	24.2	26.5	24.9	24.2	25.6	27.6	24.1	30.8	33.6	29.0	37.8
Nutritional deficiencies (E40-E64)	1.3	0.9	1.7	1.4	1.0	1.8	1.1	0.9	1.2	1.3	1.0	1.6
Malnutrition (E40-E46)	1.2	0.9	1.6	1.3	0.9	1.6	1.0	0.8	1.2	1.3	1.0	1.5
Other nutritional deficiencies (E50-E64)	0.1	0.1	0.1	0.1	0.1	0.1	0.1	*	0.1	0.1	*	*
Meningitis (G00, G03)	0.2	0.3	0.2	0.2	0.2	0.2	0.4	0.5	0.3	0.5	0.6	0.4
Parkinson's disease (G20-G21)	5.9	6.8	5.0	6.9	7.9	5.9	1.5	1.8	1.3	1.5	1.7	1.2
Alzheimer's disease (G30)	20.4	12.0	28.5	23.5	13.7	33.0	7.1	4.3	9.6	8.9	5.3	12.0

[1]Based on codes from the *International Classification of Diseases, Tenth Revision* (1992), except in cases where (*) precedes the cause of death code. Codes *U01-*U03 were added as of 2001 for deaths due to terrorism.
0.0 = Quantity more than zero but less than 0.05.
* = Figure does not meet standards of reliability or precision.
X = Not applicable.

Table II-14. Death Rates for 113 Selected Causes, by Race and Sex, 2002—*Continued*

(Rate per 100,000 population.)

Cause of death [1]	All races Both sexes	All races Male	All races Female	White Both sexes	White Male	White Female	All other Total Both sexes	All other Total Male	All other Total Female	All other Black Both sexes	All other Black Male	All other Black Female
Major cardiovascular diseases (I00-I78)	318.6	303.3	333.3	339.4	320.9	357.5	227.3	224.1	230.2	276.1	268.5	283.0
Diseases of heart (I00-I09, I11, I13, I20-I51)	241.7	240.7	242.7	258.5	256.0	261.0	168.0	171.4	164.9	205.6	206.3	205.0
Acute rheumatic fever and chronic rheumatic heart diseases (I00-I09)	1.2	0.8	1.7	1.4	0.8	1.9	0.7	0.5	0.9	0.7	0.5	0.8
Hypertensive heart disease (I11)	9.2	8.2	10.2	8.3	7.1	9.5	13.1	13.3	12.9	17.2	17.5	16.9
Hypertensive heart and renal disease (I13)	1.0	0.9	1.2	0.8	0.7	1.0	1.8	1.7	1.9	2.4	2.3	2.5
Ischemic heart diseases (I20-I25)	171.4	178.4	164.7	185.4	192.5	178.4	110.4	114.8	106.4	132.9	135.3	130.8
Acute myocardial infarction (I21-I22)	62.3	66.2	58.4	67.3	71.8	62.8	40.3	41.0	39.6	48.5	48.3	48.8
Other acute ischemic heart diseases (I24)	1.2	1.2	1.1	1.2	1.3	1.2	0.9	1.1	0.8	1.2	1.4	1.0
Other forms of chronic ischemic heart disease (I20, I25)	108.0	110.9	105.2	116.9	119.4	114.4	69.2	72.7	66.0	83.2	85.7	81.0
Atherosclerotic cardiovascular disease, so described (I25.0)	23.6	25.4	21.9	24.1	25.5	22.7	21.6	25.1	18.3	27.0	31.1	23.3
All other forms of chronic ischemic heart disease (I20, I25.1-I25.9)	84.4	85.5	83.3	92.8	93.9	91.7	47.7	47.6	47.7	56.2	54.5	57.7
Other heart diseases (I26-I51)	58.8	52.4	65.0	62.6	54.9	70.2	41.9	41.0	42.8	52.5	50.8	54.0
Acute and subacute endocarditis (I33)	0.4	0.5	0.3	0.4	0.5	0.3	0.4	0.5	0.4	0.5	0.6	0.5
Diseases of pericardium and acute myocarditis (I30-I31, I40)	0.3	0.3	0.3	0.3	0.3	0.3	0.3	0.4	0.3	0.4	0.4	0.4
Heart failure (I50)	19.6	15.3	23.7	21.6	16.7	26.4	10.9	9.2	12.4	13.7	11.5	15.8
All other forms of heart disease (I26-I28, I34-I38, I42-I49, I51)	38.5	36.3	40.6	40.4	37.5	43.2	30.3	31.0	29.7	37.8	38.3	37.4
Essential (primary) hypertension and hypertensive renal disease (I10, I12)	7.0	5.4	8.6	6.6	4.9	8.3	8.7	7.5	9.8	11.1	9.6	12.5
Cerebrovascular diseases (I60-I69)	56.4	44.2	68.2	59.5	45.7	73.0	42.8	37.6	47.6	50.0	43.5	55.8
Atherosclerosis (I70)	4.8	3.7	5.9	5.4	4.0	6.7	2.2	1.9	2.5	2.7	2.3	3.1
Other diseases of circulatory system (I71-I78)	8.6	9.4	7.9	9.3	10.2	8.5	5.6	5.8	5.4	6.7	6.7	6.6
Aortic aneurysm and dissection (I71)	5.1	6.4	4.0	5.7	7.0	4.3	2.9	3.4	2.3	3.2	3.8	2.7
Other diseases of arteries, arterioles, and capillaries (I72-I78)	3.5	3.0	4.0	3.7	3.2	4.2	2.7	2.4	3.0	3.5	3.0	3.9
Other disorders of circulatory system (I80-I99)	1.6	1.4	1.9	1.6	1.3	1.9	1.6	1.6	1.6	2.1	2.0	2.2
Influenza and pneumonia (J10-J18)	22.8	20.4	25.1	24.9	21.9	27.8	13.7	13.8	13.6	15.6	15.4	15.7
Influenza (J10-J11) [2]	0.3	0.2	0.3	0.3	0.2	0.4	0.1	*	0.1	0.1	*	*
Pneumonia (J12-J18)	22.5	20.2	24.8	24.6	21.7	27.4	13.6	13.7	13.5	15.5	15.3	15.6
Other acute lower respiratory infections (J20-J22)	0.1	0.1	0.2	0.1	0.1	0.2	0.1	0.1	0.1	0.1	0.1	0.1
Acute bronchitis and bronchiolitis (J20-J21)	0.1	0.1	0.1	0.1	0.1	0.1	0.1	0.1	0.1	0.1	0.1	*
Unspecified acute lower respiratory infection (J22)	0.0	0.0	0.1	0.0	0.0	0.1	*	*	*	*	*	*
Chronic lower respiratory diseases (J40-J47)	43.3	42.9	43.7	49.2	47.8	50.5	17.6	20.6	14.7	20.7	24.1	17.7
Bronchitis, chronic and unspecified (J40-J42)	0.3	0.3	0.4	0.4	0.3	0.4	0.1	0.2	0.1	0.2	0.2	0.2
Emphysema (J43)	5.4	5.7	5.0	6.2	6.4	5.9	1.9	2.6	1.3	2.3	3.0	1.6
Asthma (J45-J46)	1.5	1.1	1.8	1.3	0.9	1.7	2.3	2.2	2.4	2.9	2.8	3.0
Other chronic lower respiratory diseases (J44, J47)	36.1	35.7	36.5	41.3	40.2	42.5	13.2	15.7	10.9	15.4	18.2	12.9
Pneumoconioses and chemical effects (J60-J66, J68)	0.4	0.7	0.0	0.4	0.9	0.0	0.1	0.2	*	0.2	0.3	*
Pneumonitis due to solids and liquids (J69)	6.1	6.3	5.9	6.7	6.9	6.6	3.4	3.6	3.2	4.1	4.2	3.9
Other diseases of respiratory system (J00-J06, J30-J39, J67, J70-J98)	8.7	8.5	8.8	9.5	9.2	9.7	5.3	5.3	5.3	6.0	6.0	6.0
Peptic ulcer (K25-K28)	1.4	1.4	1.5	1.5	1.5	1.6	0.9	1.0	0.8	1.0	1.2	0.8
Diseases of appendix (K35-K38)	0.2	0.2	0.1	0.2	0.2	0.2	0.1	0.2	0.1	0.2	0.2	0.1
Hernia (K40-K46)	0.6	0.4	0.7	0.6	0.5	0.8	0.3	0.3	0.3	0.4	0.3	0.4
Chronic liver disease and cirrhosis (K70, K73-K74)	9.5	12.3	6.7	10.1	13.2	7.2	6.4	8.3	4.7	6.9	9.0	4.9
Alcoholic liver disease (K70)	4.2	6.2	2.3	4.4	6.6	2.3	3.2	4.4	2.0	3.2	4.4	2.0
Other chronic liver disease and cirrhosis (K73-K74)	5.2	6.1	4.5	5.7	6.5	4.9	3.3	3.9	2.7	3.7	4.6	2.9
Cholelithiasis and other disorders of gallbladder (K80-K82)	1.0	0.9	1.1	1.1	1.0	1.2	0.7	0.6	0.7	0.7	0.6	0.8
Nephritis, nephrotic syndrome, and nephrosis (N00-N07, N17-N19, N25-N27)	14.2	13.9	14.5	13.9	13.7	14.1	15.6	15.0	16.2	19.8	19.1	20.5
Acute and rapidly progressive nephritic and nephrotic syndrome (N00-N01, N04)	0.1	0.0	0.1	0.1	0.0	0.1	0.1	*	0.1	0.1	*	*
Chronic glomerulonephritis, nephritis, and nephropathy, not specified as acute or chronic, and renal sclerosis, unspecified (N02-N03, N05-N07, N26)	0.2	0.2	0.2	0.2	0.2	0.2	0.2	0.2	0.2	0.2	0.2	0.2
Renal failure (N17-N19)	13.9	13.7	14.2	13.6	13.4	13.8	15.3	14.7	15.9	19.5	18.8	20.2
Other disorders of kidney (N25, N27)	0.0	*	0.0	0.0	*	0.0	*	*	*	*	*	*
Infections of kidney (N10-N12, N13.6, N15.1)	0.3	0.2	0.4	0.3	0.2	0.4	0.2	0.1	0.2	0.2	0.1	0.3
Hyperplasia of prostate (N40)	0.2	0.3	X	0.2	0.3	X	0.1	0.2	X	0.1	0.2	X
Inflammatory diseases of female pelvic organs (N70-N76)	0.0	X	0.1	0.0	X	0.1	0.0	X	0.1	0.1	X	0.1
Pregnancy, childbirth, and the puerperium (O00-O99)	0.1	X	0.3	0.1	X	0.2	0.3	X	0.6	0.4	X	0.8
Pregnancy with abortive outcome (O00-O07)	0.0	X	0.0	*	X	*	*	X	*	*	X	*
Other complications of pregnancy, childbirth, and the puerperium (O10-O99)	0.1	X	0.2	0.1	X	0.2	0.3	X	0.6	0.4	X	0.7
Certain conditions originating in the perinatal period (P00-P96)	4.9	5.7	4.2	3.7	4.3	3.2	10.2	11.8	8.7	13.1	15.2	11.2
Congenital malformations, deformations, and chromosomal abnormalities (Q00-Q99)	3.7	3.9	3.5	3.6	3.8	3.5	4.0	4.3	3.7	4.7	5.1	4.3
Symptoms, signs, and abnormal clinical and laboratory findings, not elsewhere classified (R00-R99)	10.4	10.1	10.7	10.5	9.8	11.2	9.7	11.1	8.5	12.3	14.1	10.6
All other diseases (residual)	67.5	55.8	78.8	71.8	58.2	85.2	48.4	45.0	51.6	59.7	54.8	64.1

[1]Based on codes from the *International Classification of Diseases, Tenth Revision* (1992), except in cases where (*) precedes the cause of death code. Codes *U01-*U03 were added as of 2001 for deaths due to terrorism.
[2]Cause of death coding changes may affect comparability with the previous year's data for this cause.
0.0 = Quantity more than zero but less than 0.05.
* = Figure does not meet standards of reliability or precision.
X = Not applicable.

Table II-14. Death Rates for 113 Selected Causes, by Race and Sex, 2002—*Continued*

(Rate per 100,000 population.)

Cause of death [1]	All races			White			All other Total			All other Black		
	Both sexes	Male	Female	Both sexes	Male	Female	Both sexes	Male	Female	Both sexes	Male	Female
Accidents (unintentional injuries) (V01-X59, Y85-Y86)	37.0	48.9	25.6	38.7	50.4	27.3	29.6	42.0	18.2	33.1	47.9	19.7
Transport accidents (V01-V99, Y85)	16.8	23.7	10.1	17.3	24.2	10.5	14.5	21.1	8.4	15.4	23.1	8.3
Motor vehicle accidents (V02-V04, V09.0, V09.2, V12-V14, V19.0-V19.2, V19.4-V19.6, V20-V79, V80.3-80.5, V81.0-V81.1, V82.0-V82.1, V83-V86, V87.0-V87.8, V88.0-V88.8, V89.0, V89.2)	15.7	21.9	9.8	16.2	22.4	10.1	13.7	19.7	8.1	14.5	21.5	8.0
Other land transport accidents (V01, V05-V06, V09.1, V09.3-V09.9, V10-V11, V15-V18, V19.3, V19.8-V19.9, V80.0-V80.2, V80.6-V80.9, V81.2-V81.9, V82.2-V82.9, V87.9, V88.9, V89.1, V89.3, V89.9)	0.4	0.6	0.1	0.4	0.6	0.1	0.4	0.7	0.2	0.5	0.8	0.1
Water, air and space, and other and unspecified transport accidents and their sequelae (V90-V99, Y85)	0.7	1.1	0.2	0.7	1.2	0.2	0.4	0.7	0.1	0.4	0.8	0.1
Nontransport accidents (W00-X59, Y86)	20.2	25.2	15.4	21.4	26.2	16.8	15.2	20.9	9.8	17.8	24.8	11.4
Falls (W00-W19)	5.6	6.0	5.3	6.4	6.6	6.2	2.3	3.0	1.7	2.2	3.0	1.5
Accidental discharge of firearms (W32-W34)	0.3	0.5	0.1	0.3	0.4	0.1	0.3	0.6	*	0.4	0.8	*
Accidental drowning and submersion (W65-W74) ...	1.2	1.9	0.5	1.1	1.8	0.4	1.5	2.6	0.6	1.6	2.8	0.5
Accidental exposure to smoke, fire, and flames (X00-X09)	1.1	1.4	0.8	1.0	1.2	0.7	1.6	2.0	1.3	2.1	2.6	1.6
Accidental poisoning and exposure to noxious substances (X40-X49)	6.1	8.5	3.7	6.3	8.8	3.9	5.0	7.2	3.0	6.3	9.1	3.7
Other and unspecified nontransport accidents and their sequelae (W20-W31, W35-W64, W75-W99, X10-X39, X50-X59, Y86)	6.0	6.9	5.0	6.3	7.3	5.4	4.4	5.5	3.3	5.2	6.6	4.0
Intentional self-harm (suicide) (*U03, X60-X84, Y87.0)	11.0	17.9	4.3	12.2	19.9	4.8	5.5	9.2	2.0	5.1	9.1	1.5
Intentional self-harm (suicide) by discharge of firearms (X72-X74)	5.9	10.6	1.4	6.7	11.9	1.6	2.6	4.8	0.5	2.8	5.4	0.5
Intentional self-harm (suicide) by other and unspecified means and their sequelae (* U03, X60-X71, X75-X84, Y87.0)	5.0	7.3	2.9	5.5	8.0	3.2	2.9	4.4	1.5	2.3	3.7	1.1
Assault (homicide) (*U01-*U02, X85-Y09, Y87.1)	6.1	9.6	2.7	3.7	5.4	2.0	16.7	28.6	5.7	22.0	38.4	7.0
Assault (homicide) by discharge of firearms (*U01.4, X93-X95)	4.1	7.0	1.3	2.2	3.5	1.0	12.4	22.8	2.8	16.7	31.0	3.6
Assault (homicide) by other and unspecified means and their sequelae (*U01.0-*U01.3, *U01.5-*U01.9, *U02, X85-X92, X96-Y09, Y87.1) ..	2.0	2.6	1.4	1.5	1.9	1.1	4.3	5.9	2.9	5.3	7.3	3.4
Legal intervention (Y35, Y89.0)	0.1	0.3	*	0.1	0.2	*	0.2	0.5	*	0.3	0.6	*
Events of undetermined intent (Y10-Y34, Y87.2, Y89.9)	1.7	2.2	1.2	1.7	2.2	1.2	1.6	2.3	1.0	2.0	2.9	1.2
Discharge of firearms, undetermined intent (Y22-Y24)	0.1	0.1	0.0	0.1	0.1	0.0	0.1	0.2	*	0.1	0.2	*
Other and unspecified events of undetermined intent and their sequelae (Y10-Y21, Y25-Y34, Y87.2, Y89.9)	1.6	2.1	1.1	1.6	2.0	1.2	1.5	2.1	1.0	1.9	2.7	1.2
Operations of war and their sequelae (Y36, Y89.1)	0.0	0.0	*	*	*	*	*	*	*	*	*	*
Complications of medical and surgical care (Y40-Y84, Y88)	1.0	0.9	1.1	1.0	0.9	1.1	1.0	0.8	1.1	1.2	1.0	1.3

[1]Based on codes from the *International Classification of Diseases, Tenth Revision* (1992), except in cases where (*) precedes the cause of death code. Codes *U01-*U03 were added as of 2001 for deaths due to terrorism.
0.0 = Quantity more than zero but less than 0.05.
* = Figure does not meet standards of reliability or precision.

TABLE II-15. DEATH RATES FOR 113 SELECTED CAUSES, BY RACE, HISPANIC ORIGIN, AND SEX, 2002

As mentioned in the notes for Table II-14, crude death rates can be utilized to characterize actual measures of mortality risk. However, due to differences in age distribution between sex and racial/ethnic groups, age-adjusted death rates (see Table II-17) should be used to compare relative risk among different groups.

Table II-15. Death Rates for 113 Selected Causes, by Race, Hispanic Origin, and Sex, 2002

(Rate per 100,000 population.)

Cause of death [1]	All origins [2]			Hispanic [3]			Non-Hispanic [4]			Non-Hispanic White			Non-Hispanic Black		
	Both sexes	Male	Female	Both sexes	Male	Female	Both sexes	Male	Female	Both sexes	Male	Female	Both sexes	Male	Female
ALL CAUSES	847.3	846.6	848.0	302.2	328.7	274.0	928.8	928.0	929.5	997.5	983.9	1 010.6	792.8	842.3	748.0
Salmonella infections (A01-A02)	0.0	*	*	*	*	*	*	*	*	*	*	*	*	*	*
Shigellosis and amebiasis (A03, A06)	*	*	*	*	*	*	*	*	*	*	*	*	*	*	*
Certain other intestinal infections (A04, A07-A09)	0.9	0.7	1.0	0.2	0.2	0.3	1.0	0.8	1.1	1.1	0.9	1.3	0.4	0.4	0.5
Tuberculosis (A16-A19)	0.3	0.3	0.2	0.2	0.3	0.2	0.3	0.3	0.2	0.2	0.2	0.1	0.5	0.7	0.4
Respiratory tuberculosis (A16)	0.2	0.3	0.2	0.2	0.2	0.2	0.2	0.3	0.2	0.1	0.2	0.1	0.4	0.6	0.3
Other tuberculosis (A17-A19)	0.1	0.1	0.0	*	*	*	0.1	0.1	0.0	0.0	0.0	0.0	0.1	0.1	*
Whooping cough (A37)	*	*	*	*	*	*	*	*	*	*	*	*	*	*	*
Scarlet fever and erysipelas (A38, A46)	*	*	*	*	*	*	*	*	*	*	*	*	*	*	*
Meningococcal infection (A39)	0.1	0.1	0.1	*	*	*	0.1	0.1	0.1	0.1	0.1	0.0	0.1	*	*
Septicemia (A40-A41)	11.7	10.6	12.9	3.9	3.7	4.1	12.9	11.6	14.1	12.9	11.5	14.2	16.8	15.5	18.0
Syphilis (A50-A53)	0.0	0.0	0.0	*	*	*	0.0	0.0	*	*	*	*	0.1	*	*
Acute poliomyelitis (A80)	*	*	*	*	*	*	*	*	*	*	*	*	*	*	*
Arthropod-borne viral encephalitis (A83-A84, A85.2)	*	*	*	*	*	*	*	*	*	*	*	*	*	*	*
Measles (B05)	*	*	*	*	*	*	*	*	*	*	*	*	*	*	*
Viral hepatitis (B15-B19)	2.0	2.7	1.4	2.0	2.5	1.4	2.0	2.7	1.4	1.9	2.6	1.3	2.3	3.1	1.7
Human immunodeficiency virus (HIV) disease (B20-B24)	4.9	7.4	2.5	4.8	7.2	2.2	4.8	7.3	2.5	2.1	3.7	0.6	21.3	30.3	13.2
Malaria (B50-B54)	*	*	*	*	*	*	*	*	*	*	*	*	*	*	*
Other and unspecified infectious and parasitic diseases and their sequelae (A00, A05, A20-A36, A42-A44, A48-A49, A54-A79, A81-A82, A85.0-A85.1, A85.8, A86-B04, B06-B09, B25-B49, B55-B99)	2.3	2.6	2.1	1.5	1.8	1.2	2.4	2.7	2.2	2.5	2.7	2.3	2.6	3.0	2.2
Malignant neoplasms (C00-C97)	193.2	203.8	183.0	59.7	61.2	58.1	213.4	226.7	200.8	230.9	243.8	218.5	171.5	187.8	156.7
Malignant neoplasms of lip, oral cavity, and pharynx (C00-C14)	2.7	3.7	1.7	0.7	1.1	0.4	3.0	4.1	1.9	3.1	4.1	2.1	2.9	4.4	1.5
Malignant neoplasm of esophagus (C15)	4.4	6.9	2.0	1.1	1.6	0.4	4.9	7.8	2.2	5.3	8.4	2.3	4.3	6.5	2.4
Malignant neoplasm of stomach (C16)	4.2	5.0	3.5	3.1	3.4	2.7	4.4	5.3	3.5	4.1	5.0	3.2	5.8	6.9	4.9
Malignant neoplasm of colon, rectum, and anus (C18-C21)	19.7	20.1	19.2	6.1	6.4	5.7	21.7	22.3	21.2	23.2	23.8	22.7	18.9	19.3	18.4
Malignant neoplasms of liver and intrahepatic bile ducts (C22)	4.9	6.4	3.4	3.5	4.5	2.5	5.1	6.6	3.6	5.0	6.4	3.6	4.7	6.6	3.0
Malignant neoplasm of pancreas (C25)	10.5	10.5	10.5	3.5	3.3	3.7	11.6	11.7	11.5	12.4	12.6	12.2	9.6	9.3	9.8
Malignant neoplasm of larynx (C32)	1.3	2.1	0.5	0.4	0.7	0.1	1.4	2.3	0.6	1.4	2.3	0.6	1.9	3.1	0.7
Malignant neoplasms of trachea, bronchus, and lung (C33-C34)	54.7	63.7	46.0	10.4	13.1	7.6	61.4	71.8	51.6	67.7	77.8	57.9	44.7	58.1	32.6
Malignant melanoma of skin (C43)	2.6	3.3	1.9	0.4	0.4	0.4	2.9	3.8	2.1	3.6	4.7	2.6	0.3	0.3	0.3
Malignant neoplasm of breast (C50)	14.5	0.3	28.3	4.5	*	9.2	16.0	0.3	31.0	16.9	0.3	32.9	15.4	0.4	29.1
Malignant neoplasm of cervix uteri (C53)	1.4	X	2.7	1.0	X	2.1	1.4	X	2.8	1.3	X	2.5	2.3	X	4.3
Malignant neoplasms of corpus uteri and uterus, part unspecified (C54-C55)	2.4	X	4.7	0.9	X	1.8	2.6	X	5.1	2.6	X	5.1	3.1	X	5.8
Malignant neoplasm of ovary (C56)	5.1	X	10.0	1.6	X	3.3	5.6	X	11.0	6.3	X	12.4	3.2	X	6.1
Malignant neoplasm of prostate (C61)	10.6	21.5	X	3.1	6.0	X	11.7	24.0	X	11.9	24.3	X	14.1	29.6	X
Malignant neoplasms of kidney and renal pelvis (C64-C65)	4.2	5.4	3.1	1.7	2.1	1.2	4.6	5.9	3.4	5.1	6.5	3.8	2.9	3.6	2.3
Malignant neoplasm of bladder (C67)	4.4	6.0	2.8	1.0	1.3	0.7	4.9	6.8	3.1	5.6	7.9	3.4	2.6	2.8	2.4
Malignant neoplasms of meninges, brain, and other parts of central nervous system (C70-C72)	4.4	5.0	3.9	1.7	1.8	1.5	4.9	5.5	4.2	5.6	6.4	4.9	2.1	2.3	1.9
Malignant neoplasms of lymphoid, hematopoietic, and related tissue (C81-C96)	19.5	21.4	17.7	7.3	7.6	7.0	21.3	23.6	19.2	23.7	26.2	21.2	14.1	15.1	13.1
Hodgkin's disease (C81)	0.5	0.5	0.4	0.3	0.3	0.2	0.5	0.6	0.4	0.6	0.6	0.5	0.3	0.5	0.2
Non-Hodgkin's lymphoma (C82-C85)	7.6	8.1	7.1	2.8	2.7	2.8	8.3	9.0	7.7	9.5	10.2	8.8	4.0	4.5	3.6
Leukemia (C91-C95)	7.5	8.5	6.5	2.8	3.0	2.6	8.2	9.4	7.0	9.1	10.5	7.8	4.8	5.3	4.4
Multiple myeloma and immunoproliferative neoplasms (C88, C90)	4.0	4.2	3.7	1.5	1.6	1.4	4.3	4.6	4.0	4.5	4.8	4.1	4.8	4.8	4.9
Other and unspecified malignant neoplasms of lymphoid, hematopoietic, and related tissue (C96)	0.0	0.0	0.0	*	*	*	0.0	0.0	0.0	0.0	0.0	0.0	*	*	*
All other and unspecified malignant neoplasms (C17, C23-C24, C26-C31, C37-C41, C44-C49, C51-C52, C57-C60, C62-C63, C66, C68-C69, C73-C80, C97)	21.8	22.7	21.0	7.8	7.8	7.7	24.0	25.0	22.9	26.0	27.2	24.9	18.7	19.4	18.0
In situ neoplasms, benign neoplasms, and neoplasms of uncertain or unknown behavior (D00-D48)	4.6	4.6	4.6	1.5	1.4	1.5	5.1	5.1	5.1	5.7	5.8	5.6	3.1	2.9	3.4
Anemias (D50-D64)	1.6	1.3	1.9	0.5	0.5	0.5	1.8	1.4	2.1	1.6	1.2	2.1	2.9	2.7	3.0
Diabetes mellitus (E10-E14)	25.4	24.2	26.5	15.3	13.9	16.7	26.9	25.8	27.9	26.4	26.0	26.8	34.8	30.0	39.2
Nutritional deficiencies (E40-E64)	1.3	0.9	1.7	0.4	0.3	0.4	1.5	1.0	1.8	1.5	1.1	2.0	1.4	1.1	1.6
Malnutrition (E40-E46)	1.2	0.9	1.6	0.4	0.3	0.4	1.3	1.0	1.7	1.4	1.0	1.8	1.3	1.0	1.5
Other nutritional deficiencies (E50-E64)	0.1	0.1	0.1	*	*	*	0.1	0.1	0.1	0.1	0.1	0.2	0.2	0.1	*
Meningitis (G00, G03)	0.2	0.3	0.2	0.2	0.2	0.1	0.3	0.3	0.2	0.2	0.2	0.2	0.5	0.6	0.4
Parkinson's disease (G20-G21)	5.9	6.8	5.0	1.3	1.4	1.1	6.6	7.6	5.6	7.9	9.1	6.7	1.5	1.8	1.3
Alzheimer's disease (G30)	20.4	12.0	28.5	3.8	2.3	5.4	22.9	13.6	31.9	26.9	15.8	37.6	9.1	5.5	12.5

[1] Based on codes from the *International Classification of Diseases, Tenth Revision* (1992), except in cases where (*) precedes the cause of death code. Codes *U01-*U03 were added as of 2001 for deaths due to terrorism.
[2] Figures for origin not stated are included in "All origins" but not distributed among specified origins.
[3] May be of any race.
[4] Includes races other than White and Black.
0.0 = Quantity more than zero but less than 0.05.
* = Figure does not meet standards of reliability or precision.
X = Not applicable.

Table II-15. Death Rates for 113 Selected Causes, by Race, Hispanic Origin, and Sex, 2002—*Continued*

(Rate per 100,000 population.)

Cause of death [1]	All origins [2] Both sexes	All origins [2] Male	All origins [2] Female	Hispanic [3] Both sexes	Hispanic [3] Male	Hispanic [3] Female	Non-Hispanic [4] Both sexes	Non-Hispanic [4] Male	Non-Hispanic [4] Female	Non-Hispanic White Both sexes	Non-Hispanic White Male	Non-Hispanic White Female	Non-Hispanic Black Both sexes	Non-Hispanic Black Male	Non-Hispanic Black Female
Major cardiovascular diseases (I00-I78)	318.6	303.3	333.3	94.3	94.2	94.4	352.2	336.4	367.2	381.9	362.2	400.8	285.1	277.2	292.3
Diseases of heart (I00-I09, I11, I13, I20-I51)	241.7	240.7	242.7	71.9	74.0	69.7	267.1	267.0	267.2	290.8	289.2	292.3	212.2	212.9	211.6
Acute rheumatic fever and chronic rheumatic heart diseases (I00-I09)	1.2	0.8	1.7	0.5	0.3	0.8	1.4	0.8	1.8	1.5	0.9	2.1	0.7	0.5	0.8
Hypertensive heart disease (I11)	9.2	8.2	10.2	3.7	3.9	3.4	10.0	8.9	11.1	9.1	7.6	10.5	17.7	18.0	17.4
Hypertensive heart and renal disease (I13)	1.0	0.9	1.2	0.4	0.4	0.5	1.1	0.9	1.2	0.9	0.7	1.1	2.5	2.3	2.6
Ischemic heart diseases (I20-I25)	171.4	178.4	164.7	54.0	56.5	51.4	189.0	197.6	180.7	208.0	217.2	199.1	137.0	139.5	134.8
Acute myocardial infarction (I21-I22)	62.3	66.2	58.4	19.7	20.6	18.7	68.7	73.5	64.1	75.5	81.2	70.1	50.2	50.1	50.4
Other acute ischemic heart diseases (I24)	1.2	1.2	1.1	0.2	0.2	0.1	1.3	1.4	1.3	1.4	1.5	1.4	1.2	1.4	1.1
Other forms of chronic ischemic heart disease (I20, I25)	108.0	110.9	105.2	34.2	35.7	32.6	118.9	122.7	115.4	131.0	134.5	127.7	85.5	88.0	83.3
Atherosclerotic cardiovascular disease, so described (I25.0)	23.6	25.4	21.9	8.2	9.7	6.5	25.9	27.8	24.0	26.8	28.2	25.3	27.7	31.9	24.0
All other forms of chronic ischemic heart disease (I20, I25.1-I25.9)	84.4	85.5	83.3	26.0	25.9	26.1	93.1	94.9	91.4	104.3	106.2	102.4	57.8	56.1	59.3
Other heart diseases (I26-I51)	58.8	52.4	65.0	13.3	12.9	13.7	65.7	58.7	72.3	71.3	62.7	79.6	54.3	52.6	55.9
Acute and subacute endocarditis (I33)	0.4	0.5	0.3	0.2	0.2	0.1	0.4	0.5	0.4	0.4	0.5	0.4	0.5	0.6	0.5
Diseases of pericardium and acute myocarditis (I30-I31, I40)	0.3	0.3	0.3	0.2	0.2	0.2	0.3	0.3	0.3	0.3	0.3	0.3	0.4	0.4	0.4
Heart failure (I50)	19.6	15.3	23.7	3.6	3.0	4.4	22.0	17.3	26.5	24.7	19.2	30.0	14.2	12.0	16.3
All other forms of heart disease (I26-I28, I34-I38, I42-I49, I51)	38.5	36.3	40.6	9.3	9.6	9.0	42.9	40.6	45.1	45.8	42.7	48.9	39.1	39.6	38.7
Essential (primary) hypertension and hypertensive renal disease (I10, I12)	7.0	5.4	8.6	2.4	1.9	3.0	7.7	5.9	9.4	7.4	5.5	9.2	11.5	9.9	13.0
Cerebrovascular diseases (I60-I69)	56.4	44.2	68.2	16.6	15.0	18.4	62.4	48.9	75.3	67.0	51.3	82.1	51.7	45.1	57.7
Atherosclerosis (I70)	4.8	3.7	5.9	1.1	0.9	1.3	5.4	4.1	6.6	6.1	4.6	7.6	2.8	2.4	3.2
Other diseases of circulatory system (I71-I78)	8.6	9.4	7.9	2.2	2.3	2.0	9.6	10.5	8.8	10.6	11.6	9.6	6.9	7.0	6.9
Aortic aneurysm and dissection (I71)	5.1	6.4	4.0	1.1	1.4	0.8	5.7	7.2	4.4	6.5	8.0	4.9	3.3	3.9	2.8
Other diseases of arteries, arterioles, and capillaries (I72-I78)	3.5	3.0	4.0	1.1	0.9	1.3	3.9	3.4	4.3	4.1	3.6	4.7	3.6	3.1	4.0
Other disorders of circulatory system (I80-I99)	1.6	1.4	1.9	0.6	0.5	0.7	1.8	1.5	2.1	1.8	1.5	2.2	2.2	2.1	2.3
Influenza and pneumonia (J10-J18)	22.8	20.4	25.1	7.3	7.0	7.6	25.1	22.5	27.5	27.9	24.6	31.1	16.1	15.9	16.2
Influenza (J10-J11) [5]	0.3	0.2	0.3	*	*	*	0.3	0.2	0.3	0.3	0.3	0.4	0.1	*	*
Pneumonia (J12-J18)	22.5	20.2	24.8	7.2	6.9	7.5	24.8	22.3	27.2	27.6	24.3	30.7	16.0	15.8	16.1
Other acute lower respiratory infections (J20-J22)	0.1	0.1	0.2	0.1	*	*	0.1	0.1	0.2	0.2	0.1	0.2	0.1	0.1	0.1
Acute bronchitis and bronchiolitis (J20-J21)	0.1	0.1	0.1	*	*	*	0.1	0.1	0.1	0.1	0.1	0.1	0.1	0.1	*
Unspecified acute lower respiratory infection (J22)	0.0	0.0	0.1	*	*	*	0.0	0.0	0.1	0.0	0.0	0.1	*	*	*
Chronic lower respiratory diseases (J40-J47)	43.3	42.9	43.7	7.9	8.1	7.6	48.6	48.4	48.9	56.4	55.1	57.7	21.4	24.9	18.2
Bronchitis, chronic and unspecified (J40-J42)	0.3	0.3	0.4	0.1	0.1	0.2	0.4	0.3	0.4	0.4	0.4	0.5	0.2	0.2	0.2
Emphysema (J43)	5.4	5.7	5.0	0.8	0.8	0.7	6.1	6.5	5.7	7.1	7.4	6.8	2.3	3.1	1.6
Asthma (J45-J46)	1.5	1.1	1.8	0.7	0.6	0.9	1.6	1.2	2.0	1.4	0.9	1.8	3.0	2.8	3.1
Other chronic lower respiratory diseases (J44, J47)	36.1	35.7	36.5	6.3	6.6	5.9	40.6	40.4	40.8	47.5	46.4	48.6	15.9	18.7	13.3
Pneumoconioses and chemical effects (J60-J66, J68)	0.4	0.7	0.0	0.1	0.2	*	0.4	0.8	0.0	0.5	1.0	0.0	0.2	0.3	*
Pneumonitis due to solids and liquids (J69)	6.1	6.3	5.9	1.4	1.4	1.4	6.8	7.0	6.6	7.7	7.9	7.4	4.2	4.4	4.1
Other diseases of respiratory system (J00-J06, J30-J39, J67, J70-J98)	8.7	8.5	8.8	3.3	3.2	3.4	9.5	9.4	9.6	10.5	10.3	10.7	6.2	6.3	6.2
Peptic ulcer (K25-K28)	1.4	1.4	1.5	0.5	0.6	0.4	1.6	1.5	1.6	1.7	1.6	1.8	1.0	1.2	0.9
Diseases of appendix (K35-K38)	0.2	0.2	0.1	0.1	*	*	0.2	0.2	0.2	0.2	0.2	0.2	0.2	0.2	0.1
Hernia (K40-K46)	0.6	0.4	0.7	0.2	0.2	0.2	0.6	0.5	0.7	0.7	0.5	0.8	0.4	0.3	0.4
Chronic liver disease and cirrhosis (K70, K73-K74)	9.5	12.3	6.7	8.8	12.2	5.2	9.5	12.2	6.9	10.2	13.2	7.5	7.0	9.3	5.0
Alcoholic liver disease (K70)	4.2	6.2	2.3	4.3	7.1	1.4	4.2	6.0	2.4	4.4	6.4	2.4	3.2	4.6	2.1
Other chronic liver disease and cirrhosis (K73-K74)	5.2	6.1	4.5	4.5	5.1	3.8	5.4	6.2	4.6	5.9	6.7	5.0	3.8	4.7	3.0
Cholelithiasis and other disorders of gallbladder (K80-K82)	1.0	0.9	1.1	0.5	0.5	0.5	1.1	1.0	1.2	1.2	1.1	1.3	0.7	0.6	0.8
Nephritis, nephrotic syndrome, and nephrosis (N00-N07, N17-N19, N25-N27)	14.2	13.9	14.5	4.9	4.7	5.1	15.6	15.4	15.8	15.4	15.3	15.6	20.5	19.7	21.2
Acute and rapidly progressive nephritic and nephrotic syndrome (N00-N01, N04)	0.1	0.0	0.1	*	*	*	0.1	0.1	0.1	0.1	0.1	0.1	0.1	*	*
Chronic glomerulonephritis, nephritis, and nephropathy, not specified as acute or chronic, and renal sclerosis, unspecified (N02-N03, N05-N07, N26)	0.2	0.2	0.2	0.1	*	*	0.2	0.2	0.2	0.2	0.2	0.2	0.2	0.2	0.2
Renal failure (N17-N19)	13.9	13.7	14.2	4.8	4.6	5.0	15.3	15.1	15.5	15.2	15.0	15.3	20.2	19.4	20.9
Other disorders of kidney (N25, N27)	0.0	*	0.0	*	*	*	0.0	*	0.0	0.0	*	0.0	*	*	*
Infections of kidney (N10-N12, N13.6, N15.1)	0.3	0.2	0.4	0.1	*	0.1	0.3	0.2	0.4	0.3	0.2	0.4	0.2	0.1	0.3
Hyperplasia of prostate (N40)	0.2	0.3	X	*	*	X	0.2	0.3	X	0.2	0.4	X	0.1	0.2	X
Inflammatory diseases of female pelvic organs (N70-N76)	0.0	X	0.1	*	X	*	0.0	X	0.1	0.0	X	0.1	0.1	X	0.1
Pregnancy, childbirth, and the puerperium (O00-O99)	0.1	X	0.3	0.2	X	0.4	0.1	X	0.2	0.1	X	0.1	0.4	X	0.8
Pregnancy with abortive outcome (O00-O07)	0.0	X	0.0	*	X	*	0.0	X	0.0	*	X	*	*	X	*
Other complications of pregnancy, childbirth, and the puerperium (O10-O99)	0.1	X	0.2	0.2	X	0.4	0.1	X	0.2	0.1	X	0.1	0.4	X	0.7
Certain conditions originating in the perinatal period (P00-P96)	4.9	5.7	4.2	6.2	6.8	5.6	4.7	5.4	4.0	3.2	3.8	2.7	13.2	15.4	11.3
Congenital malformations, deformations, and chromosomal abnormalities (Q00-Q99)	3.7	3.9	3.5	4.4	4.5	4.3	3.6	3.8	3.4	3.4	3.6	3.3	4.7	5.2	4.4
Symptoms, signs, and abnormal clinical and laboratory findings, not elsewhere classified (R00-R99)	10.4	10.1	10.7	4.0	4.6	3.3	11.3	10.9	11.7	11.6	10.7	12.5	12.6	14.4	10.9
All other diseases (residual)	67.5	55.8	78.8	21.6	21.1	22.1	74.4	61.2	86.8	80.5	64.8	95.5	61.7	56.6	66.3

[1] Based on codes from the *International Classification of Diseases, Tenth Revision* (1992), except in cases where (*) precedes the cause of death code. Codes *U01-*U03 were added as of 2001 for deaths due to terrorism.
[2] Figures for origin not stated are included in "All origins" but not distributed among specified origins.
[3] May be of any race.
[4] Includes races other than White and Black.
[5] Cause of death coding changes may affect comparability with the previous year's data for this cause.
0.0 = Quantity more than zero but less than 0.05.
* = Figure does not meet standards of reliability or precision.
X = Not applicable.

Table II-15. Death Rates for 113 Selected Causes, by Race, Hispanic Origin, and Sex, 2002—*Continued*

(Rate per 100,000 population.)

Cause of death [1]	All origins [2]			Hispanic [3]			Non-Hispanic [4]			Non-Hispanic White			Non-Hispanic Black		
	Both sexes	Male	Female	Both sexes	Male	Female	Both sexes	Male	Female	Both sexes	Male	Female	Both sexes	Male	Female
Accidents (unintentional injuries) (V01-X59, Y85-Y86)	37.0	48.9	25.6	26.1	38.5	12.8	38.5	50.3	27.3	40.6	52.0	29.6	34.0	49.0	20.3
Transport accidents (V01-V99, Y85)	16.8	23.7	10.1	15.3	22.4	7.7	16.9	23.8	10.4	17.5	24.3	10.9	15.7	23.6	8.5
Motor vehicle accidents (V02-V04, V09.0, V09.2, V12-V14, V19.0-V19.2, V19.4-V19.6, V20-V79, V80.3-80.5, V81.0-V81.1, V82.0-V82.1, V83-V86, V87.0-V87.8, V88.0-V88.8, V89.0, V89.2)	15.7	21.9	9.8	14.6	21.3	7.4	15.9	21.9	10.1	16.3	22.3	10.5	14.8	22.0	8.3
Other land transport accidents (V01, V05-V06, V09.1, V09.3-V09.9, V10-V11, V15-V18, V19.3, V19.8-V19.9, V80.0-V80.2, V80.6-V80.9, V81.2-V81.9, V82.2-V82.9, V87.9, V88.9, V89.1, V89.3, V89.9)	0.4	0.6	0.1	0.4	0.6	0.1	0.4	0.6	0.1	0.4	0.6	0.1	0.5	0.8	0.1
Water, air and space, and other and unspecified transport accidents and their sequelae (V90-V99, Y85)	0.7	1.1	0.2	0.3	0.5	*	0.7	1.2	0.2	0.8	1.3	0.3	0.4	0.8	0.1
Nontransport accidents (W00-X59, Y86)	20.2	25.2	15.4	10.8	16.1	5.2	21.6	26.5	16.9	23.1	27.8	18.6	18.3	25.5	11.8
Falls (W00-W19)	5.6	6.0	5.3	2.1	2.8	1.4	6.2	6.5	5.9	7.1	7.3	7.0	2.3	3.0	1.6
Accidental discharge of firearms (W32-W34)	0.3	0.5	0.1	0.2	0.3	*	0.3	0.5	0.1	0.3	0.5	0.1	0.4	0.8	*
Accidental drowning and submersion (W65-W74)	1.2	1.9	0.5	1.2	2.0	0.3	1.2	1.9	0.5	1.1	1.7	0.5	1.7	2.9	0.5
Accidental exposure to smoke, fire, and flames (X00-X09)	1.1	1.4	0.8	0.6	0.7	0.4	1.2	1.5	0.9	1.0	1.3	0.8	2.1	2.6	1.6
Accidental poisoning and exposure to noxious substances (X40-X49)	6.1	8.5	3.7	4.3	6.6	1.7	6.3	8.8	4.0	6.6	9.1	4.3	6.4	9.3	3.8
Other and unspecified nontransport accidents and their sequelae (W20-W31, W35-W64, W75-W99, X10-X39, X50-X59, Y86)	6.0	6.9	5.0	2.5	3.6	1.2	6.5	7.5	5.6	7.0	7.9	6.1	5.4	6.8	4.2
Intentional self-harm (suicide) (*U03, X60-X84, Y87.0)	11.0	17.9	4.3	5.0	8.3	1.6	11.8	19.4	4.6	13.4	21.9	5.3	5.2	9.3	1.6
Intentional self-harm (suicide) by discharge of firearms (X72-X74)	5.9	10.6	1.4	2.2	3.8	0.4	6.5	11.7	1.6	7.5	13.4	1.8	2.9	5.5	0.5
Intentional self-harm (suicide) by other and unspecified means and their sequelae (*U03, X60-X71, X75-X84, Y87.0)	5.0	7.3	2.9	2.9	4.4	1.2	5.3	7.7	3.1	6.0	8.5	3.5	2.4	3.8	1.1
Assault (homicide) (*U01-*U02, X85-Y09, Y87.1)	6.1	9.6	2.7	8.1	13.2	2.6	5.7	8.9	2.7	2.8	3.8	1.9	22.5	39.4	7.2
Assault (homicide) by discharge of firearms (*U01.4, X93-X95)	4.1	7.0	1.3	5.6	9.7	1.2	3.8	6.5	1.3	1.5	2.2	0.9	17.1	31.9	3.7
Assault (homicide) by other and unspecified means and their sequelae (*U01.0-*U01.3, *U01.5-*U01.9, *U02, X85-X92, X96-Y09, Y87.1)	2.0	2.6	1.4	2.5	3.5	1.4	1.9	2.5	1.4	1.3	1.6	1.0	5.4	7.6	3.5
Legal intervention (Y35, Y89.0)	0.1	0.3	*	0.2	0.3	*	0.1	0.2	*	0.1	0.2	*	0.3	0.6	*
Events of undetermined intent (Y10-Y34, Y87.2, Y89.9)	1.7	2.2	1.2	0.8	1.2	0.4	1.8	2.3	1.3	1.8	2.3	1.3	2.0	2.9	1.2
Discharge of firearms, undetermined intent (Y22-Y24) ...	0.1	0.1	0.0	0.1	0.1	*	0.1	0.1	0.0	0.1	0.1	0.0	0.1	0.2	*
Other and unspecified events of undetermined intent and their sequelae (Y10-Y21, Y25-Y34, Y87.2, Y89.9)	1.6	2.1	1.1	0.8	1.1	0.4	1.7	2.2	1.2	1.7	2.2	1.3	1.9	2.7	1.2
Operations of war and their sequelae (Y36, Y89.1)	0.0	0.0	*	*	*	*	*	*	*	*	*	*	*	*	*
Complications of medical and surgical care (Y40-Y84, Y88)	1.0	0.9	1.1	0.4	0.3	0.4	1.1	1.0	1.2	1.1	1.0	1.2	1.2	1.1	1.4

[1]Based on codes from the *International Classification of Diseases, Tenth Revision* (1992), except in cases where (*) precedes the cause of death code. Codes *U01-*U03 were added as of 2001 for deaths due to terrorism.
[2]Figures for origin not stated are included in "All origins" but not distributed among specified origins.
[3]May be of any race.
[4]Includes races other than White and Black.
0.0 = Quantity more than zero but less than 0.05.
* = Figure does not meet standards of reliability or precision.

TABLE II-16. AGE-ADJUSTED DEATH RATES FOR 113 SELECTED CAUSES, BY RACE AND SEX, 2002

These age-adjusted data allow a comparison of the susceptibility of various groups to different health risks. Adjusted for age, the overall male death rate was 42 percent higher than the female death rate. As a result, males in general were more likely to have higher age-adjusted death rates for most specific causes. Two causes that did not fit this pattern were Alzheimer's disease, for which women had a higher age-adjusted death rate, and cerebrovascular disease (stroke), which was closely matched between the sexes.

Blacks had a significantly higher risk of cancer death than Whites. For cancer, White males had a 45 percent greater relative risk of death than White females, but Black males had a 68 percent higher mortality risk than Black females. Lung cancer among Black males was a major contributor to this disparity. For fatalities from diabetes, which were much smaller, the incidence rate for Blacks was more than twice the rate for Whites; for Blacks, the rates for men and women were about the same. Pneumonia hit Black men particularly heavily.

Fatal accidents occurred more than twice as often for men than women, among both Whites and Blacks. Suicide was also primarily a male phenomenon, and had twice as great a frequency among Whites as Blacks. Homicide victims were primarily men and were Black men seven times more frequently than White men.

Table II-16. Age-Adjusted Death Rates for 113 Selected Causes, by Race and Sex, 2002

(Rate per 100,000 U.S. standard population.)

Cause of death [1]	All races Both sexes	All races Male	All races Female	White Both sexes	White Male	White Female	All other Total Both sexes	All other Total Male	All other Total Female	All other Black Both sexes	All other Black Male	All other Black Female
ALL CAUSES	845.3	1 013.7	715.2	829.0	992.9	701.3	917.7	1 117.3	772.5	1 083.3	1 341.4	901.8
Salmonella infections (A01-A02)	0.0	*	*	*	*	*	*	*	*	*	*	*
Shigellosis and amebiasis (A03, A06)	*	*	*	*	*	*	*	*	*	*	*	*
Certain other intestinal infections (A04, A07-A09)	0.8	0.8	0.8	0.9	0.9	0.9	0.5	0.6	0.5	0.6	0.7	0.6
Tuberculosis (A16-A19)	0.3	0.4	0.2	0.2	0.3	0.1	0.9	1.2	0.6	0.7	1.1	0.5
Respiratory tuberculosis (A16)	0.2	0.3	0.1	0.2	0.2	0.1	0.7	1.0	0.5	0.6	0.9	0.4
Other tuberculosis (A17-A19)	0.0	0.1	0.0	0.0	0.0	0.0	0.2	0.3	0.1	0.1	0.2	*
Whooping cough (A37)	*	*	*	*	*	*	*	*	*	*	*	*
Scarlet fever and erysipelas (A38, A46)	*	*	*	*	*	*	*	*	*	*	*	*
Meningococcal infection (A39)	0.0	0.1	0.0	0.0	0.1	0.0	0.0	*	0.1	0.1	*	*
Septicemia (A40-A41)	11.7	12.9	10.9	10.7	11.7	9.9	19.2	21.6	17.6	24.2	27.8	22.1
Syphilis (A50-A53)	0.0	0.0	0.0	*	*	*	0.0	*	*	0.1	*	*
Acute poliomyelitis (A80)	*	*	*	*	*	*	*	*	*	*	*	*
Arthropod-borne viral encephalitis (A83-A84, A85.2)	*	*	*	*	*	*	*	*	*	*	*	*
Measles (B05)	*	*	*	*	*	*	*	*	*	*	*	*
Viral hepatitis (B15-B19)	2.0	2.7	1.3	1.9	2.6	1.2	2.7	3.6	1.9	2.8	3.8	1.9
Human immunodeficiency virus (HIV) disease (B20-B24)	4.9	7.4	2.5	2.6	4.3	0.9	15.8	23.3	9.3	22.5	33.3	13.4
Malaria (B50-B54)	*	*	*	*	*	*	*	*	*	*	*	*
Other and unspecified infectious and parasitic diseases and their sequelae (A00, A05, A20-A36, A42-A44, A48-A49, A54-A79, A81-A82, A85.0-A85.1, A85.8, A86-B04, B06-B09, B25-B49, B55-B99)	2.3	2.9	1.9	2.2	2.7	1.8	2.8	3.6	2.2	3.2	4.1	2.5
Malignant neoplasms (C00-C97)	193.5	238.9	163.1	191.7	235.2	162.4	203.0	263.7	164.6	238.8	319.6	190.3
Malignant neoplasms of lip, oral cavity, and pharynx (C00-C14)	2.7	4.1	1.5	2.5	3.8	1.5	3.2	5.3	1.7	3.6	6.3	1.7
Malignant neoplasm of esophagus (C15)	4.4	7.8	1.7	4.3	7.7	1.6	4.7	8.0	2.4	5.9	10.1	2.9
Malignant neoplasm of stomach (C16)	4.2	5.9	3.0	3.7	5.2	2.5	8.1	11.1	6.1	8.4	11.9	6.1
Malignant neoplasms of colon, rectum, and anus (C18-C21)	19.7	23.7	16.7	19.2	23.1	16.2	22.8	27.7	19.4	26.8	33.1	22.8
Malignant neoplasms of liver and intrahepatic bile ducts (C22)	4.9	7.1	3.0	4.5	6.5	2.8	7.2	11.3	4.2	6.3	9.9	3.6
Malignant neoplasm of pancreas (C25)	10.5	12.1	9.2	10.3	12.0	9.0	11.7	12.9	10.8	13.6	15.3	12.3
Malignant neoplasm of larynx (C32)	1.3	2.3	0.5	1.2	2.1	0.5	1.8	3.5	0.6	2.5	4.8	0.8
Malignant neoplasms of trachea, bronchus, and lung (C33-C34)	54.9	73.2	41.6	55.3	72.5	42.6	51.5	77.0	34.1	61.9	95.0	40.1
Malignant melanoma of skin (C43)	2.6	3.8	1.7	2.9	4.2	2.0	0.4	0.6	0.3	0.4	0.5	0.3
Malignant neoplasm of breast (C50)	14.5	0.3	25.6	14.1	0.3	25.0	16.4	0.5	28.0	20.2	0.6	34.0
Malignant neoplasm of cervix uteri (C53)	1.3	X	2.6	1.2	X	2.3	2.4	X	4.2	2.9	X	4.9
Malignant neoplasms of corpus uteri and uterus, part unspecified (C54-C55)	2.4	X	4.2	2.2	X	3.9	3.6	X	6.0	4.4	X	7.3
Malignant neoplasm of ovary (C56)	5.1	X	9.0	5.3	X	9.4	4.0	X	6.8	4.4	X	7.4
Malignant neoplasm of prostate (C61)	10.6	27.9	X	9.8	25.7	X	17.1	46.5	X	22.0	62.0	X
Malignant neoplasms of kidney and renal pelvis (C64-C65)	4.2	6.1	2.8	4.3	6.3	2.8	3.5	5.0	2.4	4.0	5.8	2.8
Malignant neoplasm of bladder (C67)	4.4	7.5	2.4	4.5	7.8	2.4	3.3	4.7	2.5	3.9	5.5	3.0
Malignant neoplasms of meninges, brain, and other parts of central nervous system (C70-C72)	4.4	5.5	3.6	4.8	5.8	3.9	2.4	3.1	2.0	2.6	3.2	2.2
Malignant neoplasms of lymphoid, hematopoietic, and related tissue (C81-C96)	19.5	25.1	15.5	19.9	25.6	15.7	16.7	20.7	14.1	19.4	24.4	16.1
Hodgkin's disease (C81)	0.5	0.6	0.4	0.5	0.6	0.4	0.3	0.5	0.3	0.4	0.6	0.3
Non-Hodgkin's lymphoma (C82-C85)	7.6	9.6	6.2	7.9	10.0	6.5	5.0	6.2	4.1	5.4	6.8	4.4
Leukemia (C91-C95)	7.5	10.0	5.7	7.7	10.3	5.8	5.9	7.6	4.7	6.6	8.6	5.3
Multiple myeloma and immunoproliferative neoplasms (C88, C90)	4.0	5.0	3.3	3.7	4.8	3.0	5.5	6.4	4.9	6.9	8.3	6.1
Other and unspecified malignant neoplasms of lymphoid, hematopoietic, and related tissue (C96)	0.0	0.0	0.0	0.0	0.0	0.0	*	*	*	*	*	*
All other and unspecified malignant neoplasms (C17, C23-C24, C26-C31, C37-C41, C44-C49, C51-C52, C57-C60, C62-C63, C66, C68-C69, C73-C80, C97)	21.8	26.5	18.5	21.8	26.4	18.4	21.9	26.2	18.9	25.7	31.4	21.9
In situ neoplasms, benign neoplasms, and neoplasms of uncertain or unknown behavior (D00-D48)	4.6	5.7	3.9	4.7	5.8	4.0	3.8	4.6	3.5	4.4	5.1	4.1
Anemias (D50-D64)	1.6	1.6	1.6	1.3	1.3	1.4	2.8	3.0	2.7	3.7	3.9	3.5
Diabetes mellitus (E10-E14)	25.4	28.6	23.0	23.1	26.8	20.3	41.5	41.2	41.0	49.5	49.4	48.6
Nutritional deficiencies (E40-E64)	1.3	1.2	1.3	1.2	1.2	1.3	1.8	1.8	1.7	2.1	2.1	2.1
Malnutrition (E40-E46)	1.2	1.1	1.2	1.1	1.1	1.2	1.7	1.7	1.6	2.0	2.0	2.0
Other nutritional deficiencies (E50-E64)	0.1	0.1	0.1	0.1	0.1	0.1	0.1	*	0.1	0.1	*	*
Meningitis (G00, G03)	0.2	0.3	0.2	0.2	0.3	0.2	0.4	0.6	0.3	0.5	0.7	0.4
Parkinson's disease (G20-G21)	5.9	9.0	4.1	6.3	9.5	4.3	2.7	4.2	1.8	2.5	4.0	1.7
Alzheimer's disease (G30)	20.2	16.6	22.0	21.1	17.3	22.9	12.9	10.8	13.8	15.2	13.2	15.9

[1]Based on codes from the *International Classification of Diseases, Tenth Revision* (1992), except in cases where (*) precedes the cause of death code. Codes *U01-*U03 were added as of 2001 for deaths due to terrorism.
0.0 = Quantity more than zero but less than 0.05.
* = Figure does not meet standards of reliability or precision.
X = Not applicable.

Table II-16. Age-Adjusted Death Rates for 113 Selected Causes, by Race and Sex, 2002—*Continued*

(Rate per 100,000 U.S. standard population.)

| Cause of death [1] | All races | | | White | | | All other | | | | | |
| | | | | | | | Total | | | Black | | |
	Both sexes	Male	Female	Both sexes	Male	Female	Both sexes	Male	Female	Both sexes	Male	Female
Major cardiovascular diseases (I00-I78)	317.4	377.2	270.5	310.4	370.7	262.7	353.7	410.4	310.9	416.1	487.4	363.8
Diseases of heart (I00-I09, I11, I13, I20-I51)	240.8	297.4	197.2	236.7	294.1	192.1	259.9	310.4	222.4	308.4	371.0	263.2
Acute rheumatic fever and chronic rheumatic heart diseases (I00-I09)	1.2	0.9	1.5	1.3	0.9	1.5	0.9	0.7	1.1	0.9	0.8	1.0
Hypertensive heart disease (I11)	9.1	9.5	8.3	7.6	7.8	7.0	19.0	21.3	16.9	24.4	28.0	21.2
Hypertensive heart and renal disease (I13)	1.0	1.0	0.9	0.7	0.8	0.7	2.7	3.0	2.5	3.5	3.9	3.2
Ischemic heart diseases (I20-I25)	170.8	220.4	133.6	169.8	220.5	131.2	174.1	213.8	145.4	203.0	250.6	169.7
Acute myocardial infarction (I21-I22)	62.1	80.6	48.1	61.9	81.0	47.1	63.2	76.4	53.9	73.9	89.5	63.2
Other acute ischemic heart diseases (I24)	1.2	1.5	0.9	1.1	1.4	0.9	1.4	1.7	1.1	1.7	2.3	1.3
Other forms of chronic ischemic heart disease (I20, I25)	107.6	138.3	84.5	106.8	138.0	83.2	109.5	135.6	90.5	127.5	158.9	105.2
Atherosclerotic cardiovascular disease, so described (I25.0)	23.5	30.4	17.8	22.1	28.5	16.7	32.9	43.9	24.8	40.3	54.8	30.0
All other forms of chronic ischemic heart disease (I20, I25.1-I25.9)	84.1	108.0	66.7	84.7	109.5	66.4	76.6	91.7	65.7	87.2	104.1	75.2
Other heart diseases (I26-I51)	58.5	65.5	52.8	57.3	64.1	51.7	63.1	71.6	56.5	76.6	87.8	68.1
Acute and subacute endocarditis (I33)	0.4	0.5	0.3	0.4	0.5	0.3	0.5	0.6	0.4	0.7	0.8	0.6
Diseases of pericardium and acute myocarditis (I30-I31, I40)	0.3	0.3	0.3	0.3	0.3	0.3	0.4	0.4	0.4	0.5	0.5	0.4
Heart failure (I50)	19.5	20.4	18.6	19.5	20.5	18.6	18.0	18.8	17.1	21.8	23.3	20.5
All other forms of heart disease (I26-I28, I34-I38, I42-I49, I51)	38.4	44.2	33.7	37.1	42.8	32.6	44.2	51.7	38.6	53.6	63.1	46.6
Essential (primary) hypertension and hypertensive renal disease (I10, I12)	7.0	6.8	7.0	6.0	5.8	6.0	13.7	14.0	13.3	16.9	17.7	16.1
Cerebrovascular diseases (I60-I69)	56.2	56.5	55.2	54.2	54.2	53.4	67.7	71.5	64.4	76.3	81.7	71.8
Atherosclerosis (I70)	4.7	4.9	4.6	4.8	5.0	4.7	3.8	4.0	3.6	4.4	4.9	4.0
Other diseases of circulatory system (I71-I78)	8.7	11.5	6.6	8.6	11.6	6.5	8.6	10.5	7.2	10.0	12.0	8.6
Aortic aneurysm and dissection (I71)	5.2	7.7	3.3	5.2	7.9	3.4	4.2	5.7	3.1	4.6	6.1	3.5
Other diseases of arteries, arterioles, and capillaries (I72-I78)	3.5	3.8	3.3	3.4	3.7	3.1	4.4	4.8	4.1	5.4	6.0	5.0
Other disorders of circulatory system (I80-I99)	1.6	1.6	1.6	1.5	1.5	1.6	2.2	2.4	2.0	2.9	3.2	2.6
Influenza and pneumonia (J10-J18)	22.6	27.0	19.9	22.6	26.7	19.9	22.2	28.4	18.5	24.0	30.8	20.0
Influenza (J10-J11) [2]	0.2	0.3	0.2	0.2	0.3	0.2	0.1	*	0.1	0.1	*	*
Pneumonia (J12-J18)	22.4	26.7	19.6	22.3	26.4	19.7	22.1	28.2	18.4	23.9	30.7	19.9
Other acute lower respiratory infections (J20-J22)	0.1	0.1	0.1	0.1	0.1	0.1	0.1	0.1	0.1	0.1	0.1	0.1
Acute bronchitis and bronchiolitis (J20-J21)	0.1	0.1	0.1	0.1	0.1	0.1	0.1	0.1	0.1	0.1	0.1	*
Unspecified acute lower respiratory infection (J22)	0.0	0.0	0.0	0.0	0.0	0.0	*	*	*	*	*	*
Chronic lower respiratory diseases (J40-J47)	43.5	53.5	37.4	45.4	54.9	39.7	27.3	40.3	19.6	31.2	46.3	22.6
Bronchitis, chronic and unspecified (J40-J42)	0.3	0.4	0.3	0.3	0.4	0.3	0.2	0.3	0.1	0.2	0.3	0.2
Emphysema (J43)	5.4	7.0	4.4	5.7	7.2	4.8	2.9	4.9	1.7	3.4	5.8	2.0
Asthma (J45-J46)	1.5	1.2	1.7	1.2	0.9	1.4	2.8	2.7	2.8	3.4	3.3	3.4
Other chronic lower respiratory diseases (J44, J47)	36.2	44.9	31.1	38.2	46.4	33.2	21.3	32.3	14.9	24.1	36.9	16.9
Pneumoconioses and chemical effects (J60-J66, J68)	0.4	1.0	0.0	0.4	1.0	0.0	0.2	0.5	*	0.2	0.6	*
Pneumonitis due to solids and liquids (J69)	6.1	8.4	4.7	6.1	8.5	4.7	5.7	7.9	4.5	6.6	9.2	5.1
Other diseases of respiratory system (J00-J06, J30-J39, J67, J70-J98)	8.7	10.4	7.6	8.8	10.5	7.6	7.7	9.0	6.8	8.4	9.9	7.4
Peptic ulcer (K25-K28)	1.4	1.7	1.2	1.4	1.7	1.2	1.4	1.8	1.1	1.4	2.0	1.1
Diseases of appendix (K35-K38)	0.2	0.2	0.1	0.1	0.2	0.1	0.2	0.3	0.1	0.2	0.4	0.1
Hernia (K40-K46)	0.5	0.5	0.6	0.6	0.5	0.6	0.5	0.5	0.4	0.5	0.6	0.5
Chronic liver disease and cirrhosis (K70, K73-K74)	9.4	12.9	6.3	9.6	13.2	6.3	7.9	10.8	5.5	8.5	12.0	5.7
Alcoholic liver disease (K70)	4.2	6.3	2.2	4.2	6.5	2.2	3.7	5.5	2.3	3.8	5.8	2.3
Other chronic liver disease and cirrhosis (K73-K74)	5.2	6.5	4.1	5.4	6.7	4.2	4.1	5.2	3.2	4.6	6.2	3.4
Cholelithiasis and other disorders of gallbladder (K80-K82)	1.0	1.2	0.9	1.0	1.2	0.9	1.1	1.2	1.0	1.1	1.1	1.1
Nephritis, nephrotic syndrome, and nephrosis (N00-N07, N17-N19, N25-N27)	14.2	17.6	12.1	12.7	16.1	10.7	24.0	27.8	21.6	29.7	35.3	26.3
Acute and rapidly progressive nephritic and nephrotic syndrome (N00-N01, N04)	0.0	0.1	0.0	0.0	0.1	0.0	0.1	*	0.1	0.1	*	*
Chronic glomerulonephritis, nephritis, and nephropathy, not specified as acute or chronic, and renal sclerosis, unspecified (N02-N03, N05-N07, N26)	0.2	0.2	0.2	0.2	0.2	0.1	0.3	0.3	0.3	0.3	0.4	0.3
Renal failure (N17-N19)	13.9	17.3	11.9	12.5	15.8	10.5	23.6	27.3	21.2	29.3	34.8	25.9
Other disorders of kidney (N25, N27)	0.0	*	0.0	0.0	*	0.0	*	*	*	*	*	*
Infections of kidney (N10-N12, N13.6, N15.1)	0.3	0.2	0.3	0.3	0.2	0.3	0.3	0.2	0.3	0.3	0.2	0.3
Hyperplasia of prostate (N40)	0.1	0.4	X	0.1	0.4	X	0.2	0.4	X	0.2	0.5	X
Inflammatory diseases of female pelvic organs (N70-N76)	0.0	X	0.1	0.0	X	0.0	0.0	X	0.1	0.1	X	0.1
Pregnancy, childbirth, and the puerperium (O00-O99)	0.1	X	0.3	0.1	X	0.2	0.3	X	0.6	0.4	X	0.8
Pregnancy with abortive outcome (O00-O07)	0.0	X	0.0	*	X	*	*	X	*	*	X	*
Other complications of pregnancy, childbirth, and the puerperium (O10-O99)	0.1	X	0.2	0.1	X	0.2	0.3	X	0.5	0.3	X	0.7
Certain conditions originating in the perinatal period (P00-P96)	4.9	5.4	4.3	3.9	4.3	3.4	8.4	9.1	7.6	10.1	10.9	9.2
Congenital malformations, deformations, and chromosomal abnormalities (Q00-Q99)	3.7	3.8	3.5	3.7	3.8	3.5	3.6	3.9	3.5	4.1	4.4	3.9
Symptoms, signs, and abnormal clinical and laboratory findings, not elsewhere classified (R00-R99)	10.3	11.4	9.0	9.9	10.8	8.7	11.8	14.1	9.8	14.5	18.0	11.8
All other diseases (residual)	67.1	67.3	65.2	66.1	65.9	64.3	70.5	75.1	66.4	84.7	91.5	79.1

[1]Based on codes from the *International Classification of Diseases, Tenth Revision* (1992), except in cases where (*) precedes the cause of death code. Codes *U01-*U03 were added as of 2001 for deaths due to terrorism.
[2]Cause of death coding changes may affect comparability with the previous year's data for this cause.
0.0 = Quantity more than zero but less than 0.05.
* = Figure does not meet standards of reliability or precision.
X = Not applicable.

Table II-16. Age-Adjusted Death Rates for 113 Selected Causes, by Race and Sex, 2002—*Continued*

(Rate per 100,000 U.S. standard population.)

Cause of death [1]	All races			White			All other					
							Total			Black		
	Both sexes	Male	Female	Both sexes	Male	Female	Both sexes	Male	Female	Both sexes	Male	Female
Accidents (unintentional injuries) (V01-X59, Y85-Y86)	36.9	51.5	23.5	37.5	52.0	24.0	33.0	48.9	20.0	36.9	56.2	21.3
Transport accidents (V01-V99, Y85)	16.7	23.9	9.9	17.1	24.2	10.2	14.9	22.5	8.6	16.0	25.0	8.5
Motor vehicle accidents (V02-V04, V09.0, V09.2, V12-V14, V19.0-V19.2, V19.4-V19.6, V20-V79, V80.3-80.5, V81.0-V81.1, V82.0-V82.1, V83-V86, V87.0-V87.8, V88.0-V88.8, V89.0, V89.2)	15.7	22.1	9.6	16.0	22.4	9.8	14.1	20.9	8.3	15.0	23.2	8.2
Other land transport accidents (V01, V05-V06, V09.1, V09.3-V09.9, V10-V11, V15-V18, V19.3, V19.8-V19.9, V80.0-V80.2, V80.6-V80.9, V81.2-V81.9, V82.2-V82.9, V87.9, V88.9, V89.1, V89.3, V89.9)	0.4	0.6	0.1	0.4	0.6	0.1	0.4	0.8	0.2	0.5	0.9	0.1
Water, air and space, and other and unspecified transport accidents and their sequelae (V90-V99, Y85)	0.6	1.1	0.2	0.7	1.2	0.2	0.4	0.8	0.1	0.5	0.9	0.1
Nontransport accidents (W00-X59, Y86)	20.2	27.6	13.5	20.5	27.8	13.8	18.1	26.4	11.4	20.9	31.2	12.9
Falls (W00-W19)	5.6	7.4	4.3	5.9	7.6	4.6	3.4	5.1	2.2	3.1	4.9	2.0
Accidental discharge of firearms (W32-W34)	0.3	0.4	0.1	0.2	0.4	0.1	0.3	0.6	*	0.4	0.7	*
Accidental drowning and submersion (W65-W74)	1.2	2.0	0.5	1.1	1.8	0.4	1.5	2.5	0.6	1.6	2.7	0.5
Accidental exposure to smoke, fire, and flames (X00-X09)	1.1	1.4	0.8	0.9	1.3	0.7	1.9	2.5	1.4	2.4	3.3	1.7
Accidental poisoning and exposure to noxious substances (X40-X49)	6.1	8.4	3.7	6.3	8.7	3.9	5.3	7.8	3.1	6.8	10.1	3.9
Other and unspecified nontransport accidents and their sequelae (W20-W31, W35-W64, W75-W99, X10-X39, X50-X59, Y86)	5.9	7.9	4.2	5.9	7.9	4.2	5.7	8.0	4.1	6.7	9.4	4.7
Intentional self-harm (suicide) (*U03, X60-X84, Y87.0)	10.9	18.4	4.2	12.0	20.0	4.7	5.6	9.7	2.1	5.3	9.8	1.6
Intentional self-harm (suicide) by discharge of firearms (X72-X74)	5.9	11.1	1.4	6.5	12.1	1.6	2.6	5.2	0.5	3.0	5.9	0.5
Intentional self-harm (suicide) by other and unspecified means and their sequelae (*U03, X60-X71, X75-X84, Y87.0)	5.0	7.4	2.8	5.5	7.9	3.1	3.0	4.5	1.6	2.4	3.9	1.1
Assault (homicide) (*U01-*U02, X85-Y09, Y87.1)	6.1	9.4	2.8	3.7	5.3	2.0	15.7	26.7	5.5	21.0	36.4	6.9
Assault (homicide) by discharge of firearms (*U01.4, X93-X95)	4.1	6.8	1.3	2.2	3.4	1.0	11.4	20.6	2.7	15.6	28.7	3.5
Assault (homicide) by other and unspecified means and their sequelae (*U01.0-*U01.3, *U01.5-*U01.9, *U02, X85-X92, X96-Y09, Y87.1)	2.0	2.6	1.4	1.5	1.9	1.1	4.3	6.0	2.8	5.4	7.7	3.4
Legal intervention (Y35, Y89.0)	0.1	0.3	*	0.1	0.2	*	0.2	0.4	*	0.3	0.6	*
Events of undetermined intent (Y10-Y34, Y87.2, Y89.9)	1.7	2.2	1.2	1.7	2.2	1.2	1.6	2.4	1.0	2.1	3.1	1.2
Discharge of firearms, undetermined intent (Y22-Y24)	0.1	0.1	0.0	0.1	0.1	0.0	0.1	0.2	*	0.1	0.2	*
Other and unspecified events of undetermined intent and their sequelae (Y10-Y21, Y25-Y34, Y87.2, Y89.9)	1.6	2.0	1.1	1.6	2.0	1.2	1.6	2.2	1.0	2.0	2.9	1.2
Operations of war and their sequelae (Y36, Y89.1)	0.0	0.0	*	*	*	*	*	*	*	*	*	*
Complications of medical and surgical care (Y40-Y84, Y88)	1.0	1.0	1.0	0.9	1.0	0.9	1.3	1.3	1.3	1.6	1.6	1.6

[1]Based on codes from the *International Classification of Diseases, Tenth Revision* (1992), except in cases where (*) precedes the cause of death code. Codes *U01-*U03 were added as of 2001 for deaths due to terrorism.

0.0 = Quantity more than zero but less than 0.05.

* = Figure does not meet standards of reliability or precision.

TABLE II-17. AGE-ADJUSTED DEATH RATES FOR 113 SELECTED CAUSES, BY RACE, HISPANIC ORIGIN, AND SEX, 2002

The overall age-adjusted Hispanic death rate amounted to only 73 percent of the non-Hispanic rate. Average death rates for Hispanic males were 52 percent greater than those for Hispanic females, as compared to a 42 percent difference between non-Hispanic males and females. Cancer mortality rates were significantly lower for Hispanics than for non-Hispanics. Hispanics were more affected by diabetes than non-Hispanic Whites, but an even larger death rate for this disease occurred among non-Hispanic Blacks.

Suicide occurred only about half as often among Hispanics as non-Hispanics. The low Hispanic suicide rate was about the same as the rate for non-Hispanic Blacks. Hispanics were victims of homicide more than twice as frequently as non-Hispanic Whites, but much less frequently than non-Hispanic Blacks.

Table II-17. Age-Adjusted Death Rates for 113 Selected Causes, by Race, Hispanic Origin, and Sex, 2002

(Rate per 100,000 U.S. standard population.)

Cause of death [1]	All origins [2] Both sexes	Male	Female	Hispanic [3] Both sexes	Male	Female	Non-Hispanic [4] Both sexes	Male	Female	Non-Hispanic White Both sexes	Male	Female	Non-Hispanic Black Both sexes	Male	Female
ALL CAUSES	845.3	1 013.7	715.2	629.3	766.7	518.3	856.5	1 026.5	725.8	837.5	1 002.2	709.9	1 099.2	1 360.6	915.3
Salmonella infections (A01-A02)	0.0	*	*	*	*	*	*	*	*	*	*	*	*	*	*
Shigellosis and amebiasis (A03, A06)	*	*	*	*	*	*	*	*	*	*	*	*	*	*	*
Certain other intestinal infections (A04, A07-A09)	0.8	0.8	0.8	0.5	0.5	0.5	0.9	0.9	0.8	0.9	0.9	0.9	0.6	0.7	0.6
Tuberculosis (A16-A19)	0.3	0.4	0.2	0.5	0.6	0.4	0.3	0.4	0.2	0.1	0.2	0.1	0.8	1.1	0.5
Respiratory tuberculosis (A16)	0.2	0.3	0.1	0.4	0.5	0.3	0.2	0.3	0.1	0.1	0.2	0.1	0.6	0.9	0.4
Other tuberculosis (A17-A19)	0.0	0.1	0.0	*	*	*	0.0	0.1	0.0	0.0	0.0	0.0	0.1	0.2	*
Whooping cough (A37)	*	*	*	*	*	*	*	*	*	*	*	*	*	*	*
Scarlet fever and erysipelas (A38, A46)	*	*	*	*	*	*	*	*	*	*	*	*	*	*	*
Meningococcal infection (A39)	0.0	0.1	0.0	*	*	*	0.0	0.1	0.0	0.0	0.1	0.0	0.1	*	*
Septicemia (A40-A41)	11.7	12.9	10.9	8.9	9.8	8.1	11.9	13.0	11.1	10.7	11.7	10.0	24.6	28.1	22.4
Syphilis (A50-A53)	0.0	0.0	0.0	*	*	*	0.0	0.0	*	*	*	*	0.1	*	*
Acute poliomyelitis (A80)	*	*	*	*	*	*	*	*	*	*	*	*	*	*	*
Arthropod-borne viral encephalitis (A83-A84, A85.2)	*	*	*	*	*	*	*	*	*	*	*	*	*	*	*
Measles (B05)	*	*	*	*	*	*	*	*	*	*	*	*	*	*	*
Viral hepatitis (B15-B19)	2.0	2.7	1.3	3.3	4.2	2.4	1.9	2.6	1.2	1.7	2.4	1.1	2.8	3.9	1.9
Human immunodeficiency virus (HIV) disease (B20-B24)	4.9	7.4	2.5	5.8	9.1	2.6	4.8	7.2	2.5	2.1	3.5	0.6	23.0	33.9	13.8
Malaria (B50-B54)	*	*	*	*	*	*	*	*	*	*	*	*	*	*	*
Other and unspecified infectious and parasitic diseases and their sequelae (A00, A05, A20-A36, A42-A44, A48-A49, A54-A79, A81-A82, A85.0-A85.1, A85.8, A86-B04, B06-B09, B25-B49, B55-B99)	2.3	2.9	1.9	2.5	3.2	1.9	2.3	2.8	1.9	2.2	2.6	1.8	3.2	4.1	2.5
Malignant neoplasms (C00-C97)	193.5	238.9	163.1	128.4	161.4	106.1	197.4	243.4	166.6	195.6	239.6	165.9	242.5	324.4	193.4
Malignant neoplasms of lip, oral cavity, and pharynx (C00-C14)	2.7	4.1	1.5	1.5	2.6	0.7	2.8	4.1	1.6	2.6	3.9	1.5	3.7	6.4	1.7
Malignant neoplasm of esophagus (C15)	4.4	7.8	1.7	2.3	4.2	0.9	4.5	8.0	1.8	4.5	8.0	1.7	6.0	10.3	3.0
Malignant neoplasm of stomach (C16)	4.2	5.9	3.0	6.6	8.8	5.0	4.1	5.7	2.8	3.5	4.9	2.3	8.5	12.1	6.2
Malignant neoplasms of colon, rectum, and anus (C18-C21)	19.7	23.7	16.7	13.7	16.9	11.2	20.0	24.1	17.0	19.5	23.5	16.5	27.2	33.6	23.1
Malignant neoplasms of liver and intrahepatic bile ducts (C22)	4.9	7.1	3.0	7.5	10.7	4.9	4.7	6.9	2.9	4.2	6.2	2.7	6.4	10.0	3.7
Malignant neoplasm of pancreas (C25)	10.5	12.1	9.2	7.9	8.4	7.4	10.7	12.3	9.3	10.5	12.2	9.0	13.8	15.5	12.5
Malignant neoplasm of larynx (C32)	1.3	2.3	0.5	0.9	1.7	0.3	1.3	2.4	0.5	1.2	2.2	0.5	2.5	4.9	0.9
Malignant neoplasms of trachea, bronchus, and lung (C33-C34)	54.9	73.2	41.6	23.7	36.2	14.6	56.9	75.6	43.3	57.5	75.0	44.6	62.9	96.6	40.8
Malignant melanoma of skin (C43)	2.6	3.8	1.7	0.8	0.8	0.7	2.7	4.0	1.8	3.1	4.5	2.1	0.4	0.5	0.3
Malignant neoplasm of breast (C50)	14.5	0.3	25.6	8.6	*	15.5	14.8	0.3	26.2	14.4	0.3	25.6	20.5	0.6	34.6
Malignant neoplasm of cervix uteri (C53)	1.3	X	2.6	1.7	X	3.1	1.3	X	2.5	1.1	X	2.2	2.9	X	5.0
Malignant neoplasms of corpus uteri and uterus, part unspecified (C54-C55)	2.4	X	4.2	1.9	X	3.3	2.4	X	4.2	2.2	X	3.9	4.5	X	7.4
Malignant neoplasm of ovary (C56)	5.1	X	9.0	3.3	X	6.0	5.2	X	9.2	5.4	X	9.6	4.5	X	7.5
Malignant neoplasm of prostate (C61)	10.6	27.9	X	8.4	21.6	X	10.7	28.2	X	9.8	25.8	X	22.2	62.8	X
Malignant neoplasms of kidney and renal pelvis (C64-C65)	4.2	6.1	2.8	3.6	5.3	2.3	4.2	6.2	2.8	4.4	6.3	2.9	4.1	5.9	2.9
Malignant neoplasms of bladder (C67)	4.4	7.5	2.4	2.5	4.2	1.5	4.5	7.7	2.4	4.6	8.0	2.4	4.0	5.5	3.1
Malignant neoplasms of meninges, brain, and other parts of central nervous system (C70-C72)	4.4	5.5	3.6	2.9	3.4	2.4	4.6	5.6	3.7	4.9	6.1	4.0	2.6	3.2	2.2
Malignant neoplasms of lymphoid, hematopoietic, and related tissue (C81-C96)	19.5	25.1	15.5	14.5	17.4	12.4	19.8	25.5	15.7	20.1	26.0	15.8	19.6	24.8	16.2
Hodgkin's disease (C81)	0.5	0.6	0.4	0.4	0.5	0.4	0.5	0.6	0.4	0.5	0.6	0.4	0.4	0.6	0.3
Non-Hodgkin's lymphoma (C82-C85)	7.6	9.6	6.2	5.8	6.6	5.2	7.7	9.7	6.2	8.0	10.1	6.5	5.4	6.9	4.4
Leukemia (C91-C95)	7.5	10.0	5.7	4.9	6.0	4.1	7.6	10.2	5.7	7.8	10.5	5.9	6.7	8.8	5.4
Multiple myeloma and immunoproliferative neoplasms (C88, C90)	4.0	5.0	3.3	3.4	4.3	2.7	4.0	5.0	3.3	3.7	4.8	3.0	7.0	8.4	6.1
Other and unspecified malignant neoplasms of lymphoid, hematopoietic, and related tissue (C96)	0.0	0.0	0.0	*	*	*	0.0	0.0	0.0	0.0	0.0	0.0	*	*	*
All other and unspecified malignant neoplasms (C17, C23-C24, C26-C31, C37-C41, C44-C49, C51-C52, C57-C60, C62-C63, C66, C68-C69, C73-C80, C97)	21.8	26.5	18.5	16.2	19.1	14.0	22.2	26.9	18.7	22.1	26.8	18.6	26.1	31.8	22.3
In situ neoplasms, benign neoplasms, and neoplasms of uncertain or unknown behavior (D00-D48)	4.6	5.7	3.9	3.2	3.7	2.8	4.7	5.8	4.0	4.8	5.9	4.0	4.5	5.2	4.1
Anemias (D50-D64)	1.6	1.6	1.6	1.3	1.6	1.1	1.6	1.6	1.6	1.3	1.3	1.4	3.7	4.0	3.5
Diabetes mellitus (E10-E14)	25.4	28.6	23.0	35.6	38.1	33.6	24.8	28.0	22.3	22.2	25.9	19.3	50.3	50.3	49.4
Nutritional deficiencies (E40-E64)	1.3	1.2	1.3	1.0	1.0	1.0	1.3	1.2	1.3	1.2	1.2	1.3	2.2	2.1	2.1
Malnutrition (E40-E46)	1.2	1.1	1.2	1.0	1.0	0.9	1.2	1.2	1.2	1.1	1.1	1.2	2.0	2.0	2.0
Other nutritional deficiencies (E50-E64)	0.1	0.1	0.1	*	*	*	0.1	0.1	0.1	0.1	0.1	0.1	0.1	*	*
Meningitis (G00, G03)	0.2	0.3	0.2	0.3	0.3	0.2	0.2	0.3	0.2	0.2	0.2	0.2	0.6	0.8	0.4
Parkinson's disease (G20-G21)	5.9	9.0	4.1	3.5	5.1	2.6	6.0	9.2	4.1	6.4	9.7	4.4	2.5	4.0	1.7
Alzheimer's disease (G30)	20.2	16.6	22.0	11.6	9.7	12.6	20.6	17.0	22.4	21.5	17.7	23.4	15.3	13.2	16.1

[1] Based on codes from the *International Classification of Diseases, Tenth Revision* (1992), except in cases where (*) precedes the cause of death code. Codes *U01-*U03 were added as of 2001 for deaths due to terrorism.
[2] Figures for origin not stated are included in "All origins" but not distributed among specified origins.
[3] May be of any race.
[4] Includes races other than White and Black.
0.0 = Quantity more than zero but less than 0.05.
* = Figure does not meet standards of reliability or precision.
X = Not applicable.

Table II-17. Age-Adjusted Death Rates for 113 Selected Causes, by Race, Hispanic Origin, and Sex, 2002—Continued

(Rate per 100,000 U.S. standard population.)

Cause of death [1]	All origins [2] Both sexes	Male	Female	Hispanic [3] Both sexes	Male	Female	Non-Hispanic [4] Both sexes	Male	Female	Non-Hispanic White Both sexes	Male	Female	Non-Hispanic Black Both sexes	Male	Female
Major cardiovascular diseases (I00-I78)	317.4	377.2	270.5	236.3	280.1	201.7	321.1	382.0	273.4	313.4	374.8	264.9	421.3	493.6	368.4
Diseases of heart (I00-I09, I11, I13, I20-I51)	240.8	297.4	197.2	180.5	219.8	149.7	243.7	301.4	199.3	239.2	297.7	193.7	312.1	375.5	266.4
Acute rheumatic fever and chronic rheumatic heart diseases (I00-I09)	1.2	0.9	1.5	1.1	0.6	1.4	1.2	0.9	1.5	1.3	0.9	1.5	0.9	0.8	1.0
Hypertensive heart disease (I11)	9.1	9.5	8.3	8.4	9.7	7.1	9.2	9.5	8.4	7.5	7.6	7.0	24.7	28.2	21.5
Hypertensive heart and renal disease (I13)	1.0	1.0	0.9	1.1	1.2	1.0	1.0	1.0	0.9	0.7	0.7	0.7	3.6	3.9	3.2
Ischemic heart diseases (I20-I25)	170.8	220.4	133.6	138.3	172.2	112.2	172.3	222.7	134.4	171.0	222.7	131.7	205.1	253.2	171.4
Acute myocardial infarction (I21-I22)	62.1	80.6	48.1	49.5	61.6	40.2	62.8	81.7	48.5	62.5	82.1	47.4	75.0	90.9	64.1
Other acute ischemic heart diseases (I24)	1.2	1.5	0.9	0.4	0.5	0.3	1.2	1.5	1.0	1.2	1.5	0.9	1.7	2.3	1.3
Other forms of chronic ischemic heart disease (I20, I25)	107.6	138.3	84.5	88.4	110.0	71.8	108.3	139.5	84.9	107.3	139.1	83.4	128.5	160.0	106.1
Atherosclerotic cardiovascular disease, so described (I25.0)	23.5	30.4	17.8	19.3	26.2	13.9	23.6	30.4	17.9	22.1	28.4	16.8	40.6	55.2	30.3
All other forms of chronic ischemic heart disease (I20, I25.1-I25.9)	84.1	108.0	66.7	69.1	83.9	57.9	84.7	109.1	66.9	85.2	110.7	66.6	87.9	104.8	75.8
Other heart diseases (I26-I51)	58.5	65.5	52.8	31.5	36.1	27.9	60.0	67.2	54.1	58.6	65.7	52.9	77.8	89.3	69.2
Acute and subacute endocarditis (I33)	0.4	0.5	0.3	0.3	0.5	0.2	0.4	0.5	0.3	0.4	0.5	0.3	0.7	0.8	0.6
Diseases of pericardium and acute myocarditis (I30-I31, I40)	0.3	0.3	0.3	0.3	0.3	0.2	0.3	0.3	0.3	0.3	0.3	0.2	0.5	0.5	0.5
Heart failure (I50)	19.5	20.4	18.6	10.2	10.7	9.8	19.9	20.9	18.9	19.9	21.0	19.0	22.1	23.7	20.7
All other forms of heart disease (I26-I28, I34-I38, I42-I49, I51)	38.4	44.2	33.7	20.7	24.7	17.7	39.4	45.5	34.6	38.1	43.9	33.4	54.6	64.2	47.5
Essential (primary) hypertension and hypertensive renal disease (I10, I12)	7.0	6.8	7.0	6.2	6.0	6.3	7.0	6.8	7.0	6.0	5.8	6.0	17.2	18.0	16.4
Cerebrovascular diseases (I60-I69)	56.2	56.5	55.2	41.3	44.3	38.6	56.8	57.0	55.9	54.6	54.4	53.9	77.5	83.0	72.8
Atherosclerosis (I70)	4.7	4.9	4.6	3.1	3.3	3.0	4.8	5.0	4.6	4.9	5.1	4.7	4.5	5.0	4.1
Other diseases of circulatory system (I71-I78)	8.7	11.5	6.6	5.2	6.6	4.1	8.8	11.8	6.7	8.8	11.9	6.6	10.1	12.2	8.7
Aortic aneurysm and dissection (I71)	5.2	7.7	3.3	2.5	3.8	1.6	5.3	7.9	3.4	5.4	8.1	3.5	4.7	6.1	3.6
Other diseases of arteries, arterioles, and capillaries (I72-I78)	3.5	3.8	3.3	2.7	2.9	2.6	3.5	3.9	3.3	3.4	3.7	3.2	5.5	6.1	5.1
Other disorders of circulatory system (I80-I99)	1.6	1.6	1.6	1.1	1.0	1.2	1.7	1.6	1.6	1.6	1.5	1.6	2.9	3.2	2.7
Influenza and pneumonia (J10-J18)	22.6	27.0	19.9	19.2	23.3	16.5	22.7	27.1	20.0	22.6	26.8	20.0	24.3	31.2	20.3
Influenza (J10-J11) [5]	0.2	0.3	0.2	*	*	*	0.2	0.3	0.2	0.3	0.3	0.2	0.1	*	*
Pneumonia (J12-J18)	22.4	26.7	19.6	19.2	23.2	16.4	22.5	26.9	19.8	22.4	26.5	19.8	24.2	31.1	20.2
Other acute lower respiratory infections (J20-J22)	0.1	0.1	0.1	0.1	*	*	0.1	0.1	0.1	0.1	0.1	0.1	0.1	0.1	0.1
Acute bronchitis and bronchiolitis (J20-J21)	0.1	0.1	0.1	*	*	*	0.1	0.1	0.1	0.1	0.1	0.1	0.1	0.1	*
Unspecified acute lower respiratory infection (J22)	0.0	0.0	0.0	*	*	*	0.0	0.0	0.0	0.0	0.0	0.0	*	*	*
Chronic lower respiratory diseases (J40-J47)	43.5	53.5	37.4	20.6	27.2	16.2	44.8	54.9	38.6	46.9	56.5	41.2	31.5	46.8	22.9
Bronchitis, chronic and unspecified (J40-J42)	0.3	0.4	0.3	0.3	0.3	0.3	0.3	0.4	0.3	0.3	0.4	0.3	0.2	0.3	0.2
Emphysema (J43)	5.4	7.0	4.4	2.0	2.8	1.5	5.6	7.2	4.6	6.0	7.5	5.0	3.5	5.9	2.1
Asthma (J45-J46)	1.5	1.2	1.7	1.3	1.0	1.5	1.5	1.2	1.7	1.2	0.9	1.4	3.5	3.4	3.5
Other chronic lower respiratory diseases (J44, J47)	36.2	44.9	31.1	16.9	23.1	12.9	37.3	46.0	32.1	39.4	47.7	34.5	24.3	37.3	17.1
Pneumoconioses and chemical effects (J60-J66, J68)	0.4	1.0	0.0	0.2	0.5	*	0.4	1.0	0.0	0.4	1.0	0.0	0.2	0.6	*
Pneumonitis due to solids and liquids (J69)	6.1	8.4	4.7	3.9	5.3	3.1	6.2	8.6	4.8	6.2	8.7	4.8	6.7	9.4	5.2
Other diseases of respiratory system (J00-J06, J30-J39, J67, J70-J98)	8.7	10.4	7.6	7.5	8.4	6.7	8.7	10.5	7.6	8.8	10.5	7.6	8.6	10.1	7.5
Peptic ulcer (K25-K28)	1.4	1.7	1.2	1.2	1.6	0.8	1.4	1.7	1.2	1.4	1.7	1.2	1.4	2.0	1.1
Diseases of appendix (K35-K38)	0.2	0.2	0.1	0.1	*	*	0.2	0.2	0.1	0.1	0.2	0.1	0.2	0.4	0.1
Hernia (K40-K46)	0.5	0.5	0.6	0.5	0.4	0.5	0.5	0.5	0.6	0.6	0.5	0.6	0.5	0.6	0.5
Chronic liver disease and cirrhosis (K70, K73-K74)	9.4	12.9	6.3	15.4	22.3	9.0	8.9	12.0	6.1	9.0	12.2	6.1	8.6	12.1	5.8
Alcoholic liver disease (K70)	4.2	6.3	2.2	6.9	12.1	2.1	3.9	5.8	2.2	3.9	5.8	2.2	3.9	5.9	2.3
Other chronic liver disease and cirrhosis (K73-K74)	5.2	6.5	4.1	8.5	10.2	6.9	5.0	6.2	3.9	5.1	6.3	4.0	4.7	6.2	3.5
Cholelithiasis and other disorders of gallbladder (K80-K82)	1.0	1.2	0.9	1.2	1.3	1.1	1.0	1.2	0.9	1.0	1.2	0.9	1.1	1.1	1.1
Nephritis, nephrotic syndrome, and nephrosis (N00-N07, N17-N19, N25-N27)	14.2	17.6	12.1	11.6	13.7	10.2	14.3	17.8	12.2	12.7	16.1	10.6	30.1	35.8	26.7
Acute and rapidly progressive nephritic and nephrotic syndrome (N00-N01, N04)	0.0	0.1	0.0	*	*	*	0.0	0.1	0.0	0.0	0.0	0.0	0.1	*	*
Chronic glomerulonephritis, nephritis, and nephropathy, not specified as acute or chronic, and renal sclerosis, unspecified (N02-N03, N05-N07, N26)	0.2	0.2	0.2	0.2	*	*	0.2	0.2	0.2	0.2	0.2	0.1	0.3	0.4	0.3
Renal failure (N17-N19)	13.9	17.3	11.9	11.4	13.4	9.9	14.0	17.4	11.9	12.5	15.9	10.4	29.7	35.3	26.3
Other disorders of kidney (N25, N27)	0.0	*	0.0	*	*	*	0.0	*	0.0	0.0	*	0.0	*	*	*
Infections of kidney (N10-N12, N13.6, N15.1)	0.3	0.2	0.3	0.3	*	0.3	0.3	0.2	0.3	0.3	0.2	0.3	0.3	0.3	0.3
Hyperplasia of prostate (N40)	0.1	0.4	X	*	*	X	0.1	0.4	X	0.1	0.4	X	0.2	0.5	X
Inflammatory diseases of female pelvic organs (N70-N76)	0.0	X	0.1	*	X	*	0.0	X	0.1	0.0	X	0.0	0.1	X	0.1
Pregnancy, childbirth, and the puerperium (O00-O99)	0.1	X	0.3	0.2	X	0.3	0.1	X	0.2	0.1	X	0.2	0.4	X	0.8
Pregnancy with abortive outcome (O00-O07)	0.0	X	0.0	*	X	*	0.0	X	0.0	*	X	*	*	X	*
Other complications of pregnancy, childbirth, and the puerperium (O10-O99)	0.1	X	0.2	0.2	X	0.3	0.1	X	0.2	0.1	X	0.1	0.4	X	0.7
Certain conditions originating in the perinatal period (P00-P96)	4.9	5.4	4.3	4.0	4.4	3.6	5.0	5.6	4.5	3.8	4.2	3.3	10.2	11.1	9.3
Congenital malformations, deformations, and chromosomal abnormalities (Q00-Q99)	3.7	3.8	3.5	3.4	3.6	3.2	3.7	3.8	3.5	3.6	3.8	3.4	4.2	4.5	4.0
Symptoms, signs, and abnormal clinical and laboratory findings, not elsewhere classified (R00-R99)	10.3	11.4	9.0	5.5	6.6	4.5	10.7	11.8	9.3	10.2	11.1	9.0	14.8	18.2	12.0
All other diseases (residual)	67.1	67.3	65.2	45.2	48.8	41.7	68.2	68.3	66.3	67.1	66.7	65.3	86.1	92.8	80.5

[1] Based on codes from the *International Classification of Diseases, Tenth Revision* (1992), except in cases where (*) precedes the cause of death code. Codes *U01-*U03 were added as of 2001 for deaths due to terrorism.
[2] Figures for origin not stated are included in "All origins" but not distributed among specified origins.
[3] May be of any race.
[4] Includes races other than White and Black.
[5] Cause of death coding changes may affect comparability with the previous year's data for this cause.
0.0 = Quantity more than zero but less than 0.05.
* = Figure does not meet standards of reliability or precision.
X = Not applicable.

Table II-17. Age-Adjusted Death Rates for 113 Selected Causes, by Race, Hispanic Origin, and Sex, 2002—*Continued*

(Rate per 100,000 U.S. standard population.)

Cause of death [1]	All origins [2] Both sexes	Male	Female	Hispanic [3] Both sexes	Male	Female	Non-Hispanic [4] Both sexes	Male	Female	Non-Hispanic White Both sexes	Male	Female	Non-Hispanic Black Both sexes	Male	Female
Accidents (unintentional injuries) (V01-X59, Y85-Y86)	36.9	51.5	23.5	30.7	45.6	16.1	37.3	51.8	24.2	38.0	52.3	24.8	37.6	57.2	21.8
Transport accidents (V01-V99, Y85)	16.7	23.9	9.9	16.0	23.4	8.4	16.7	23.8	10.1	17.1	24.1	10.5	16.2	25.4	8.6
Motor vehicle accidents (V02-V04, V09.0, V09.2, V12-V14, V19.0-V19.2, V19.4-V19.6, V20-V79, V80.3-80.5, V81.0-V81.1, V82.0-V82.1, V83-V86, V87.0-V87.8, V88.0-V88.8, V89.0, V89.2)	15.7	22.1	9.6	15.2	22.2	8.1	15.7	22.0	9.8	16.0	22.2	10.1	15.2	23.5	8.4
Other land transport accidents (V01, V05-V06, V09.1, V09.3-V09.9, V10-V11, V15-V18, V19.3, V19.8-V19.9, V80.0-V80.2, V80.6-V80.9, V81.2-V81.9, V82.2-V82.9, V87.9, V88.9, V89.1, V89.3, V89.9)	0.4	0.6	0.1	0.4	0.7	0.1	0.4	0.6	0.1	0.4	0.6	0.1	0.5	1.0	0.1
Water, air and space, and other and unspecified transport accidents and their sequelae (V90-V99, Y85)	0.6	1.1	0.2	0.3	0.6	*	0.7	1.2	0.2	0.8	1.3	0.2	0.5	0.9	0.1
Nontransport accidents (W00-X59, Y86)	20.2	27.6	13.5	14.7	22.1	7.7	20.6	28.0	14.0	20.9	28.2	14.3	21.3	31.7	13.2
Falls (W00-W19)	5.6	7.4	4.3	4.3	6.1	2.9	5.6	7.4	4.4	5.9	7.6	4.6	3.1	4.9	2.0
Accidental discharge of firearms (W32-W34)	0.3	0.4	0.1	0.2	0.2	*	0.3	0.5	0.1	0.3	0.5	0.1	0.4	0.8	*
Accidental drowning and submersion (W65-W74)	1.2	2.0	0.5	1.1	1.9	0.3	1.2	1.9	0.5	1.1	1.7	0.5	1.6	2.8	0.5
Accidental exposure to smoke, fire, and flames (X00-X09)	1.1	1.4	0.8	0.8	1.0	0.5	1.2	1.5	0.8	1.0	1.3	0.7	2.5	3.3	1.8
Accidental poisoning and exposure to noxious substances (X40-X49)	6.1	8.4	3.7	4.7	7.3	2.0	6.3	8.6	4.0	6.6	9.0	4.2	6.9	10.3	4.0
Other and unspecified nontransport accidents and their sequelae (W20-W31, W35-W64, W75-W99, X10-X39, X50-X59, Y86)	5.9	7.9	4.2	3.6	5.5	2.0	6.1	8.1	4.3	6.1	8.1	4.3	6.8	9.6	4.8
Intentional self-harm (suicide) (*U03, X60-X84, Y87.0)	10.9	18.4	4.2	5.7	9.9	1.8	11.6	19.5	4.5	12.9	21.4	5.1	5.4	10.0	1.6
Intentional self-harm (suicide) by discharge of firearms (X72-X74)	5.9	11.1	1.4	2.5	4.8	0.4	6.3	11.8	1.5	7.0	13.0	1.8	3.0	6.0	0.5
Intentional self-harm (suicide) by other and unspecified means and their sequelae (*U03, X60-X71, X75-X84, Y87.0)	5.0	7.4	2.8	3.2	5.1	1.4	5.3	7.7	3.0	5.8	8.4	3.3	2.4	3.9	1.1
Assault (homicide) (*U01-*U02, X85-Y09, Y87.1)	6.1	9.4	2.8	7.3	11.6	2.5	5.8	8.9	2.8	2.8	3.7	1.9	21.6	37.4	7.0
Assault (homicide) by discharge of firearms (*U01.4, X93-X95)	4.1	6.8	1.3	4.8	8.1	1.2	3.9	6.5	1.3	1.6	2.2	0.9	16.1	29.5	3.6
Assault (homicide) by other and unspecified means and their sequelae (*U01.0-*U01.3, *U01.5-*U01.9, *U02, X85-X92, X96-Y09, Y87.1)	2.0	2.6	1.4	2.4	3.5	1.4	1.9	2.4	1.4	1.3	1.6	1.0	5.5	7.9	3.5
Legal intervention (Y35, Y89.0)	0.1	0.3	*	0.2	0.3	*	0.1	0.3	*	0.1	0.2	*	0.3	0.6	*
Events of undetermined intent (Y10-Y34, Y87.2, Y89.9)	1.7	2.2	1.2	0.8	1.3	0.4	1.8	2.3	1.3	1.8	2.3	1.3	2.1	3.1	1.3
Discharge of firearms, undetermined intent (Y22-Y24)	0.1	0.1	0.0	0.1	0.1	*	0.1	0.1	0.0	0.1	0.1	0.0	0.1	0.2	*
Other and unspecified events of undetermined intent and their sequelae (Y10-Y21, Y25-Y34, Y87.2, Y89.9)	1.6	2.0	1.1	0.8	1.2	0.4	1.7	2.2	1.2	1.7	2.2	1.3	2.0	2.9	1.2
Operations of war and their sequelae (Y36, Y89.1)	*	0.0	*	*	*	*	*	*	*	*	*	*	*	*	*
Complications of medical and surgical care (Y40-Y84, Y88)	1.0	1.0	1.0	0.7	0.6	0.7	1.0	1.0	1.0	0.9	1.0	0.9	1.6	1.7	1.6

[1]Based on codes from the *International Classification of Diseases, Tenth Revision* (1992), except in cases where (*) precedes the cause of death code. Codes *U01-*U03 were added as of 2001 for deaths due to terrorism.
[2]Figures for origin not stated are included in "All origins" but not distributed among specified origins.
[3]May be of any race.
[4]Includes races other than White and Black.
0.0 = Quantity more than zero but less than 0.05.
* = Figure does not meet standards of reliability or precision.

TABLE II-18. NUMBER OF DEATHS, DEATH RATES, AND AGE-ADJUSTED DEATH RATES FOR INJURY DEATHS, ACCORDING TO MECHANISM AND INTENT OF DEATH, 1999–2002

This table classifies deaths from injury from 1999 to 2002 in two different ways: by type of hazard (drowning, firearms, etc.), and by whether the injury was inflicted intentionally (by homicide or suicide) or accidentally (this classification also includes injuries of undetermined intent). There were 161,269 deaths due to injury in 2002. The five leading mechanisms of injury death were motor vehicle traffic accidents (27 percent), firearms (19 percent), poisoning (16 percent), falls (11 percent), and suffocation (8 percent), which together accounted for 81 percent of all injury deaths in 2002.

For all injuries combined in 2002, 106,000 deaths (66 percent) were unintentional, 32,000 (20 percent) were classified as suicides, 18,000 (11 percent) were homicides, 4,830 (3 percent) were of undetermined intent, and 404 were caused by legal intervention or war. Motor vehicle traffic accidents caused 44,065 deaths in 2002, including those of 3,153 motorcyclists, 550 bicyclists, and 5,041 pedestrians. Firearms caused more than 30,200 fatalities in 2002; 17,100 (57 percent) of these were suicides. The next largest category was poisoning, which caused 26,400 deaths in 2002. Although the majority of these fatalities were unintentional, one-fifth represented suicides. Falls, mostly unintentional, were also a major cause of death in 2002, claiming 17,100 lives.

The age-adjusted rate for all injury deaths increased by over 5 percent between 2000 and 2002. This trend was

Table II-18. Number of Deaths, Death Rates, and Age-Adjusted Death Rates for Injury Deaths, According to Mechanism and Intent of Death, 1999–2002

(Number, rate per 100,000 population.)

Mechanism and intent of death [1]	Deaths				Death rate				Age-adjusted death rate			
	2002	2001	2000	1999	2002	2001	2000	1999	2002	2001	2000	1999
ALL INJURY (*U01-*U03, V01-Y36, Y85-Y87, Y89) [2]	161 269	157 078	148 209	148 286	55.9	55.2	52.7	53.1	55.7	55.1	52.8	53.3
Unintentional (V01-X59, Y85-Y86)	106 742	101 537	97 900	97 860	37.0	35.7	34.8	35.1	36.9	35.7	34.9	35.3
Suicide (*U03, X60-X84, Y87.0) [2]	31 655	30 622	29 350	29 199	11.0	10.8	10.4	10.5	10.9	10.7	10.4	10.5
Homicide (*U01-*U02, X85-Y09, Y87.1) [2]	17 638	20 308	16 765	16 889	6.1	7.1	6.0	6.1	6.1	7.1	5.9	6.0
Undetermined (Y10-Y34, Y87.2, Y89.9)	4 830	4 198	3 819	3 917	1.7	1.5	1.4	1.4	1.7	1.5	1.3	1.4
Legal intervention/war (Y35-Y36, Y89 [.0, .1])	404	413	375	421	0.1	0.1	0.1	0.2	0.1	0.2	0.1	0.2
Cut/Pierce (W25-W29, W45, X78, X99, Y28, Y35.4)	2 762	2 532	2 288	2 369	1.0	0.9	0.8	0.8	1.0	0.9	0.8	0.8
Unintentional (W25-W29, W45)	109	85	85	74	0.0	0.0	0.0	0.0	0.0	0.0	0.0	0.0
Suicide (X78)	566	458	383	404	0.2	0.2	0.1	0.1	0.2	0.2	0.1	0.1
Homicide (X99)	2 074	1 971	1 805	1 879	0.7	0.7	0.6	0.7	0.7	0.7	0.6	0.7
Undetermined (Y28)	13	18	15	12	*	*	*	*	*	*	*	*
Legal intervention/war (Y35.4)	-	-	-	-								
Drowning (W65-W74, X71, X92, Y21)	4 146	3 923	4 073	4 153	1.4	1.4	1.4	1.5	1.4	1.4	1.4	1.5
Unintentional (W65-W74)	3 447	3 281	3 482	3 529	1.2	1.2	1.2	1.3	1.2	1.1	1.2	1.3
Suicide (X71)	368	339	321	311	0.1	0.1	0.1	0.1	0.1	0.1	0.1	0.1
Homicide (X92)	72	68	39	70	0.0	0.0	0.0	0.0	0.0	0.0	0.0	0.0
Undetermined (Y21)	259	235	231	243	0.1	0.1	0.1	0.1	0.1	0.1	0.1	0.1
Fall (W00-W19, X80, Y01, Y30)	17 116	15 764	14 002	13 931	5.9	5.5	5.0	5.0	5.9	5.6	5.1	5.1
Unintentional (W00-W19)	16 257	15 019	13 322	13 162	5.6	5.3	4.7	4.7	5.6	5.3	4.8	4.8
Suicide (X80)	740	651	607	693	0.3	0.2	0.2	0.2	0.2	0.2	0.2	0.3
Homicide (Y01)	16	17	18	17	*	*	*	*	*	*	*	*
Undetermined (Y30)	103	77	55	59	0.0	0.0	0.0	0.0	0.0	0.0	0.0	0.0
Fire/Hot Object or Substance (*U01.3, X00-X19, X76-X77, X97-X98, Y26-Y27, Y36.3) [3]	3 645	3 796	3 907	3 910	1.3	1.3	1.4	1.4	1.3	1.3	1.4	1.4
Unintentional (X00-X19)	3 261	3 423	3 487	3 471	1.1	1.2	1.2	1.2	1.1	1.2	1.2	1.2
Suicide (X76-X77)	150	148	162	171	0.1	0.1	0.1	0.1	0.1	0.1	0.1	0.1
Homicide (*U01.3, X97-X98)	134	148	181	197	0.0	0.1	0.1	0.1	0.0	0.0	0.1	0.1
Undetermined (Y26-Y27)	100	77	77	71	0.0	0.0	0.0	0.0	0.0	0.0	0.0	0.0
Legal intervention/war (Y36.3)	-	-	-	-	*	*	*	*	*	*	*	*
Fire/Flame (X00-X09, X76, X97, Y26)	3 539	3 673	3 789	3 779	1.2	1.3	1.3	1.4	1.2	1.3	1.4	1.3
Unintentional (X00-X09)	3 159	3 309	3 377	3 348	1.1	1.2	1.2	1.2	1.1	1.2	1.2	1.2
Suicide (X76)	150	147	162	171	0.1	0.1	0.1	0.1	0.1	0.1	0.1	0.1
Homicide (X97)	131	141	174	190	0.0	0.0	0.1	0.1	0.0	0.0	0.1	0.1
Undetermined (Y26)	99	76	76	70	0.0	0.0	0.0	0.0	0.0	0.0	0.0	0.0
Hot Object/Substance (X10-X19, X77, X98, Y27)	106	123	118	131	0.0	0.0	0.0	0.0	0.0	0.0	0.0	0.0
Unintentional (X10-X19)	102	114	110	123	0.0	0.0	0.0	0.0	0.0	0.0	0.0	0.0
Suicide (X77)	-	1	-	-	*	*	*	*	*	*	*	*
Homicide (X98)	3	7	7	7	*	*	*	*	*	*	*	*
Undetermined (Y27)	1	1	1	1	*	*	*	*	*	*	*	*
Firearm (*U01.4, W32-W34, X72-X74, X93-X95, Y22-Y24, Y35.0)	30 242	29 573	28 663	28 874	10.5	10.4	10.2	10.3	10.4	10.3	10.2	10.3
Unintentional (W32-W34)	762	802	776	824	0.3	0.3	0.3	0.3	0.3	0.3	0.3	0.3
Suicide (X72-X74)	17 108	16 869	16 586	16 599	5.9	5.9	5.9	5.9	5.9	5.9	5.9	6.0
Homicide (*U01.4, X93-X95)	11 829	11 348	10 801	10 828	4.1	4.0	3.8	3.9	4.1	3.9	3.8	3.8
Undetermined (Y22-Y24)	243	231	230	324	0.1	0.1	0.1	0.1	0.1	0.1	0.1	0.1
Legal intervention/war (Y35.0)	300	323	270	299	0.1	0.1	0.1	0.1	0.1	0.1	0.1	0.1
Machinery (W24, W30-W31) [4]	652	648	676	622	0.2	0.2	0.2	0.2	0.2	0.2	0.2	0.2

[1] Based on codes from the *International Classification of Diseases, Tenth Revision* (1992), except in cases where (*) precedes the cause of death code. Codes *U01-*U03 were added as of 2001 for deaths due to terrorism.
[2] 2001 and 2002 figures include September 11, 2001-related deaths for which death certificates were filed as of October 24, 2002.
[3] Codes *U01.3 and Y36.3 cannot be divided separately into the subcategories shown below; therefore, subcategories may not add to the total.
[4] Intent of death is unintentional.
0.0 = Quantity more than zero but less than 0.05.
* = Figure does not meet standards of reliability or precision.
- = Quantity zero.

influenced by increases in the rates of unintentional injury deaths and suicides, as well as fluctuations in homicide rates. Rate increases were observed for deaths due to motor-vehicle traffic, firearms, poisoning, and falls. The rate of poisoning deaths increased by 17.9 percent between 2001 and 2002 (continuing an upward trend from 2000), but a portion of this increase was due to coding changes implemented in 2002. The spike in homicide deaths in 2001 represented the terror attacks of September 11, 2001, which were coded as transport injury deaths. (For further detailed data on injury deaths in 2002, see: Miniño, A.M., R.N. Anderson, et al. 2006. Deaths: Injuries, 2002. *National Vital Statistics Reports* 54 (10). Hyattsville, MD: National Center for Health Statistics.)

Table II-18. Number of Deaths, Death Rates, and Age-Adjusted Death Rates for Injury Deaths, According to Mechanism and Intent of Death, 1999–2002—*Continued*

(Number, rate per 100,000 population.)

Mechanism and intent of death [1]	Deaths				Death rate				Age-adjusted death rate			
	2002	2001	2000	1999	2002	2001	2000	1999	2002	2001	2000	1999
All Transport (*U01.1, V01-V99, X82, Y03, Y32, Y36.1) [2]	47 939	49 827	46 509	46 150	16.6	17.5	16.5	16.5	16.5	17.4	16.5	16.5
Unintentional (V01-V99)	47 739	46 706	46 259	45 927	16.6	16.4	16.4	16.5	16.5	16.3	16.4	16.4
Suicide (X82)	112	91	103	87	0.0	0.0	0.0	0.0	0.0	0.0	0.0	0.0
Homicide (*U01.1, Y03) [2]	61	3 008	106	106	0.0	1.1	0.0	0.0	0.0	1.0	0.0	0.0
Undetermined (Y32)	27	22	41	30	0.0	0.0	0.0	0.0	0.0	0.0	0.0	0.0
Legal intervention/war (Y36.1)	-	-	-	-	*	*	*	*	*	*	*	*
Motor vehicle traffic (V02-V04 [.1, .9], V09.2, V12-V14 [.3-.9], V19 [.4-.6], V20-V28 [.3-.9], V29-V79 [.4-.9], V80 [.3-.5], V81.1, V82.1, V83-V86 [.0-.3], V87 [.0-.8], V89.2) [4]	44 065	42 443	41 994	40 965	15.3	14.9	14.9	14.7	15.2	14.9	14.9	14.7
Occupant (V30-V79 [.4-.9], V83-V86 [.0-.3]) [4]	21 344	19 270	18 649	18 326	7.4	6.8	6.6	6.6	7.4	6.8	6.6	6.6
Motorcyclist (V20-V28 [.3-.9], V29 [.4-.9]) [4]	3 153	2 976	2 704	2 254	1.1	1.0	1.0	0.8	1.1	1.0	1.0	0.8
Pedal cyclist (V12-V14 [.3-.9], V19 [.4-.6]) [4]	550	585	572	615	0.2	0.2	0.2	0.2	0.2	0.2	0.2	0.2
Pedestrian (V02-V04 [.1, .9], V09.2) [4]	5 041	4 822	4 598	4 545	1.7	1.7	1.6	1.6	1.7	1.7	1.6	1.7
Other (V80 [.3-.5], V81.1, V82.1) [4]	16	15	12	9	*	*	*	*	*	*	*	*
Unspecified (V87 [.0-.8], V89.2) [4]	13 961	14 775	15 459	15 216	4.8	5.2	5.5	5.5	4.8	5.2	5.5	5.4
Pedal cyclist, other (V10-V11, V12-V14 [.0-.2], V15-V18, V19 [.0-.3, .8, .9]) [4]	217	207	168	185	0.1	0.1	0.1	0.1	0.1	0.1	0.1	0.1
Pedestrian, other (V01, V02-V04 [.0], V05, V06, V09 [.0, .1, .3, .9]) [4]	1 050	1 249	1 272	1 502	0.4	0.4	0.5	0.5	0.4	0.4	0.5	0.5
Other land transport (V20-V28 [.0-.2], V29-V79 [.0-.3], V80 [.0-.2, .6-.9], V81-V82 [.0, .2-.9], V83-V86 [.4-.9], V87.9, V88 [.0-.9], V89 [.0, .1, .3, .9], X82, Y03, Y32, V83-V86 [.4-.9], V87.9, V88 [.0-.9], V89 [.0, .1, .3, .9])	1 333	1 493	1 662	2 090	0.5	0.5	0.6	0.7	0.4	0.5	0.6	0.7
Unintentional (V20-V28 [.0-.2], V29-V79 [.0-.3], V80 [.0-.2, .6-.9], V81-V82 [.0, .2-.9])	1 134	1 294	1 412	1 867	0.4	0.5	0.5	0.7	0.4	0.5	0.5	0.7
Suicide (X82)	112	91	103	87	0.0	0.0	0.0	0.0	0.1	0.0	0.0	0.0
Homicide (Y03)	60	86	106	106	0.0	0.0	0.0	0.0	0.0	0.0	0.0	0.0
Undetermined (Y32)	27	22	41	30	0.0	0.0	0.0	0.0	0.0	0.0	0.0	0.0
Other transport (*U01.1, V90-V99, Y36.1) [2]	1 274	4 435	1 413	1 408	0.4	1.6	0.5	0.5	0.5	1.5	0.5	0.5
Unintentional (V90-V99)	1 273	1 513	1 413	1 408	0.4	0.5	0.5	0.5	0.4	0.5	0.5	0.5
Homicide (*U01.1) [2]	1	2 922	-	-	*	1.0	*	*	*	1.0	*	*
Legal intervention/war (Y36.1)	-	-	-	-	*	*	*	*	*	*	*	*
Natural/Environmental (W42-W43, W53-W64, W92-W99, X20-X39, X51-X57) [4]	1 554	1 427	1 643	1 923	0.5	0.5	0.6	0.7	0.5	0.5	0.6	0.7
Overexertion (X50) [4]	10	8	13	21	*	*	*	0.0	*	*	*	0.0
Poisoning (*U01 [.6-.7], X40-X49, X60-X69, X85-X90, Y10-Y19, Y35.2)	26 435	22 242	20 230	19 741	9.2	7.8	7.2	7.1	9.2	7.8	7.2	7.1
Unintentional (X40-X49)	17 550	14 078	12 757	12 186	6.1	4.9	4.5	4.4	6.1	4.9	4.5	4.4
Suicide (X60-X69)	5 486	5 191	4 859	4 893	1.9	1.8	1.7	1.8	1.9	1.8	1.7	1.8
Homicide (*U01 [.6-.7], X85-X90)	63	64	56	67	0.0	0.0	0.0	0.0	0.0	0.0	0.0	0.0
Undetermined (Y10-Y19)	3 336	2 909	2 557	2 595	1.2	1.0	0.9	0.9	1.2	1.0	0.9	0.9
Legal intervention/war (Y35.2)	-	-	-	1	*	*	*	*	*	*	*	*
Struck By or Against (W20-W22, W50-W52, X79, Y00, Y04, Y29, Y35.3) [4]	1 182	1 244	1 292	1 309	0.4	0.4	0.5	0.5	0.4	0.4	0.5	0.5
Unintentional (W20-W22, W50-W52)	890	898	938	894	0.3	0.3	0.3	0.3	0.3	0.3	0.3	0.3
Suicide (X79)	3	2	2	3	*	*	*	*	*	*	*	*
Homicide (Y00, Y04)	287	341	349	408	0.1	0.1	0.1	0.1	0.1	0.1	0.1	0.2
Undetermined (Y29)	2	3	3	3	*	*	*	*	*	*	*	*
Legal intervention/war (Y35.3)	-	-	-	1	*	*	*	*	*	*	*	*
Suffocation (W75-W84, X70, X91, Y20)	12 791	12 574	12 098	11 748	4.4	4.4	4.3	4.2	4.4	4.4	4.3	4.2
Unintentional (W75-W84)	5 517	5 555	5 648	5 503	1.9	2.0	2.0	2.0	1.9	2.0	2.1	2.0
Suicide (X70)	6 462	6 198	5 688	5 427	2.2	2.2	2.0	1.9	2.2	2.2	2.0	1.9
Homicide (X91)	679	690	658	708	0.2	0.2	0.2	0.3	0.2	0.2	0.2	0.2
Undetermined (Y20)	133	131	104	110	0.0	0.0	0.0	0.0	0.0	0.0	0.0	0.0
Other Specified, Classifiable (*U01 [.0, .2, .5], *U03.0, W23, W35-W41, W44, W49, W85-W91, X75, X81, X96, Y02, Y05-Y07, Y25, Y31, Y35 [.1, .5], Y36 [.0, .2, .4-.8], Y85) [2]	2 073	2 061	1 970	2 047	0.7	0.7	0.7	0.7	0.7	0.7	0.7	0.7
Unintentional (W23, W35-W41, W44, W49, W85-W91, Y85)	1 398	1 355	1 238	1 310	0.5	0.5	0.4	0.5	0.5	0.5	0.4	0.5
Suicide (*U03, X75, X81) [2]	315	283	278	280	0.1	0.1	0.1	0.1	0.1	0.1	0.1	0.1
Homicide (*U01 [.0, .2, .5], X96, Y02, Y05-Y07)	267	316	325	317	0.1	0.1	0.1	0.1	0.1	0.1	0.1	0.1
Undetermined (Y25, Y31)	26	42	48	51	0.0	0.0	0.0	0.0	0.0	0.0	0.0	0.0
Legal intervention/war (Y35 [.1, .5], Y36 [.0, .2, .4-.8])	67	65	81	89	0.0	0.0	0.0	0.0	0.0	0.0	0.0	0.0
Other Specified, Not Elsewhere Classified (*U01.8, *U02, X58, X83, Y08, Y33, Y35.6, Y86-Y87, Y89 [.0-.1])	2 066	2 299	2 261	2 230	0.7	0.8	0.8	0.8	0.7	0.8	0.8	0.8
Unintentional (X58, Y86)	1 046	1 034	903	955	0.4	0.4	0.3	0.3	0.3	0.4	0.3	0.4
Suicide (X83, Y87.0)	200	246	216	215	0.1	0.1	0.1	0.1	0.1	0.1	0.1	0.1
Homicide (*U01.8, *U02, Y08, Y87.1)	623	831	964	881	0.2	0.3	0.3	0.3	0.2	0.3	0.3	0.3
Undetermined (Y33, Y87.2)	163	163	156	149	0.1	0.1	0.1	0.1	0.1	0.1	0.1	0.1
Legal intervention/war (Y35.6, Y89 [.0, .1])	34	25	22	30	0.0	0.0	0.0	0.0	0.0	0.0	0.0	0.0
Unspecified (*U01.9, *U03.9, X59, X84, Y09, Y34, Y35.7, Y36.9, Y89.9)	8 656	9 160	8 584	9 258	3.0	3.2	3.1	3.3	3.0	3.2	3.1	3.4
Unintentional (X59)	6 550	7 218	6 673	7 459	2.3	2.5	2.4	2.7	2.3	2.5	2.4	2.7
Suicide (*U03.9, X84)	145	146	145	116	0.1	0.1	0.1	0.0	0.1	0.1	0.1	0.0
Homicide (*U01.9, Y09)	1 533	1 506	1 463	1 411	0.5	0.5	0.5	0.5	0.5	0.5	0.5	0.5
Undetermined (Y34, Y89.9)	425	290	302	270	0.1	0.1	0.1	0.1	0.2	0.1	0.1	0.1
Legal intervention/war (Y35.7, Y36.9)	3	-	1	2	*	*	*	*	*	*	*	*

[1]Based on codes from the *International Classification of Diseases, Tenth Revision* (1992), except in cases where (*) precedes the cause of death code. Codes *U01-*U03 were added as of 2001 for deaths due to terrorism.
[2]2001 and 2002 figures include September 11, 2001-related deaths for which death certificates were filed as of October 24, 2002.
[4]Intent of death is unintentional.
0.0 = Quantity more than zero but less than 0.05.
* = Figure does not meet standards of reliability or precision.
- = Quantity zero.

TABLE II-18A. DEATH RATES DUE TO INJURY, ACCORDING TO MECHANISM AND INTENT OF DEATH, BY AGE, 2002

Injury mortality in 2002 had three different age-specific patterns. (See Figure II-9.) For the population under 21 years old, the distribution was J-shaped, with rates nearly as high for infants (33.5 per 100,000 persons) as for 16-year-old teenagers (43.6 per 100,000 persons). Within this group, the injury death rates ranged from lows of 6.3 per 100,000 persons for 7-year-olds to 76.1 per 100,000 persons for 21-year-olds. The second age group, persons age 22–74 years, had a long W-shaped distribution, with relatively high death rates at both ends of the range. The third age group, persons 75 years old and over, had the highest injury death rates, which had increased steadily with age. The death rate for people age 75 years and over was 86.1 per 100,000 persons; those 85 years old and over had the highest injury death rates of any age group, at 296.9 per 100,000 persons.

Death rates were higher for males than for females at each year of age. (See Figure II-9, data not shown.) For children under 12 years of age, injury death rates for males were not quite twice the rates for females. Starting in the teenage years, however, there was a sharp increase in the difference between male and female death rates; this difference peaked at age 23. After age 23, it fell sharply until the age of 39, and decreased slowly thereafter.

(For further detailed data on injury deaths in 2002, see: Miniño, A.M., R.N. Anderson, et al. 2006. Deaths: Injuries, 2002. *National Vital Statistics Reports* 54 (10). Hyattsville, MD: National Center for Health Statistics.)

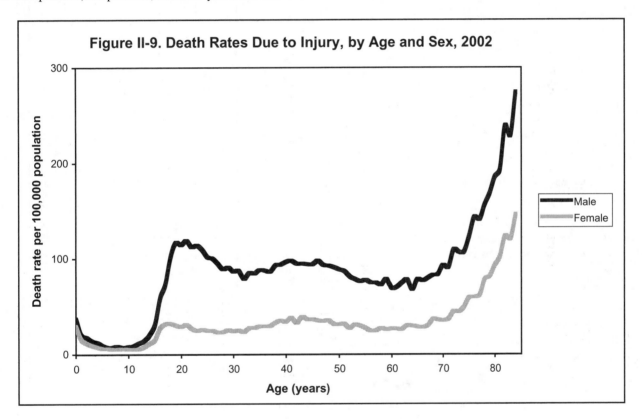

Figure II-9. Death Rates Due to Injury, by Age and Sex, 2002

Table II-18A. Death Rates Due to Injury, According to Mechanism and Intent of Death, by Age, 2002

(Rate per 100,000 population.)

Mechanism and intent of death [1]	All ages [2]	Under 1 year	1–4 years	5–9 years	10–14 years	15–19 years	20–24 years	25–34 years
ALL INJURY (*U01-*U03, V01-Y36, Y85-Y87, Y89) [3]	55.9	33.5	13.6	6.8	9.8	52.6	71.8	57.7
Unintentional (V01-X59, Y85-Y86)	37.0	23.5	10.5	5.9	7.3	35.0	40.9	31.5
Suicide (*U03, X60-X84, Y87.0) [3]	11.0	X	X	*	1.2	7.4	12.4	12.6
Homicide (*U01-*U02, X85-Y09, Y87.1) [3]	6.1	7.5	2.7	0.7	1.0	9.3	16.5	11.2
Undetermined (Y10-Y34, Y87.2, Y89.9)	1.7	2.5	0.4	0.1	0.2	0.7	1.7	2.1
Legal intervention/war (Y35-Y36, Y89 [.0, .1])	0.1	*	*	*	*	0.1	0.3	0.3
Cut/Pierce (W25-W29, W45, X78, X99, Y28, Y35.4)	1.0	*	*	0.1	0.1	0.8	1.5	1.5
Unintentional (W25-W29, W45)	0.0	*	*	*	*	*	*	*
Suicide (X78)	0.2	X	X	*	*	*	*	0.2
Homicide (X99)	0.7	*	*	0.1	*	0.7	1.4	1.2
Undetermined (Y28)	*	*	*	*	*	*	*	*
Legal intervention/war (Y35.4)	*	*	*	*	*	*	*	*
Drowning (W65-W74, X71, X92, Y21)	1.4	2.0	3.1	0.8	0.8	1.6	1.8	1.3
Unintentional (W65-W74)	1.2	1.6	2.9	0.8	0.8	1.6	1.5	1.1
Suicide (X71)	0.1	X	X	*	*	*	0.1	0.2
Homicide (X92)	0.0	*	0.1	*	*	*	*	*
Undetermined (Y21)	0.1	*	*	*	*	*	0.1	0.1
Fall (W00-W19, X80, Y01, Y30)	5.9	0.7	0.3	*	0.1	0.6	1.3	1.2
Unintentional (W00-W19)	5.6	*	0.2	*	0.1	0.4	0.8	0.8
Suicide (X80)	0.3	X	X	*	*	0.2	0.4	0.4
Homicide (Y01)	*	*	*	*	*	*	*	*
Undetermined (Y30)	0.0	*	*	*	*	*	*	*
Fire/Hot Object or Substance (*U01.3, X00-X19, X76-X77, X97-X98, Y26-Y27, Y36.3) [4]	1.3	1.1	1.6	0.9	0.5	0.5	0.7	0.8
Unintentional (X00-X19)	1.1	1.0	1.5	0.8	0.5	0.4	0.5	0.7
Suicide (X76-X77)	0.1	X	X	*	*	*	*	0.1
Homicide (*U01.3, X97-X98)	0.0	*	*	*	*	*	*	0.1
Undetermined (Y26-Y27)	0.0	*	*	*	*	*	*	*
Legal intervention/war (Y36.3)	*	*	*	*	*	*	*	*
Fire/Flame (X00-X09, X76, X97, Y26)	1.2	1.0	1.6	0.9	0.5	0.5	0.7	0.8
Unintentional (X00-X09)	1.1	0.9	1.4	0.8	0.5	0.4	0.5	0.7
Suicide (X76)	0.1	X	X	*	*	*	*	0.1
Homicide (X97)	0.0	*	*	*	*	*	*	0.1
Undetermined (Y26)	0.0	*	*	*	*	*	*	*
Hot Object/Substance (X10-X19, X77, X98, Y27)	0.0	*	*	*	*	*	*	*
Unintentional (X10-X19)	0.0	*	*	*	*	*	*	*
Suicide (X77)	*	X	X	*	*	*	*	*
Homicide (X98)	*	*	*	*	*	*	*	*
Undetermined (Y27)	*	*	*	*	*	*	*	*
Firearm (*U01.4, W32-W34, X72-X74, X93-X95, Y22-Y24, Y35.0)	10.5	*	0.4	0.4	1.3	12.1	21.3	15.4
Unintentional (W32-W34)	0.3	*	*	*	0.2	0.5	0.5	0.4
Suicide (X72-X74)	5.9	X	X	*	0.4	3.6	6.7	6.0
Homicide (*U01.4, X93-X95)	4.1	*	0.3	0.3	0.7	7.7	13.6	8.7
Undetermined (Y22-Y24)	0.1	*	*	*	*	0.2	0.2	0.1
Legal intervention/war (Y35.0)	0.1	*	*	*	*	0.1	0.3	0.2
Machinery (W24, W30-W31) [5]	0.2	*	*	*	*	*	0.1	0.2
All Transport (*U01.1, V01-V99, X82, Y03, Y32, Y36.1) [3]	16.6	3.2	4.1	3.5	4.9	28.4	29.8	18.6
Unintentional (V01-V99)	16.6	3.1	4.1	3.5	4.9	28.3	29.7	18.5
Suicide (X82)	0.0	X	X	*	*	*	*	0.1
Homicide (*U01.1, Y03) [3]	0.0	*	*	*	*	*	*	*
Undetermined (Y32)	0.0	*	*	*	*	*	*	*
Legal intervention/war (Y36.1)	*	*	*	*	*	*	*	*
Motor vehicle traffic (V02-V04 [.1, .9], V09.2, V12-V14 [.3-.9], V19 [.4-.6], V20-V28 [.3-.9], V29-V79 [.4-.9], V80 [.3-.5], V81.1, V82.1, V83-V86 [.0-.3], V87 [.0-.8], V89.2) [5]	15.3	3.0	3.4	3.1	4.1	27.1	28.3	17.4
Occupant (V30-V79 [.4-.9], V83-V86 [.0-.3]) [5]	7.4	1.8	1.5	1.4	2.0	15.3	15.0	8.4
Motorcyclist (V20-V28 [.3-.9], V29 [.4-.9]) [5]	1.1	*	*	*	*	0.8	2.2	1.9
Pedal cyclist (V12-V14 [.3-.9], V19 [.4-.6]) [5]	0.2	*	*	0.2	0.3	0.2	0.1	0.2
Pedestrian (V02-V04 [.1, .9], V09.2) [5]	1.7	*	1.0	0.7	0.7	1.4	1.5	1.5
Other (V80 [.3-.5], V81.1, V82.1) [5]	*	*	*	*	*	*	*	*
Unspecified (V87 [.0-.8], V89.2) [5]	4.8	1.0	0.9	0.8	1.1	9.4	9.4	5.4
Pedal cyclist, other (V10-V11, V12-V14 [.0-.2], V15-V18, V19 [.0-.3, .8, .9]) [5]	0.1	*	*	*	*	*	*	0.1
Pedestrian, other (V01, V02-V04 [.0], V05, V06, V09 [.0, .1, .3, .9]) [5]	0.4	*	0.5	0.1	0.1	0.3	0.4	0.3
Other land transport (V20-V28 [.0-.2], V29-V79 [.0-.3], V80 [.0-.2, .6-.9], V81-V82 [.0, .2-.9], V83-V86 [.4-.9], V87.9, V88 [.0-.9], V89 [.0, .1, .3, .9], X82, Y03, Y32, V83-V86 [.4-.9], V87.9, V88 [.0-.9], V89 [.0, .1, .3, .9])	0.5	*	*	0.2	0.4	0.6	0.7	0.4
Unintentional (V20-V28 [.0-.2], V29-V79 [.0-.3], V80 [.0-.2, .6-.9], V81-V82 [.0, .2-.9])	0.4	*	*	0.2	0.4	0.5	0.6	0.3
Suicide (X82)	0.0	X	X	*	*	*	*	0.1
Homicide (Y03)	0.0	*	*	*	*	*	*	*
Undetermined (Y32)	0.0	*	*	*	*	*	*	*
Other transport (*U01.1, V90-V99, Y36.1) [3]	0.4	*	*	*	0.1	0.3	0.4	0.4
Unintentional (V90-V99)	0.4	*	*	*	0.1	0.3	0.4	0.4
Homicide (*U01.1) [3]	*	*	*	*	*	*	*	*
Legal intervention/war (Y36.1) .	*	*	*	*	*	*	*	*
Natural/Environmental (W42-W43, W53-W64, W92-W99, X20-X39, X51-X57) [5]	0.5	*	0.2	*	*	0.1	0.1	0.2
Overexertion (X50) [5]	*	*	*	*	*	*	*	*
Poisoning (*U01 [.6-.7], X40-X49, X60-X69, X85-X90, Y10-Y19, Y35.2)	9.2	0.9	0.3	0.1	0.2	3.4	8.0	11.4
Unintentional (X40-X49)	6.1	0.6	0.2	*	0.1	2.4	5.9	7.8
Suicide (X60-X69)	1.9	X	X	*	*	0.6	1.0	2.0
Homicide (*U01 [.6-.7], X85-X90)	0.0	*	*	*	*	*	*	*
Undetermined (Y10-Y19)	1.2	*	*	*	*	0.4	1.1	1.6
Legal intervention/war (Y35.2)	*	*	*	*	*	*	*	*

[1]Based on codes from the *International Classification of Diseases, Tenth Revision* (1992), except in cases where (*) precedes the cause of death code. Codes *U01-*U03 were added as of 2001 for deaths due to terrorism.
[2]Figures for age not stated are included in "All ages" but not distributed among age groups.
[3]Includes September 11, 2001-related deaths for which death certificates were filed as of October 24, 2002.
[4]Codes *U01.3 and Y36.3 cannot be divided separately into the subcategories shown below; therefore, subcategories may not add to the total.
[5]Intent of death is unintentional.
0.0 = Quantity more than zero but less than 0.05.
* = Figure does not meet standards of reliability or precision.
X = Not applicable.

Table II-18A. Death Rates Due to Injury, According to Mechanism and Intent of Death, by Age, 2002
—Continued

(Rate per 100,000 population.)

Mechanism and intent of death [1]	35–44 years	45–54 years	55–64 years	65 years and over	65–74 years	75–84 years	85 years and over
ALL INJURY (*U01-*U03, V01-Y36, Y85-Y87, Y89) [3]	63.3	60.1	49.4	113.3	60.8	122.2	296.9
Unintentional (V01-X59, Y85-Y86)	37.2	36.6	31.4	94.5	44.2	101.3	275.4
Suicide (*U03, X60-X84, Y87.0) [3]	15.3	15.7	13.6	15.6	13.5	17.7	18.0
Homicide (*U01-*U02, X85-Y09, Y87.1) [3]	7.2	4.8	3.2	2.3	2.3	2.3	2.1
Undetermined (Y10-Y34, Y87.2, Y89.9)	3.4	2.8	1.2	0.8	0.8	0.7	1.4
Legal intervention/war (Y35-Y36, Y89 [.0, .1])	0.2	0.1	*	0.1	*	*	*
Cut/Pierce (W25-W29, W45, X78, X99, Y28, Y35.4)	1.4	1.1	0.9	0.8	0.8	0.9	1.0
Unintentional (W25-W29, W45)	*	*	0.1	0.1	*	*	*
Suicide (X78)	0.3	0.3	0.3	0.3	0.2	0.4	0.5
Homicide (X99)	1.1	0.8	0.5	0.4	0.4	0.4	*
Undetermined (Y28)	*	*	*	*	*	*	*
Legal intervention/war (Y35.4)	*	*	*	*	*	*	*
Drowning (W65-W74, X71, X92, Y21)	1.5	1.2	1.1	1.5	1.2	1.6	2.2
Unintentional (W65-W74)	1.2	0.9	0.8	1.2	0.9	1.3	1.7
Suicide (X71)	0.2	0.1	0.2	0.2	0.2	0.3	*
Homicide (X92)	*	*	*	*	*	*	*
Undetermined (Y21)	0.1	0.1	0.1	0.1	*	*	*
Fall (W00-W19, X80, Y01, Y30)	1.9	2.9	4.4	36.4	11.0	38.7	131.1
Unintentional (W00-W19)	1.5	2.5	4.1	36.1	10.8	38.3	130.4
Suicide (X80)	0.3	0.3	0.3	0.3	0.2	0.3	0.6
Homicide (Y01)	*	*	*	*	*	*	*
Undetermined (Y30)	0.1	*	*	*	*	*	*
Fire/Hot Object or Substance (*U01.3, X00-X19, X76-X77, X97-X98, Y26-Y27, Y36.3) [4]	1.0	1.3	1.5	3.2	2.3	3.7	5.4
Unintentional (X00-X19)	0.8	1.1	1.3	3.1	2.2	3.6	5.2
Suicide (X76-X77)	0.1	0.1	0.1	*	*	*	*
Homicide (*U01.3, X97-X98)	0.0	*	*	*	*	*	*
Undetermined (Y26-Y27)	*	*	*	*	*	*	*
Legal intervention/war (Y36.3)	*	*	*	*	*	*	*
Fire/Flame (X00-X09, X76, X97, Y26)	1.0	1.3	1.4	3.0	2.2	3.5	5.0
Unintentional (X00-X09)	0.8	1.1	1.3	2.9	2.1	3.4	4.8
Suicide (X76)	0.1	0.1	0.1	*	*	*	*
Homicide (X97)	0.0	*	*	*	*	*	*
Undetermined (Y26)	*	*	*	*	*	*	*
Hot Object/Substance (X10-X19, X77, X98, Y27)	*	*	*	0.2	*	0.2	*
Unintentional (X10-X19)	*	*	*	0.2	*	0.2	*
Suicide (X77)	*	*	*	*	*	*	*
Homicide (X98)	*	*	*	*	*	*	*
Undetermined (Y27)	*	*	*	*	*	*	*
Firearm (*U01.4, W32-W34, X72-X74, X93-X95, Y22-Y24, Y35.0)	12.1	10.8	10.2	12.4	10.9	14.4	12.5
Unintentional (W32-W34)	0.3	0.2	0.2	0.2	0.2	0.3	*
Suicide (X72-X74)	7.0	7.8	8.4	11.3	9.7	13.2	12.0
Homicide (*U01.4, X93-X95)	4.5	2.6	1.5	0.8	0.9	0.9	*
Undetermined (Y22-Y24)	0.1	0.1	*	0.1	*	*	*
Legal intervention/war (Y35.0)	0.2	0.1	*	*	*	*	*
Machinery (W24, W30-W31) [5]	0.2	0.3	0.4	0.5	0.5	0.5	*
All Transport (*U01.1, V01-V99, X82, Y03, Y32, Y36.1) [3]	16.9	16.1	15.4	22.5	18.2	26.6	28.5
Unintentional (V01-V99)	16.8	16.0	15.3	22.5	18.1	26.5	28.4
Suicide (X82)	0.1	0.1	*	*	*	*	*
Homicide (*U01.1, Y03) [3]	*	*	*	*	*	*	*
Undetermined (Y32)	*	*	*	*	*	*	*
Legal intervention/war (Y36.1)							
Motor vehicle traffic (V02-V04 [.1, .9], V09.2, V12-V14 [.3-.9], V19 [.4-.6], V20-V28 [.3-.9], V29-V79 [.4-.9], V80 [.3-.5], V81.1, V82.1, V83-V86 [.0-.3], V87 [.0-.8], V89.2) [5]	15.3	14.4	13.7	20.8	16.4	24.9	27.1
Occupant (V30-V79 [.4-.9], V83-V86 [.0-.3]) [5]	7.0	6.2	6.5	9.8	7.6	12.0	12.6
Motorcyclist (V20-V28 [.3-.9], V29 [.4-.9]) [5]	1.7	1.6	1.0	0.3	0.4	0.2	*
Pedal cyclist (V12-V14 [.3-.9], V19 [.4-.6]) [5]	0.2	0.3	0.2	0.1	0.1	0.2	*
Pedestrian (V02-V04 [.1, .9], V09.2) [5]	1.9	2.0	1.9	3.3	2.7	3.8	4.4
Other (V80 [.3-.5], V81.1, V82.1) [5]	*	*	*	*	*	*	*
Unspecified (V87 [.0-.8], V89.2) [5]	4.5	4.3	4.1	7.3	5.6	8.8	9.7
Pedal cyclist, other (V10-V11, V12-V14 [.0-.2], V15-V18, V19 [.0-.3, .8, .9]) [5]	0.1	0.1	0.1	0.1	0.1	*	*
Pedestrian, other (V01, V02-V04 [.0], V05, V06, V09 [.0, .1, .3, .9]) [5]	0.4	0.4	0.4	0.5	0.4	0.5	0.7
Other land transport (V20-V28 [.0-.2], V29-V79 [.0-.3], V80 [.0-.2, .6-.9], V81-V82 [.0, .2-.9], V83-V86 [.4-.9], V87.9, V88 [.0-.9], V89 [.0, .1, .3, .9], X82, Y03, Y32, V83-V86 [.4-.9], V87.9, V88 [.0-.9], V89 [.0, .1, .3, .9])	0.5	0.5	0.4	0.6	0.5	0.7	0.6
Unintentional (V20-V28 [.0-.2], V29-V79 [.0-.3], V80 [.0-.2, .6-.9], V81-V82 [.0, .2-.9])	0.4	0.4	0.4	0.6	0.5	0.7	0.6
Suicide (X82)	0.1	0.1	*	*	*	*	*
Homicide (Y03)	*	*	*	*	*	*	*
Undetermined (Y32)	*	*	*	*	*	*	*
Other transport (*U01.1, V90-V99, Y36.1) [3]	0.6	0.7	0.8	0.5	0.7	0.4	*
Unintentional (V90-V99)	0.6	0.7	0.8	0.5	0.7	0.3	*
Homicide (*U01.1) [3]	*	*	*	*	*	*	*
Legal intervention/war (Y36.1) .	*	*	*	*	*	*	*
Natural/Environmental (W42-W43, W53-W64, W92-W99, X20-X39, X51-X57) [5]	0.5	0.6	0.8	1.8	1.0	2.1	4.4
Overexertion (X50) [5]	*	*	*	*	*	*	*
Poisoning (*U01 [.6-.7], X40-X49, X60-X69, X85-X90, Y10-Y19, Y35.2)	19.6	17.9	7.3	4.3	3.9	4.3	5.9
Unintentional (X40-X49)	13.4	11.7	4.1	2.4	2.1	2.3	3.9
Suicide (X60-X69)	3.5	3.9	2.4	1.6	1.5	1.8	1.7
Homicide (*U01 [.6-.7], X85-X90)	*	*	*	*	*	*	*
Undetermined (Y10-Y19)	2.7	2.3	0.7	0.2	0.3	*	*
Legal intervention/war (Y35.2)	*	*	*	*	*	*	*

[1]Based on codes from the *International Classification of Diseases, Tenth Revision* (1992), except in cases where (*) precedes the cause of death code. Codes *U01-*U03 were added as of 2001 for deaths due to terrorism.
[3]Includes September 11, 2001-related deaths for which death certificates were filed as of October 24, 2002.
[4]Codes *U01.3 and Y36.3 cannot be divided separately into the subcategories shown below; therefore, subcategories may not add to the total.
[5]Intent of death is unintentional.
0.0 = Quantity more than zero but less than 0.05.
* = Figure does not meet standards of reliability or precision.

Table II-18A. Death Rates Due to Injury, According to Mechanism and Intent of Death, by Age, 2002 —Continued

(Rate per 100,000 population.)

Mechanism and intent of death [1]	All ages [2]	Under 1 year	1–4 years	5–9 years	10–14 years	15–19 years	20–24 years	25–34 years
Struck By or Against (W20-W22, W50-W52, X79, Y00, Y04, Y29, Y35.3)	0.4	*	0.3	0.1	0.1	0.2	0.4	0.4
Unintentional (W20-W22, W50-W52)	0.3	*	0.2	0.1	0.1	0.1	0.2	0.3
Suicide (X79)	*	X	X	*	*	*	*	*
Homicide (Y00, Y04)	0.1	*	*	*	*	*	0.1	0.1
Undetermined (Y29)	*	*	*	*	*	*	*	*
Legal intervention/war (Y35.3)	*	*	*	*	*	*	*	*
Suffocation (W75-W84, X70, X91, Y20)	4.4	17.9	1.1	0.3	1.2	3.3	4.4	4.4
Unintentional (W75-W84)	1.9	15.8	0.9	0.2	0.3	0.3	0.4	0.5
Suicide (X70)	2.2	X	X	*	0.7	2.7	3.6	3.5
Homicide (X91)	0.2	0.8	0.2	*	*	0.2	0.3	0.3
Undetermined (Y20)	0.0	1.4	*	*	*	*	*	*
Other Specified, Classifiable (*U01 [.0, .2, .5], *U03.0, W23, W35-W41, W44, W49, W85-W91, X75, X81, X96, Y02, Y05-Y07, Y25, Y31, Y35 [.1, .5], Y36 [.0, .2, .4-.8], Y85) [3]	0.7	2.5	0.7	0.2	0.1	0.4	0.7	0.7
Unintentional (W23, W35-W41, W44, W49, W85-W91, Y85)	0.5	*	0.1	*	0.1	0.3	0.5	0.5
Suicide (*U03, X75, X81) [3]	0.1	X	X	*	*	0.1	0.2	0.1
Homicide (*U01 [.0, .2, .5], X96, Y02, Y05-Y07)	0.1	2.4	0.6	*	*	*	*	*
Undetermined (Y25, Y31)	0.0	*	*	*	*	*	*	*
Legal intervention/war (Y35 [.1, .5], Y36 [.0, .2, .4-.8])	0.0	*	*	*	*	*	*	*
Other Specified, Not Elsewhere Classified (*U01.8, *U02, X58, X83, Y08, Y33, Y35.6, Y86-Y87, Y89 [.0-.1])	0.7	*	0.3	*	0.1	0.3	0.5	0.5
Unintentional (X58, Y86)	0.4	*	*	*	*	*	0.1	0.1
Suicide (X83, Y87.0)	0.1	X	X	*	*	*	*	*
Homicide (*U01.8, * U02, Y08, Y87.1)	0.2	*	0.2	*	*	0.2	0.2	0.2
Undetermined (Y33, Y87.2)	0.1	*	*	*	*	*	*	0.1
Legal intervention/war (Y35.6, Y89 [.0, .1])	0.0	*	*	*	*	*	*	*
Unspecified (*U01.9, *U03.9, X59, X84, Y09, Y34, Y35.7, Y36.9, Y89.9)	3.0	3.7	1.1	0.2	0.2	0.8	1.1	1.0
Unintentional (X59)	2.3	*	*	0.1	*	0.4	0.4	0.4
Suicide (*U03.9, X84)	0.1	X	X	*	*	*	*	0.1
Homicide (*U01.9, Y09)	0.5	3.0	1.0	*	*	0.3	0.6	0.5
Undetermined (Y34, Y89.9)	0.1	*	*	*	*	*	0.1	0.1
Legal intervention/war (Y35.7, Y36.9)	*	*	*	*	*	*	0.1	0.1

[1]Based on codes from the *International Classification of Diseases, Tenth Revision* (1992), except in cases where (*) precedes the cause of death code. Codes *U01-*U03 were added as of 2001 for deaths due to terrorism.
[2]Figures for age not stated are included in "All ages" but not distributed among age groups.
[3]Includes September 11, 2001-related deaths for which death certificates were filed as of October 24, 2002.
0.0 = Quantity more than zero but less than 0.05.
* = Figure does not meet standards of reliability or precision.
X = Not applicable.

Table II-18A. Death Rates Due to Injury, According to Mechanism and Intent of Death, by Age, 2002 —Continued

(Rate per 100,000 population.)

Mechanism and intent of death [1]	35–44 years	45–54 years	55–64 years	65 years and over	65–74 years	75–84 years	85 years and over
Struck By or Against (W20-W22, W50-W52, X79, Y00, Y04, Y29, Y35.3)	0.5	0.6	0.5	0.6	0.5	0.6	0.7
Unintentional (W20-W22, W50-W52)	0.4	0.4	0.4	0.5	0.5	0.5	0.6
Suicide (X79)	*	*	*	*	*	*	*
Homicide (Y00, Y04)	0.1	0.1	0.1	0.1	*	*	*
Undetermined (Y29)	*	*	*	*	*	*	*
Legal intervention/war (Y35.3)	*	*	*	*	*	*	*
Suffocation (W75-W84, X70, X91, Y20)	4.4	3.9	3.3	10.7	4.9	11.6	31.9
Unintentional (W75-W84)	0.7	0.9	1.5	9.0	3.3	9.9	29.4
Suicide (X70)	3.4	2.7	1.7	1.6	1.4	1.6	2.3
Homicide (X91)	0.3	0.3	0.1	0.1	0.2	*	*
Undetermined (Y20)	*	*	*	*	*	*	*
Other Specified, Classifiable (*U01 [.0, .2, .5], *U03.0, W23, W35-W41, W44, W49, W85-W91, X75, X81, X96, Y02, Y05-Y07, Y25, Y31, Y35 [.1, .5], Y36 [.0, .2, .4-.8], Y85) [3]	1.0	1.0	0.8	0.7	0.5	0.8	0.8
Unintentional (W23, W35-W41, W44, W49, W85-W91, Y85)	0.7	0.7	0.6	0.5	0.4	0.7	0.7
Suicide (*U03, X75, X81) [3]	0.2	0.2	0.1	*	*	*	*
Homicide (*U01 [.0, .2, .5], X96, Y02, Y05-Y07)	*	*	*	0.1	*	*	*
Undetermined (Y25, Y31)	*	*	*	*	*	*	*
Legal intervention/war (Y35 [.1, .5], Y36 [.0, .2, .4-.8])	0.1	*	*	*	*	*	*
Other Specified, Not Elsewhere Classified (*U01.8, *U02, X58, X83, Y08, Y33, Y35.6, Y86-Y87, Y89 [.0-.1])	0.7	0.8	0.8	2.2	1.1	2.4	6.2
Unintentional (X58, Y86)	0.2	0.3	0.4	1.7	0.7	1.9	5.6
Suicide (X83, Y87.0)	0.1	0.1	0.1	0.1	*	*	*
Homicide (*U01.8, * U02, Y08, Y87.1)	0.3	0.3	0.3	0.2	0.2	0.3	*
Undetermined (Y33, Y87.2)	0.1	0.1	*	0.1	*	*	*
Legal intervention/war (Y35.6, Y89 [.0, .1])	*	*	*	*	*	*	*
Unspecified (*U01.9, *U03.9, X59, X84, Y09, Y34, Y35.7, Y36.9, Y89.9)	1.5	1.7	2.1	15.6	4.1	14.1	65.9
Unintentional (X59)	0.6	0.7	1.3	14.8	3.4	13.4	64.4
Suicide (*U03.9, X84)	0.1	0.1	*	0.1	*	*	*
Homicide (*U01.9, Y09)	0.6	0.6	0.5	0.5	0.5	0.4	0.6
Undetermined (Y34, Y89.9)	0.2	0.2	0.2	0.3	0.2	0.3	0.7
Legal intervention/war (Y35.7, Y36.9)	*	*	*	*	*	*	*

[1]Based on codes from the *International Classification of Diseases, Tenth Revision* (1992), except in cases where (*) precedes the cause of death code. Codes *U01-*U03 were added as of 2001 for deaths due to terrorism.
[3]Includes September 11, 2001-related deaths for which death certificates were filed as of October 24, 2002.
* = Figure does not meet standards of reliability or precision.

TABLE II-19. NUMBER OF DEATHS, DEATH RATES, AND AGE-ADJUSTED DEATH RATES FOR INJURY BY FIREARMS, BY RACE AND SEX, 1999–2002

Firearms injuries accounted for 18.8 percent of all injury deaths in 2002. Fatality rates from firearms injuries were 10.5 per 100,000 persons in 2002, representing a gradual uptick from the previous three years. However, these rates differed according to sex and race. For White females, the death rate was 2.7 per 100,000 persons, while White males had a death rate of 16.1 per 100,000 persons. For Blacks, the female fatality rate was 4.2 per 100,000 persons and the male fatality rate was 37.8 per 100,000 persons.

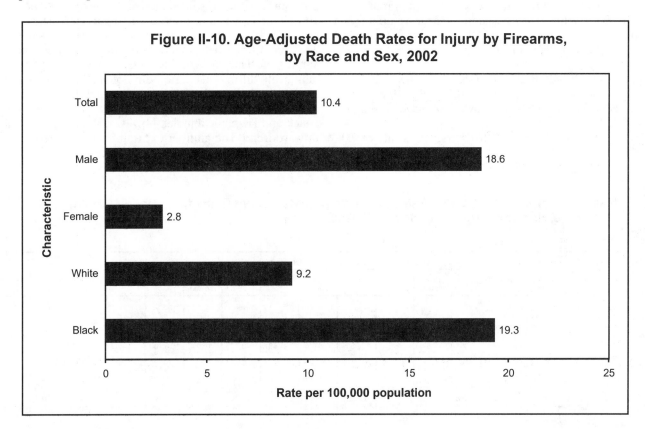

Figure II-10. Age-Adjusted Death Rates for Injury by Firearms, by Race and Sex, 2002

Table II-19. Number of Deaths, Death Rates, and Age-Adjusted Death Rates for Injury by Firearms, by Race and Sex, 1999–2002

(Number, rate per 100,000 population.)

Year	All races			White			All other					
							Total			Black		
	Both sexes	Male	Female	Both sexes	Male	Female	Both sexes	Male	Female	Both sexes	Male	Female
Number												
2002	30 242	26 098	4 144	21 902	18 714	3 188	8 340	7 384	956	7 623	6 798	825
2001	29 573	25 480	4 093	21 760	18 527	3 233	7 813	6 953	860	7 184	6 438	746
2000	28 663	24 582	4 081	20 945	17 750	3 195	7 718	6 832	886	7 054	6 284	770
1999	28 874	24 700	4 174	21 143	17 942	3 201	7 731	6 758	973	7 017	6 184	833
Rate												
2002	10.5	18.4	2.8	9.3	16.1	2.7	15.6	28.7	3.4	20.2	37.8	4.2
2001	10.4	18.2	2.8	9.4	16.2	2.7	14.9	27.6	3.2	19.3	36.4	3.8
2000	10.2	17.8	2.8	9.1	15.6	2.7	15.0	27.8	3.3	19.3	36.1	4.0
1999	10.3	18.1	2.9	9.2	15.9	2.8	15.4	28.0	3.7	19.4	36.0	4.4
Age-Adjusted Rate												
2002	10.4	18.6	2.8	9.2	16.2	2.7	14.6	26.9	3.3	19.3	36.0	4.1
2001	10.3	18.5	2.8	9.2	16.3	2.7	14.0	25.9	3.1	18.4	34.5	3.8
2000	10.2	18.1	2.8	9.0	15.9	2.7	14.1	26.0	3.2	18.4	34.2	3.9
1999	10.3	18.4	2.9	9.1	16.2	2.7	14.4	26.3	3.6	18.4	34.1	4.3

TABLE II-20. NUMBER OF DEATHS, DEATH RATES, AND AGE-ADJUSTED DEATH RATES FOR INJURY BY FIREARMS, BY RACE, HISPANIC ORIGIN, AND SEX, 1999–2002

For Hispanics, the firearms-related fatality rate was lower than the rate for the population as a whole. The rate for Hispanics was also moderately lower than the rate for non-Hispanic Whites. The Hispanic firearms-related death rate in 2002 was 14.2 per 100,000 persons for males and 1.6 per 100,000 persons for females.

TABLE II-21. NUMBER OF DEATHS, DEATH RATES, AND AGE-ADJUSTED DEATH RATES FOR DRUG-INDUCED CAUSES, BY RACE AND SEX, 1999–2002

Drug-induced deaths totaled 26,018 in 2002, a rate of 9.0 per 100,000 persons. This category consists of accidental poisoning by legal and illegal drugs, including medically prescribed drugs and biological substances, as well as the direct use of items for intentional self-poisoning and for homicidal assaults. The latter two categories are classified under intentional self-harm and assault in the tables detailing causes of death. This table does not include newborn deaths associated with the mother's drug use.

Drug-induced deaths have increased every year since 1999, with a particular jump occurring in 2002. The age-adjusted death rate for drug-induced causes has climbed 32 percent since 1999, mainly reflecting increases among Whites, particularly White females. The age-adjusted death rate during this period did not change significantly for Black males (although it was at a high level), and declined somewhat for Hispanic males. (See Table II-22.) Black and Hispanic females, however, shared in the upward trend. The number of fatalities for White males was nearly twice the number of fatalities for White females in 2002.

Table II-20. Number of Deaths, Death Rates, and Age-Adjusted Death Rates for Injury by Firearms, by Race, Hispanic Origin, and Sex, 1999–2002

(Number, rate per 100,000 population.)

Year	All origins [1]			Hispanic [2]			Non-Hispanic [3]			Non-Hispanic White			Non-Hispanic Black		
	Both sexes	Male	Female	Both sexes	Male	Female	Both sexes	Male	Female	Both sexes	Male	Female	Both sexes	Male	Female
Number															
2002	30 242	26 098	4 144	3 143	2 834	309	26 944	23 127	3 817	18 762	15 881	2 881	7 494	6 681	813
2001	29 573	25 480	4 093	3 087	2 774	313	26 341	22 573	3 768	18 676	15 760	2 916	7 063	6 323	740
2000	28 663	24 582	4 081	2 891	2 582	309	25 637	21 881	3 756	18 042	15 160	2 882	6 958	6 193	765
1999	28 874	24 700	4 174	2 878	2 549	329	25 877	22 050	3 827	18 260	15 384	2 876	6 933	6 114	819
Rate															
2002	10.5	18.4	2.8	8.1	14.2	1.6	10.8	19.0	3.0	9.4	16.3	2.8	20.7	38.9	4.3
2001	10.4	18.2	2.8	8.3	14.6	1.7	10.6	18.7	3.0	9.4	16.3	2.9	19.8	37.3	4.0
2000	10.2	17.8	2.8	8.2	14.2	1.8	10.4	18.3	3.0	9.1	15.7	2.9	19.8	37.1	4.2
1999	10.3	18.1	2.9	8.5	14.6	2.0	10.6	18.5	3.0	9.3	15.9	2.9	20.0	37.1	4.5
Age-Adjusted Rate															
2002	10.4	18.6	2.8	7.6	13.4	1.6	10.7	19.1	3.0	9.0	16.0	2.8	19.8	37.0	4.2
2001	10.3	18.5	2.8	7.8	13.7	1.7	10.5	18.8	3.0	9.1	16.0	2.8	18.9	35.4	3.9
2000	10.2	18.1	2.8	7.8	13.6	1.8	10.3	18.4	3.0	8.8	15.5	2.8	18.9	35.2	4.1
1999	10.3	18.4	2.9	8.2	14.2	2.0	10.5	18.7	3.0	8.9	15.8	2.8	19.0	35.2	4.4

[1]Figures for origin not stated are included in "All origins" but are not distributed among specified origins.
[2]May be of any race.
[3]Includes races other than White and Black.

Table II-21. Number of Deaths, Death Rates, and Age-Adjusted Death Rates for Drug-Induced Causes, by Race and Sex, 1999–2002

(Number, rate per 100,000 population.)

Year	All races			White			All other					
							Total			Black		
	Both sexes	Male	Female	Both sexes	Male	Female	Both sexes	Male	Female	Both sexes	Male	Female
Number												
2002	26 018	16 724	9 294	22 126	14 160	7 966	3 892	2 564	1 328	3 461	2 307	1 154
2001	21 683	14 244	7 439	18 176	11 873	6 303	3 507	2 371	1 136	3 163	2 163	1 000
2000	19 698	13 125	6 573	16 371	10 849	5 522	3 327	2 276	1 051	3 032	2 093	939
1999	19 102	12 873	6 229	15 694	10 497	5 197	3 408	2 376	1 032	3 094	2 188	906
Rate												
2002	9.0	11.8	6.3	9.4	12.2	6.7	7.3	10.0	4.8	9.2	12.8	5.8
2001	7.6	10.2	5.1	7.8	10.4	5.4	6.7	9.4	4.2	8.5	12.2	5.1
2000	7.0	9.5	4.6	7.1	9.6	4.7	6.5	9.2	3.9	8.3	12.0	4.9
1999	6.8	9.4	4.4	6.9	9.3	4.5	6.8	9.9	3.9	8.6	12.7	4.8
Age-Adjusted Rate												
2002	9.0	11.7	6.3	9.4	12.1	6.7	7.6	10.8	4.9	9.9	14.2	6.1
2001	7.6	10.1	5.1	7.8	10.2	5.3	7.1	10.3	4.3	9.2	13.6	5.4
2000	7.0	9.5	4.6	7.1	9.4	4.7	6.9	10.2	4.1	9.0	13.5	5.2
1999	6.8	9.4	4.4	6.8	9.2	4.4	7.2	10.8	4.1	9.3	14.3	5.0

TABLE II-22. NUMBER OF DEATHS, DEATH RATES, AND AGE-ADJUSTED DEATH RATES FOR DRUG-INDUCED CAUSES, BY RACE, HISPANIC ORIGIN, AND SEX, 1999–2002

See the notes for Table II-21 for the definition of drug-induced causes. The rates of drug-induced deaths among Hispanics were considerably lower than the rates for non-Hispanic Whites. In 2002, the age-adjusted death rate per 100,000 persons was 3.0 for Hispanic women, compared to 7.2 for non-Hispanic White women. For Hispanic men, the death rate was 9.3 per 100,000 persons, while the rate for non-Hispanic White men was 12.6 per 100,000 persons.

TABLE II-23. NUMBER OF DEATHS, DEATH RATES, AND AGE-ADJUSTED DEATH RATES FOR ALCOHOL-INDUCED CAUSES, BY RACE AND SEX, 1999–2002

In 2002, a total of 19,928 persons died from alcohol-induced causes in the United States. This category includes deaths from the direct use of alcohol, including diseases due to alcoholism and accidental poisonings from alcohol. However, it excludes causes (such as accidents) that are indirectly related to alcohol and newborn deaths associated with maternal alcohol use.

The age-adjusted death rate for alcohol-induced causes for males in 2002 was 3.4 times the rate for females, which can be compared to the less than 2 to 1 male excess for drug-induced fatalities. The rate for alcohol-induced deaths for Black men was somewhat higher than the rate for White men, but among females, the fatality rate for Whites slightly exceeded the rate for Blacks. Between 1999 and 2002, the age-adjusted death rate due to alcohol-induced causes for the total population increased each year.

Table II-22. Number of Deaths, Death Rates, and Age-Adjusted Death Rates for Drug-Induced Causes, by Race, Hispanic Origin, and Sex, 1999–2002

(Number, rate per 100,000 population.)

Year	All origins [1]			Hispanic [2]			Non-Hispanic [3]			Non-Hispanic White			Non-Hispanic Black		
	Both sexes	Male	Female	Both sexes	Male	Female	Both sexes	Male	Female	Both sexes	Male	Female	Both sexes	Male	Female
Number															
2002	26 018	16 724	9 294	2 137	1 647	490	23 734	14 968	8 766	19 929	12 468	7 461	3 402	2 264	1 138
2001	21 683	14 244	7 439	1 731	1 335	396	19 778	12 769	7 009	16 349	10 456	5 893	3 097	2 113	984
2000	19 698	13 125	6 573	1 700	1 348	352	17 813	11 644	6 169	14 568	9 431	5 137	2 975	2 049	926
1999	19 102	12 873	6 229	1 965	1 605	360	16 940	11 124	5 816	13 624	8 822	4 802	3 024	2 131	893
Rate															
2002	9.0	11.8	6.3	5.5	8.2	2.6	9.5	12.3	6.9	10.0	12.8	7.4	9.4	13.2	6.0
2001	7.6	10.2	5.1	4.7	7.0	2.2	8.0	10.6	5.5	8.3	10.8	5.8	8.7	12.5	5.3
2000	7.0	9.5	4.6	4.8	7.4	2.1	7.2	9.7	4.9	7.4	9.8	5.1	8.5	12.3	5.0
1999	6.8	9.4	4.4	5.8	9.2	2.2	6.9	9.3	4.6	6.9	9.1	4.8	8.7	12.9	4.9
Age-Adjusted Rate															
2002	9.0	11.7	6.3	6.2	9.3	3.0	9.4	12.1	6.7	9.9	12.6	7.2	10.0	14.5	6.3
2001	7.6	10.1	5.1	5.3	8.0	2.5	7.9	10.4	5.4	8.1	10.6	5.7	9.3	13.8	5.5
2000	7.0	9.5	4.6	5.4	8.3	2.4	7.1	9.5	4.8	7.2	9.6	4.9	9.1	13.6	5.3
1999	6.8	9.4	4.4	6.4	10.3	2.5	6.8	9.2	4.5	6.8	8.9	4.6	9.4	14.4	5.1

[1]Figures for origin not stated are included in "All origins" but are not distributed among specified origins.
[2]May be of any race.
[3]Includes races other than White and Black.

Table II-23. Number of Deaths, Death Rates, and Age-Adjusted Death Rates for Alcohol-Induced Causes, by Race and Sex, 1999–2002

(Number, rate per 100,000 population.)

Year	All races			White			All other					
							Total			Black		
	Both sexes	Male	Female	Both sexes	Male	Female	Both sexes	Male	Female	Both sexes	Male	Female
Number												
2002	19 928	15 036	4 892	16 762	12 741	4 021	3 166	2 295	871	2 373	1 749	624
2001	19 817	14 923	4 894	16 428	12 426	4 002	3 389	2 497	892	2 643	1 988	655
2000	19 358	14 770	4 588	16 019	12 349	3 670	3 339	2 421	918	2 636	1 933	703
1999	19 171	14 665	4 506	15 686	12 110	3 576	3 485	2 555	930	2 757	2 042	715
Rate												
2002	6.9	10.6	3.3	7.1	11.0	3.4	5.9	8.9	3.1	6.3	9.7	3.2
2001	7.0	10.7	3.4	7.1	10.8	3.4	6.5	9.9	3.3	7.1	11.2	3.4
2000	6.9	10.7	3.2	7.0	10.9	3.1	6.5	9.8	3.4	7.2	11.1	3.7
1999	6.9	10.7	3.2	6.9	10.7	3.1	6.9	10.6	3.5	7.6	11.9	3.8
Age-Adjusted Rate												
2002	6.9	10.9	3.2	6.9	10.8	3.2	6.9	11.4	3.4	7.6	12.8	3.6
2001	6.9	11.0	3.3	6.8	10.8	3.2	7.7	12.6	3.6	8.6	14.7	3.8
2000	6.9	11.2	3.2	6.8	10.9	3.0	7.8	12.8	4.0	8.8	14.8	4.2
1999	7.0	11.3	3.1	6.7	10.9	2.9	8.5	14.1	4.1	9.6	16.2	4.4

TABLE II-24. NUMBER OF DEATHS, DEATH RATES, AND AGE-ADJUSTED DEATH RATES FOR ALCOHOL-INDUCED CAUSES, BY RACE, HISPANIC ORIGIN, AND SEX, 1999–2002

On an age-adjusted basis, the alcohol-induced fatality rate for Hispanics was 1.4 times the rate for non-Hispanic Whites. The Hispanic rate also exceeded the rate for non-Hispanic Blacks, but by a smaller margin. (See the notes to Table II-23 for the definition of alcohol-induced fatalities.)

Table II-24. Number of Deaths, Death Rates, and Age-Adjusted Death Rates for Alcohol-Induced Causes, by Race, Hispanic Origin, and Sex, 1999–2002

(Number, rate per 100,000 population.)

Year	All origins [1]			Hispanic [2]			Non-Hispanic [3]			Non-Hispanic White			Non-Hispanic Black		
	Both sexes	Male	Female	Both sexes	Male	Female	Both sexes	Male	Female	Both sexes	Male	Female	Both sexes	Male	Female
Number															
2002	19 928	15 036	4 892	2 381	2 040	341	17 401	12 870	4 531	14 297	10 625	3 672	2 336	1 720	616
2001	19 817	14 923	4 894	2 363	2 009	354	17 315	12 801	4 514	13 991	10 351	3 640	2 598	1 957	641
2000	19 358	14 770	4 588	2 290	1 994	296	16 929	12 654	4 275	13 645	10 280	3 365	2 598	1 901	697
1999	19 171	14 665	4 506	2 166	1 849	317	16 863	12 691	4 172	13 434	10 185	3 249	2 719	2 008	711
Rate															
2002	6.9	10.6	3.3	6.1	10.2	1.8	7.0	10.6	3.5	7.2	10.9	3.6	6.5	10.0	3.3
2001	7.0	10.7	3.4	6.4	10.6	2.0	7.0	10.6	3.6	7.1	10.7	3.6	7.3	11.6	3.4
2000	6.9	10.7	3.2	6.5	11.0	1.7	6.9	10.6	3.4	6.9	10.6	3.3	7.4	11.4	3.8
1999	6.9	10.7	3.2	6.4	10.6	1.9	6.9	10.6	3.3	6.8	10.6	3.2	7.8	12.2	3.9
Age-Adjusted Rate															
2002	6.9	10.9	3.2	9.4	16.9	2.7	6.6	10.2	3.3	6.5	10.0	3.2	7.7	13.0	3.6
2001	6.9	11.0	3.3	10.0	18.0	2.9	6.6	10.3	3.3	6.4	9.9	3.2	8.7	14.9	3.8
2000	6.9	11.2	3.2	10.4	19.2	2.5	6.6	10.5	3.2	6.4	10.0	3.0	9.0	15.0	4.3
1999	7.0	11.3	3.1	10.3	18.5	2.9	6.7	10.6	3.1	6.3	10.0	2.9	9.7	16.4	4.5

[1]Figures for origin not stated are included in "All origins" but are not distributed among specified origins.
[2]May be of any race.
[3]Includes races other than White and Black.

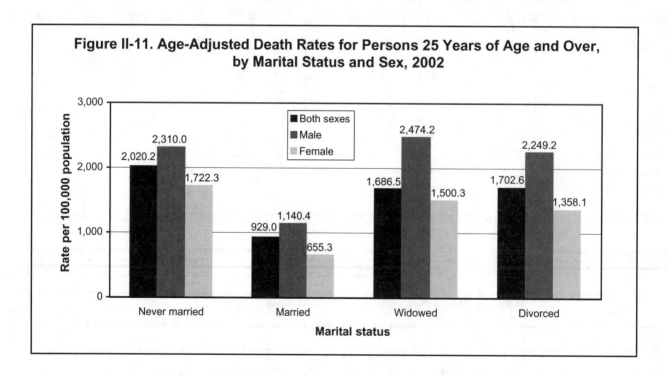

Figure II-11. Age-Adjusted Death Rates for Persons 25 Years of Age and Over, by Marital Status and Sex, 2002

TABLE II-25. NUMBER OF DEATHS, DEATH RATES, AND AGE-ADJUSTED DEATH RATES FOR PERSONS 15 YEARS OF AGE AND OVER, BY MARITAL STATUS AND SEX, 2002

The number of deaths of currently married persons (over 15 years of age) was 946,000 in 2002; for widowed persons, it was 926,000; for divorced persons, 274,000; and for persons who never married, 248,000. On an age-adjusted basis, the death rate was lowest for currently married persons. It was 82 percent higher for widowed persons and 83 percent higher for divorced persons. Individuals who were never married had an age-adjusted death rate that was 2.2 times higher than the rate for currently married persons.

For women of all races, the age-adjusted death rate for those who were never married was 2.6 times higher than the rate for currently married women. In the case of men, the age-adjusted rate for those who were never married was 2.0 times greater than the rate for currently married men.

For all age groups, age 15 years and over, death rates for married persons were much lower than those for persons who had never married. For the 25- to 34-year-old age group, widowed persons had the highest death rates; however, beginning at age 35, those who had never married had the highest death rates.

Table II-25. Number of Deaths, Death Rates, and Age-Adjusted Death Rates for Persons 15 Years of Age and Over, by Marital Status and Sex, 2002

(Number, rate per 100,000 population.)

Marital status and sex	15 years and over [1]	15–24 years	25–34 years	35–44 years	45–54 years	55–64 years	65–74 years	75 years and over	Age-adjusted rate [2]
NUMBER									
Both Sexes	2 402 988	33 046	41 355	91 140	172 385	253 342	422 990	1 388 730	X
Never married	247 823	30 320	23 382	31 839	34 650	26 058	28 050	73 524	X
Ever married	2 145 377	2 623	17 712	58 453	136 089	225 371	392 960	1 312 169	X
Married	945 795	2 246	13 077	37 164	82 873	140 486	230 473	439 476	X
Widowed	925 609	56	311	1 688	6 648	25 091	100 445	791 370	X
Divorced	273 973	321	4 324	19 601	46 568	59 794	62 042	81 323	X
Not stated	9 788	103	261	848	1 646	1 913	1 980	3 037	X
Male	1 176 261	24 416	28 736	57 593	107 722	151 363	237 021	569 410	X
Never married	149 569	22 734	17 431	22 597	23 900	16 889	17 567	28 451	X
Ever married	1 019 670	1 612	11 106	34 344	82 510	132 894	217 925	539 279	X
Married	643 439	1 395	8 287	21 726	50 364	89 527	154 626	317 514	X
Widowed	228 577	34	129	654	2 278	7 365	29 005	189 112	X
Divorced	147 654	183	2 690	11 964	29 868	36 002	34 294	32 653	X
Not stated	7 022	70	199	652	1 312	1 580	1 529	1 680	X
Female	1 226 727	8 630	12 619	33 547	64 663	101 979	185 969	819 320	X
Never married	98 254	7 586	5 951	9 242	10 750	9 169	10 483	45 073	X
Ever married	1 125 707	1 011	6 606	24 109	53 579	92 477	175 035	772 890	X
Married	302 356	851	4 790	15 438	32 509	50 959	75 847	121 962	X
Widowed	697 032	22	182	1 034	4 370	17 726	71 440	602 258	X
Divorced	126 319	138	1 634	7 637	16 700	23 792	27 748	48 670	X
Not stated	2 766	33	62	196	334	333	451	1 357	X
RATE [3]									
Both Sexes	1 055.2	81.4	103.6	202.9	430.1	952.4	2 314.7	8 014.5	1 275.3
Never married	380.6	84.0	156.7	439.6	875.2	1 666.4	4 128.1	11 228.4	2 020.2
Ever married	1 319.3	58.3	70.8	155.2	376.7	900.1	2 233.4	7 870.1	1 216.4
Married	750.3	53.9	58.4	117.3	287.5	729.8	1 907.3	5 722.7	929.0
Widowed	6 146.4	*	236.5	405.3	758.0	1 428.1	2 692.1	9 743.7	1 686.5
Divorced	1 274.7	106.3	172.5	351.6	724.5	1 483.6	3 485.9	9 330.9	1 702.6
Male	1 063.3	117.3	142.2	257.5	547.5	1 184.0	2 855.3	8 799.6	1 481.3
Never married	418.3	118.6	198.8	528.1	1 110.7	2 078.3	5 292.0	11 605.7	2 310.0
Ever married	1 362.0	97.7	97.1	189.9	470.8	1 110.1	2 734.6	8 662.1	1 403.7
Married	1 019.7	90.6	79.9	139.6	347.6	890.4	2 359.8	7 017.4	1 140.4
Widowed	8 210.0	*	*	676.1	1 069.1	2 346.1	4 047.8	13 413.7	2 474.2
Divorced	1 644.7	177.7	260.6	492.9	1 058.9	2 245.9	4 899.7	11 212.5	2 249.2
Female	1 047.6	43.7	64.0	148.8	316.9	738.0	1 864.7	7 546.6	1 111.2
Never married	334.7	44.8	96.8	311.7	594.9	1 220.8	3 016.4	11 002.6	1 722.3
Ever married	1 282.9	35.5	48.7	123.1	288.1	707.7	1 818.4	7 398.1	1 072.9
Married	480.3	32.4	39.9	95.8	226.9	554.1	1 371.3	3 865.8	655.3
Widowed	5 678.3	*	174.4	323.4	658.2	1 228.4	2 369.8	8 972.9	1 500.3
Divorced	1 009.3	69.3	110.8	242.6	463.0	980.2	2 569.5	8 386.7	1 358.1

[1]Excludes figures for age not stated.
[2]Calculated based on ages 25 years and over.
[3]Figures for marital status are included in totals but not distributed among specified marital status groups.
* = Figure does not meet standards of reliability or precision.
X = Not applicable.

TABLE II-26. NUMBER OF DEATHS, DEATH RATES, AND AGE-ADJUSTED DEATH RATES FOR PERSONS 25–64 YEARS OF AGE, BY EDUCATIONAL ATTAINMENT AND SEX: UNITED STATES EXCLUDING GEORGIA, RHODE ISLAND, AND SOUTH DAKOTA, 2002

The data in this table show that the higher the level of educational attainment, the lower the corresponding death rate. In this table, three levels of educational achievement are compared: under 12 years of school, 12 years of school, and 13 years or more of school. The drop in death rates was particularly sharp between 12 years and 13 years or more of school.

This table is limited to the population between 25 and 64 years of age, as total educational attainment may not have been achieved by persons under 25 years of age. The level of educational attainment reported on the death certificates of older persons has also proved to be less reliable than the reports for younger persons.

Table II-26. Number of Deaths, Death Rates, and Age-Adjusted Death Rates for Persons 25–64 Years of Age, by Educational Attainment and Sex: United States Excluding Georgia, Rhode Island, and South Dakota, 2002

(Number, rate per 100,000 population.)

Years of school completed and sex	25–64 years [1]	25–34 years	35–44 years	45–54 years	55–64 years	Age-adjusted rate [2]
NUMBER						
Both Sexes	536 089	39 646	87 357	165 549	243 537	X
Under 12 years	113 291	9 125	18 658	29 910	55 598	X
12 years	234 768	18 022	40 594	71 659	104 493	X
13 years or more	170 749	11 413	25 445	58 531	75 360	X
Not stated	17 281	1 086	2 660	5 449	8 086	X
Male	331 703	27 589	55 230	103 474	145 410	X
Under 12 years	72 604	6 646	12 425	19 525	34 008	X
12 years	144 385	12 992	26 372	45 105	59 916	X
13 years or more	102 796	7 200	14 590	35 044	45 962	X
Not stated	11 918	751	1 843	3 800	5 524	X
Female	204 386	12 057	32 127	62 075	98 127	X
Under 12 years	40 687	2 479	6 233	10 385	21 590	X
12 years	90 383	5 030	14 222	26 554	44 577	X
13 years or more	67 953	4 213	10 855	23 487	29 398	X
Not stated	5 363	335	817	1 649	2 562	X
RATE [3]						
Both Sexes	367.2	103.3	201.9	428.4	947.6	360.0
Under 12 years	615.6	180.6	368.0	711.0	1 364.3	575.1
12 years	516.2	164.7	293.3	596.5	1 202.7	490.9
13 years or more	207.9	51.0	104.4	261.1	582.5	211.3
Male	458.6	141.9	256.1	546.0	1 175.9	455.7
Under 12 years	744.5	230.9	450.2	914.6	1 718.4	726.1
12 years	646.4	222.5	372.2	790.8	1 615.5	650.2
13 years or more	255.5	67.1	124.4	315.4	688.2	253.5
Female	277.4	63.7	148.0	315.3	735.8	268.0
Under 12 years	470.2	114.1	269.7	501.2	1 029.9	416.6
12 years	390.5	98.6	210.6	420.9	895.2	350.7
13 years or more	162.3	36.1	85.9	207.7	469.6	168.8

Note: Georgia, Rhode Island, and South Dakota were excluded because educational attainment was not included on their death certificates.

[1] Excludes figures for age not stated.
[2] Calculated based on ages 25–64 years.
[3] Figures for education not stated are included in totals for "Both sexes," "Male," and "Female," but are not distributed among specified years of education.
X = Not applicable.

TABLE II-27. NUMBER OF DEATHS, DEATH RATES, AND AGE-ADJUSTED DEATH RATES FOR INJURY AT WORK, BY AGE, RACE, AND SEX, 2002

Deaths due to job-related injuries totaled 5,307 in 2002, a sharp decrease from the previous year (which included 2,826 victims of the September 11, 2001, terror attacks).

The risk of work-related death in 2002 was much higher for males than for females. White males had an age-adjusted death rate of 4.5 per 100,000 persons, while the rate for females was 0.4 per 100,000 persons. The rates for Blacks were not notably different. By age group, the highest risk for death on the job occurred for workers between 45 and 65 years of age.

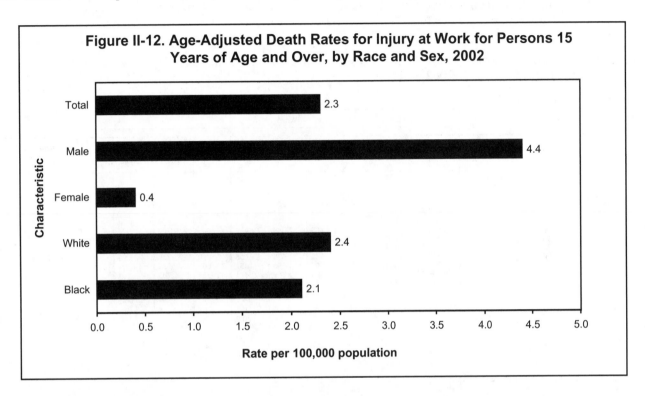

Figure II-12. Age-Adjusted Death Rates for Injury at Work for Persons 15 Years of Age and Over, by Race and Sex, 2002

Table II-27. Number of Deaths, Death Rates, and Age-Adjusted Death Rates for Injury at Work, by Age, Race, and Sex, 2002

(Number, rate per 100,000 population.)

Race and sex	15 years and over [1]	15–24 years	25–34 years	35–44 years	45–54 years	55–64 years	65 years and over	Age-adjusted rate [2]
NUMBER								
All Races, Both Sexes [3]	5 307	518	928	1 280	1 174	778	627	X
Male	4 861	486	851	1 190	1 081	721	530	X
Female	446	32	77	90	93	57	97	X
White, Both Sexes	4 569	456	797	1 086	990	672	567	X
Male	4 200	427	738	1 017	917	623	477	X
Female	369	29	59	69	73	49	90	X
Black, Both Sexes	560	49	94	148	141	79	48	X
Male	501	46	80	135	123	73	43	X
Female	59	3	14	13	18	6	5	X
RATE								
All Races, Both Sexes [3]	2.3	1.3	2.3	2.8	2.9	2.9	1.8	2.3
Male	4.4	2.3	4.2	5.3	5.5	5.6	3.6	4.4
Female	0.4	0.2	0.4	0.4	0.5	0.4	0.5	0.4
White, Both Sexes	2.4	1.4	2.5	3.0	3.0	3.0	1.8	2.4
Male	4.6	2.6	4.6	5.5	5.5	5.6	3.6	4.5
Female	0.4	0.2	0.4	0.4	0.4	0.4	0.5	0.4
Black, Both Sexes	2.0	0.8	1.7	2.5	3.0	3.0	1.6	2.1
Male	3.9	1.5	3.1	5.0	5.7	6.2	3.8	4.1
Female	0.4	*	*	*	*	*	*	0.4

[1] Excludes figures for age not stated.
[2] Calculated based on ages 15 years and over.
[3] Includes races other than White and Black.
* = Figure does not meet standards of reliability or precision.
X = Not applicable.

TABLE II-28. NUMBER OF DEATHS, DEATH RATES, AND AGE-ADJUSTED DEATH RATES FOR INJURY AT WORK, BY RACE AND SEX, 1993–2002

The number of deaths from job-related injuries, as well as the related death rate, has been declining gradually since 1993 (despite the sharp spike in 2001 caused by the terror attacks on September 11, 2001). For the total population, the age-adjusted death rate was 2.9 per 100,000 persons in 1993 and 2.3 per 100,000 persons in 2002. The unadjusted death rate remained the same.

In most years, the rates for males were about 11 times higher than the rates for females. In the 1990s, the work-related death rates for Black males were somewhat greater than those for White males. However, since then, this relationship has reversed.

Table II-28. Number of Deaths, Death Rates, and Age-Adjusted Death Rates for Injury at Work, by Race and Sex, 1993–2002

(Number, rate per 100,000 population.)

Year	All races			White			All other					
							Total			Black		
	Both sexes	Male	Female	Both sexes	Male	Female	Both sexes	Male	Female	Both sexes	Male	Female
Number												
2002	5 307	4 861	446	4 569	4 200	369	738	661	77	560	501	59
2001 [1]	8 303	7 181	1 122	7 093	6 211	882	1 210	970	240	849	680	169
2000	5 430	4 969	461	4 657	4 270	387	773	699	74	591	536	55
1999	5 651	5 152	499	4 805	4 385	420	846	767	79	659	598	61
1998	5 543	5 036	507	4 804	4 366	438	739	670	69	587	535	52
1997	5 666	5 144	522	4 785	4 352	433	881	792	89	684	626	58
1996	5 778	5 280	498	4 940	4 535	405	838	745	93	649	582	67
1995	5 872	5 334	538	5 007	4 550	457	865	784	81	692	627	65
1994	5 987	5 425	562	5 103	4 642	461	884	783	101	710	632	78
1993	5 847	5 352	495	4 979	4 581	398	868	771	97	677	608	69
Rate												
2002	2.3	4.4	0.4	2.4	4.6	0.4	1.8	3.5	0.4	2.0	3.9	0.4
2001 [1]	3.7	6.6	1.0	3.8	6.9	0.9	3.1	5.3	1.2	3.1	5.4	1.2
2000	2.5	4.6	0.4	2.5	4.8	0.4	2.0	3.7	0.4	2.2	4.3	0.4
1999	2.6	4.9	0.4	2.6	4.9	0.5	2.3	4.4	0.4	2.5	4.9	0.4
1998	2.6	4.8	0.5	2.7	5.0	0.5	2.0	3.9	0.4	2.3	4.5	0.4
1997	2.7	5.0	0.5	2.7	5.0	0.5	2.5	4.8	0.5	2.7	5.3	0.4
1996	2.7	5.2	0.5	2.8	5.3	0.4	2.4	4.6	0.5	2.6	5.1	0.5
1995	2.8	5.3	0.5	2.9	5.4	0.5	2.6	5.0	0.5	2.8	5.5	0.5
1994	2.9	5.5	0.5	3.0	5.5	0.5	2.7	5.1	0.6	3.0	5.7	0.6
1993	2.9	5.5	0.5	2.9	5.5	0.5	2.7	5.2	0.6	2.9	5.6	0.5
Age-Adjusted Rate [2]												
2002	2.3	4.4	0.4	2.4	4.5	0.4	1.9	3.7	0.4	2.1	4.1	0.4
2001 [1]	3.7	6.6	1.0	3.8	6.8	0.9	3.1	5.3	1.1	3.1	5.5	1.1
2000	2.5	4.6	0.4	2.5	4.8	0.4	2.1	3.9	0.4	2.3	4.6	0.4
1999	2.6	4.9	0.4	2.6	4.9	0.4	2.3	4.5	0.4	2.6	5.1	0.4
1998	2.6	4.8	0.5	2.7	5.0	0.5	2.1	4.1	0.4	2.3	4.7	0.4
1997	2.7	5.0	0.5	2.7	5.0	0.5	2.6	5.0	0.5	2.8	5.5	0.4
1996	2.8	5.2	0.5	2.8	5.3	0.4	2.5	4.8	0.5	2.6	5.3	0.5
1995	2.8	5.3	0.5	2.9	5.4	0.5	2.7	5.3	0.5	3.0	6.0	0.5
1994	2.9	5.5	0.5	3.0	5.6	0.5	2.8	5.4	0.6	3.1	6.0	0.6
1993	2.9	5.5	0.5	2.9	5.5	0.5	2.8	5.4	0.6	3.0	6.0	0.5

[1]Figures include September 11, 2001, terrorism-related deaths for which death certificates were filed as of October 24, 2002.
[2]Calculated based on ages 15 years and over.

TABLE II-29. NUMBER OF DEATHS, DEATH RATES, AND AGE-ADJUSTED DEATH RATES FOR MAJOR CAUSES OF DEATH, FOR EACH STATE AND TERRITORY, 2002

This table includes combined statistics for all causes of death, as well as details on most of the leading 15 causes of death. In addition, death rates are given for HIV, motor vehicle accidents, and injury by firearms, all of which were causes of death with significant public health policy implications. (HIV was among the 15 leading causes of death until 1997.)

The 2.4 million deaths in the United States in 2002 represented an age-adjusted death rate of 845.3 per 100,000 persons. Age-adjusted rates differed considerably among states. The four states with the lowest death rates were Hawaii (660.6 per 100,000 persons), Minnesota (747.5),

Table II-29. Number of Deaths, Death Rates, and Age-Adjusted Death Rates for Major Causes of Death, for Each State and Territory, 2002

(Number, rate per 100,000 population.)

State	All causes			Human inmmunodeficiency virus (HIV) disease (B20-B24)			Malignant neoplasms (C00-C97)			Diabetes mellitus (E1-E14)		
	Number	Rate	Age-adjusted rate [1]	Number	Rate	Age-adjusted rate [1]	Number	Rate	Age-adjusted rate [1]	Number	Rate	Age-adjusted rate [1]
UNITED STATES [2]	2 443 387	847.3	845.3	14 095	4.9	4.9	557 271	193.2	193.5	73 249	25.4	25.4
Alabama	46 069	1 026.8	998.1	190	4.2	4.3	9 698	216.2	207.5	1 486	33.1	31.9
Alaska	3 030	470.7	789.1	16	*	*	715	111.1	185.9	86	13.4	21.7
Arizona	42 816	784.7	795.7	165	3.0	3.3	9 359	171.5	171.6	1 231	22.6	22.7
Arkansas	28 513	1 052.1	964.4	81	3.0	3.2	6 282	231.8	212.1	793	29.3	26.8
California	234 565	668.0	757.8	1 435	4.1	4.2	54 143	154.2	176.0	6 807	19.4	22.2
Colorado	29 210	648.2	790.2	105	2.3	2.3	6 384	141.7	171.8	659	14.6	17.7
Connecticut	30 122	870.5	762.4	186	5.4	5.2	7 163	207.0	186.4	675	19.5	17.2
Delaware	6 861	849.8	838.2	70	8.7	8.5	1 621	200.8	193.8	215	26.6	25.9
District of Columbia	5 851	1 024.9	1 021.4	233	40.8	40.8	1 298	227.4	230.0	191	33.5	33.7
Florida	167 814	1 004.1	786.4	1 719	10.3	10.4	39 140	234.2	183.4	4 583	27.4	21.4
Georgia	65 449	764.6	949.1	708	8.3	8.2	13 975	163.3	199.6	1 576	18.4	22.9
Hawaii	8 801	707.0	660.6	26	2.1	2.1	1 945	156.2	145.4	204	16.4	15.2
Idaho	9 923	739.9	793.0	11	*	*	2 138	159.4	172.2	322	24.0	26.0
Illinois	106 667	846.5	856.0	490	3.9	3.9	24 737	196.3	201.9	3 011	23.9	24.4
Indiana	55 396	899.4	899.6	118	1.9	2.0	12 865	208.9	209.8	1 688	27.4	27.5
Iowa	27 978	952.7	774.5	29	1.0	1.0	6 473	220.4	189.0	734	25.0	20.7
Kansas	25 021	921.3	843.5	37	1.4	1.4	5 362	197.4	188.1	765	28.2	26.3
Kentucky	40 697	994.3	993.9	98	2.4	2.3	9 438	230.6	226.3	1 265	30.9	30.7
Louisiana	41 984	936.6	1 000.5	364	8.1	8.4	9 441	210.6	222.9	1 774	39.6	42.1
Maine	12 694	980.6	846.5	12	*	*	3 206	247.7	214.2	404	31.2	27.0
Maryland	43 970	805.6	864.1	610	11.2	10.7	10 395	190.4	201.6	1 519	27.8	29.9
Massachusetts	56 928	885.7	791.9	232	3.6	3.5	13 914	216.5	199.2	1 423	22.1	20.1
Michigan	87 795	873.5	876.2	240	2.4	2.4	19 985	198.8	199.2	2 785	27.7	27.8
Minnesota	38 510	767.2	747.5	53	1.1	1.0	9 210	183.5	185.0	1 317	26.2	25.9
Mississippi	28 853	1 004.7	1 036.3	185	6.4	6.8	6 069	211.3	218.3	671	23.4	24.2
Missouri	55 940	986.1	916.7	123	2.2	2.2	12 322	217.2	204.3	1 625	28.6	26.7
Montana	8 506	935.3	849.7	8	*	*	1 911	210.1	190.7	210	23.1	21.0
Nebraska	15 738	910.1	814.8	21	1.2	1.3	3 433	198.5	185.9	393	22.7	20.6
Nevada	16 927	778.8	916.5	76	3.5	3.5	3 937	181.1	202.0	343	15.8	17.5
New Hampshire	9 853	772.8	781.7	13	*	*	2 529	198.3	199.5	311	24.4	24.6
New Jersey	74 009	861.5	808.7	762	8.9	8.5	17 827	207.5	196.3	2 532	29.5	27.8
New Mexico	14 344	773.2	815.0	35	1.9	2.0	3 067	165.3	172.5	582	31.4	32.9
New York	158 118	825.4	783.3	1 980	10.3	10.2	36 661	191.4	184.0	3 934	20.5	19.6
North Carolina	72 027	865.7	906.1	486	5.8	5.8	16 210	194.8	200.4	2 205	26.5	27.5
North Dakota	5 892	929.2	749.8	1	*	*	1 293	203.9	175.0	214	33.7	26.9
Ohio	109 766	961.1	908.2	241	2.1	2.2	25 173	220.4	208.8	3 846	33.7	31.8
Oklahoma	35 502	1 016.2	973.2	91	2.6	2.7	7 474	213.9	204.2	1 064	30.5	29.2
Oregon	31 119	883.7	834.2	91	2.6	2.6	7 249	205.8	197.8	1 041	29.6	28.2
Pennsylvania	130 223	1 055.7	862.1	497	4.0	4.0	29 849	242.0	200.8	3 708	30.1	24.6
Rhode Island	10 246	957.8	809.5	23	2.2	2.1	2 404	224.7	196.9	263	24.6	21.2
South Carolina	37 736	918.8	946.9	301	7.3	7.4	8 333	202.9	203.7	1 112	27.1	27.4
South Dakota	6 898	906.4	771.2	5	*	*	1 562	205.2	182.4	195	25.6	22.6
Tennessee	56 606	976.4	981.5	347	6.0	5.9	12 518	215.9	213.6	1 749	30.2	30.1
Texas	155 524	714.1	870.0	1 075	4.9	5.1	34 164	156.9	189.6	5 654	26.0	31.7
Utah	13 116	566.3	782.0	19	*	*	2 376	102.6	143.3	514	22.2	31.4
Vermont	5 075	823.1	775.0	8	*	*	1 224	198.5	186.7	174	28.2	26.6
Virginia	57 196	784.2	856.6	261	3.6	3.5	13 602	186.5	199.8	1 558	21.4	23.1
Washington	45 338	747.0	785.3	119	2.0	1.9	10 858	178.9	189.9	1 494	24.6	26.2
West Virginia	21 016	1 166.3	991.7	20	1.1	1.1	4 652	258.2	215.3	846	47.0	39.3
Wisconsin	46 981	863.4	799.8	77	1.4	1.4	10 828	199.0	189.5	1 353	24.9	23.3
Wyoming	4 174	837.0	864.3	2	*	*	859	172.2	175.1	145	29.1	30.0
Puerto Rico [3]	27 924	723.6	790.8	580	15.0	16.4	4 664	120.9	130.9	2 465	63.9	69.5
Virgin Islands [3]	617	567.0	734.3	7	*	*	129	118.6	147.1	26	23.9	33.1
Guam [3]	638	396.1	736.6	2	*	*	118	73.3	136.1	18	*	*
American Samoa [3]	290	502.5	1 467.9	-	*	*	34	58.9	187.9	31	53.7	159.7
Northern Marianas [3]	161	217.6	1 057.4	-	*	*	19	*	*	7	*	*

[1]Death rates are affected by the population composition of the area. Age-adjusted death rates should be used for comparisons between areas.
[2]Excludes data for Puerto Rico, Virgin Islands, Guam, American Samoa, and Northern Marianas.
[3]Age-adjusted death rates for Puerto Rico, Virgin Islands, Guam, American Samoa, and Northern Marianas are calculated using different age groups in the weighting procedure.
* = Figure does not meet standards of reliability or precision.
- = Quantity zero.

California (757.8), and Connecticut (762.4). The four highest death rates were reported for Mississippi (1,036.3 per 100,000 persons), Louisiana (1,000.5), Alabama (998.1), and Kentucky (993.9). The District of Columbia, which, as a city, cannot be fully compared to the states, showed a high rate of 1,021.4 deaths per 100,000 persons.

Turning to specific causes of death, age-adjusted death rates for HIV ranked highest in the District of Columbia and Puerto Rico. Such deaths also amounted to more than 10 per 100,000 persons in New York, Florida, and Maryland. Death rates from cancer were lowest in Utah, Hawaii, Arizona, and Colorado, and highest in the District of Columbia, Kentucky, Louisiana, Mississippi, and West Virginia. Diabetes death rates were highest in Louisiana, West Virginia, New Mexico, Alabama, and the District of Columbia.

Table II-29. Number of Deaths, Death Rates, and Age-Adjusted Death Rates for Major Causes of Death, for Each State and Territory, 2002—*Continued*

(Number, rate per 100,000 population.)

State	Alzheimer's disease (G30)			Diseases of heart (I00-I09, I11, I13, I20-I51)			Cerebrovascular diseases (I60-I69)			Influenza and pneumonia (J10-J18)		
	Number	Rate	Age-adjusted rate[1]	Number	Rate	Age-adjusted rate[1]	Number	Rate	Age-adjusted rate[1]	Number	Rate	Age-adjusted rate[1]
UNITED STATES[2]	58 866	20.4	20.2	696 947	241.7	240.8	162 672	56.4	56.2	65 681	22.8	22.6
Alabama	1 189	26.5	26.1	13 197	294.1	285.8	3 201	71.3	69.6	1 218	27.1	26.6
Alaska	61	9.5	25.4	567	88.1	166.0	158	24.5	55.1	51	7.9	19.2
Arizona	1 433	26.3	27.5	10 852	198.9	202.9	2 535	46.5	47.7	1 319	24.2	24.9
Arkansas	551	20.3	18.2	8 330	307.4	278.7	2 232	82.4	74.3	776	28.6	25.7
California	5 421	15.4	18.0	68 797	195.9	225.7	17 626	50.2	58.0	8 128	23.1	26.8
Colorado	954	21.2	28.0	6 425	142.6	178.9	1 915	42.5	54.4	752	16.7	21.3
Connecticut	570	16.5	13.4	8 815	254.7	217.6	1 861	53.8	45.6	888	25.7	21.2
Delaware	128	15.9	16.2	1 918	237.6	236.0	405	50.2	50.4	168	20.8	20.9
District of Columbia	107	18.7	18.3	1 666	291.8	291.7	279	48.9	48.7	81	14.2	14.1
Florida	4 052	24.2	17.5	49 235	294.6	222.0	10 269	61.4	46.0	3 290	19.7	14.8
Georgia	1 525	17.8	24.7	17 529	204.8	261.8	4 261	49.8	65.3	1 791	20.9	27.8
Hawaii	141	11.3	10.6	2 512	201.8	188.3	812	65.2	60.6	246	19.8	18.4
Idaho	318	23.7	25.6	2 532	188.8	203.0	736	54.9	59.4	265	19.8	21.3
Illinois	2 398	19.0	18.8	30 821	244.6	246.4	7 183	57.0	57.2	2 940	23.3	23.2
Indiana	1 475	23.9	23.7	15 321	248.8	248.4	3 717	60.4	60.1	1 360	22.1	21.9
Iowa	899	30.6	22.2	8 181	278.6	219.5	2 226	75.8	57.9	942	32.1	24.0
Kansas	755	27.8	23.6	6 680	246.0	220.6	1 845	67.9	59.5	698	25.7	22.3
Kentucky	1 013	24.8	25.6	11 696	285.8	287.0	2 554	62.4	63.5	1 236	30.2	30.8
Louisiana	1 111	24.8	27.8	11 185	249.5	269.6	2 595	57.9	63.0	956	21.3	23.5
Maine	513	39.6	33.0	3 170	244.9	208.5	823	63.6	53.7	317	24.5	20.5
Maryland	866	15.9	18.0	12 008	220.0	239.6	2 811	51.5	56.7	1 121	20.5	22.7
Massachusetts	1 570	24.4	20.6	14 736	229.3	201.3	3 559	55.4	48.1	2 087	32.5	27.8
Michigan	1 958	19.5	19.6	26 659	265.3	266.0	5 814	57.8	58.1	2 029	20.2	20.3
Minnesota	1 192	23.7	22.0	8 602	171.4	164.7	2 706	53.9	51.3	900	17.9	16.7
Mississippi	574	20.0	21.0	9 061	315.5	326.6	1 926	67.1	69.5	801	27.9	28.9
Missouri	1 187	20.9	18.7	16 708	294.5	270.3	3 885	68.5	62.5	1 619	28.5	25.9
Montana	285	31.3	27.6	1 944	213.8	191.6	639	70.3	62.4	255	28.0	25.0
Nebraska	460	26.6	21.9	4 242	245.3	213.5	1 103	63.8	54.7	418	24.2	20.4
Nevada	253	11.6	16.7	4 421	203.4	245.1	976	44.9	56.8	368	16.9	22.1
New Hampshire	311	24.4	24.7	2 776	217.7	220.2	627	49.2	50.1	237	18.6	18.9
New Jersey	1 522	17.7	16.2	22 510	262.0	243.5	4 016	46.8	43.4	1 973	23.0	21.3
New Mexico	325	17.5	19.4	3 360	181.1	193.3	715	38.5	41.5	372	20.1	21.7
New York	1 803	9.4	8.6	56 672	295.8	277.4	7 625	39.8	37.4	5 368	28.0	26.1
North Carolina	1 962	23.6	25.9	18 524	222.6	235.2	5 259	63.2	67.8	1 898	22.8	24.6
North Dakota	294	46.4	33.2	1 623	255.9	201.3	469	74.0	54.6	162	25.5	18.4
Ohio	2 599	22.8	21.2	31 388	274.8	258.2	7 252	63.5	59.4	2 487	21.8	20.4
Oklahoma	754	21.6	20.5	11 230	321.4	306.0	2 427	69.5	66.2	914	26.2	24.9
Oregon	1 124	31.9	29.0	7 262	206.2	192.3	2 645	75.1	69.5	666	18.9	17.3
Pennsylvania	2 823	22.9	17.3	38 852	315.0	250.1	8 579	69.5	54.4	2 957	24.0	18.6
Rhode Island	264	24.7	19.0	3 109	290.6	239.1	605	56.6	45.8	319	29.8	23.9
South Carolina	967	23.5	26.1	9 659	235.2	244.4	2 822	68.7	72.7	910	22.2	23.8
South Dakota	167	21.9	16.6	1 937	254.5	209.7	518	68.1	54.2	240	31.5	25.0
Tennessee	1 299	22.4	23.3	16 226	279.9	282.4	3 980	68.7	70.1	1 710	29.5	30.2
Texas	3 793	17.4	23.0	43 452	199.5	249.8	10 548	48.4	61.8	3 673	16.9	21.6
Utah	303	13.1	19.4	2 977	128.5	185.1	903	39.0	56.8	424	18.3	26.6
Vermont	163	26.4	24.6	1 370	222.2	208.3	335	54.3	50.9	111	18.0	16.7
Virginia	1 368	18.8	21.7	14 952	205.0	226.8	3 960	54.3	61.2	1 480	20.3	23.1
Washington	2 195	36.2	37.9	11 141	183.6	193.3	3 753	61.8	65.2	907	14.9	15.6
West Virginia	405	22.5	18.7	6 189	343.5	287.3	1 260	69.9	58.3	427	23.7	19.8
Wisconsin	1 344	24.7	21.6	12 923	237.5	216.5	3 479	63.9	57.7	1 291	23.7	21.0
Wyoming	122	24.5	26.3	1 005	201.5	210.0	243	48.7	51.5	135	27.1	28.5
Puerto Rico[3]	943	24.4	28.5	5 950	154.2	170.2	1 574	40.8	46.1	1 021	26.5	29.9
Virgin Islands[3]	3	*	*	190	174.6	238.6	41	37.7	49.8	16	*	*
Guam[3]	3	*	*	201	124.8	253.6	49	30.4	60.4	20	12.4	23.8
American Samoa[3]	-	*	*	54	93.6	307.1	21	36.4	128.0	11	*	*
Northern Marianas[3]	-	*	*	27	36.5	226.8	12	*	*	3	*	*

[1] Death rates are affected by the population composition of the area. Age-adjusted death rates should be used for comparisons between areas.
[2] Excludes data for Puerto Rico, Virgin Islands, Guam, American Samoa, and Northern Marianas.
[3] Age-adjusted death rates for Puerto Rico, Virgin Islands, Guam, American Samoa, and Northern Marianas are calculated using different age groups in the weighting procedure.
* = Figure does not meet standards of reliability or precision.
- = Quantity zero.

Washington, North Dakota, Maine, and Oregon ranked highest for death rates from Alzheimer's disease. Minnesota, Alaska, Colorado, and Utah had the lowest death rates from heart diseases, while Mississippi, Oklahoma, West Virginia, Kentucky, and the District of Columbia had the highest death rates from cardiovascular disease.

The impact of age on accidents, suicides, homicides, and firearms deaths (examined in Table II-11) were less pronounced than the effect of age on diseases, but were still influenced enough to warrant comparisons of age-adjusted rates. For motor vehicle accidents, the states with the lowest fatality rates were Rhode Island, New York, Massachusetts, New Jersey, and the District of Columbia. Those with the highest death rates were Wyoming, Mississippi, Montana, and Arkansas. When all types of accidents were considered, Alaska stood out with the highest rate of fatalities, followed by New Mexico, Mississippi, Wyoming, and Montana. The lowest rates of completed suicides were found in the District of Columbia, New York, New Jersey, Massachusetts, and

Table II-29. Number of Deaths, Death Rates, and Age-Adjusted Death Rates for Major Causes of Death, for Each State and Territory, 2002—*Continued*

(Number, rate per 100,000 population.)

State	Chronic lower respiratory diseases (J40-J47)			Chronic liver disease and cirrhosis (K70, K73-K74)			Nephritis, nephrotic syndrome, and nephrosis (N00-N07, N17-N19, N25-N27)			Accidents (V01-X59, Y85-Y86)		
	Number	Rate	Age-adjusted rate [1]	Number	Rate	Age-adjusted rate [1]	Number	Rate	Age-adjusted rate [1]	Number	Rate	Age-adjusted rate [1]
UNITED STATES [2]	124 816	43.3	43.5	27 257	9.5	9.4	40 974	14.2	14.2	106 742	37.0	36.9
Alabama	2 328	51.9	50.3	425	9.5	9.1	1 032	23.0	22.4	2 228	49.7	49.2
Alaska	142	22.1	46.9	55	8.5	9.3	21	3.3	6.7	346	53.7	59.0
Arizona	2 575	47.2	47.4	671	12.3	12.6	622	11.4	11.6	2 577	47.2	48.1
Arkansas	1 441	53.2	48.2	222	8.2	7.7	601	22.2	20.2	1 311	48.4	47.3
California	12 684	36.1	42.0	3 747	10.7	11.6	2 164	6.2	7.1	10 107	28.8	29.9
Colorado	1 848	41.0	52.2	415	9.2	9.9	417	9.3	11.7	1 812	40.2	42.8
Connecticut	1 453	42.0	36.7	318	9.2	8.5	554	16.0	13.9	1 182	34.2	32.5
Delaware	350	43.3	42.7	88	10.9	10.4	117	14.5	14.3	292	36.2	35.9
District of Columbia	133	23.3	23.5	88	15.4	15.5	70	12.3	12.4	200	35.0	34.5
Florida	9 062	54.2	40.5	2 151	12.9	11.2	2 201	13.2	10.0	7 396	44.3	41.9
Georgia	3 163	36.9	47.8	696	8.1	9.0	1 335	15.6	20.1	3 333	38.9	41.8
Hawaii	265	21.3	19.7	79	6.3	6.0	136	10.9	10.1	393	31.6	30.4
Idaho	595	44.4	48.6	105	7.8	8.2	86	6.4	6.9	611	45.6	46.8
Illinois	4 827	38.3	39.3	1 068	8.5	8.7	2 328	18.5	18.7	4 222	33.5	33.5
Indiana	3 138	50.9	51.3	514	8.3	8.4	1 222	19.8	19.8	2 148	34.9	34.8
Iowa	1 580	53.8	44.3	220	7.5	6.8	261	8.9	7.0	1 093	37.2	33.3
Kansas	1 367	50.3	46.9	187	6.9	6.8	517	19.0	17.1	1 139	41.9	40.6
Kentucky	2 401	58.7	58.7	377	9.2	8.8	813	19.9	20.1	2 090	51.1	50.5
Louisiana	1 696	37.8	41.0	365	8.1	8.4	983	21.9	23.7	2 115	47.2	48.0
Maine	791	61.1	52.7	116	9.0	7.9	232	17.9	15.3	511	39.5	37.6
Maryland	1 944	35.6	39.1	443	8.1	8.1	630	11.5	12.5	1 332	24.4	25.1
Massachusetts	2 745	42.7	38.3	602	9.4	8.8	1 297	20.2	17.8	1 413	22.0	20.5
Michigan	4 431	44.1	44.5	993	9.9	9.7	1 618	16.1	16.2	3 285	32.7	32.7
Minnesota	1 971	39.3	39.1	320	6.4	6.5	649	12.9	12.5	1 928	38.4	37.3
Mississippi	1 378	48.0	50.0	229	8.0	8.2	580	20.2	20.9	1 642	57.2	57.9
Missouri	2 867	50.5	47.1	433	7.6	7.3	1 076	19.0	17.4	2 641	46.6	45.3
Montana	576	63.3	57.7	127	14.0	12.8	105	11.5	10.4	524	57.6	55.2
Nebraska	934	54.0	48.8	127	7.3	7.3	277	16.0	14.1	762	44.1	41.4
Nevada	1 174	54.0	65.5	268	12.3	12.4	372	17.1	20.6	860	39.6	41.9
New Hampshire	577	45.3	46.6	105	8.2	8.1	141	11.1	11.3	357	28.0	28.1
New Jersey	2 885	33.6	31.5	730	8.5	8.0	1 662	19.3	18.1	2 599	30.3	29.5
New Mexico	857	46.2	49.3	317	17.1	17.1	220	11.9	12.7	1 105	59.6	61.1
New York	6 966	36.4	34.6	1 338	7.0	6.7	2 465	12.9	12.2	4 663	24.3	23.7
North Carolina	3 674	44.2	46.5	735	8.8	8.8	1 437	17.3	18.3	3 700	44.5	45.2
North Dakota	322	50.8	41.6	63	9.9	9.3	57	9.0	6.8	246	38.8	35.0
Ohio	6 063	53.1	49.9	1 047	9.2	8.8	2 027	17.7	16.7	4 146	36.3	35.6
Oklahoma	1 988	56.9	54.3	428	12.3	11.9	500	14.3	13.7	1 580	45.2	44.6
Oregon	1 845	52.4	50.2	367	10.4	10.0	266	7.6	7.1	1 397	39.7	38.1
Pennsylvania	6 017	48.8	38.9	1 156	9.4	8.2	2 944	23.9	19.0	4 728	38.3	35.6
Rhode Island	521	48.7	40.9	128	12.0	11.1	142	13.3	11.1	277	25.9	23.1
South Carolina	1 889	46.0	47.4	386	9.4	9.1	781	19.0	19.8	1 972	48.0	48.2
South Dakota	383	50.3	43.0	75	9.9	9.7	128	16.8	13.7	348	45.7	43.3
Tennessee	3 011	51.9	52.2	611	10.5	10.2	586	10.1	10.2	2 744	47.3	47.4
Texas	7 720	35.4	44.9	2 284	10.5	11.7	2 166	9.9	12.4	8 232	37.8	40.1
Utah	603	26.0	37.7	133	5.7	7.7	184	7.9	11.5	714	30.8	35.6
Vermont	276	44.8	42.5	66	10.7	9.9	53	8.6	8.2	240	38.9	37.2
Virginia	2 752	37.7	41.9	598	8.2	8.4	1 236	16.9	18.8	2 479	34.0	35.0
Washington	2 721	44.8	48.3	525	8.7	8.8	306	5.0	5.3	2 203	36.3	36.5
West Virginia	1 228	68.2	56.4	209	11.6	10.1	462	25.6	21.4	956	53.1	50.7
Wisconsin	2 335	42.9	40.1	437	8.0	7.8	852	15.7	14.3	2 274	41.8	39.7
Wyoming	324	65.0	67.7	70	14.0	13.4	43	8.6	9.0	289	58.0	57.9
Puerto Rico [3]	1 075	27.9	31.6	265	6.9	7.2	829	21.5	23.4	1 123	29.1	29.2
Virgin Islands [3]	8	*	*	12	*	*	12	*	*	26	23.9	28.1
Guam [3]	27	16.8	44.5	12	*	*	12	*	*	31	19.2	21.8
American Samoa [3]	14	*	*	1	*	*	9	*	*	18	*	*
Northern Marianas [3]	6	*	*	3	*	*	5	*	*	15	*	*

[1]Death rates are affected by the population composition of the area. Age-adjusted death rates should be used for comparisons between areas.
[2]Excludes data for Puerto Rico, Virgin Islands, Guam, American Samoa, and Northern Marianas.
[3]Age-adjusted death rates for Puerto Rico, Virgin Islands, Guam, American Samoa, and Northern Marianas are calculated using different age groups in the weighting procedure.
* = Figure does not meet standards of reliability or precision.

Connecticut. The highest rates of completed suicides occurred in Alaska, Wyoming, Montana, and Nevada.

The highest rates of homicides occurred in the District of Columbia, Louisiana, Mississippi, Maryland, and Alabama. The lowest rates were recorded in Iowa, Utah, Idaho, and Nebraska. However, there were four states in which the absolute numbers of homicide deaths were too low to calculate reliable rates. These states, Maine, New Hampshire, North Dakota, and Vermont, were candidates for the lowest homicide death rates.

Age-adjusted death rates were high in American Samoa and the Northern Mariana Islands, but were somewhat below the U.S. average in Puerto Rico, the Virgin Islands, and Guam. In regard to specific causes of death, fatality

Table II-29. Number of Deaths, Death Rates, and Age-Adjusted Death Rates for Major Causes of Death, for Each State and Territory, 2002—Continued

(Number, rate per 100,000 population.)

State	Motor vehicle accidents [4]			Intentional self-harm (suicide) (*U03, X60-X84, Y87.0)			Assault (homicide) (*U01-*U02, X85-Y09, Y87.1)			Injury by firearms [5]		
	Number	Rate	Age-adjusted rate [1]	Number	Rate	Age-adjusted rate [1]	Number	Rate	Age-adjusted rate [1]	Number	Rate	Age-adjusted rate [1]
UNITED STATES [2]	45 380	15.7	15.7	31 655	11.0	10.9	17 638	6.1	6.1	30 242	10.5	10.4
Alabama	1 115	24.9	24.7	514	11.5	11.4	416	9.3	9.2	724	16.1	16.0
Alaska	112	17.4	19.1	132	20.5	21.0	40	6.2	6.0	127	19.7	20.0
Arizona	1 105	20.3	20.5	886	16.2	16.5	504	9.2	9.2	968	17.7	17.9
Arkansas	693	25.6	25.4	377	13.9	14.0	194	7.2	7.2	441	16.3	16.3
California	4 248	12.1	12.2	3 228	9.2	9.6	2 485	7.1	6.8	3 410	9.7	9.7
Colorado	781	17.3	17.4	727	16.1	16.2	184	4.1	4.0	517	11.5	11.5
Connecticut	348	10.1	10.2	260	7.5	7.4	98	2.8	3.0	147	4.2	4.3
Delaware	121	15.0	14.8	74	9.2	9.0	38	4.7	4.7	74	9.2	9.0
District of Columbia	58	10.2	9.4	31	5.4	5.1	229	40.1	37.2	195	34.2	31.3
Florida	3 196	19.1	18.9	2 338	14.0	13.4	1 008	6.0	6.3	1 886	11.3	11.1
Georgia	1 526	17.8	18.1	909	10.6	11.0	672	7.9	7.5	1 133	13.2	13.4
Hawaii	121	9.7	9.5	120	9.6	9.5	38	3.1	3.1	36	2.9	2.8
Idaho	296	22.1	22.2	202	15.1	15.5	32	2.4	2.4	163	12.2	12.4
Illinois	1 579	12.5	12.5	1 145	9.1	9.1	1 016	8.1	7.9	1 231	9.8	9.7
Indiana	963	15.6	15.5	743	12.1	12.1	385	6.3	6.2	723	11.7	11.7
Iowa	426	14.5	13.9	314	10.7	10.5	56	1.9	1.9	201	6.8	6.7
Kansas	563	20.7	20.3	345	12.7	12.6	129	4.7	4.7	268	9.9	9.7
Kentucky	923	22.6	22.1	540	13.2	12.8	195	4.8	4.7	544	13.3	12.9
Louisiana	959	21.4	21.3	499	11.1	11.2	607	13.5	13.3	876	19.5	19.4
Maine	215	16.6	16.1	166	12.8	12.3	11	*	*	88	6.8	6.5
Maryland	718	13.2	13.3	477	8.7	8.7	540	9.9	10.0	615	11.3	11.4
Massachusetts	565	8.8	8.6	436	6.8	6.5	185	2.9	2.9	204	3.2	3.1
Michigan	1 386	13.8	13.8	1 106	11.0	11.0	696	6.9	7.0	1 092	10.9	10.9
Minnesota	744	14.8	14.6	497	9.9	9.7	127	2.5	2.5	306	6.1	6.0
Mississippi	879	30.6	30.6	343	11.9	12.1	305	10.6	10.7	492	17.1	17.2
Missouri	1 213	21.4	21.1	693	12.2	12.1	366	6.5	6.5	696	12.3	12.2
Montana	255	28.0	27.4	184	20.2	19.99	23	2.5	2.5	134	14.7	14.5
Nebraska	337	19.5	18.9	201	11.6	11.7	50	2.9	2.9	140	8.1	8.1
Nevada	386	17.8	18.3	423	19.5	19.8	175	8.1	8.1	370	17.0	17.3
New Hampshire	125	9.8	9.8	132	10.4	10.2	9	*	*	76	6.0	5.8
New Jersey	786	9.1	9.2	553	6.4	6.3	333	3.9	4.0	415	4.8	4.9
New Mexico	423	22.8	22.7	349	18.8	19.1	161	8.7	8.7	304	16.4	16.6
New York	1 695	8.8	8.7	1 228	6.4	6.3	929	4.8	4.8	994	5.2	5.1
North Carolina	1 690	20.3	20.3	986	11.9	11.8	644	7.7	7.6	1 136	13.7	13.6
North Dakota	111	17.5	16.6	91	14.4	14.2	7	*	*	58	9.1	9.0
Ohio	1 602	14.0	13.9	1 287	11.3	11.2	549	4.8	4.9	1 069	9.4	9.3
Oklahoma	766	21.9	21.6	501	14.3	14.3	196	5.6	5.6	452	12.9	12.8
Oregon	462	13.1	12.8	518	14.7	14.4	106	3.0	3.1	374	10.6	10.5
Pennsylvania	1 739	14.1	13.8	1 341	10.9	10.7	640	5.2	5.4	1 220	9.9	9.9
Rhode Island	95	8.9	8.5	86	8.0	7.9	43	4.0	4.0	55	5.1	5.0
South Carolina	1 024	24.9	24.6	440	10.7	10.6	326	7.9	7.8	566	13.8	13.6
South Dakota	186	24.4	23.9	94	12.4	12.2	22	2.9	3.0	61	8.0	7.9
Tennessee	1 250	21.6	21.5	778	13.4	13.2	467	8.1	8.0	905	15.6	15.4
Texas	4 024	18.5	18.7	2 311	10.6	11.0	1 421	6.5	6.4	2 301	10.6	10.8
Utah	329	14.2	14.7	340	14.7	16.1	54	2.3	2.3	207	8.9	9.6
Vermont	78	12.7	12.5	92	14.9	14.1	8	*	*	62	10.1	9.6
Virginia	963	13.2	13.2	799	11.0	10.9	397	5.4	5.4	806	11.1	11.0
Washington	760	12.5	12.5	811	13.4	13.3	213	3.5	3.5	568	9.4	9.4
West Virginia	414	23.0	22.4	276	15.3	14.8	95	5.3	5.5	271	15.0	14.7
Wisconsin	870	16.0	15.6	627	11.5	11.3	191	3.5	3.5	446	8.2	8.0
Wyoming	157	31.5	31.2	105	21.1	20.7	23	4.6	4.7	95	19.0	18.8
Puerto Rico [3]	533	13.8	13.6	240	6.2	6.5	733	19.0	18.5	698	18.1	17.6
Virgin Islands [3]	12	*	*	2	*	*	41	37.7	39.8	36	33.1	35.2
Guam [3]	12	*	*	21	13.0	13.2	1	*	*	2	*	*
American Samoa [3]	3	*	*	1	*	*	10	*	*	1	*	*
Northern Marianas [3]	4	*	*	4	*	*	4	*	*	2	*	*

[1]Death rates are affected by the population composition of the area. Age-adjusted death rates should be used for comparisons between areas.
[2]Excludes data for Puerto Rico, Virgin Islands, Guam, American Samoa, and Northern Marianas.
[3]Age-adjusted death rates for Puerto Rico, Virgin Islands, Guam, American Samoa, and Northern Marianas are calculated using different age groups in the weighting procedure.
[4]*International Classification of Diseases, Tenth Revision* (1992), *ICD-10* codes for motor vehicle accidents are V02-V04, V09.0, V09.2, V12-V14, V19.0-V19.2, V19.4-V19.6, V20-V79, V80.3-V80.5, V81.0-V81.1, V82.0-V82.1, V83-V86, V87.0-V87.8, V88.0-V88.8, V89.0, V89.2.
[5]*ICD-10* codes for injury by firearms are *U01.4, W32-W34, X72-X74, X93-X95, Y22-Y24, Y35.0.
* = Figure does not meet standards of reliability or precision.

rates for diabetes were very high in American Samoa and Puerto Rico, and relatively high in the Virgin Islands. Also noticeably high were death rates from nephritis in Puerto Rico and from homicides in the Virgin Islands.

TABLE II-29A. NUMBER OF DEATHS, DEATH RATES, AND AGE-ADJUSTED DEATH RATES, FOR EACH STATE AND TERRITORY, 2002 AND PRELIMINARY 2003

The preliminary age-adjusted death rate in 2003 was 831.2 per 100,000 persons, but this was adjusted upward in the final 2003 data release to 832.7 per 100,000 persons. This compares with the final 2002 rate of 845.3 per 100,000 persons. The states that had the lowest death rates in 2002 also had the lowest preliminary rates in 2003. These were Hawaii, Minnesota, and Connecticut. In each of these states, there was a noticeable drop in the death rates for 2003. Rates for California, which were also among the lowest in 2002, were not available for 2003.

The states with the highest age-adjusted death rates in 2002 also ranked high in 2003. At the top in the preliminary 2003 release were Mississippi (1,015.2 per 100,000 persons), Louisiana (1,007.4), Alabama (1,001.9), and West Virginia (994.5).

Table II-29A. Number of Deaths, Death Rates, and Age-Adjusted Death Rates, for Each State and Territory, 2002 and Preliminary 2003

(Number, rate per 100,000 population.)

State	2003			2002		
	Number	Rate	Age-adjusted rate	Number	Rate	Age-adjusted rate
UNITED STATES [1]	2 443 908	840.4	831.2	2 443 387	847.3	845.3
Alabama	46 726	1 038.2	1 001.9	46 069	1 026.8	998.1
Alaska	3 185	490.9	831.3	3 030	470.7	789.1
Arizona	43 496	779.4	788.9	42 816	784.7	795.7
Arkansas	27 924	1 024.5	937.6	28 513	1 052.1	964.4
California [2]	. . .	. . .	. . .	234 565	668.0	757.8
Colorado	29 542	649.2	785.3	29 210	648.2	790.2
Connecticut	29 432	844.9	729.5	30 122	870.5	762.4
Delaware	7 070	864.8	844.3	6 861	849.8	838.2
District of Columbia	5 513	976.9	968.2	5 851	1 024.9	1 021.4
Florida	168 607	990.7	775.7	167 814	1 004.1	786.4
Georgia	66 473	765.4	946.4	65 449	764.6	949.1
Hawaii	8 987	714.6	650.1	8 801	707.0	660.6
Idaho	10 385	760.1	797.5	9 923	739.9	793.0
Illinois [2]	. . .	. . .	. . .	106 667	846.5	856.0
Indiana	56 193	907.0	898.1	55 396	899.4	899.6
Iowa	28 080	953.8	769.0	27 978	952.7	774.5
Kansas	24 596	903.1	824.0	25 021	921.3	843.5
Kentucky	40 236	977.1	976.9	40 697	994.3	993.9
Louisiana	42 893	954.0	1 007.4	41 984	936.6	1 000.5
Maine	12 534	959.9	821.9	12 694	980.6	846.5
Maryland	44 500	807.8	852.9	43 970	805.6	864.1
Massachusetts	56 297	875.1	778.8	56 928	885.7	791.9
Michigan	86 710	860.2	850.3	87 795	873.5	876.2
Minnesota	37 636	743.9	713.4	38 510	767.2	747.5
Mississippi	28 535	990.4	1 015.2	28 853	1 004.7	1 036.3
Missouri	55 569	974.1	902.4	55 940	986.1	916.7
Montana	8 467	922.7	828.3	8 506	935.3	849.7
Nebraska	15 466	889.2	790.6	15 738	910.1	814.8
Nevada	17 864	797.1	925.0	16 927	778.8	916.5
New Hampshire	9 691	752.6	748.4	9 853	772.8	781.7
New Jersey	73 683	853.0	794.7	74 009	861.5	808.7
New Mexico	14 877	793.6	827.7	14 344	773.2	815.0
New York	155 852	812.1	759.8	158 118	825.4	783.3
North Carolina	73 548	874.8	906.8	72 027	865.7	906.1
North Dakota	6 095	961.6	767.5	5 892	929.2	749.8
Ohio	108 660	950.2	886.2	109 766	961.1	908.2
Oklahoma	35 733	1 017.6	973.9	35 502	1 016.2	973.2
Oregon	30 934	869.0	808.9	31 119	883.7	834.2
Pennsylvania	129 767	1 049.4	849.1	130 223	1 055.7	862.1
Rhode Island	10 038	932.8	786.6	10 246	957.8	809.5
South Carolina	38 111	919.0	934.8	37 736	918.8	946.9
South Dakota	7 133	933.3	790.5	6 898	906.4	771.2
Tennessee	57 306	981.0	982.1	56 606	976.4	981.5
Texas	155 171	701.5	857.2	155 524	714.1	870.0
Utah	13 408	570.2	782.1	13 116	566.3	782.0
Vermont	5 112	825.7	764.1	5 075	823.1	775.0
Virginia	58 415	790.9	852.8	57 196	784.2	856.6
Washington	45 964	749.6	776.6	45 338	747.0	785.3
West Virginia	21 299	1 176.5	994.5	21 016	1 166.3	991.7
Wisconsin	46 174	843.8	772.3	46 981	863.4	799.8
Wyoming	4 173	832.5	850.6	4 174	837.0	864.3
Puerto Rico	28 243	728.2	782.0	27 924	723.6	790.8
Virgin Islands	628	577.1	712.8	617	567.0	734.3
Guam	672	410.8	748.3	638	396.1	736.6
American Samoa	. . .	. . .	. . .	290	502.5	1 467.9
Northern Marianas	143	187.8	808.5	161	217.6	1 057.4

[1] Excludes data for U.S. territories.
[2] California and Illinois data are not shown separately but are included in U.S. totals.
. . . = Not available.

TABLE II-30. NUMBER OF INFANT, NEONATAL, AND POSTNEONATAL DEATHS AND MORTALITY, 2002–2003

While the number of infant deaths (deaths of children under 1 year of age) declined by only 9 in 2003, the rate per 1,000 live births fell more significantly, dropping by 0.12 to reach 6.85. This drop reflected a larger number of births. Female babies experienced a greater decline in their mortality rate than male babies. The reduction was stronger during the postneonatal period (28 days to 1 year) than during the neonatal period (under 28 days of life), with males showing no decline in mortality during the neonatal period. As a result, the neonatal mortality increase of 2002 was only partly reversed.

Table II-30. Number of Infant, Neonatal, and Postneonatal Deaths and Mortality, 2002–2003

(Number, rate per 1,000 live births.)

Sex	2003		2002	
	Number	Rate	Number	Rate
Infant				
Total	28 025	6.9	28 034	7.0
Male	15 902	7.6	15 717	7.6
Female	12 123	6.1	12 317	6.3
Neonatal				
Total	18 893	4.6	18 747	4.7
Male	10 636	5.1	10 408	5.1
Female	8 257	4.1	8 339	4.3
Postneonatal				
Total	9 132	2.2	9 287	2.3
Male	5 266	2.5	5 309	2.6
Female	3 866	1.9	3 978	2.0

Note: Infant age = under 1 year; neonatal age = under 28 days; and postneonatal age = 28 days to 1 year.

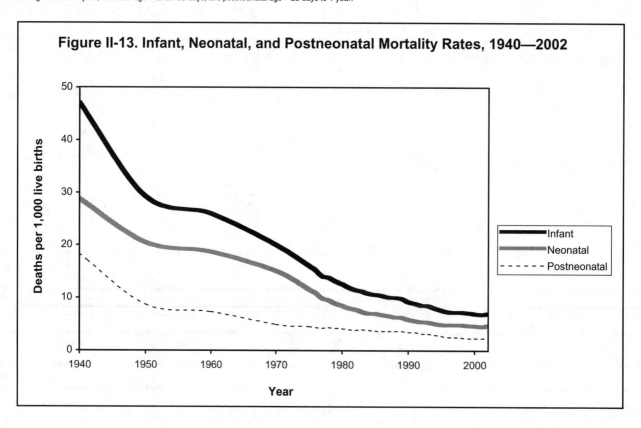

Figure II-13. Infant, Neonatal, and Postneonatal Mortality Rates, 1940—2002

TABLE II-30A. INFANT, NEONATAL, AND POSTNEONATAL MORTALITY RATES, BY RACE AND SEX, SELECTED YEARS, 1940–2002

Infant death rates, presented in some of the previous tables that showed data by age, used the estimated mid-year population under 1 year of age, based on the 2000 census, as denominators. (Tables II-9 and II-11 were constructed in this fashion.) However, the most commonly used index for measuring the risk of dying during the first year of life is the "infant mortality rate" (shown here), which is calculated by dividing the number of infant deaths in a calendar year by the number of live births registered for that year. Due to the different denominators, infant mortality rates may differ from infant death rates.

Infant mortality rates declined from 47.0 per 1,000 live births in 1940 to 12.6 per 1,000 live births in 1980 and 7.0 per 1,000 live births in 2002. However, the 2001 rate of 6.8 per 1,000 live births was the lowest rate ever recorded for the United States. For babies born to White mothers, the infant mortality rate was 5.8 per 1,000 live births in 2002. This rate was as high as 14.4 per 1,000 live births for those born to Black mothers. (However, this represented a fall from the death rate of 72.9 per 1,000 live births

recorded for Blacks in 1940.) The ratio of the infant mortality rates for Blacks to Whites was 2.5 in 2002. The infant mortality rate tended to be about 20 percent greater for males than for females.

The increase in infant mortality in 2002 represented the first time in more than 40 years that the rate had not gone down or remained steady. The increase was concentrated in neonatal deaths (those occurring among infants less than 28 days old). This was associated with an abrupt increase of about 660 in the number of newborns with very low birthweights, who were born weighing less than 1,500 grams (3.3 lbs.) The major components of this increase were a gain of 330 in newborns who weighed less than 500 grams at birth (less than 1.1 lbs), and an increase of 209 in babies who weighed between 500 and 750 grams (1.1–1.7 lbs) at birth. The majority of infants with such low birthweights tended to die within the first year of life. Non-Hispanic White, non-Hispanic Black, and Hispanic mothers all experienced some of this increase. In 2002, there were tendencies towards shorter periods of gestation. Preterm or very preterm deliveries were important risk factors for low birthweight babies. On the basis of statistical analysis, the shifts described above would explain about 60 percent of the increase in early infant deaths.

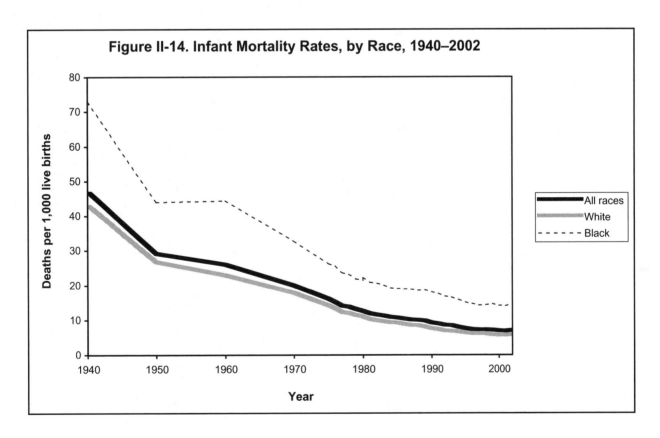

Figure II-14. Infant Mortality Rates, by Race, 1940–2002

(See: MacDorman, Marion F., et al. 2005. Explaining the 2001–02 infant mortality increase: Data from the linked birth/infant death data set. *National Vital Statistics Report* 53 (12). Hyattsville, MD: National Center for Health Statistics.)

In 2002, neonatal deaths accounted for two-thirds of all infant deaths within the first year of life, and post-neonatal deaths accounted for the remaining one-third of the total.

Table II-30A. Infant, Neonatal, and Postneonatal Mortality Rates, by Race and Sex, Selected Years, 1940–2002

(Rates per 1,000 live births in specified group.)

Year	All races			White			All other					
							Total			Black		
	Both sexes	Male	Female	Both sexes	Male	Female	Both sexes	Male	Female	Both sexes	Male	Female
INFANT MORTALITY RATE												
Race of Mother [1]												
2002	7.0	7.6	6.3	5.8	6.4	5.1	11.4	12.2	10.5	14.4	15.4	13.3
2001	6.8	7.5	6.1	5.7	6.2	5.1	11.3	12.4	10.2	14.0	15.5	12.5
2000	6.9	7.6	6.2	5.7	6.2	5.1	11.4	12.6	10.3	14.1	15.5	12.6
1999	7.1	7.7	6.4	5.8	6.4	5.2	11.9	12.9	10.9	14.6	15.9	13.2
1998	7.2	7.8	6.5	6.0	6.5	5.4	11.9	13.0	10.8	14.3	15.7	12.8
1997	7.2	8.0	6.5	6.0	6.7	5.4	11.8	12.8	10.7	14.2	15.5	12.8
1996	7.3	8.0	6.6	6.1	6.7	5.4	12.2	13.3	11.0	14.7	16.0	13.3
1995	7.6	8.3	6.8	6.3	7.0	5.6	12.6	13.5	11.6	15.1	16.3	13.9
1994	8.0	8.8	7.2	6.6	7.2	5.9	13.5	14.8	12.1	15.8	17.5	14.1
1993	8.4	9.3	7.4	6.8	7.6	6.0	14.1	15.6	12.5	16.5	18.3	14.7
1992	8.5	9.4	7.6	6.9	7.7	6.1	14.4	15.7	13.1	16.8	18.4	15.3
1991	8.9	10.0	7.8	7.3	8.3	6.3	15.1	16.5	13.6	17.6	19.4	15.7
1990	9.2	10.3	8.1	7.6	8.5	6.6	15.5	17.0	14.0	18.0	19.6	16.2
1989	9.8	10.8	8.8	8.1	9.0	7.1	16.3	17.6	15.0	18.6	20.0	17.2
1988	10.0	11.0	8.9	8.4	9.4	7.3	16.1	17.3	14.8	18.5	20.0	17.0
1987	10.1	11.2	8.9	8.5	9.5	7.5	16.5	18.1	14.8	18.8	20.6	16.8
1986	10.4	11.5	9.1	8.8	9.9	7.7	16.7	18.5	14.9	18.9	20.9	16.8
1985	10.6	11.9	9.3	9.2	10.4	7.9	16.8	18.3	15.3	19.0	20.8	17.2
1984	10.8	11.9	9.6	9.3	10.4	8.2	17.1	18.4	15.7	19.2	20.7	17.6
1983	11.2	12.3	10.0	9.6	10.7	8.5	17.8	19.4	16.1	20.0	22.0	18.0
1982	11.5	12.8	10.2	9.9	11.1	8.7	18.3	20.1	16.5	20.5	22.5	18.4
1981	11.9	13.1	10.7	10.3	11.5	9.1	18.8	20.4	17.2	20.8	22.5	19.0
1980	12.6	13.9	11.2	10.9	12.1	9.5	20.2	21.9	18.4	22.2	24.2	20.2
Race of Child [2]												
1980	12.6	13.9	11.2	11.0	12.3	9.6	19.1	20.7	17.5	21.4	23.3	19.4
1979	13.1	14.5	11.6	11.4	12.8	9.9	19.8	21.5	18.1	21.8	23.7	19.8
1978	13.8	15.3	12.2	12.0	13.4	10.6	21.1	23.1	18.9	23.1	25.4	20.8
1977	14.1	15.8	12.4	12.3	13.9	10.7	21.7	23.7	19.6	23.6	25.9	21.3
1976	15.2	16.8	13.6	13.3	14.8	11.7	23.5	25.5	21.4	25.5	27.8	23.2
1975	16.1	17.9	14.2	14.2	15.9	12.3	24.2	26.2	22.2	26.2	28.3	24.0
1970	20.0	22.4	17.5	17.8	20.0	15.4	30.9	34.2	27.5	32.6	36.2	29.0
1960	26.0	29.3	22.6	22.9	26.0	19.6	43.2	47.9	38.5	44.3	49.1	39.4
1950	29.2	32.8	25.5	26.8	30.2	23.1	44.5	48.9	39.9	43.9	48.3	39.4
1940	47.0	52.5	41.3	43.2	48.3	37.8	73.8	82.2	65.2	72.9	81.1	64.6
NEONATAL MORTALITY RATE												
Race of Mother [1]												
2002	4.7	5.1	4.2	3.9	4.3	3.5	7.5	8.0	7.0	9.5	10.1	8.9
2001	4.5	5.0	4.1	3.8	4.2	3.4	7.4	8.1	6.6	9.2	10.2	8.2
2000	4.6	5.1	4.2	3.8	4.2	3.5	7.6	8.4	6.8	9.4	10.4	8.3
1999	4.7	5.1	4.3	3.9	4.2	3.6	7.9	8.6	7.3	9.8	10.7	8.8
1998	4.8	5.2	4.4	4.0	4.3	3.6	7.9	8.6	7.2	9.5	10.5	8.6
1997	4.8	5.2	4.3	4.0	4.4	3.6	7.7	8.4	7.1	9.4	10.1	8.6
1996	4.8	5.2	4.3	4.0	4.3	3.6	7.9	8.6	7.1	9.6	10.4	8.7
1995	4.9	5.4	4.4	4.1	4.5	3.6	8.1	8.7	7.5	9.8	10.6	9.0
1994	5.1	5.6	4.6	4.2	4.5	3.8	8.6	9.5	7.7	10.2	11.3	9.1
1993	5.3	5.7	4.8	4.3	4.6	3.9	9.0	9.9	8.1	10.7	11.8	9.6
1992	5.4	5.8	4.9	4.3	4.7	4.0	9.2	10.0	8.3	10.8	11.8	9.8
1991	5.6	6.2	5.0	4.5	5.0	4.0	9.5	10.5	8.5	11.2	12.6	9.9
1990	5.8	6.5	5.2	4.8	5.4	4.2	9.9	10.8	8.9	11.6	12.7	10.4
1989	6.2	6.8	5.6	5.1	5.7	4.6	10.3	11.1	9.5	11.9	12.8	11.0
1988	6.3	6.9	5.7	5.3	5.8	4.7	10.3	11.2	9.4	12.1	13.1	10.9
1987	6.5	7.1	5.8	5.4	6.0	4.8	10.7	11.7	9.6	12.3	13.5	11.0
1986	6.7	7.4	6.0	5.7	6.3	5.1	10.8	11.8	9.7	12.3	13.6	11.0
1985	7.0	7.8	6.1	6.0	6.8	5.2	11.0	12.0	10.0	12.6	13.8	11.4
1984	7.0	7.7	6.3	6.1	6.7	5.4	10.9	11.7	10.1	12.3	13.2	11.4
1983	7.3	8.0	6.5	6.3	7.0	5.6	11.4	12.5	10.3	12.9	14.2	11.6
1982	7.7	8.5	6.9	6.7	7.4	5.9	12.0	13.2	10.9	13.6	14.9	12.3
1981	8.0	8.8	7.2	7.0	7.7	6.2	12.5	13.5	11.5	14.0	15.2	12.8
1980	8.5	9.3	7.6	7.4	8.2	6.5	13.2	14.3	12.1	14.6	15.9	13.3

Note: Infant age = under 1 year; neonatal age = under 28 days; and postneonatal age = 28 days to 1 year.

[1] Infant deaths based on race of child as stated on the death certificate; live births based on race of mother as stated on the birth certificate.
[2] Infant deaths based on race of child as stated on the death certificate; live births based on race of parents as stated on the birth certificate.

Table II-30A. Infant, Neonatal, and Postneonatal Mortality Rates, by Race and Sex, Selected Years, 1940–2002—*Continued*

(Rates per 1,000 live births in specified group.)

Year	All races			White			All other					
							Total			Black		
	Both sexes	Male	Female	Both sexes	Male	Female	Both sexes	Male	Female	Both sexes	Male	Female
Race of Child [2]												
1980	8.5	9.3	7.6	7.5	8.3	6.6	12.5	13.5	11.5	14.1	15.3	12.8
1979	8.9	9.8	7.9	7.9	8.8	6.9	12.9	13.9	11.8	14.3	15.5	13.1
1978	9.5	10.5	8.4	8.4	9.3	7.4	14.0	15.5	12.4	15.5	17.2	13.7
1977	9.9	11.0	8.7	8.7	9.8	7.6	14.7	16.0	13.3	16.1	17.6	14.5
1976	10.9	12.0	9.7	9.7	10.7	8.5	16.3	17.7	14.9	17.9	19.5	16.3
1975	11.6	12.9	10.2	10.4	11.7	9.0	16.8	18.2	15.3	18.3	19.8	16.8
1970	15.1	17.0	13.1	13.8	15.5	11.9	21.4	23.9	18.9	22.8	25.4	20.1
1960	18.7	21.2	16.1	17.2	19.7	14.7	26.9	30.0	23.6	27.8	31.1	24.5
1950	20.5	23.3	17.5	19.4	22.2	16.4	27.5	30.8	24.2	27.8	31.1	24.4
1940	28.8	32.6	24.7	27.2	30.9	23.3	39.7	44.9	34.5	39.9	44.8	34.9
POSTNEONATAL MORTALITY RATE												
Race of Mother [1]												
2002	2.3	2.6	2.0	1.9	2.1	1.6	3.9	4.2	3.5	4.8	5.3	4.4
2001	2.3	2.5	2.1	1.9	2.1	1.7	4.0	4.4	3.5	4.8	5.3	4.3
2000	2.3	2.5	2.0	1.9	2.1	1.7	3.8	4.2	3.5	4.7	5.1	4.3
1999	2.3	2.6	2.0	1.9	2.2	1.6	4.0	4.3	3.6	4.8	5.2	4.4
1998	2.4	2.6	2.2	2.0	2.2	1.8	4.0	4.4	3.6	4.8	5.2	4.3
1997	2.5	2.8	2.1	2.0	2.3	1.8	4.0	4.5	3.6	4.8	5.3	4.2
1996	2.5	2.8	2.2	2.1	2.4	1.8	4.3	4.7	3.9	5.1	5.6	4.6
1995	2.7	3.0	2.4	2.2	2.5	1.9	4.5	4.8	4.1	5.3	5.7	4.8
1994	2.9	3.2	2.6	2.4	2.7	2.1	4.9	5.3	4.4	5.6	6.2	5.0
1993	3.1	3.5	2.6	2.5	2.9	2.1	5.1	5.7	4.4	5.8	6.6	5.1
1992	3.1	3.5	2.7	2.6	3.0	2.2	5.2	5.7	4.8	6.0	6.5	5.5
1991	3.4	3.8	2.9	2.8	3.2	2.3	5.6	6.0	5.1	6.3	6.8	5.8
1990	3.4	3.8	3.0	2.8	3.1	2.4	5.7	6.2	5.1	6.4	6.9	5.9
1989	3.6	4.0	3.1	2.9	3.4	2.5	6.0	6.5	5.5	6.7	7.2	6.2
1988	3.6	4.0	3.2	3.1	3.5	2.6	5.7	6.1	5.4	6.5	6.9	6.1
1987	3.6	4.1	3.2	3.1	3.5	2.6	5.8	6.3	5.2	6.4	7.1	5.8
1986	3.6	4.1	3.1	3.1	3.5	2.6	5.9	6.6	5.2	6.6	7.3	5.8
1985	3.7	4.2	3.2	3.2	3.6	2.7	5.8	6.3	5.3	6.4	7.0	5.8
1984	3.8	4.2	3.3	3.2	3.7	2.8	6.2	6.7	5.6	6.8	7.5	6.2
1983	3.9	4.3	3.4	3.3	3.7	2.9	6.4	7.0	5.8	7.0	7.8	6.3
1982	3.8	4.3	3.3	3.2	3.7	2.8	6.3	6.9	5.6	6.9	7.6	6.1
1981	3.9	4.3	3.5	3.4	3.8	2.9	6.3	6.8	5.8	6.8	7.4	6.3
1980	4.1	4.6	3.6	3.5	3.9	3.0	7.0	7.6	6.3	7.6	8.3	6.9
Race of Child [2]												
1980	4.1	4.6	3.6	3.5	4.0	3.0	6.6	7.2	6.0	7.3	7.9	6.6
1979	4.2	4.7	3.7	3.5	4.0	3.0	6.9	7.6	6.3	7.5	8.2	6.7
1978	4.3	4.7	3.9	3.6	4.0	3.2	7.0	7.6	6.5	7.6	8.2	7.0
1977	4.2	4.8	3.7	3.6	4.1	3.1	7.0	7.7	6.3	7.6	8.3	6.8
1976	4.3	4.8	3.8	3.6	4.1	3.2	7.2	7.8	6.5	7.6	8.4	6.9
1975	4.5	4.9	4.0	3.8	4.2	3.3	7.5	8.0	6.9	7.9	8.5	7.2
1970	4.9	5.4	4.4	4.0	4.4	3.5	9.5	10.3	8.6	9.9	10.8	8.9
1960	7.3	8.1	6.5	5.7	6.3	4.9	16.4	17.8	14.8	16.5	18.0	14.9
1950	8.7	9.4	8.0	7.4	8.0	6.7	16.9	18.1	15.7	16.1	17.2	15.0
1940	18.3	19.9	16.6	16.0	17.5	14.5	34.1	37.3	30.7	33.0	36.4	29.7

Note: Infant age = under 1 year; neonatal age = under 28 days; and postneonatal age = 28 days to 1 year.

[1] Infant deaths based on race of child as stated on the death certificate; live births based on race of mother as stated on the birth certificate.
[2] Infant deaths based on race of child as stated on the death certificate; live births based on race of parents as stated on the birth certificate.

TABLE II-30B. NUMBER OF INFANT, NEONATAL, AND POSTNEONATAL DEATHS, BY SEX, 2001–2002

This table summarizes infant deaths for 2001 and 2002 by sex. Infants are defined as children under 1 year old, neonates as infants less than 28 days old, and postneonates as infants 28 days up to 1 year old. The infant mortality rate is the number of infant deaths in a calendar year divided by the number of live births registered in that year, with analogous definitions for neonatal and post-neonatal mortality rates. (See comments for Table II-30A.)

In 2002, there were 28,034 infant deaths, 466 more than in 2001. (See comments for Table II-30A.) Roughly two-thirds of infant deaths occurred during the neonatal period. Male infants had higher mortality rates than female infants.

TABLE II-31. NUMBER OF INFANT DEATHS, INFANT MORTALITY RATES, AND PERCENT CHANGE IN RATE FROM PREVIOUS YEAR, FOR 10 LEADING CAUSES OF INFANT DEATH, 2003

The four most frequent causes of death were congenital malformations, disorders related to short gestation and low birthweight, sudden infant death syndrome, and effects from maternal complications of pregnancy. These factors combined accounted for 51 percent of all infant deaths in 2003. Deaths in over half of the 10 categories listed in this table declined in 2003, but deaths caused by complications of the placenta, cord, and membranes increased 5 percent.

Table II-30B. Number of Infant, Neonatal, and Postneonatal Deaths, by Sex, 2001–2002

(Number, rate per 1,000 live births.)

Sex	2002		2001	
	Number	Rate	Number	Rate
Infant				
Total	28 034	7.0	27 568	6.8
Male	15 717	7.6	15 477	7.5
Female	12 317	6.3	12 091	6.1
Neonatal				
Total	18 747	4.7	18 265	4.5
Male	10 408	5.1	10 237	5.0
Female	8 339	4.2	8 028	4.1
Postneonatal				
Total	9 287	2.3	9 303	2.3
Male	5 309	2.5	5 240	2.5
Female	3 978	2.1	4 063	2.1

Note: Infant age = under 1 year; neonatal age = under 28 days; and postneonatal age = 28 days to 1 year.

Table II-31. Number of Infant Deaths, Infant Mortality Rates, and Percent Change in Rate from Previous Year, for 10 Leading Causes of Infant Death, 2003

(Number, percent, rate per 100,000 live births.)

Rank [1]	Cause of death [2]	Number	Percent of total deaths	Rate	Percent change, 2002–2003 [3]
	All Causes	28 025	100.0	685.2	-1.7
1	Congenital malformations, deformations, and chromosomal abnormalities (Q00–Q99)	5 621	20.1	137.4	-1.7
2	Disorders related to short gestation and low birthweight, not elsewhere classified (P07)	4 849	17.3	118.6	2.9
3	Sudden infant death syndrome (R95)	2 162	7.7	52.9	-7.4
4	Newborn affected by maternal complications of pregnancy (P01)	1 710	6.1	41.8	-1.6
5	Newborn affected by complications of placenta, cord, and membranes (P02)	1 099	3.9	26.9	5.1
6	Accidents (unintentional injuries) (V01–X59)	945	3.4	23.1	-1.7
7	Respiratory distress of newborn (P22)	831	3.0	20.3	-13.2
8	Bacterial sepsis of newborn (P36)	772	2.8	18.9	1.6
9	Neonatal hemorrhage (P50–P52, P54) [4]	649	2.3	15.9	65.6
10	Diseases of the circulatory system (I00–I99)	591	2.1	14.5	-12.7
	All other causes (residual)	8 796	31.4	215.1	X

[1]Rank based on number of deaths.
[2]Based on codes from the *International Classification of Diseases, Tenth Revision* (1992).
[3]Percent change based on a comparison of the 2003 infant mortality rate with the 2002 infant mortality rate.
[4]Cause of death coding changes may affect comparability with the previous year's data for this cause.
X = Not applicable.

TABLE II-31A. NUMBER OF INFANT DEATHS, INFANT MORTALITY RATES, AND PERCENT CHANGE IN RATE FROM PREVIOUS YEAR, FOR 10 LEADING CAUSES OF INFANT DEATH, 2002

The infant mortality rates in this table are expressed as deaths per 100,000 live births. The 10 leading causes of death accounted for 61 percent of all infant fatalities. The top cause, representing 20.1 percent of all infant deaths in 2002, was congenital malformations, deformations, and chromosomal abnormalities. Disorders related to short gestation and low birthweight, not elsewhere classified, were second in importance, causing 16.5 percent of all deaths. Sudden infant death syndrome ranked third, accounting for 8.2 percent of deaths. Newborns affected by maternal complications of pregnancy accounted for 6.1 percent of all infant deaths. Accidents (unintentional injuries) made up 3.4 percent of fatalities. Respiratory distress of the newborn accounted for another 3.4 percent of deaths.

There were a number of significant percentage changes in the rates for the 10 leading causes of infant death between 2001 and 2002. The largest increase occurred for newborns affected by maternal complications of pregnancy, which rose 14.2 percent. However, this increase was partly due to a cause of death coding change, which shifted some cases from atelectasis (in "other respiratory conditions originating in the perinatal period," Table II-31B) to the category of maternal complications of pregnancy. Intrauterine hypoxia and birth asphyxia also showed a large increase of 9.0 percent. There were only two reductions in mortality causes; the largest was a 6.8 percent decline in deaths due to respiratory distress of newborn.

TABLE II-31B. NUMBER OF INFANT DEATHS AND INFANT MORTALITY RATES FOR 130 SELECTED CAUSES, 2002 AND PRELIMINARY 2003

This table shows 130 selected causes of infant death for 2003 (preliminary) and 2002 (final). Rates are shown per 100,000 live births. Age adjustment was not necessary, as the data were confined to infants less than 1 year of age.

Table II-31A. Number of Infant Deaths, Infant Mortality Rates, and Percent Change in Rate from Previous Year, for 10 Leading Causes of Infant Death, 2002

(Number, percent, rate per 100,000 live births.)

Rank [1]	Cause of death [2]	Number	Percent of total deaths	Rate	Percent change, 2001–2002 [3]
	All Causes	28 034	100.0	697.1	1.8
1	Congenital malformations, deformations, and chromosomal abnormalities (Q00–Q99)	5 623	20.1	139.8	2.1
2	Disorders related to short gestation and low birthweight, not elsewhere classified (P07)	4 637	16.5	115.3	5.3
3	Sudden infant death syndrome (R95)	2 295	8.2	57.1	2.9
4	Newborn affected by maternal complications of pregnancy (P01) [4]	1 708	6.1	42.5	14.2
5	Newborn affected by complications of placenta, cord, and membranes (P02)	1 028	3.7	25.6	1.2
6	Accidents (unintentional injuries) (V01–X59)	946	3.4	23.5	-2.9
7	Respiratory distress of newborn (P22)	943	3.4	23.4	-6.8
8	Bacterial sepsis of newborn (P36)	749	2.7	18.6	7.5
9	Diseases of the circulatory system (I00–I99)	667	2.4	16.6	7.8
10	Intrauterine hypoxia and birth asphyxia (P20–P21)	583	2.1	14.5	9.0
	All other causes (residual)	8 855	31.6	220.2	X

[1] Rank based on number of deaths.
[2] Based on codes from the *International Classification of Diseases, Tenth Revision* (1992).
[3] Percent change based on a comparison of the 2002 infant mortality rate with the 2001 infant mortality rate.
[4] Cause of death coding changes may affect comparability with the previous year's data for this cause.
X = Not applicable.

Table II-31B. Number of Infant Deaths and Infant Mortality Rates for 130 Selected Causes, 2002 and Preliminary 2003

(Number, rate per 100,000 live births.)

Cause of death[1]	2003		2002	
	Number	Rate	Number	Rate
ALL CAUSES	28 422	694.7	28 034	697.1
Certain infectious and parasitic diseases (A00-B99)	495	12.1	582	14.5
Certain intestinal infectious diseases (A00-A08)	9	*	13	*
Diarrhea and gastroenteritis of infectious origin (A09)	1	*	3	*
Tuberculosis (A16-A19)	-	*	1	*
Tetanus (A33, A35)	-	*	-	*
Diphtheria (A36)	-	*	-	*
Whooping cough (A37)	9	*	18	*
Meningococcal infection (A39)	10	*	17	*
Septicemia (A40-A41)	279	6.8	296	7.4
Congenital syphilis (A50)	-	*	1	*
Gonococcal infection (A54)	-	*	1	*
Viral diseases (A80-B34)	117	2.9	164	4.1
Acute poliomyelitis (A80)	-	*	-	*
Varicella (chickenpox) (B01)	1	*	1	*
Measles (B05)	-	*	-	*
Human immunodeficiency virus (HIV) disease (B20-B24)	5	*	7	*
Mumps (B26)	-	*	-	*
Other and unspecified viral diseases (A81-B00, B02-B04, B06-B19, B25, B27-B34)	110	2.7	156	3.9
Candidiasis (B37)	23	0.6	19	*
Malaria (B50-B54)	-	*	-	*
Pneumocystosis (B59)	3	*	2	*
All other and unspecified infectious and parasitic diseases (A20-A32, A38, A42-A49, A51-A53, A55-A79, B35-B36, B38-B49, B55-B58, B60-B99)	43	1.1	47	1.2
Neoplasms (C00-D48)	152	3.7	143	3.6
Malignant neoplasms (C00-C97)	83	2.0	74	1.8
Hodgkin's disease and non-Hodgkin's lymphomas (C81-C85)	-	*	2	*
Leukemia (C91-C95)	33	0.8	21	0.5
Other and unspecified malignant neoplasms (C00-C80, C88-C90, C96-C97)	50	1.2	51	1.3
In situ neoplasms, benign neoplasms, and neoplasms of uncertain or unknown behavior (D00-D48)	70	1.7	69	1.7
Diseases of the blood and blood-forming organs and certain disorders involving the immune mechanism (D50-D89)	105	2.6	82	2.0
Anemias (D50-D64)	21	0.5	18	*
Hemorrhagic conditions and other diseases of blood and blood-forming organs (D65-D76)	66	1.6	43	1.1
Certain disorders involving the immune mechanism (D80-D89)	17	*	21	0.5
Endocrine, nutritional, and metabolic diseases (E00-E88)	264	6.5	266	6.6
Short stature, not elsewhere classified (E34.3)	10	*	26	0.6
Nutritional deficiencies (E40-E64)	10	*	4	*
Cystic fibrosis (E84)	5	*	10	*
Volume depletion, disorders of fluid, electrolyte, and acid-base balance (E86-E87)	86	2.1	74	1.8
All other endocrine, nutritional, and metabolic diseases (E00-E32, E34.0-E34.2, E34.4-E34.9, E65-E83, E85, E88)	152	3.7	152	3.8
Diseases of the nervous system (G00-G98)	424	10.4	382	9.5
Meningitis (G00, G03)	69	1.7	74	1.8
Infantile spinal muscular atrophy, type I (Werdnig-Hoffman) (G12.0)	21	0.5	25	0.6
Infantile cerebral palsy (G80)	14	*	9	*
Anoxic brain damage, not elsewhere classified (G93.1)	51	1.2	39	1.0
Other diseases of nervous system (G04, G06-G11, G12.1-G12.9, G20-G72, G81-G92, G93.0, G93.2-G93.9, G95-G98)	268	6.6	235	5.8
Diseases of the ear and mastoid process (H60-H93)	5	*	6	*
Diseases of the circulatory system (I00-I99)	834	20.4	667	16.6
Pulmonary heart disease and diseases of pulmonary circulation (I26-I28)	361	8.8	186	4.6
Pericarditis, endocarditis, and myocarditis (I30, I33, I40)	22	0.5	22	0.5
Cardiomyopathy (I42)	129	3.2	118	2.9
Cardiac arrest (I46)	21	0.5	34	0.8
Cerebrovascular diseases (I60-I69)	111	2.7	117	2.9
All other diseases of circulatory system (I00-I25, I31, I34-I38, I44-I45, I47-I51, I70-I99)	189	4.6	190	4.7
Diseases of the respiratory system (J00-J98)	671	16.4	636	15.8
Acute upper respiratory infections (J00-J06)	8	*	9	*
Influenza and pneumonia (J10-J18)	314	7.7	263	6.5
Influenza (J10-J11)	30	0.7	7	*
Pneumonia (J12-J18)	284	6.9	256	6.4
Acute bronchitis and acute bronchiolitis (J20-J21)	51	1.2	49	1.2
Bronchitis, chronic and unspecified (J40-J42)	19	*	24	0.6
Asthma (J45-J46)	6	*	4	*
Pneumonitis due to solids and liquids (J69)	12	*	2	*
Other and unspecified diseases of respiratory system (J22, J30-J39, J43-J44, J47-J68, J70-J98)	260	6.4	285	7.1
Diseases of the digestive system (K00-K92)	567	13.9	509	12.7
Gastritis, duodenitis, and noninfective enteritis and colitis (K29, K50-K55)	317	7.7	268	6.7
Hernia of abdominal cavity and intestinal obstruction without hernia (K40-K46, K56)	68	1.7	50	1.2
All other and unspecified diseases of digestive system (K00-K28, K30-K38, K57-K92)	182	4.4	191	4.7

[1]Based on codes from the *International Classification of Diseases, Tenth Revision* (1992), except in cases where (*) precedes the cause of death code. Codes *U01-*U03 were added as of 2001 for deaths due to terrorism.
* = Figure does not meet standards of reliability or precision.
- = Quantity zero.

Table II-31B. Number of Infant Deaths and Infant Mortality Rates for 130 Selected Causes, 2002 and Preliminary 2003—*Continued*

(Number, rate per 100,000 live births.)

Cause of death[1]	2003 Number	2003 Rate	2002 Number	2002 Rate
Diseases of the genitourinary system (N00-N98)	185	4.5	187	4.6
Renal failure and other disorders of kidney (N17-N19, N25, N27)	151	3.7	165	4.1
Other and unspecified diseases of genitourinary system (N00-N15, N20-N23, N26, N28-N98)	34	0.8	22	0.5
Certain conditions originating in the perinatal period (P00-P96)	14 173	346.4	14 106	350.7
Newborn affected by maternal factors and by complications of pregnancy, labor, and delivery (P00-P04)	3 186	77.9	3 063	76.2
Newborn affected by maternal hypertensive disorders (P00.0)	69	1.7	71	1.8
Newborn affected by other maternal conditions which may be unrelated to present pregnancy (P00.1-P00.9)	80	2.0	76	1.9
Newborn affected by maternal complications of pregnancy (P01)	1 734	42.4	1 708	42.5
Newborn affected by incompetent cervix (P01.0)	437	10.7	475	11.8
Newborn affected by premature rupture of membranes (P01.1)	744	18.2	764	19.0
Newborn affected by multiple pregnancy (P01.5)	319	7.8	252	6.3
Newborn affected by other maternal complications of pregnancy (P01.2-P01.4, P01.6-P01.9)	233	5.7	217	5.4
Newborn affected by complications of placenta, cord, and membranes (P02)	1 112	27.2	1 028	25.6
Newborn affected by complications involving placenta (P02.0-P02.3)	610	14.9	512	12.7
Newborn affected by complications involving cord (P02.4-P02.6)	42	1.0	55	1.4
Newborn affected by chorioamnionitis (P02.7)	457	11.2	460	11.4
Newborn affected by other and unspecified abnormalities of membranes (P02.8-P02.9)	3	*	1	*
Newborn affected by other complications of labor and delivery (P03)	161	3.9	144	3.6
Newborn affected by noxious influences transmitted via placenta or breast milk (P04)	31	0.8	36	0.9
Disorders related to length of gestation and fetal malnutrition (P05-P08)	4 905	119.9	4 714	117.2
Slow fetal growth and fetal malnutrition (P05)	60	1.5	77	1.9
Disorders related to short gestation and low birthweight, not elsewhere classified (P07)	4 844	118.4	4 637	115.3
Extremely low birthweight or extreme immaturity (P07.0, P07.2)	3 668	89.7	3 543	88.1
Other low birthweight or preterm (P07.1, P07.3)	1 177	28.8	1 094	27.2
Disorders related to long gestation and high birthweight (P08)	-	*	-	*
Birth trauma (P10-P15)	28	0.7	345	8.6
Intrauterine hypoxia and birth asphyxia (P20-P21)	567	13.9	583	14.5
Intrauterine hypoxia (P20)	113	2.8	110	2.7
Birth asphyxia (P21)	454	11.1	473	11.8
Respiratory distress of newborn (P22)	819	20.0	943	23.4
Other respiratory conditions originating in the perinatal period (P23-P28)	1 221	29.8	1 245	31.0
Congenital pneumonia (P23)	76	1.9	78	1.9
Neonatal aspiration syndromes (P24)	54	1.3	54	1.3
Interstitial emphysema and related conditions originating in the perinatal period (P25)	160	3.9	164	4.1
Pulmonary hemorrhage originating in the perinatal period (P26)	168	4.1	191	4.7
Chronic respiratory disease originating in the perinatal period (P27)	252	6.2	314	7.8
Atelectasis (P28.0-P28.1)	450	11.0	400	9.9
All other respiratory conditions originating in the perinatal period (P28.2-P28.9)	62	1.5	44	1.1
Infections specific to the perinatal period (P35-P39)	958	23.4	948	23.6
Bacterial sepsis of newborn (P36)	766	18.7	749	18.6
Omphalitis of newborn with or without mild hemorrhage (P38)	4	*	1	*
All other infections specific to the perinatal period (P35, P37, P39)	188	4.6	198	4.9
Hemorrhagic and hematological disorders of newborn (P50-P61)	745	18.2	509	12.7
Neonatal hemorrhage (P50-P52, P54)	648	15.8	387	9.6
Hemorrhagic disease of newborn (P53)	-	*	1	*
Hemolytic disease of newborn due to isoimmunization and other perinatal jaundice (P55-P59)	10	*	19	*
Hematological disorders (P60-P61)	87	2.1	102	2.5
Syndrome of infant of a diabetic mother and neonatal diabetes mellitus (P70.0-P70.2)	5	*	10	*
Necrotizing enterocolitis of newborn (P77)	397	9.7	352	8.8
Hydrops fetalis not due to hemolytic disease (P83.2)	190	4.6	192	4.8
Other perinatal conditions (P29, P70.3-P76, P78-P81, P83.0-P83.1, P83.3-P96)	1 153	28.2	1 202	29.9
Congenital malformations, deformations, and chromosomal abnormalities (Q00-Q99)	5 714	139.7	5 623	139.8
Anencephaly and similar malformations (Q00)	330	8.1	297	7.4
Congenital hydrocephalus (Q03)	97	2.4	90	2.2
Spina bifida (Q05)	10	*	20	0.5
Other congenital malformations of nervous system (Q01-Q02, Q04, Q06-Q07)	334	8.2	286	7.1
Congenital malformations of heart (Q20-Q24)	1 507	36.8	1 510	37.5
Other congenital malformations of circulatory system (Q25-Q28)	239	5.8	223	5.5
Congenital malformations of respiratory system (Q30-Q34)	641	15.7	638	15.9
Congenital malformations of digestive system (Q35-Q45)	92	2.2	103	2.6
Congenital malformations of genitourinary system (Q50-Q64)	338	8.3	351	8.7
Congenital malformations and deformations of musculoskeletal system, limbs, and integument (Q65-Q85)	509	12.4	460	11.4
Down's syndrome (Q90)	115	2.8	118	2.9
Edward's syndrome (Q91.0-Q91.3)	474	11.6	494	12.3
Patau's syndrome (Q91.4-Q91.7)	284	6.9	295	7.3
Other congenital malformations and deformations (Q10-Q18, Q86-Q89)	547	13.4	548	13.6
Other chromosomal abnormalities, not elsewhere classified (Q92-Q99)	197	4.8	190	4.7

[1]Based on codes from the *International Classification of Diseases, Tenth Revision* (1992), except in cases where (*) precedes the cause of death code. Codes *U01-*U03 were added as of 2001 for deaths due to terrorism.

* = Figure does not meet standards of reliability or precision.

- = Quantity zero.

Table II-31B. Number of Infant Deaths and Infant Mortality Rates for 130 Selected Causes, 2002 and Preliminary 2003—*Continued*

(Number, rate per 100,000 live births.)

Cause of death[1]	2003		2002	
	Number	Rate	Number	Rate
Symptoms, signs and abnormal clinical and laboratory findings, not elsewhere classified (R00-R99)	3 477	85.0	3 456	85.9
Sudden infant death syndrome (R95)	1 994	48.7	2 295	57.1
Other symptoms, signs and abnormal clinical and laboratory findings, not elsewhere classified (R00-R53, R55-R94, R96-R99)	1 483	36.2	1 161	28.9
All other diseases (residual)	32	0.8	24	0.6
External causes of mortality (*U01, V01-Y84)	1 324	32.4	1 365	33.9
Accidents (unintentional injuries) (V01-X59)	928	22.7	946	23.5
Transport accidents (V01-V99)	150	3.7	127	3.2
Motor vehicle accidents (V02-V04, V09.0, V09.2, V12-V14, V19.0-V19.2, V19.4-V19.6, V20-V79, V80.3-V80.5, V81.0-V81.1, V82.0-V82.1, V83-V86, V87.0-V87.8, V88.0-V88.8, V89.0, V89.2)	147	3.6	123	3.1
Other and unspecified transport accidents (V01, V05-V06, V09.1, V09.3-V09.9, V10-V11, V15-V18, V19.3, V19.8, V19.9, V80.0-V80.2, V80.6-V80.9, V81.2-V81.9, V82.2-V82.9, V87.9, V88.9, V89.1, V89.3, V89.9, V90-V99)	3	*	4	*
Falls (W00-W19)	13	*	16	*
Accidental discharge of firearms (W32-W34)	-	*	1	*
Accidental drowning and submersion (W65-W74)	57	1.4	63	1.6
Accidental suffocation and strangulation in bed (W75)	409	10.0	425	10.6
Other accidental suffocation and strangulation (W76-W77, W81-W84)	138	3.4	150	3.7
Accidental inhalation and ingestion of food or other objects causing obstruction of respiratory tract (W78-W80)	56	1.4	61	1.5
Accidents caused by exposure to smoke, fire, and flames (X00-X09)	32	0.8	36	0.9
Accidental poisoning and exposure to noxious substances (X40-X49)	16	*	26	0.6
Other and unspecified accidents (W20-W31, W35-W64, W85-W99, X10-X39, X50-X59)	56	1.4	41	1.0
Assault (homicide) (*U01, X85-Y09)	318	7.8	303	7.5
Assault (homicide) by hanging, strangulation, and suffocation (X91)	41	1.0	32	0.8
Assault (homicide) by discharge of firearms (*U01.4, X93-X95)	7	*	9	*
Neglect, abandonment, and other maltreatment syndromes (Y06-Y07)	94	2.3	98	2.4
Assault (homicide) by other and unspecified means (*U01.0-*U01.3, *U01.5-*U01.9, X85-X90, X92, X96-X99, Y00-Y05, Y08-Y09)	176	4.3	164	4.1
Complications of medical and surgical care (Y40-Y84)	12	*	15	*
Other external causes and their sequelae (X60-X84, Y10-Y36)	65	1.6	101	2.5

[1]Based on codes from the *International Classification of Diseases, Tenth Revision* (1992), except in cases where (*) precedes the cause of death code. Codes *U01-*U03 were added as of 2001 for deaths due to terrorism.
* = Figure does not meet standards of reliability or precision.
- = Quantity zero.

TABLE II-31C. NUMBER OF INFANT DEATHS AND INFANT MORTALITY RATES FOR 130 SELECTED CAUSES, BY RACE, 2002

This table presents the number of deaths and the mortality rates by race for 130 selected causes of death. Specific causes are indented under more general summary group-

ings. Rates are not considered reliable or precise when less than 20 deaths occurred for the cause; therefore, these causes are not presented.

See Table II-31A for a summary of the 10 leading causes of infant death, which together accounted for 68 percent of all fatalities.

Table II-31C. Number of Infant Deaths and Infant Mortality Rates for 130 Selected Causes, by Race, 2002

(Number, rate per 100,000 live births in specified group.)

Cause of death [1]	Number			Rate		
	All races [2]	White	Black	All races [2]	White	Black
ALL CAUSES	28 034	18 369	8 524	697.1	578.6	1 435.8
Certain infectious and parasitic diseases (A00-B99)	582	389	166	14.5	12.3	28.0
Certain intestinal infectious diseases (A00-A08)	13	8	5	*	*	*
Diarrhea and gastroenteritis of infectious origin (A09)	3	1	1	*	*	*
Tuberculosis (A16-A19)	1	-	1	*	*	*
Tetanus (A33, A35)	-	-	-	*	*	*
Diphtheria (A36)	-	-	-	*	*	*
Whooping cough (A37)	18	15	2	*	*	*
Meningococcal infection (A39)	17	14	3	*	*	*
Septicemia (A40-A41)	296	191	91	7.4	6.0	15.3
Congenital syphilis (A50)	1	-	1	*	*	*
Gonococcal infection (A54)	1	-	1	*	*	*
Viral diseases (A80-B34)	164	116	39	4.1	3.7	6.6
Acute poliomyelitis (A80)	-	-	-	*	*	*
Varicella (chickenpox) (B01)	1	1	-	*	*	*
Measles (B05)	-	-	-	*	*	*
Human immunodeficiency virus (HIV) disease (B20-B24)	7	4	3	*	*	*
Mumps (B26)	-	-	-	*	*	*
Other and unspecified viral diseases (A81-B00, B02-B04, B06-B19, B25, B27-B34)	156	111	36	3.9	3.5	6.1
Candidiasis (B37)	19	14	5	*	*	*
Malaria (B50-B54)	-	-	-	*	*	*
Pneumocystosis (B59)	2	2	-	*	*	*
All other and unspecified infectious and parasitic diseases (A20-A32, A38, A42-A49, A51-A53, A55-A79, B35-B36, B38-B49, B55-B58, B60-B99)	47	28	18	1.2	0.9	*
Neoplasms (C00-D48)	143	115	21	3.6	3.6	3.5
Malignant neoplasms (C00-C97)	74	56	12	1.8	1.8	*
Hodgkin's disease and non-Hodgkin's lymphomas (C81-C85)	2	1	1	*	*	*
Leukemia (C91-C95)	21	16	4	0.5	*	*
Other and unspecified malignant neoplasms (C00-C80, C88-C90, C96-C97)	51	39	7	1.3	1.2	*
In situ neoplasms, benign neoplasms, and neoplasms of uncertain or unknown behavior (D00-D48)	69	59	9	1.7	1.9	*
Diseases of the blood and blood-forming organs and certain disorders involving the immune mechanism (D50-D89)	82	58	17	2.0	1.8	*
Anemias (D50-D64)	18	8	6	*	*	*
Hemorrhagic conditions and other diseases of blood and blood-forming organs (D65-D76)	43	32	8	1.1	1.0	*
Certain disorders involving the immune mechanism (D80-D89)	21	18	3	0.5	*	*
Endocrine, nutritional, and metabolic diseases (E00-E88)	266	194	56	6.6	6.1	9.4
Short stature, not elsewhere classified (E34.3)	26	23	2	0.6	0.7	*
Nutritional deficiencies (E40-E64)	4	3	-	*	*	*
Cystic fibrosis (E84)	10	9	1	*	*	*
Volume depletion, disorders of fluid, electrolyte and acid-base balance (E86-E87)	74	45	24	1.8	1.4	4.0
All other endocrine, nutritional, and metabolic diseases (E00-E32, E34.0-E34.2, E34.4-E34.9, E65-E83, E85, E88)	152	114	29	3.8	3.6	4.9
Diseases of the nervous system (G00-G98)	382	290	78	9.5	9.1	13.1
Meningitis (G00, G03)	74	52	20	1.8	1.6	3.4
Infantile spinal muscular atrophy, type I (Werdnig-Hoffman) (G12.0)	25	22	2	0.6	0.7	*
Infantile cerebral palsy (G80)	9	5	3	*	*	*
Anoxic brain damage, not elsewhere classified (G93.1)	39	22	16	1.0	0.7	*
Other diseases of nervous system (G04, G06-G11, G12.1-G12.9, G20-G72, G81-G92, G93.0, G93.2-G93.9, G95-G98)	235	189	37	5.8	6.0	6.2
Diseases of the ear and mastoid process (H60-H93)	6	2	3	*	*	*
Diseases of the circulatory system (I00-I99)	667	441	193	16.6	13.9	32.5
Pulmonary heart disease and diseases of pulmonary circulation (I26-I28)	186	121	55	4.6	3.8	9.3
Pericarditis, endocarditis, and myocarditis (I30, I33, I40)	22	10	10	0.5	*	*
Cardiomyopathy (I42)	118	88	23	2.9	2.8	3.9
Cardiac arrest (I46)	34	22	9	0.8	0.7	*
Cerebrovascular diseases (I60-I69)	117	71	37	2.9	2.2	6.2
All other diseases of circulatory system (I00-I25, I31, I34-I38, I44-I45, I47-I51, I70-I99)	190	129	59	4.7	4.1	9.9
Diseases of the respiratory system (J00-J98)	636	375	230	15.8	11.8	38.7
Acute upper respiratory infections (J00-J06)	9	4	4	*	*	*
Influenza and pneumonia (J10-J18)	263	162	87	6.5	5.1	14.7
Influenza (J10-J11) [3]	7	5	1	*	*	*
Pneumonia (J12-J18)	256	157	86	6.4	4.9	14.5
Acute bronchitis and acute bronchiolitis (J20-J21)	49	31	16	1.2	1.0	*
Bronchitis, chronic and unspecified (J40-J42)	24	16	8	0.6	*	*
Asthma (J45-J46)	4	2	2	*	*	*
Pneumonitis due to solids and liquids (J69)	2	2	-	*	*	*
Other and unspecified diseases of respiratory system (J22, J30-J39, J43-J44, J47-J68, J70-J98)	285	158	113	7.1	5.0	19.0
Diseases of the digestive system (K00-K92)	509	315	175	12.7	9.9	29.5
Gastritis, duodenitis, and noninfective enteritis and colitis (K29, K50-K55)	268	153	103	6.7	4.8	17.3
Hernia of abdominal cavity and intestinal obstruction without hernia (K40-K46, K56)	50	34	15	1.2	1.1	*
All other and unspecified diseases of digestive system (K00-K28, K30-K38, K57-K92)	191	128	57	4.7	4.0	9.6

[1]Based on codes from the *International Classification of Diseases, Tenth Revision* (1992), except in cases where (*) precedes the cause of death code. Codes *U01-*U03 were added as of 2001 for deaths due to terrorism.
[2]Includes races other than White and Black.
[3]Cause of death coding changes may affect comparability with the previous year's data for this cause.
* = Figure does not meet standards of reliability or precision.
- = Quantity zero.

Table II-31C. Number of Infant Deaths and Infant Mortality Rates for 130 Selected Causes, by Race, 2002—*Continued*

(Number, rate per 100,000 live births in specified group.)

Cause of death [1]	Number			Rate		
	All races [2]	White	Black	All races [2]	White	Black
Diseases of the genitourinary system (N00-N95)	187	124	56	4.6	3.9	9.4
Renal failure and other disorders of kidney (N17-N19, N25, N27)	165	107	52	4.1	3.4	8.8
Other and unspecified diseases of genitourinary system (N00-N15, N20-N23, N26, N28-N95)	22	17	4	0.5	*	*
Certain conditions originating in the perinatal period (P00-P96)	14 106	8 679	4 889	350.7	273.4	823.5
Newborn affected by maternal factors and by complications of pregnancy, labor, and delivery (P00-P04)	3 063	1 912	1 019	76.2	60.2	171.6
Newborn affected by maternal hypertensive disorders (P00.0)	71	38	30	1.8	1.2	5.1
Newborn affected by other maternal conditions which may be unrelated to present pregnancy (P00.1-P00.9)	76	43	27	1.9	1.4	4.5
Newborn affected by maternal complications of pregnancy (P01) [3]	1 708	1 055	572	42.5	33.2	96.3
Newborn affected by incompetent cervix (P01.0)	475	276	170	11.8	8.7	28.6
Newborn affected by premature rupture of membranes (P01.1)	764	463	266	19.0	14.6	44.8
Newborn affected by multiple pregnancy (P01.5)	252	164	82	6.3	5.2	13.8
Newborn affected by other maternal complications of pregnancy (P01.2-P01.4, P01.6-P01.9)	217	152	54	5.4	4.8	9.1
Newborn affected by complications of placenta, cord, and membranes (P02)	1 028	668	329	25.6	21.0	55.4
Newborn affected by complications involving placenta (P02.0-P02.3)	512	364	139	12.7	11.5	23.4
Newborn affected by complications involving cord (P02.4-P02.6)	55	33	17	1.4	1.0	*
Newborn affected by chorioamnionitis (P02.7)	460	271	173	11.4	8.5	29.1
Newborn affected by other and unspecified abnormalities of membranes (P02.8-P02.9)	1	-	-	*	*	*
Newborn affected by other complications of labor and delivery (P03)	144	93	41	3.6	2.9	6.9
Newborn affected by noxious influences transmitted via placenta or breast milk (P04)	36	15	20	0.9	*	3.4
Disorders related to length of gestation and fetal malnutrition (P05-P08)	4 714	2 629	1 904	117.2	82.8	320.7
Slow fetal growth and fetal malnutrition (P05)	77	58	19	1.9	1.8	*
Disorders related to short gestation and low birthweight, not elsewhere classified (P07)	4 637	2 571	1 885	115.3	81.0	317.5
Extremely low birthweight or extreme immaturity (P07.0, P07.2)	3 543	1 944	1 466	88.1	61.2	246.9
Other low birthweight or preterm (P07.1, P07.3)	1 094	627	419	27.2	19.7	70.6
Disorders related to long gestation and high birthweight (P08)	-	-	-	*	*	*
Birth trauma (P10-P15) [3]	345	245	85	8.6	7.7	14.3
Intrauterine hypoxia and birth asphyxia (P20-P21)	583	413	149	14.5	13.0	25.1
Intrauterine hypoxia (P20)	110	79	26	2.7	2.5	4.4
Birth asphyxia (P21)	473	334	123	11.8	10.5	20.7
Respiratory distress of newborn (P22)	943	584	338	23.4	18.4	56.9
Other respiratory conditions originating in the perinatal period (P23-P28)	1 245	798	408	31.0	25.1	68.7
Congenital pneumonia (P23)	78	56	21	1.9	1.8	3.5
Neonatal aspiration syndromes (P24) [3]	54	35	16	1.3	1.1	*
Interstitial emphysema and related conditions originating in the perinatal period (P25)	164	116	43	4.1	3.7	7.2
Pulmonary hemorrhage originating in the perinatal period (P26)	191	118	64	4.7	3.7	10.8
Chronic respiratory disease originating in the perinatal period (P27)	314	181	123	7.8	5.7	20.7
Atelectasis (P28.0-P28.1) [3]	400	262	128	9.9	8.3	21.6
All other respiratory conditions originating in the perinatal period (P28.2-P28.9)	44	30	13	1.1	0.9	*
Infections specific to the perinatal period (P35-P39)	948	621	304	23.6	19.6	51.2
Bacterial sepsis of newborn (P36)	749	493	239	18.6	15.5	40.3
Omphalitis of newborn with or without mild hemorrhage (P38)	1	1	-	*	*	*
All other infections specific to the perinatal period (P35, P37, P39)	198	127	65	4.9	4.0	10.9
Hemorrhagic and hematological disorders of newborn (P50-P61)	509	348	140	12.7	11.0	23.6
Neonatal hemorrhage (P50-P52, P54) [3]	387	271	101	9.6	8.5	17.0
Hemorrhagic disease of newborn (P53)	1	1	-	*	*	*
Hemolytic disease of newborn due to isoimmunization and other perinatal jaundice (P55-P59)	19	11	8	*	*	*
Hematological disorders (P60-P61)	102	65	31	2.5	2.0	5.2
Syndrome of infant of a diabetic mother and neonatal diabetes mellitus (P70.0-P70.2)	10	4	5	*	*	*
Necrotizing enterocolitis of newborn (P77)	352	203	135	8.8	6.4	22.7
Hydrops fetalis not due to hemolytic disease (P83.2)	192	163	14	4.8	5.1	*
Other perinatal conditions (P29, P70.3-P70.9, P71-P76, P78-P81, P83.0-P83.1, P83.3-P83.9, P90-P96) [3]	1 202	759	388	29.9	23.9	65.4
Congenital malformations, deformations, and chromosomal abnormalities (Q00-Q99)	5 623	4 330	1 047	139.8	136.4	176.4
Anencephaly and similar malformations (Q00)	297	239	41	7.4	7.5	6.9
Congenital hydrocephalus (Q03)	90	70	20	2.2	2.2	3.4
Spina bifida (Q05)	20	15	4	0.5	*	*
Other congenital malformations of nervous system (Q01-Q02, Q04, Q06-Q07)	286	225	46	7.1	7.1	7.7
Congenital malformations of heart (Q20-Q24)	1 510	1 140	299	37.5	35.9	50.4
Other congenital malformations of circulatory system (Q25-Q28)	223	158	50	5.5	5.0	8.4
Congenital malformations of respiratory system (Q30-Q34)	638	459	152	15.9	14.5	25.6
Congenital malformations of digestive system (Q35-Q45)	103	72	25	2.6	2.3	4.2
Congenital malformations of genitourinary system (Q50-Q64)	351	300	41	8.7	9.4	6.9
Congenital malformations and deformations of musculoskeletal system, limbs, and integument (Q65-Q85)	460	374	73	11.4	11.8	12.3
Down's syndrome (Q90)	118	98	16	2.9	3.1	*
Edward's syndrome (Q91.0-Q91.3)	494	378	96	12.3	11.9	16.2
Patau's syndrome (Q91.4-Q91.7)	295	243	40	7.3	7.7	6.7
Other congenital malformations and deformations (Q10-Q18, Q86-Q89)	548	411	111	13.6	12.9	18.7
Other chromosomal abnormalities, not elsewhere classified (Q92-Q99)	190	148	33	4.7	4.7	5.6

[1]Based on codes from the *International Classification of Diseases, Tenth Revision* (1992), except in cases where (*) precedes the cause of death code. Codes *U01-*U03 were added as of 2001 for deaths due to terrorism.
[2]Includes races other than White and Black.
[3]Cause of death coding changes may affect comparability with the previous year's data for this cause.
* = Figure does not meet standards of reliability or precision.
- = Quantity zero.

Table II-31C. Number of Infant Deaths and Infant Mortality Rates for 130 Selected Causes, by Race, 2002—*Continued*

(Number, rate per 100,000 live births in specified group.)

Cause of death [1]	Number			Rate		
	All races [2]	White	Black	All races [2]	White	Black
Symptoms, signs and abnormal clinical and laboratory findings, not elsewhere classified (R00-R99)	3 456	2 224	1 095	85.9	70.1	184.4
Sudden infant death syndrome (R95)	2 295	1 494	703	57.1	47.1	118.4
Other symptoms, signs and abnormal clinical and laboratory findings, not elsewhere classified (R00-R53, R55-R94, R96-R99)	1 161	730	392	28.9	23.0	66.0
All other diseases (residual)	24	16	7	0.6	*	*
External causes of mortality (*U01, V01-Y84)	1 365	817	491	33.9	25.7	82.7
Accidents (unintentional injuries) (V01-X59)	946	583	330	23.5	18.4	55.6
Transport accidents (V01-V99)	127	84	36	3.2	2.6	6.1
Motor vehicle accidents (V02-V04, V09.0, V09.2, V12-V14, V19.0-V19.2, V19.4-V19.6, V20-V79, V80.3-V80.5, V81.0-V81.1, V82.0-V82.1, V83-V86, V87.0-V87.8, V88.0-V88.8, V89.0, V89.2)	123	81	35	3.1	2.6	5.9
Other and unspecified transport accidents (V01, V05-V06, V09.1, V09.3-V09.9, V10-V11, V15-V18, V19.3, V19.8, V19.9, V80.0-V80.2, V80.6-V80.9, V81.2-V81.9, V82.2-V82.9, V87.9, V88.9, V89.1, V89.3, V89.9, V90-V99)	4	3	1	*	*	*
Falls (W00-W19)	16	12	3	*	*	*
Accidental discharge of firearms (W32-W34)	1	1	-	*	*	*
Accidental drowning and submersion (W65-W74)	63	49	11	1.6	1.5	*
Accidental suffocation and strangulation in bed (W75)	425	247	165	10.6	7.8	27.8
Other accidental suffocation and strangulation (W76-W77, W81-W84)	150	87	59	3.7	2.7	9.9
Accidental inhalation and ingestion of food or other objects causing obstruction of respiratory tract (W78-W80)	61	43	16	1.5	1.4	*
Accidents caused by exposure to smoke, fire, and flames (X00-X09)	36	19	15	0.9	*	*
Accidental poisoning and exposure to noxious substances (X40-X49)	26	13	12	0.6	*	*
Other and unspecified accidents (W20-W31, W35-W64, W85-W99, X10-X39, X50-X59)	41	28	13	1.0	0.9	*
Assault (homicide) (*U01, X85-Y09)	303	170	117	7.5	5.4	19.7
Assault (homicide) by hanging, strangulation, and suffocation (X91)	32	20	7	0.8	0.6	*
Assault (homicide) by discharge of firearms (*U01.4, X93-X95)	9	3	6	*	*	*
Neglect, abandonment, and other maltreatment syndromes (Y06-Y07)	98	58	38	2.4	1.8	6.4
Assault (homicide) by other and unspecified means (*U01.0-*U01.3, *U01.5-*U01.9, X85-X90, X92, X96-X99, Y00-Y05, Y08-Y09)	164	89	66	4.1	2.8	11.1
Complications of medical and surgical care (Y40-Y84)	15	8	7	*	*	*
Other external causes (X60-X84, Y10-Y36)	101	56	37	2.5	1.8	6.2

[1]Based on codes from the *International Classification of Diseases, Tenth Revision* (1992), except in cases where (*) precedes the cause of death code. Codes *U01-*U03 were added as of 2001 for deaths due to terrorism.
[2]Includes races other than White and Black.
* = Figure does not meet standards of reliability or precision.
- = Quantity zero.

TABLE II-31D. INFANT DEATHS AND INFANT MORTALITY RATES FOR THE 10 LEADING CAUSES OF INFANT DEATH, BY RACE AND HISPANIC ORIGIN, PRELIMINARY 2003

The Black infant mortality rate, at 14 per 1,000 live births, was more than twice the rate for White infants. The rate for Hispanic infants, at 5.9 per 1,000 live births, was only slightly higher than the rate for non-Hispanic Whites. For the various groups other than Blacks, the leading cause of death was congenital malformations, deformations, and chromosomal abnormalities. However, for Black infants, the leading cause of death (accounting for 23 percent of fatalities) was "disorders related to short gestation and low birthweight, not elsewhere classified." As shown in Chapter I, Black mothers had a greater risk of shorter gestational periods and low birthweight babies.

Table II-31D. Infant Deaths and Infant Mortality Rates for the 10 Leading Causes of Infant Death, by Race and Hispanic Origin, Preliminary 2003

(Number, rate per 100,000 live births in specified group.)

Rank [1] and race	Cause of death [2]	Number	Rate
All Races [3]			
	All Causes	28 422	694.7
1	Congenital malformations, deformations, and chromosomal abnormalities (Q00-Q99)	5 714	139.7
2	Disorders related to short gestation and low birthweight, not elsewhere classified (P07)	4 844	118.4
3	Sudden infant death syndrome (R95)	1 994	48.7
4	Newborn affected by maternal complications of pregnancy (P01)	1 734	42.4
5	Newborn affected by complications of placenta, cord, and membranes (P02)	1 112	27.2
6	Accidents (unintentional injuries) (V01-X59)	928	22.7
7	Diseases of the circulatory system (I00-I99)	834	20.4
8	Respiratory distress of newborn (P22)	819	20.0
9	Bacterial sepsis of newborn (P36)	766	18.7
10	Neonatal hemorrhage (P50-P52, P54)	648	15.8
	All other causes (residual)	9 029	220.7
White [4]			
	All Causes	18 800	582.4
1	Congenital malformations, deformations, and chromosomal abnormalities (Q00-Q99)	4 378	135.6
2	Disorders related to short gestation and low birthweight, not elsewhere classified (P07)	2 769	85.8
3	Sudden infant death syndrome (R95)	1 246	38.6
4	Newborn affected by maternal complications of pregnancy (P01)	1 117	34.6
5	Newborn affected by complications of placenta, cord, and membranes (P02)	756	23.4
6	Accidents (unintentional injuries) (V01-X59)	621	19.2
7	Diseases of the circulatory system (I00-I99)	539	16.7
8	Respiratory distress of newborn (P22)	537	16.6
9	Neonatal hemorrhage (P50-P52, P54)	476	14.8
10	Bacterial sepsis of newborn (P36)	465	14.4
	All other causes (residual)	5 896	182.7
Non-Hispanic White			
	All Causes	13 454	579.7
1	Congenital malformations, deformations, and chromosomal abnormalities (Q00-Q99)	3 002	129.3
2	Disorders related to short gestation and low birthweight, not elsewhere classified (P07)	1 894	81.6
3	Sudden infant death syndrome (R95)	1 025	44.2
4	Newborn affected by maternal complications of pregnancy (P01)	803	34.6
5	Newborn affected by complications of placenta, cord, and membranes (P02)	559	24.1
6	Accidents (unintentional injuries) (V01-X59)	501	21.6
7	Diseases of the circulatory system (I00-I99)	398	17.1
8	Respiratory distress of newborn (P22)	388	16.7
9	Neonatal hemorrhage (P50-P52, P54)	359	15.5
10	Bacterial sepsis of newborn (P36)	346	14.9
	All other causes (residual)	4 179	180.1
Black [4]			
	All Causes	8 400	1 401.4
1	Disorders related to short gestation and low birthweight, not elsewhere classified (P07)	1 903	317.4
2	Congenital malformations, deformations, and chromosomal abnormalities (Q00-Q99)	1 041	173.7
3	Sudden infant death syndrome (R95)	656	109.5
4	Newborn affected by maternal complications of pregnancy (P01)	563	93.9
5	Newborn affected by complications of placenta, cord, and membranes (P02)	311	51.9
6	Bacterial sepsis of newborn (P36)	279	46.6
7	Accidents (unintentional injuries) (V01-X59)	272	45.4
8	Respiratory distress of newborn (P22)	255	42.6
9	Diseases of the circulatory system (I00-I99)	241	40.3
10	Necrotizing enterocolitis of newborn (P77)	158	26.4
	All other causes (residual)	2 721	453.9
Hispanic [5]			
	All Causes	5 425	594.7
1	Congenital malformations, deformations, and chromosomal abnormalities (Q00-Q99)	1 381	151.4
2	Disorders related to short gestation and low birthweight, not elsewhere classified (P07)	888	97.4
3	Newborn affected by maternal complications of pregnancy (P01)	319	35.0
4	Sudden infant death syndrome (R95)	245	26.9
5	Newborn affected by complications of placenta, cord, and membranes (P02)	201	22.1
6	Respiratory distress of newborn (P22)	152	16.6
7	Diseases of the circulatory system (I00-I99)	142	15.5
8	Accidents (unintentional injuries) (V01-X59)	123	13.5
9	Bacterial sepsis of newborn (P36)	120	13.1
10	Neonatal hemorrhage (P50-P52, P54)	120	13.1
	All other causes (residual)	1 734	190.1

[1] Rank based on number of deaths in specified group.
[2] Based on codes from the *International Classification of Diseases, Tenth Revision* (1992).
[3] Includes races other than White and Black.
[4] Race and Hispanic origin are reported separately on both the birth and death certificate.
[5] May be of any race.

TABLE II-32. NUMBER OF INFANT AND NEONATAL DEATHS AND MORTALITY RATES, BY RACE, FOR EACH STATE AND TERRITORY, 2002

Louisiana and Mississippi recorded the highest infant mortality rates, each with 10.3 deaths per 1,000 live births in 2002, compared to the U.S. average of 7.0 per 1,000 live births. The rate for the District of Columbia, as expected, was even higher at 11.3 per 1,000 live births. Rates in Tennessee and South Carolina were 9.4 and 9.3 per 1,000 live births, respectively. Mississippi, South Carolina, and the District of Columbia also had high rates of neonatal deaths. On the low side, Vermont and Maine each had infant mortality rates of 4.4 per 1,000

Table II-32. Number of Infant and Neonatal Deaths and Mortality Rates, by Race, for Each State and Territory, 2002

(Number, rate per 1,000 live births in specified group.)

State	Infant deaths						Neonatal deaths					
	All races [1]		White		Black		All races [1]		White		Black	
	Number	Rate	Number	Rate	Number	Rate	Number	Rate	Number	Rate	Number	Rate
UNITED STATES [2]	28 034	7.0	18 369	5.8	8 524	14.4	18 747	4.7	12 354	3.9	5 646	9.5
Male	15 717	7.6	10 433	6.4	4 652	15.4	10 408	5.1	6 941	4.3	3 054	10.1
Female	12 317	6.3	7 936	5.1	3 872	13.3	8 339	4.2	5 413	3.5	2 592	8.9
Alabama	539	9.1	283	7.1	255	13.9	345	5.9	182	4.6	163	8.9
Alaska	55	5.5	27	4.2	6	*	20	2.0	11	*	1	*
Arizona	559	6.4	475	6.2	36	13.0	361	4.1	318	4.1	16	*
Arkansas	312	8.3	201	6.9	103	13.9	191	5.1	123	4.2	62	8.3
California	2 889	5.5	2 212	5.2	420	12.9	1 934	3.7	1 505	3.5	260	8.0
Colorado	415	6.1	342	5.5	62	21.1	275	4.0	227	3.6	40	13.6
Connecticut	274	6.5	191	5.5	74	14.2	198	4.7	144	4.2	47	9.0
Delaware	96	8.7	58	7.3	35	12.9	78	7.0	48	6.1	28	10.3
District of Columbia	85	11.3	16	*	67	14.5	57	7.6	14	*	43	9.3
Florida	1 548	7.5	893	5.8	629	13.6	1 032	5.0	596	3.9	419	9.1
Georgia	1 192	8.9	569	6.6	588	13.7	792	5.9	360	4.2	404	9.4
Hawaii	127	7.3	18	*	7	*	83	4.7	12	*	5	*
Idaho	128	6.1	123	6.1	1	*	84	4.0	82	4.1	-	*
Illinois	1 339	7.4	780	5.6	519	16.3	911	5.0	557	4.0	324	10.2
Indiana	657	7.7	503	6.8	143	15.3	448	5.3	347	4.7	90	9.6
Iowa	199	5.3	179	5.1	17	*	134	3.6	123	3.5	9	*
Kansas	281	7.1	228	6.5	44	15.2	191	4.8	155	4.4	29	10.0
Kentucky	392	7.2	318	6.6	70	14.2	228	4.2	193	4.0	33	6.7
Louisiana	665	10.3	253	6.9	401	15.0	429	6.6	162	4.4	259	9.7
Maine	59	4.4	56	4.3	1	*	43	3.2	41	3.1	-	*
Maryland	551	7.5	240	5.3	298	12.3	394	5.4	178	3.9	206	8.5
Massachusetts	395	4.9	302	4.5	76	9.1	298	3.7	234	3.5	51	6.1
Michigan	1 057	8.1	619	6.0	416	18.5	720	5.5	430	4.2	272	12.1
Minnesota	364	5.4	290	5.0	50	10.3	240	3.5	205	3.5	24	4.9
Mississippi	428	10.3	155	6.9	269	14.8	281	6.8	99	4.4	178	9.8
Missouri	637	8.5	443	7.1	189	17.1	417	5.5	292	4.7	121	11.0
Montana	83	7.5	68	7.1	3	*	54	4.9	45	4.7	2	*
Nebraska	178	7.0	141	6.1	30	20.8	121	4.8	96	4.2	22	15.3
Nevada	197	6.0	138	5.1	48	18.4	126	3.9	90	3.3	28	10.7
New Hampshire	72	5.0	72	5.3	*	*	51	3.5	51	3.7	-	*
New Jersey	655	5.7	382	4.5	255	12.8	471	4.1	273	3.2	184	9.2
New Mexico	174	6.3	132	5.7	11	*	120	4.3	92	4.0	7	*
New York	1 519	6.0	977	5.4	493	9.9	1 074	4.3	709	3.9	334	6.7
North Carolina	959	8.2	505	5.9	430	15.6	659	5.6	326	3.8	318	11.5
North Dakota	49	6.3	38	5.6	2	*	32	4.1	25	3.7	2	*
Ohio	1 180	7.9	761	6.2	400	17.7	800	5.4	512	4.2	272	12.1
Oklahoma	410	8.1	279	7.1	81	17.2	257	5.1	172	4.4	52	11.1
Oregon	260	5.8	229	5.6	13	*	172	3.8	158	3.8	5	*
Pennsylvania	1 091	7.6	772	6.6	305	15.1	800	5.6	581	4.9	206	10.2
Rhode Island	90	7.0	71	6.4	15	*	62	4.8	48	4.3	11	*
South Carolina	507	9.3	213	6.0	287	15.8	346	6.3	138	3.9	203	11.2
South Dakota	70	6.5	42	4.9	3	*	38	3.6	25	2.9	2	*
Tennessee	727	9.4	419	7.0	299	18.3	456	5.9	250	4.2	203	12.5
Texas	2 368	6.4	1 773	5.6	561	13.5	1 451	3.9	1 082	3.4	347	8.3
Utah	273	5.6	255	5.5	6	*	186	3.8	176	3.8	3	*
Vermont	28	4.4	28	4.5	-	*	19	*	19	*	-	*
Virginia	741	7.4	394	5.5	323	14.6	513	5.1	260	3.6	239	10.8
Washington	456	5.8	366	5.5	43	12.7	291	3.7	230	3.5	30	8.8
West Virginia	188	9.1	169	8.5	19	*	109	5.3	100	5.0	9	*
Wisconsin	472	6.9	329	5.6	121	18.9	330	4.8	234	4.0	83	12.9
Wyoming	44	6.7	42	6.8	-	*	25	3.8	24	3.9	-	*
Puerto Rico	511	9.7	498	10.4	13	*	376	7.1	365	7.6	11	*
Virgin Islands	8	*	4	*	3	*	6	*	3	*	2	*
Guam	19	*	1	*	-	*	11	*	1	*	-	*
American Samoa	22	13.5	-	*	-	*	9	*	-	*	-	*
Northern Marianas	8	*	1	*	-	*	6	*	1	*	-	*

Note: Infant deaths based on race of decedent; live births based on race of mother.

[1] Includes races other than White and Black.
[2] Excludes data for Puerto Rico, Virgin Islands, Guam, American Samoa, and Northern Marianas.
* = Figure does not meet standards of reliability or precision.
- = Quantity zero.

live births, Massachusetts experienced 4.9 deaths per 1,000 live births, and New Hampshire totaled 5.0 deaths per 1,000 live births.

The Black infant mortality rate, which averaged 14.4 per 1,000 live births for the United States, was more than 20 per 1,000 live births in Colorado and Nebraska, and reached rates of 18.9 per 1,000 live births in Wisconsin and 18.5 per 1,000 live births in Michigan. However, these rates appeared to fluctuate considerably from year to year, and these four states did not stand out in terms of Black infant mortality rates in 2001. Massachusetts and New York had low Black infant mortality rates.

TABLE II-33. NUMBER OF MATERNAL DEATHS AND MATERNAL MORTALITY RATES FOR SELECTED CAUSES, BY RACE, 2002

Maternal mortality does not include all deaths occurring during pregnancy, but only those related to physical conditions aggravated by pregnancy or pregnancy management. Deaths occurring more than 42 days after the termination of pregnancy are excluded. The mortality rate was computed on the basis of the number of live births. In 2002, a total of 357 women were reported to have died of maternal causes, a rate of 8.9 per 100,000 live births. Final maternal mortality data for 2003 are shown and discussed in Table II-1.

There was a big difference in the maternal mortality rates for White and for Black mothers. The rate for White mothers was 8.0 deaths per 100,000 live births, while that for Black mothers was 24.9 deaths per 100,000 live births.

Table II-33. Number of Maternal Deaths and Maternal Mortality Rates for Selected Causes, by Race, 2002

(Number, rate per 100,000 live births in specified group.)

Cause of death [1]	Number				Rate			
			All other				All other	
	All races	White	Total	Black	All races	White	Total	Black
Maternal causes (A34, O00-O95, O98-O99)	357	190	167	148	8.9	6.0	19.7	24.9
Pregnancy with abortive outcome (O00-O07)	22	7	15	12	0.5	*	*	*
Ectopic pregnancy (O00)	12	3	9	8	*	*	*	*
Spontaneous abortion (O03)	2	1	1	1	*	*	*	*
Medical abortion (O04)	1	-	1	1	*	*	*	*
Other abortion (O05)	-	-	-	-	*	*	*	*
Other and unspecified pregnancy with abortive outcome (O01-O02, O06-O07)	7	3	4	2	*	*	*	*
Other direct obstetric causes (A34, O10-O92)	285	154	131	117	7.1	4.9	15.5	19.7
Eclampsia and pre-eclampsia (O11, O13-O16)	56	32	24	23	1.4	1.0	2.8	3.9
Hemorrhage of pregnancy and childbirth and placenta previa (O20, O44-O46, O67, O72)	26	16	10	9	0.6	*	*	*
Complications predominantly related to the puerperium (A34, O85-O92)	82	39	43	38	2.0	1.2	5.1	6.4
Obstetrical tetanus (A34)	-	-	-	-	*	*	*	*
Obstetric embolism (O88)	47	26	21	16	1.2	0.8	2.5	*
Other complications predominantly related to the puerperium (O85-O87, O89-O92)	35	13	22	22	0.9	*	2.6	3.7
All other direct obstetric causes (O10, O12, O21-O43, O47-O66, O68-O71, O73-O75)	121	67	54	47	3.0	2.1	6.4	7.9
Obstetric death of unspecified cause (O95)	4	1	3	3	*	*	*	*
Indirect obstetric causes (O98-O99)	46	28	18	16	1.1	0.9	*	*
Maternal causes more than 42 days after delivery or termination of pregnancy (O96-O97)	22	13	9	9	0.5	*	*	*
Death from any obstetric cause occurring more than 42 days but less than one year after delivery (O96)	9	3	6	6	*	*	*	*
Death from sequelae of direct obstetric causes (O97)	13	10	3	3	*	*	*	*

[1] Based on codes from the *International Classification of Diseases, Tenth Revision* (1992).
* = Figure does not meet standards of reliability or precision.
- = Quantity zero.

TABLE II-34. NUMBER OF MATERNAL DEATHS AND MATERNAL MORTALITY RATES FOR SELECTED CAUSES, BY RACE AND HISPANIC ORIGIN, 2002

The maternal mortality rate for Hispanic women was 7.1 deaths per 100,000 live births. This was somewhat higher than the rate of 5.6 per 100,000 live births for non-Hispanic White mothers. However, non-Hispanic Black mothers had a higher rate of 24.9 deaths per 100,000 live births.

Table II-34. Number of Maternal Deaths and Maternal Mortality Rates for Selected Causes, by Race and Hispanic Origin, 2002

(Number, rate per 100,000 live births in specified group.)

Cause of death [1]	Number					Rate				
	All origins [2]	Hispanic [3]	Non-Hispanic [4]	Non-Hispanic White	Non-Hispanic Black	All origins [2]	Hispanic [3]	Non-Hispanic [4]	Non-Hispanic White	Non-Hispanic Black
Maternal causes (A34, O00-O95, O98-O99)	357	62	291	128	144	8.9	7.1	9.3	5.6	24.9
Pregnancy with abortive outcome (O00-O07)	22	1	20	6	11	0.5	*	0.6	*	*
Ectopic pregnancy (O00)	12	-	12	3	8	*	*	*	*	*
Spontaneous abortion (O03)	2	-	2	1	1	*	*	*	*	*
Medical abortion (O04)	1	-	1	-	1	*	*	*	*	*
Other abortion (O05)	-	-	-	-	-	*	*	*	*	*
Other and unspecified pregnancy with abortive outcome (O01-O02, O06-O07)	7	1	5	2	1	*	*	*	*	*
Other direct obstetric causes (A34, O10-O92)	285	55	228	99	115	7.1	6.3	7.3	4.3	19.9
Eclampsia and pre-eclampsia (O11, O13-O16)	56	18	37	14	22	1.4	*	1.2	*	3.8
Hemorrhage of pregnancy and childbirth and placenta previa (O20, O44-O46, O67, O72)	26	6	20	10	9	0.6	*	0.6	*	*
Complications predominantly related to the puerperium (A34, O85-O92)	82	8	73	31	37	2.0	*	2.3	1.3	6.4
Obstetrical tetanus (A34)	-	-	-	-	-	*	*	*	*	*
Obstetric embolism (O88)	47	4	43	22	16	1.2	*	1.4	1.0	*
Other complications predominantly related to the puerperium (O85-O87, O89-O92)	35	4	30	9	21	0.9	*	1.0	*	3.6
All other direct obstetric causes (O10, O12, O21-O43, O47-O66, O68-O71, O73-O75)	121	23	98	44	47	3.0	2.6	3.1	1.9	8.1
Obstetric death of unspecified cause (O95)	4	-	3	1	2	*	*	*	*	*
Indirect obstetric causes (O98-O99)	46	6	40	22	16	1.1	*	1.3	1.0	*
Maternal causes more than 42 days after delivery or termination of pregnancy (O96-O97)	22	8	14	5	9	0.5	*	*	*	*
Death from any obstetric cause occurring more than 42 days but less than one year after delivery (O96)	9	2	7	1	6	*	*	*	*	*
Death from sequelae of direct obstetric causes (O97)	13	6	7	4	3	*	*	*	*	*

[1]Based on codes from the *International Classification of Diseases, Tenth Revision,* (1992).
[2]All origins includes origin not stated; specified origins exclude origin not stated.
[3]May be of any race.
[4]Includes races other than White and Black.
* = Figure does not meet standards of reliability or precision.
- = Quantity zero.

CHAPTER III: HEALTH

In view of the multitude of health data available, only a few major topics have been selected for this chapter. They are presented under the following headings: Determinants and Measures of Health, Use of Addictive Substances, Ambulatory Care, Inpatient Care, Health Personnel, Health Expenditures, and Health Insurance.

DETERMINANTS AND MEASURES OF HEALTH

TABLES III-1, 1A. OCCUPATIONAL INJURIES AND ILLNESSES WITH DAYS AWAY FROM WORK, JOB TRANSFER, OR RESTRICTION IN THE PRIVATE SECTOR, ACCORDING TO INDUSTRY, SELECTED YEARS, 1980–2003

(Data are based on employer records from a sample of business establishments.)

The number of injuries and illnesses with lost workdays totaled 2.3 million in 2003, representing 2.6 percent of full-time employees. The percentages of illnesses and injuries with lost workdays were highest in transportation and warehousing (5.4 percent), manufacturing (3.8 percent), and construction (3.8 percent). In the mining sector, the illness and injury rate had climbed as high as 6.5 percent in 1980, but was reported at 2.0 percent in 2003. Injuries and illnesses with lost workdays were least frequent in financial activities (0.8 percent).

The frequency of injuries and illnesses has declined considerably since 1980 and 1990, years in which the overall injury and illness rate was about 4.0 percent. By 2003, these rates had dropped to 2.6 percent. Declines took place in most industries.

Table III-1. Occupational Injuries and Illnesses with Days Away from Work, Job Transfer, or Restriction in the Private Sector, According to Industry, Selected Years, 1980–2002

(Number in thousands, percent.)

Characteristic	2002 [1]	2001	2000	1999	1998	1995	1990	1985	1980
Per Full-Time Equivalents [2, 3]									
Total private sector [4]	2.8	2.8	3.0	3.0	3.1	3.6	4.1	3.6	4.0
Agriculture, fishing, and forestry [4]	3.3	3.6	3.6	3.4	3.9	4.3	5.9	5.7	5.8
Mining	2.6	2.4	3.0	2.7	2.9	3.9	5.0	4.8	6.5
Construction	3.8	4.0	4.1	4.2	4.0	4.9	6.7	6.8	6.5
Manufacturing	4.1	4.1	4.5	4.6	4.7	5.3	5.8	4.6	5.4
Transportation, communication, and public utilities	4.0	4.3	4.3	4.4	4.3	5.2	5.5	5.0	5.5
Wholesale trade	3.1	2.8	3.1	3.3	3.3	3.6	3.7	3.5	3.9
Retail trade	2.5	2.4	2.5	2.5	2.7	3.0	3.4	3.1	2.9
Finance, insurance, and real estate	0.8	0.7	0.8	0.8	0.7	1.0	1.1	0.9	0.8
Services	2.2	2.2	2.2	2.2	2.4	2.8	2.8	2.6	2.3
Services									
Total private sector [4]	2 494.3	2 559.1	2 752.1	2 742.8	2 780.7	2 972.1	3 123.8	2 537.0	2 539.9
Agriculture, fishing, and forestry [4]	49.3	54.4	54.2	48.8	55.4	53.5	58.8	46.1	40.4
Mining	15.1	14.4	17.5	14.9	17.6	23.4	36.1	44.3	66.9
Construction	226.8	240.9	249.1	243.8	220.0	221.9	299.4	275.0	245.2
Manufacturing	656.4	702.4	829.5	848.0	891.2	970.7	1 072.8	857.1	1 038.7
Transportation, communication, and public utilities	251.8	285.1	283.1	284.1	268.8	299.3	298.1	246.2	266.5
Wholesale trade	190.5	183.0	207.6	217.1	216.9	221.6	215.5	189.7	193.7
Retail trade	435.1	421.6	432.7	431.7	445.8	472.2	490.2	403.2	332.3
Finance, insurance, and real estate	52.3	51.1	53.3	51.6	45.3	59.3	67.1	47.0	38.8
Services	617.1	606.2	625.2	602.8	619.8	650.2	585.7	428.3	317.4

[1]Data for 2002, except for mining and transportation, are not comparable with those from previous years because of changes to the Occupational Safety and Health Administration (OSHA) recordkeeping requirements. The mining and transportation industries did not adopt OSHA recordkeeping requirements for 2002.

[2]Data for 1980–2001 include injuries and illnesses with lost workdays.

[3]Incidence rate calculated as (N/EH) x 200,000, where N = total number of injuries and illnesses, EH = total hours worked by all employees during the calendar year, and 200,000 = base for 100 full-time equivalent employees working 40 hours per week, 50 weeks per year.

[4]Excludes farms with fewer than 11 employees.

Table III-1A. Occupational Injuries and Illnesses with Days Away from Work, Job Transfer, or Restriction in the Private Sector, According to Industry, 2003

(Per 100 full-time equivalents, number of events in thousands.)

Industry	Injuries and illnesses with days away from work, job transfer, or restriction	
	Cases per 100 full-time workers [1]	Number of cases in thousands [2]
Total private industry [3]	2.6	2 301.9
Goods-producing	3.7	796.5
Natural resources and mining [4]	2.8	40.5
Agriculture, forestry, fishing, and hunting [4]	3.3	29.3
Mining	2.0	11.2
Construction	3.6	218.0
Manufacturing	3.8	538.0
Service-providing	2.3	1 505.4
Trade, transportation, and utilities	3.2	683.2
Wholesale trade	2.8	147.4
Retail trade	2.7	319.6
Transportation and warehousing	5.4	204.0
Utilities	2.2	12.2
Information	1.1	30.8
Financial activities	0.8	56.9
Finance and insurance	0.4	21.3
Real estate and rental and leasing	2.1	35.6
Professional and business services	1.4	157.7
Professional, scientific, and technical services	0.6	36.0
Management of companies and enterprises	1.6	25.1
Administrative and support and waste management and remediation services	2.4	96.7
Educational and health services	2.9	355.8
Educational services	1.2	17.9
Health care and social assistance	3.1	337.9
Leisure and hospitality	2.1	169.3
Arts, entertainment, and recreation	2.9	34.1
Accommodation and food services	2.0	135.2
Other services, except public administration	1.7	51.7

[1]Incidence rate calculated as (N/EH) x 200,000, where N = total number of injuries and illnesses, EH = total hours worked by all employees during the calendar year, and 200,000 = base for 100 full-time equivalent employees working 40 hours per week, 50 weeks per year.

[2]Due to rounding, components may not add to totals.

[3]Totals include data for industries not shown separately. Excludes self-employed, private households, and employers in federal, state, and local government agencies.

[4]Excludes farms with fewer than 11 employees.

TABLE III-2. SELECTED NOTIFIABLE DISEASE RATES, ACCORDING TO DISEASE, SELECTED YEARS, 1950–2003

(Data are based on reporting by state health departments.)

Chlamydial infections, with 877,000 cases in 2003, had the most frequent occurrence of diseases requiring official notification. Chlamydia can lead to pelvic inflammatory disease, which can cause further serious complications. Reported chlamydia has been increasing annually since the late 1980s, when public programs for the screening and treatment of women were first established. About 335,000 cases of gonorrhea were reported in 2003. Hepatitis A and B each had less than 10,000 reported cases. Reported cases of Lyme disease increased from 17,000 in 2001 to nearly 24,000 in 2002; they receded to 21,000 in 2003. Although the rates of some reportable childhood infectious diseases, such as mumps and measles, have all but disappeared, the incidence of pertussis (whooping cough) in children and adults has increased since 1980, with epidemics occurring every 3 to 5 years. More than 11,600 new cases of pertussis were reported in 2003 (an incidence rate of 4.0 per 100,000 people), the highest number of cases since 1964.

Table III-2. Selected Notifiable Disease Rates, According to Disease, Selected Years, 1950–2003

(Cases per 100,000 population, number.)

Disease	2003	2002	2001	2000	1995	1990	1980	1970	1960	1950
Rate										
Diphtheria	0.00	0.00	0.00	0.00	-	0.00	0.00	0.21	0.51	3.83
Haemophilus influenzae, invasive	0.70	0.62	0.57	0.51	0.45	...	...	...	...	...
Hepatitis A	2.66	3.13	3.77	4.91	12.13	12.64	12.84	27.87	...	...
Hepatitis B	2.61	2.84	2.79	2.95	4.19	8.48	8.39	4.08	...	...
Lyme disease	7.39	8.44	6.05	6.53	4.49	...	...	...	...	...
Meningococcal disease	0.61	0.64	0.83	0.83	1.25	0.99	1.25	1.23	...	...
Mumps	0.08	0.10	0.10	0.13	0.35	2.17	3.86	55.55	...	...
Pertussis (whooping cough)	4.04	3.47	2.69	2.88	1.97	1.84	0.76	2.08	8.23	79.82
Poliomyelitis, total	-	-	-	-	0.00	0.00	0.00	0.02	1.77	22.02
Paralytic [1]	-	-	-	-	0.00	0.00	0.00	0.02	1.40	...
Rocky Mountain spotted fever	0.38	0.39	0.25	0.18	0.23	0.26	0.52	0.19	...	...
Rubella (German measles)	0.00	0.01	0.01	0.06	0.05	0.45	1.72	27.75	...	...
Rubeola (measles)	0.02	0.02	0.04	0.03	0.12	11.17	5.96	23.23	245.42	211.01
Salmonellosis, excluding typhoid fever	15.16	15.73	14.39	14.51	17.66	19.54	14.88	10.84	3.85	...
Shigellosis	8.19	8.37	7.19	8.41	12.32	10.89	8.41	6.79	6.94	15.45
Tuberculosis [2]	5.17	5.36	5.68	6.01	8.70	10.33	12.25	18.28	30.83	...
Sexually transmitted diseases [3]										
Syphilis [4]	11.89	11.41	11.31	11.20	26.05	54.32	30.51	45.26	68.78	146.02
Primary and secondary	2.49	2.38	2.14	2.12	6.21	20.26	12.06	10.89	9.06	16.73
Early latent	2.90	2.92	3.05	3.35	10.01	22.19	9.00	8.08	10.11	39.71
Late and late latent [5]	6.35	6.00	5.95	5.53	9.12	10.32	9.30	24.94	45.91	70.22
Congenital [6]	0.14	0.16	0.18	0.21	0.70	1.55	0.12	0.97	2.48	8.97
Chlamydia [7]	304.29	289.41	274.52	251.38	187.84	160.19	...	...	...	...
Gonorrhea [8]	116.21	122.01	126.77	128.67	147.46	276.43	445.10	297.22	145.40	192.50
Chancroid	0.02	0.02	0.01	0.03	0.23	1.69	0.30	0.70	0.94	3.34
Number										
Diphtheria	1	1	2	1	-	4	3	435	918	5 796
Haemophilus influenzae, invasive	2 013	1 743	1 597	1 398	1 180	...	...	...	...	...
Hepatitis A	7 653	8 795	10 609	13 397	31 582	31 441	29 087	56 797	...	...
Hepatitis B	7 526	7 996	7 843	8 036	10 805	21 102	19 015	8 310	...	...
Lyme disease	21 273	23 763	17 029	17 730	11 700	...	...	...	...	...
Meningococcal disease	1 756	1 814	2 333	2 256	3 243	2 451	2 840	2 505	...	...
Mumps	231	270	266	338	906	5 292	8 576	104 953	...	...
Pertussis (whooping cough)	11 647	9 771	7 580	7 867	5 137	4 570	1 730	4 249	14 809	120 718
Poliomyelitis, total	-	-	-	-	7	6	9	33	3 190	33 300
Paralytic [1]	-	-	-	-	7	6	9	31	2 525	...
Rocky Mountain spotted fever	1 091	1 104	695	495	590	651	1 163	380	...	...
Rubella (German measles)	7	18	23	176	128	1 125	3 904	56 552	...	...
Rubeola (measles)	56	44	116	86	309	27 786	13 506	47 351	441 703	319 124
Salmonellosis, excluding typhoid fever	43 657	44 264	40 495	39 574	45 970	48 603	33 715	22 096	6 929	...
Shigellosis	23 581	23 541	20 221	22 922	32 080	27 077	19 041	13 845	12 487	23 367
Tuberculosis [2]	14 874	15 075	15 989	16 377	22 860	25 701	27 749	37 137	55 494	...
Sexually transmitted diseases [3]										
Syphilis [4]	34 270	32 912	32 278	31 616	69 356	135 590	68 832	91 382	122 538	217 558
Primary and secondary	7 177	6 862	6 103	5 979	16 543	50 578	27 204	21 982	16 145	23 939
Early latent	8 361	8 429	8 701	9 465	26 657	55 397	20 297	16 311	18 017	59 256
Late and late latent [5]	18 319	17 168	16 976	15 594	24 296	25 750	20 979	50 348	81 798	113 569
Congenital [6]	413	453	498	578	1 861	3 865	277	1 953	4 416	13 377
Chlamydia [7]	877 478	834 555	783 242	709 452	478 577	323 663	...	...	...	...
Gonorrhea [8]	335 104	351 852	361 705	363 136	392 651	690 042	1 004 029	600 072	258 933	286 746
Chancroid	54	48	38	78	607	4 212	788	1 416	1 680	4 977

Note: The total resident population was used to calculate all rates except those for sexually transmitted diseases, which used the civilian resident population. For sexually transmitted diseases, 2000 population estimates were used to calculate 2001 and 2002 rates. Population data from those states where diseases were not notifiable or not available were excluded from rate calculation.

[1] Data beginning in 1986 may be updated due to retrospective case evaluations or late reports.
[2] Case reporting for tuberculosis began in 1953. Data prior to 1975 are not comparable with subsequent years' data because of changes in reporting criteria effective in 1975. Data for 2002 were updated through the Division of Tuberculosis Elimination, National Center for HIV, STD, and TB Prevention (NCHSTP), as of March 28, 2003.
[3] Newly reported civilian cases prior to 1991; includes military cases beginning in 1991. Adjustments to the number of cases from state health departments were made for hard copy forms and for electronic data submissions through May 2, 2003. For 1950, data for Alaska and Hawaii were not included.
[4] Includes stage of syphilis not stated.
[5] Includes cases of unknown duration.
[6] Data reported for 1989 and later years reflect change in case definition introduced in 1988. Through 1994, all cases of congenitally acquired syphilis; as of 1995, congenital syphilis less than 1 year of age. See STD Surveillance Report for congenital syphilis rates per 100,000 live births. In 2002, the rate was 10.2 congenital syphilis cases per 100,000 live births.
[7] Chlamydia was nonnotifiable in 1994 and earlier years. From 1994–1999, cases for New York based exclusively on those reported by New York City. Starting in 2000, includes cases for New York State.
[8] Data for 1994 do not include cases from Georgia.
0.00 = Quantity more than zero but less than 0.05.
- = Quantity zero.
... = Not available.

TABLE III-3. ACQUIRED IMMUNODEFICIENCY SYNDROME (AIDS) CASES, ACCORDING TO AGE AT DIAGNOSIS, SEX, RACE, AND HISPANIC ORIGIN, SELECTED YEARS, 1999–2003

It is estimated that between 1.04 and 1.19 million persons in the United States were living with HIV/AIDS by the end of 2003, with 24–27 percent of sufferers undiagnosed and unaware of their HIV infection. In 2003, 43,200 new cases of AIDS were reported, reflecting an increasing trend since 2000. However, rates were still 40 percent less than those in the mid-1990s. Since the mid-1990s, prevention measures have reduced the infection rates of certain at-risk groups. Effective medicines have also reduced or delayed the onset of AIDS in HIV-infected people.

Black males had the highest rate of new AIDS cases in 2003, accounting for 49.3 percent of all new cases. Females represented considerably fewer cases than

males. For children under 13 years of age, only 59 new AIDS cases were reported in 2003. Such cases have declined steadily since 1994, when U.S. Public Health Service guidelines recommended testing and treatment during pregnancy. The vast majority of pediatric AIDS cases occurred through perinatal exposure.

Table III-3. Acquired Immunodeficiency Syndrome (AIDS) Cases, According to Age at Diagnosis, Sex, Race, and Hispanic Origin, Selected Years, 1999–2003

(Number, percent.)

Age at diagnosis, sex, race, and Hispanic origin	All years [1]	Year of diagnosis				
		2003	2002	2001	2000	1999
ESTIMATED NUMBER OF CASES [2]						
All Persons [3]	929 985	43 171	41 289	40 833	41 267	41 356
Sex						
Male, 13 years and over	749 887	31 614	30 517	30 074	30 387	31 159
Female, 13 years and over	170 679	11 498	10 666	10 639	10 763	10 010
Children, under 13 years	9 419	59	105	119	117	187
Not Hispanic or Latino						
White	376 834	12 222	11 960	11 620	12 047	12 626
Black or African American	368 169	21 304	20 476	20 291	20 312	19 960
American Indian or Alaska Native	3 026	196	196	179	186	162
Asian or Pacific Islander	7 166	497	452	409	373	369
Hispanic or Latino [4]	172 993	8 757	8 021	8 204	8 233	8 141
Age of Diagnosis						
Under 13 years	9 419	59	105	119	117	187
13–14 years	891	59	68	76	56	57
15–24 years	37 599	1 991	1 810	1 625	1 642	1 541
25–34 years	311 137	9 605	9 504	9 947	10 385	11 349
35–44 years	365 432	17 633	17 008	16 890	17 295	17 165
45–54 years	148 347	10 051	9 310	8 929	8 566	8 099
55–64 years	43 451	2 888	2 724	2 468	2 422	2 218
65 years and over	13 711	886	759	779	783	739
Region of Residence						
Northeast	285 040	11 461	10 551	11 350	12 516	11 885
Midwest	91 926	4 498	4 337	4 094	4 139	4 069
South	337 409	19 609	18 482	17 693	16 757	17 224
West	186 100	6 667	6 843	6 468	6 661	6 892
U.S. dependencies, possessions, and associated nations	29 511	935	1 075	1 228	1 194	1 286
PERCENT DISTRIBUTION [5]						
All persons [3]	100.0	100.0	100.0	100.0	100.0	100.0
Sex						
Male, 13 years and over	80.6	73.2	73.9	73.7	73.6	75.3
Female, 13 years and over	18.4	26.6	25.8	26.1	26.1	24.2
Children, under 13 years	1.0	0.1	0.3	0.3	0.3	0.5
Not Hispanic or Latino						
White	40.5	28.3	29.0	28.5	29.2	30.5
Black or African American	39.6	49.3	49.6	49.7	49.2	48.3
American Indian or Alaska Native	0.3	0.5	0.5	0.4	0.5	0.4
Asian or Pacific Islander	0.8	1.2	1.1	1.0	0.9	0.9
Hispanic or Latino [4]	18.6	20.3	19.4	20.1	20.0	19.7
Age at Diagnosis						
Under 13 years	1.0	0.1	0.3	0.3	0.3	0.5
13–14 years	0.1	0.1	0.2	0.2	0.1	0.1
15–24 years	4.0	4.6	4.4	4.0	4.0	3.7
25–34 years	33.5	22.2	23.0	24.4	25.2	27.4
35–44 years	39.3	40.8	41.2	41.4	41.9	41.5
45–54 years	16.0	23.3	22.5	21.9	20.8	19.6
55–64 years	4.7	6.7	6.6	6.0	5.9	5.4
65 years and over	1.5	2.1	1.8	1.9	1.9	1.8
Region of Residence						
Northeast	30.6	26.5	25.6	27.8	30.3	28.7
Midwest	9.9	10.4	10.5	10.0	10.0	9.8
South	36.3	45.4	44.8	43.3	40.6	41.6
West	20.0	15.4	16.6	15.8	16.1	16.7
U.S. dependencies, possessions, and associated nations	3.2	2.2	2.6	3.0	2.9	3.1

[1]Based on cases reported to the Centers for Disease Control and Prevention from the beginning of the epidemic through 2003.
[2]Numbers are point estimates that result from adjustments for reporting delays to AIDS case counts. The estimates do not include adjustments for incomplete reporting. Data are provisional.
[3]Total for all years includes 1,796 persons of unknown race or multiple races and 1 person of unknown sex. All persons totals were calculated independent of values for subpopulations. Consequently, sums of subpopulations may not equal total for all persons.
[4]May be of any race.
[5]Percents may not sum to 100 percent due to rounding and because 0.2 percent of respondents are of unknown race and Hispanic origin.

TABLE III-4. AGE-ADJUSTED CANCER INCIDENCE RATES FOR SELECTED CANCER SITES, ACCORDING TO SEX, RACE, AND HISPANIC ORIGIN: LARGE U.S. SAMPLE, SELECTED YEARS, 1990–2001

According to the National Cancer Institute, 1.4 million new cases of cancer were expected to be diagnosed in 2005 in the United States. Measured per 100,000 persons, there were 457 new cancer cases in 2001, the latest date for

Table III-4. Age-Adjusted [1] Cancer Incidence Rates for Selected Cancer Sites, According to Sex, Race, and Hispanic Origin: Large U.S. Sample, Selected Years, 1990–2001

(Number of new cases per 100,000 population.)

Site, sex, race, and Hispanic origin	1990–2001 APC [2]	2001	2000	1999	1998	1997	1996	1995	1990
All Sites									
All persons	-0.5	457.1	465.9	476.1	477.0	476.5	471.0	469.9	476.0
White	-0.4	468.0	476.2	485.1	485.8	483.7	477.7	475.9	483.3
Black or African American	-0.7	486.2	511.6	526.1	523.7	533.3	528.4	532.6	514.9
American Indian or Alaska Native	-2.0	212.7	213.0	252.2	249.7	269.7	254.3	269.6	263.8
Asian or Pacific Islander	-0.4	331.6	331.7	339.6	337.1	345.1	333.6	337.8	335.8
Hispanic or Latino [3]	-0.2	334.5	346.7	362.8	363.2	352.6	357.3	361.1	343.0
White, not Hispanic or Latino	-0.3	480.1	488.9	496.9	494.2	495.1	488.5	485.0	490.9
Male	-1.3	537.3	552.5	561.4	558.8	562.9	560.5	562.3	584.4
White	-1.3	542.2	555.7	560.5	560.5	562.4	561.9	561.1	590.8
Black or African American	-1.2	642.9	686.6	701.3	701.8	717.1	707.4	729.5	690.1
American Indian or Alaska Native	-3.0	244.9	217.1	292.9	258.6	312.8	276.5	320.0	313.9
Asian or Pacific Islander	-0.8	374.7	387.0	391.6	381.6	397.1	385.3	396.0	387.6
Hispanic or Latino [3]	-0.6	399.5	416.7	432.9	430.4	423.2	433.2	442.1	407.2
White, not Hispanic or Latino	-1.3	549.4	564.6	569.7	563.6	569.5	568.6	566.8	598.9
Female	0.0	402.0	407.3	419.8	424.1	420.1	412.8	409.6	411.7
White	0.2	418.2	423.6	434.9	439.0	433.9	424.4	422.2	421.6
Black or African American	-0.3	378.4	393.7	410.6	408.1	411.7	410.5	400.9	404.4
American Indian or Alaska Native	-1.0	191.3	215.9	226.4	245.3	241.0	241.6	237.2	229.8
Asian or Pacific Islander	0.2	302.9	293.4	304.1	307.0	308.3	296.6	295.1	295.2
Hispanic or Latino [3]	0.0	294.3	305.4	320.5	322.3	309.6	311.7	311.5	307.7
White, not Hispanic or Latino	0.4	433.0	437.7	449.6	450.9	447.9	437.3	433.0	428.2
Lung and Bronchus									
Male	-2.2	73.6	76.5	80.0	83.2	82.7	84.4	87.0	95.4
White	-2.2	72.8	75.3	78.6	82.1	81.1	82.9	85.2	94.6
Black or African American	-2.2	108.2	109.2	119.4	123.5	126.4	128.9	136.8	134.8
Asian or Pacific Islander	-1.1	54.7	62.2	62.1	61.3	62.5	61.1	60.4	64.5
Hispanic or Latino [3]	-2.6	39.6	44.7	44.2	50.5	48.4	48.3	52.6	59.3
White, not Hispanic or Latino	-2.1	74.0	76.6	80.1	83.1	81.8	84.4	85.6	95.2
Female	0.0	46.4	48.0	50.2	50.8	50.3	50.2	49.4	47.4
White	0.2	48.3	50.2	52.2	53.1	53.0	52.5	51.8	48.7
Black or African American	0.2	52.5	54.3	58.0	56.9	50.8	53.9	50.4	53.4
Asian or Pacific Islander	0.1	28.3	27.2	29.0	28.5	29.9	27.8	27.8	28.4
Hispanic or Latino [3]	-1.0	21.3	22.9	24.4	26.0	25.7	25.6	24.4	24.7
White, not Hispanic or Latino	0.3	50.1	52.1	54.8	54.8	55.3	54.7	54.1	49.9
Colon and Rectum									
Male	-1.4	59.5	61.9	63.8	65.7	66.3	64.5	63.1	72.4
White	-1.5	58.9	61.6	63.8	65.6	66.1	64.9	62.5	73.1
Black or African American	-0.6	68.3	72.0	73.8	76.8	74.1	67.4	73.4	73.1
Asian or Pacific Islander	-0.8	54.7	56.4	54.1	57.5	59.6	56.1	58.3	61.4
Hispanic or Latino [3]	0.4	47.3	48.9	50.1	52.0	50.5	51.0	46.4	46.0
White, not Hispanic or Latino	-1.4	59.6	62.7	65.2	66.1	65.8	65.2	63.0	74.4
Female	-0.8	44.1	45.5	46.8	48.5	47.1	46.0	45.8	50.2
White	-0.8	43.3	45.1	46.1	48.2	47.0	45.6	45.5	49.8
Black or African American	-0.4	54.0	57.2	57.5	56.3	57.5	54.1	54.7	61.1
Asian or Pacific Islander	-0.4	39.7	36.7	40.2	40.5	35.6	39.1	38.5	38.1
Hispanic or Latino [3]	-0.1	29.7	32.9	34.4	34.1	32.1	32.1	33.1	32.6
White, not Hispanic or Latino	-0.7	44.2	46.6	47.3	49.5	48.5	46.8	46.0	50.8
Prostate									
Male	-1.8	171.4	174.6	177.7	167.6	170.4	165.4	165.5	166.7
White	-2.1	167.8	169.5	172.2	161.9	165.6	160.8	160.1	168.1
Black or African American	-0.7	251.3	281.2	278.1	275.3	271.0	268.8	272.4	219.2
American Indian or Alaska Native	-6.7	48.4	29.8	59.8	50.6	71.0	76.6	65.4	84.8
Asian or Pacific Islander	-0.9	103.9	104.3	105.1	92.8	96.9	94.0	103.3	88.9
Hispanic or Latino [3]	0.0	136.2	140.6	144.7	140.7	138.2	135.4	139.2	115.7
White, not Hispanic or Latino	2.1	167.5	169.4	171.3	159.1	166.1	161.1	160.3	169.6
Breast									
Female	0.5	132.1	132.9	137.4	138.3	135.4	131.8	130.6	129.3
White	0.6	139.0	139.8	144.1	144.6	141.1	136.9	136.1	134.3
Black or African American	0.0	111.9	119.5	122.7	122.8	123.5	122.4	122.4	116.6
American Indian or Alaska Native	-1.1	49.5	53.0	55.2	57.9	57.1	76.3	65.4	46.0
Asian or Pacific Islander	1.5	97.8	91.7	97.5	99.0	98.6	89.9	86.7	87.0
Hispanic or Latino [3]	0.5	85.4	92.1	92.0	91.9	87.0	91.2	89.1	84.7
White, not Hispanic or Latino	0.9	148.3	147.5	152.9	152.2	148.6	144.1	142.1	138.6
Cervix Uteri									
Female	-2.5	8.6	8.8	9.3	9.8	9.8	10.6	9.9	11.9
White	-2.2	8.3	8.8	9.0	9.3	9.2	9.9	9.2	11.2
Black or African American	-3.3	10.5	10.6	12.9	12.4	13.1	13.6	14.4	16.2
Asian or Pacific Islander	-3.2	9.8	8.0	8.3	10.9	11.1	13.0	10.9	12.1
Hispanic or Latino [3]	-2.9	14.9	16.8	17.3	15.7	16.2	18.5	18.1	21.2
White, not Hispanic or Latino	-2.5	6.7	6.7	7.5	8.0	7.8	8.3	7.7	9.5

[1] Age adjusted by 5-year age groups to the U.S. standard population in 2000. Age-adjusted rates are based on at least 25 cases.
[2] Annual percent change (APC) has been calculated by fitting a linear regression model to the natural logarithm of yearly rates from 1990 to 2001.
[3] May be of any race.
0.0 = Quantity more than zero but less than 0.05.

which detailed information is available for a large sample covering 12 geographic areas. The rate for men was one-third higher than that for women. However, new cancer cases in men have been declining slowly since 1990, at a trend rate of 1.4 percent per year. The trend rate for women has not declined, partly due to an increased number of breast cancer cases. From 1998 to 2001, however, breast cancer cases for women did decline, and total new cancer cases for women dropped by 5 percent.

For men, prostate cancer had by far the highest incidence of new cases, followed by lung and colon or rectal cancer.

Black men had the highest rates of these cancers. Colon and rectal cancer rates have declined significantly since 1990 for non-Hispanic White men, but Black men have experienced little or no decline for this type of cancer. Lung cancer rates have declined significantly since 1990 for men in all racial groups. For women, breast cancer has been the clear leader in new cases, followed by lung and colon cancer; the rate for the latter two cancers is lower for women than for men. Black women, as well as Asian and Hispanic women, had a lower rate of breast cancer than non-Hispanic White women.

Table III-4. Age-Adjusted [1] Cancer Incidence Rates for Selected Cancer Sites, According to Sex, Race, and Hispanic Origin: Large U.S. Sample, Selected Years, 1990–2001—*Continued*

(Number of new cases per 100,000 population.)

Site, sex, race, and Hispanic origin	1990–2001 APC [2]	2001	2000	1999	1998	1997	1996	1995	1990
Corpus Uteri									
Female	-0.1	24.2	23.7	24.5	24.9	25.2	24.5	24.9	24.7
White	-0.1	25.6	25.4	26.2	26.5	26.9	25.9	26.4	26.4
Black or African American	-1.0	19.7	16.9	18.0	18.3	18.0	19.2	17.9	17.0
Asian or Pacific Islander	1.8	17.7	16.4	17.5	17.2	17.5	16.6	17.7	13.2
Hispanic or Latino [3]	0.2	16.9	15.3	16.6	18.0	17.3	16.2	17.2	16.3
White, not Hispanic or Latino	0.0	26.6	26.5	27.1	27.6	27.9	27.0	27.4	27.0
Ovary									
Female	-1.2	13.6	13.8	14.1	14.0	14.2	14.0	14.5	15.6
White	-1.0	14.7	14.7	15.0	14.9	14.9	15.1	15.4	16.4
Black or African American	-1.2	8.7	10.4	10.3	10.7	10.3	9.1	10.8	11.1
Asian or Pacific Islander	-0.8	9.5	9.9	10.8	10.2	11.3	9.4	10.4	11.1
Hispanic or Latino [3]	-0.6	11.9	10.6	11.0	12.2	11.2	12.4	11.6	12.1
White, not Hispanic or Latino	-1.0	15.0	15.3	15.6	15.2	15.3	15.4	15.7	17.0
Oral Cavity and Pharynx									
Male	-2.2	14.6	15.7	15.2	16.4	16.9	17.4	16.9	19.2
White	-2.1	14.8	15.5	15.1	16.2	16.7	17.0	16.8	18.7
Black or African American	-2.9	17.7	19.2	19.3	21.7	19.8	23.3	22.4	26.3
Asian or Pacific Islander	-2.1	9.7	13.0	11.1	12.9	14.7	14.2	11.8	15.1
Hispanic or Latino [3]	-2.4	9.0	8.7	10.2	10.1	10.5	11.5	13.1	11.0
White, not Hispanic or Latino	-2.0	15.3	16.2	15.9	16.7	17.4	17.4	16.7	19.2
Female	-1.4	6.4	6.1	6.3	6.6	6.9	6.9	7.0	7.3
White	-1.5	6.4	6.1	6.1	6.7	6.9	6.9	7.1	7.4
Black or African American	-1.3	6.3	5.4	5.9	6.4	7.1	7.3	6.7	6.3
Asian or Pacific Islander	-0.7	5.5	6.1	6.5	4.5	6.5	5.7	5.2	6.0
Hispanic or Latino [3]	-0.3	3.9	3.6	4.5	3.5	3.9	3.7	3.8	3.7
White, not Hispanic or Latino	-1.7	6.4	6.4	6.3	7.2	7.3	7.3	7.3	7.7
Stomach									
Male	-2.0	11.5	12.5	12.9	12.9	13.5	13.8	13.6	14.7
White	-2.1	10.0	10.6	11.2	11.1	11.4	12.0	12.0	12.9
Black or African American	-2.5	16.3	18.7	17.1	20.4	22.0	22.5	18.5	21.9
Asian or Pacific Islander	-2.9	19.1	22.2	22.6	21.1	24.7	23.7	23.9	26.9
Hispanic or Latino [3]	-2.1	15.1	16.1	20.1	19.5	19.0	17.8	19.8	20.1
White, not Hispanic or Latino	-2.4	8.9	9.9	9.7	9.8	10.1	11.1	10.8	11.9
Female	-1.2	5.6	6.0	6.5	6.4	6.1	6.1	6.2	6.7
White	-1.6	4.5	5.0	5.4	5.2	4.9	5.1	5.2	5.7
Black or African American	-0.6	9.0	8.5	10.5	10.9	10.9	9.3	9.9	9.9
Asian or Pacific Islander	-2.6	11.9	12.8	12.2	12.8	12.2	13.7	13.1	15.5
Hispanic or Latino [3]	-1.1	9.3	10.4	9.4	11.0	10.1	10.1	11.2	10.9
White, not Hispanic or Latino	-2.4	3.5	4.1	4.7	4.3	4.0	4.3	4.4	5.0
Pancreas									
Male	-0.4	12.0	12.6	12.5	12.9	12.9	12.6	12.7	13.1
White	-0.1	12.2	12.4	12.3	12.9	12.5	12.3	12.4	12.7
Black or African American	-1.4	14.1	18.0	18.4	17.2	18.2	19.1	18.9	19.7
Asian or Pacific Islander	-1.7	9.3	10.4	9.2	10.5	12.1	10.6	10.5	11.2
Hispanic or Latino [3]	-0.5	9.4	11.5	9.7	9.8	12.0	11.4	12.5	11.1
White, not Hispanic or Latino	0.1	12.1	12.4	12.7	13.0	12.5	12.1	12.1	12.4
Female	-0.6	9.2	9.7	9.6	10.1	10.2	10.0	10.0	10.1
White	-0.6	8.9	9.5	9.3	9.9	9.7	9.7	9.7	9.8
Black or African American	-1.4	13.0	12.7	13.4	13.8	17.0	15.1	15.7	13.0
Asian or Pacific Islander	0.5	8.8	9.1	8.5	8.4	8.4	7.9	8.1	9.9
Hispanic or Latino [3]	-0.7	8.4	9.1	10.0	9.8	10.0	9.1	8.7	9.7
White, not Hispanic or Latino	-0.7	8.5	9.4	9.0	9.8	9.3	9.7	9.6	9.6

[1] Age adjusted by 5-year age groups to the U.S. standard population in 2000. Age-adjusted rates are based on at least 25 cases.
[2] Annual percent change (APC) has been calculated by fitting a linear regression model to the natural logarithm of yearly rates from 1990 to 2001.
[3] May be of any race.
0.0 = Quantity more than zero but less than 0.05.

Table III-4.   Age-Adjusted [1] Cancer Incidence Rates for Selected Cancer Sites, According to Sex, Race, and Hispanic Origin: Large U.S. Sample, Selected Years, 1990–2001—*Continued*

(Number of new cases per 100,000 population.)

Site, sex, race, and Hispanic origin	1990–2001 APC [2]	2001	2000	1999	1998	1997	1996	1995	1990
Urinary Bladder									
Male	-0.3	35.5	36.4	36.2	36.7	35.8	35.6	35.3	37.2
White	-0.2	39.4	40.3	39.8	40.5	39.5	39.2	38.7	40.7
Black or African American	-0.3	18.5	19.6	22.3	20.5	21.0	19.3	19.5	19.8
Asian or Pacific Islander	0.8	16.6	16.5	16.8	16.0	15.3	15.6	16.7	15.6
Hispanic or Latino [3]	-0.8	18.7	19.2	18.2	18.5	18.4	18.4	18.6	21.5
White, not Hispanic or Latino	-0.1	40.9	41.4	41.3	41.7	40.9	40.7	39.8	41.8
Female	-0.5	8.8	9.0	9.3	9.0	9.3	9.0	9.3	9.5
White	-0.2	9.7	9.7	10.0	9.8	9.9	9.8	10.1	9.9
Black or African American	-0.7	7.0	7.8	8.6	6.7	8.1	7.2	7.4	8.6
Asian or Pacific Islander	-0.4	4.5	4.1	4.1	4.7	5.1	3.9	4.5	5.3
Hispanic or Latino [3]	-0.7	5.0	5.4	4.4	4.8	5.1	5.5	5.3	5.4
White, not Hispanic or Latino	0.0	10.0	10.0	10.5	10.2	10.6	10.1	10.4	10.1
Non-Hodgkins Lymphoma									
Male	-0.1	22.8	23.0	23.9	22.8	23.9	24.6	25.0	22.7
White	-0.1	23.8	24.3	25.0	24.0	24.7	25.7	26.2	23.8
Black or African American	-0.5	17.1	16.9	17.9	17.0	22.9	18.9	21.5	17.6
Asian or Pacific Islander	0.3	17.0	16.0	18.9	15.3	16.2	16.8	16.3	16.5
Hispanic or Latino [3]	-0.1	17.2	19.8	18.1	19.8	17.7	21.9	21.8	17.2
White, not Hispanic or Latino	-0.1	24.6	24.6	26.0	24.8	25.2	26.4	27.0	24.6
Female	0.9	15.4	15.5	15.8	16.1	15.9	15.2	15.1	14.6
White	0.8	16.1	16.3	16.9	16.9	16.7	15.9	15.8	15.4
Black or African American	1.9	11.7	11.8	10.6	12.5	11.9	11.4	10.0	10.4
Asian or Pacific Islander	1.7	12.5	11.0	11.1	11.0	11.0	9.5	11.7	9.1
Hispanic or Latino [3]	0.8	13.7	12.5	13.8	13.4	14.4	13.5	12.7	13.1
White, not Hispanic or Latino	0.9	16.5	16.6	17.1	17.3	16.9	16.0	16.0	15.4
Leukemia									
Male	-1.0	15.2	15.3	15.9	16.5	16.6	16.3	17.4	17.0
White	-0.9	16.1	16.2	16.8	17.5	17.7	17.1	18.7	17.9
Black or African American	-1.4	11.4	12.9	12.8	13.3	13.8	13.5	13.0	15.6
Asian or Pacific Islander	-0.1	9.4	9.5	10.5	9.9	8.8	11.0	10.0	8.5
Hispanic or Latino [3]	-0.5	9.8	12.2	11.2	11.7	12.3	12.4	15.6	11.6
White, not Hispanic or Latino	-0.8	16.4	16.2	17.0	17.7	17.9	17.1	19.0	17.7
Female	-0.8	9.0	9.6	8.9	9.7	9.6	9.8	10.0	9.8
White	-0.5	9.5	10.1	9.4	10.3	10.3	10.3	10.6	10.2
Black or African American	-0.9	8.2	8.7	7.5	7.4	7.9	8.1	8.1	8.3
Asian or Pacific Islander	-1.4	4.9	6.0	6.2	6.7	5.7	6.5	6.3	6.1
Hispanic or Latino [3]	-1.0	6.2	7.5	7.7	8.3	8.4	7.2	8.2	8.3
White, not Hispanic or Latino	-0.7	9.4	9.7	9.3	10.0	10.2	10.3	10.4	10.1

[1]Age adjusted by 5-year age groups to the U.S. standard population in 2000. Age-adjusted rates are based on at least 25 cases.
[2]Annual percent change (APC) has been calculated by fitting a linear regression model to the natural logarithm of yearly rates from 1990 to 2001.
[3]May be of any race.
0.0 = Quantity more than zero but less than 0.05.

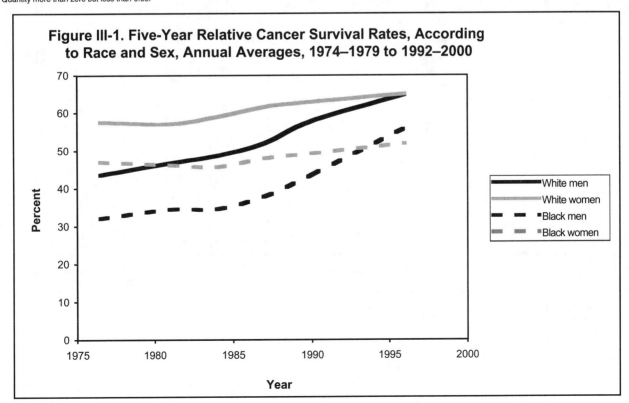

Figure III-1. Five-Year Relative Cancer Survival Rates, According to Race and Sex, Annual Averages, 1974–1979 to 1992–2000

TABLE III-5. FIVE-YEAR RELATIVE CANCER SURVIVAL RATES FOR SELECTED CANCER SITES, ACCORDING TO RACE AND SEX, SELECTED YEARS, 1974–2000

From 1992–2000, White male cancer patients achieved a 64.8 percent 5-year survival rate for all cancers, and White women attained a similar survival rate of 64.9 percent. For Black males, the 5-year survival rate was 55.8 percent; for Black women, this rate was 51.8 percent. Survival rates have risen substantially since 1974–1979. They have particularly increased for prostate cancer, leading to a greater overall percentage of improvement for men than for women.

The highest cancer survival rates for men were for prostate and bladder cancer; for women, rates were highest for melanoma and breast cancer. The lowest 5-year survival rates for both men and women were for pancreatic, lung, and esophageal cancer.

The observed survival rate is adjusted to factor out expected normal deaths during the 5-year period. Without such adjustment, survival rates for young patients would be overstated relative to older patients, who have higher general mortality rates. To make the adjustment, the observed survival rate is divided by the expected survival rate of the same group in the general population. Thus, if 50 percent of the patient group survived, and if the survival rate of that same group in the general population for the same 5 years was 90 percent, the adjusted cancer survival rate would be $50 \div 90 = 55.6$.

Table III-5. Five-Year Relative Cancer Survival Rates for Selected Cancer Sites, According to Race and Sex, Selected Years, 1974–2000

(Percent.)

Sex and site of cancer	White						Black or African American					
	1992–2000	1989–1991	1986–1988	1983–1985	1980–1982	1974–1979	1992–2000	1989–1991	1986–1988	1983–1985	1980–1982	1974–1979
BOTH SEXES												
All Sites	64.8	60.3	56.8	53.9	52.1	50.9	54.0	46.2	42.7	39.8	39.8	39.3
Oral cavity and pharynx	60.1	55.6	55.4	55.4	55.7	55.0	37.0	33.3	34.8	35.2	31.1	36.6
Esophagus	15.7	11.7	10.7	9.3	7.3	5.5	9.4	8.9	7.2	5.9	5.4	3.2
Stomach	21.4	18.4	19.2	16.3	16.5	15.2	21.8	24.8	19.3	18.9	19.1	15.6
Colon	63.5	63.2	61.6	58.5	55.6	51.9	53.2	53.9	53.1	49.5	49.4	47.3
Rectum	63.6	60.5	59.2	55.9	53.1	49.8	54.3	54.5	51.3	44.1	38.3	40.3
Pancreas	4.5	4.1	3.2	2.9	2.8	2.4	3.8	3.9	6.0	5.0	4.5	3.3
Lung and bronchus	15.3	14.4	13.5	13.8	13.5	13.1	12.6	10.8	11.9	11.4	12.1	11.3
Urinary bladder	82.6	82.2	80.7	78.3	78.9	75.0	63.4	62.0	62.8	59.8	58.5	51.6
Non-Hodgkin's lymphoma	58.2	52.1	52.8	54.5	51.9	48.3	47.9	43.7	50.4	45.1	50.5	50.3
Leukemia	48.3	46.4	44.3	42.1	39.5	36.7	38.9	34.9	38.0	33.6	32.9	30.8
MALE												
All Sites	64.8	57.8	51.9	48.6	46.7	43.5	55.8	43.5	37.8	34.5	34.4	32.1
Oral cavity and pharynx	59.2	52.2	52.3	54.5	54.6	54.5	31.5	28.9	29.6	29.9	26.5	31.2
Esophagus	15.4	11.8	11.3	7.7	6.4	5.2	9.5	8.0	7.0	4.7	4.6	2.1
Stomach	20.0	15.1	16.2	14.6	15.6	13.8	20.0	22.3	15.3	18.4	18.2	15.2
Colon	64.2	63.8	62.5	59.0	55.9	51.0	53.8	53.8	52.8	48.3	46.9	45.5
Rectum	62.6	60.3	58.9	55.2	51.7	48.9	52.7	56.4	46.7	43.1	36.4	36.7
Pancreas	4.3	3.9	3.0	2.6	2.5	2.6	3.4	3.1	6.1	4.4	3.2	2.6
Lung and bronchus	13.5	12.8	12.0	12.1	12.2	11.6	11.3	9.6	12.0	10.2	10.9	9.9
Prostate gland	99.0	92.0	82.7	76.2	74.5	70.3	94.3	80.8	69.3	63.9	64.8	60.7
Urinary bladder	84.6	84.4	82.3	79.6	79.9	76.0	68.4	65.7	67.6	64.8	63.0	59.1
Non-Hodgkin's lymphoma	55.3	47.8	50.1	53.5	51.0	47.3	43.2	38.3	47.0	43.6	47.8	44.7
Leukemia	49.2	46.9	45.7	41.7	39.6	35.6	38.7	30.1	36.3	32.3	30.1	30.7
FEMALE												
All Sites	64.9	62.8	61.5	58.9	57.1	57.5	51.8	49.2	47.9	45.6	46.1	46.9
Colon	63.0	62.6	60.7	58.0	55.4	52.6	52.8	54.1	53.4	50.3	51.4	48.8
Rectum	64.9	60.8	59.5	56.8	54.7	50.8	56.0	52.6	56.0	44.9	40.6	43.8
Pancreas	4.6	4.4	3.4	3.2	3.0	2.3	4.2	4.6	6.0	5.5	5.8	4.1
Lung and bronchus	17.5	16.6	15.8	17.0	16.2	16.7	14.8	13.0	11.7	14.2	15.6	15.7
Melanoma of skin	92.2	91.8	91.5	89.6	88.3	86.0	71.9	94.0	*	70.1	*	69.9
Breast	88.3	86.2	83.9	79.3	77.1	75.4	74.1	71.2	69.2	63.6	65.8	63.1
Cervix uteri	73.3	72.5	71.9	70.6	68.2	69.8	62.6	62.6	55.7	60.8	61.5	63.1
Corpus uteri	86.3	85.7	84.4	84.5	82.8	87.7	60.8	57.8	57.5	54.3	55.2	59.5
Ovary	43.4	41.2	39.4	40.3	38.7	37.2	42.0	30.7	36.6	41.5	39.3	40.5
Non-Hodgkin's lymphoma	61.7	57.4	56.2	55.5	52.9	49.3	55.4	51.2	54.8	46.9	53.7	57.5

Note: Rates are based on follow-up of patients through 2002. The rate is the ratio of the observed survival rate for the patient group to the expected survival rate for persons in the general population similar to the patient group with respect to age, sex, race, and calendar year of observation. It estimates the chance of surviving the effects of cancer. The race groups White and Black include persons of Hispanic and non-Hispanic origin.

* = Figure too small to meet standards of reliability and precison.

TABLE III-6. DIABETES AMONG PERSONS 20 YEARS OF AGE AND OVER, ACCORDING TO SEX, AGE, RACE, AND HISPANIC ORIGIN, 1988–1994 AND 1999–2002

From 1999–2002, more than 9 percent of persons age 20 years old and over were estimated to have diabetes, including diabetes previously diagnosed by a physician and previously undiagnosed diabetes that was diagnosed by testing blood sugar after fasting. Diabetes became more prevalent during the 1992–2002 period. Type 2 diabetes, which accounted for 90–95 percent of all cases, is associated with older age, obesity, family history of diabetes, physical inactivity, and race/ethnicity. It is more common among Black adults than non-Hispanic White adults. The incidence of diabetes rises sharply with age.

TABLE III-7. LIMITATION OF ACTIVITY CAUSED BY CHRONIC CONDITIONS, ACCORDING TO SELECTED CHARACTERISTICS, SELECTED YEARS, 1997–2003

In 2003, as many as 12.1 percent of interview respondents reported limitations of activity. In the 18- to 44-year-old age group, this incidence rate was 6.0 percent, but it rose to 34.6 percent for persons age 65 years and over. Among races,

American Indians had the highest rates of activity limitations.

The term "limitation of activity" refers to a long-term reduction in a person's performance of activities associated with his or her age group, due to chronic physical or mental conditions. For persons age 65 years and over, additional detail is presented in the second part of the table in order to establish more stringent criteria of limitations of activities. Two different types of activities are established: those pertaining to activities of daily living (ADL) and those pertaining to instrumental activities of daily living (IADL). ADL relates to personal care and includes bathing, dressing, or eating. IADL focuses on persons living independently and includes meal preparation, shopping, and using a telephone. In this survey, persons are considered to have an IADL limitation if they report needing help with an independent living activity due to a chronic problem. The 2003 survey shows 6.4 percent of persons age 65 years and over with ADL limitations and 12.2 percent with IADL limitation. When poverty status is considered, 21.6 percent of poor persons age 65 years and over are reported to have IADL limitations, while the incidence rate for nonpoor adults was 9.4 percent.

Table III-6. Diabetes Among Persons 20 Years of Age and Over, According to Sex, Age, Race, and Hispanic Origin, 1988–1994 and 1999–2002

(Percent.)

Sex, age, race, and Hispanic origin [1]	Physician-diagnosed and undiagnosed diabetes [2,3]		Physician-diagnosed diabetes [2]		Undiagnosed diabetes [3]	
	1999–2002	1988–1994	1999–2002	1988–1994 [4]	1999–2002	1988–1994
20 Years and Over, Age-Adjusted [4]						
All persons [5]	9.4	8.4	6.6	5.4	2.9	3.0
Male	10.7	8.8	7.1	5.4	3.8	3.5
Female	8.3	8.0	6.2	5.4	2.2	2.6
Not Hispanic or Latino						
White	8.0	7.5	5.3	5.0	2.8	2.6
Black or African American	14.8	12.6	11.2	8.6	*3.9	4.2
Mexican	13.6	14.1	10.5	9.7	3.5	4.7
20 Years and Over, Crude						
All persons [5]	9.3	7.8	6.5	5.1	2.8	2.7
Male	10.2	7.9	6.7	4.8	3.5	3.0
Female	8.5	7.8	6.3	5.4	2.2	2.4
Not Hispanic or Latino						
White	8.5	7.5	5.6	5.0	2.9	2.5
Black or African American	13.2	10.4	9.9	6.9	*3.3	3.4
Mexican	8.3	9.0	6.5	5.6	1.8	3.4
Age						
20–39 years	*	1.6	1.7	1.1	*	0.6
40–59 years	9.8	8.9	6.6	5.5	3.3	3.4
60 years and over	20.9	18.9	15.1	12.8	5.8	6.1

Note: Data are based on physical examinations of a sample of the civilian noninstitutional population.

[1] Persons of Mexican origin may be of any race. Starting with data year 1999, race-specific estimates are tabulated according to 1997 standards for Federal Data on Race and Ethnicity and are not strictly comparable with estimates for earlier years. The two non-Hispanic race categories shown in the table conform to 1997 standards. The 1999–2002 race-specific estimates are for persons who reported only one racial group. Data for 1988–1994 were tabulated according to 1977 standards. Estimates for single race categories prior to 1999 included persons who reported one race or, if they reported more than one race, identified one race as best representing their race.
[2] Physician-diagnosed diabetes was obtained by self-report and excludes women who reported diabetes only during pregnancy.
[3] Undiagnosed diabetes is defined as a fasting blood glucose of at least 126 mg/dL and no reported physician diagnosis.
[4] Estimates are age adjusted to the year 2000 standard population using three age groups: 20–39 years, 40–59 years, and 60 years and over. Age-adjusted estimates in this table may differ from other age-adjusted estimates based on the same data and presented elsewhere if different age groups are used in the adjustment procedure.
[5] Includes all other races and Hispanic origins not shown separately.
* = Figure does not meet standards of reliability or precision.

Table III-7. Limitation of Activity Caused by Chronic Conditions, According to Selected Characteristics, Selected Years, 1997–2003

(Percent.)

Characteristic	Persons with any activity limitation [1]				Persons with ADL limitation [2]				Persons with IADL limitation [2]			
	2003	2002	2001	1997	2003	2002	2001	1997	2003	2002	2001	1997
All Ages												
Total [3]	12.1	12.3	12.1	13.3	X	X	X	X	X	X	X	X
Age												
Under 18 years	6.9	7.1	6.8	6.6	X	X	X	X	X	X	X	X
Under 5 years	3.6	3.2	3.3	3.5	X	X	X	X	X	X	X	X
5–17 years	8.1	8.5	8.0	7.8	X	X	X	X	X	X	X	X
18–44 years	6.0	6.2	6.0	7.0	X	X	X	X	X	X	X	X
18–24 years	4.1	4.3	4.6	5.1	X	X	X	X	X	X	X	X
25–44 years	6.6	6.8	6.5	7.6	X	X	X	X	X	X	X	X
45–54 years	13.0	13.8	13.1	14.2	X	X	X	X	X	X	X	X
55–64 years	21.1	21.1	20.7	22.2	X	X	X	X	X	X	X	X
65 years and over	34.6	34.5	34.6	38.7	6.4	6.1	6.4	6.7	12.2	12.2	12.6	13.7
65–74 years	26.3	25.2	26.0	30.0	3.1	2.7	3.4	3.4	6.5	6.0	6.7	6.9
75 years and over	44.0	45.2	44.7	50.2	9.9	9.8	9.6	10.4	18.4	19.1	18.9	21.2
Sex												
Male	11.9	12.3	12.2	13.1	5.2	4.7	6.0	5.2	8.6	7.8	9.6	9.1
Female	12.2	12.3	11.9	13.4	7.2	7.0	6.5	7.7	14.6	15.2	14.6	16.9
Race [4]												
White only	11.8	12.1	11.8	13.1	5.9	5.6	5.7	6.3	11.5	11.5	11.8	13.1
Black or African American only	15.3	14.9	15.6	17.1	10.5	10.0	11.8	11.7	19.2	18.5	18.8	21.3
American Indian and Alaska Native only	21.2	19.5	18.9	23.1	*	*	*	*	*	*	*	*
Asian only	6.4	6.4	6.7	7.5	*	*	*9.2	*	*11.8	*11.2	15.9	*9.1
Native Hawaiian and Other Pacific Islander only	*	*	*	...	*	*	*	...	*	*	*	...
Two or more races	20.2	22.0	19.8	...	*	*	*	...	*20.4	*20.8	*16.0	...
Black or African American; White	*16.8	*8.3	14.8	...	...	...	...	...	...	...	...	...
American Indian and Alaska Native; White	24.8	30.0	22.0	...	...	...	...	...	...	...	...	...
Hispanic Origin and Race [4]												
Hispanic or Latino	10.2	10.7	10.5	12.8	10.3	9.2	11.2	10.8	13.8	13.1	17.0	16.3
Mexican	9.7	10.8	10.3	12.5	9.8	10.2	10.6	11.4	15.1	14.0	17.0	18.8
Not Hispanic or Latino	12.4	12.6	12.4	13.5	6.1	5.9	6.1	6.5	12.1	12.2	12.3	13.6
White only	12.2	12.4	12.1	13.2	5.7	5.5	5.5	6.1	11.4	11.5	11.6	13.0
Black or African American only	15.4	15.0	15.5	17.0	10.4	10.1	11.9	11.7	19.0	18.7	18.8	21.2
Poverty Status [5]												
Poor	23.1	22.9	22.3	25.4	10.4	9.5	11.2	12.5	21.6	21.1	22.9	25.3
Near poor	17.0	17.4	17.1	17.9	7.0	6.9	7.5	7.4	15.0	14.7	14.9	15.8
Nonpoor	9.2	9.5	9.5	10.1	5.5	5.1	5.0	5.3	9.4	9.5	9.7	10.4
Hispanic Origin and Race and Poverty Status [4,5]												
Hispanic or Latino												
Poor	15.5	16.3	16.2	19.2	*15.2	12.5	13.5	16.0	20.1	17.3	24.0	25.5
Near poor	9.9	12.2	10.9	12.7	*8.4	10.0	11.3	11.1	12.3	15.6	16.4	15.5
Nonpoor	8.2	7.7	7.9	9.2	*8.5	*6.7	8.8	*6.6	*11.1	8.7	12.2	10.2
Not Hispanic or Latino												
White only												
Poor	26.2	25.4	24.8	27.8	8.9	8.2	9.9	11.8	20.7	20.4	23.0	24.9
Near poor	19.3	19.5	18.8	19.2	6.4	6.3	6.5	6.6	14.8	14.2	14.1	15.2
Nonpoor	9.4	9.7	9.7	10.4	5.1	4.8	4.6	5.0	9.0	9.2	9.2	10.3
Black or African American												
Poor	26.1	25.0	24.8	28.2	14.0	13.8	15.9	13.5	28.3	26.6	25.8	27.8
Near poor	19.0	17.9	20.1	19.5	10.4	*9.8	12.3	12.4	18.9	19.3	18.6	22.4
Nonpoor	9.7	10.0	10.0	10.7	8.4	8.1	9.3	9.8	13.9	13.4	14.9	15.1
Geographic Region												
Northeast	11.3	11.8	11.1	13.0	6.6	6.3	6.5	6.1	11.4	11.0	11.3	12.2
Midwest	13.3	13.1	13.3	13.1	4.7	5.2	4.9	5.8	11.3	11.7	12.6	13.1
South	12.4	12.6	12.3	13.9	7.2	6.3	7.5	8.2	13.1	13.0	13.3	15.8
West	11.1	11.5	11.5	13.0	6.5	6.5	6.0	5.9	12.1	12.7	12.6	12.4
Location of Residence												
Within MSA [6]	11.2	11.4	11.3	12.7	6.3	6.2	6.1	6.6	12.0	12.1	12.2	13.5
Outside MSA [6]	15.7	15.9	15.3	15.5	6.7	5.6	7.3	7.2	12.8	12.6	13.8	14.4

[1]Limitation of activity is assessed by asking respondents a series of questions about limitations in their ability to perform activities usual for their age group due to a physical, mental, or emotional problem.

[2]These estimates are for noninstitutionalized persons and are age-adjusted to the year 2000 standard population using two age groups: 65–74 years and 75 years and over. ADL is activities of daily living and IADL is instrumental activities of daily living. Respondents were asked about needing the help of another person with personal care (ADL) and routine needs such as chores and shopping (IADL) because of physical, mental, or emotional problems. The first four columns show percentages for the indicated population groups. The last eight columns show percentages for the elderly noninstitutionalized populations only.

[3]Includes all other races not shown separately and unknown poverty status.

[4]The race groups, White, Black, American Indian and Alaska Native (AI/AN), Asian, Native Hawaiian and Other Pacific Islander, and two or more races, include persons of Hispanic and non-Hispanic origin. Persons of Hispanic origin may be of any race.

[5]Poor persons are defined as having a total income below the poverty threshold. Near poor persons have incomes of 100 percent to less than 200 percent of the poverty threshold. Nonpoor persons have incomes of 200 percent or more than the poverty threshold.

[6]MSA = Metropolitan Statistical Area.

* = Figure does not meet standards of reliability or precision.

X = Not applicable.

. . . = Not available.

TABLE III-8. SELECTED CHRONIC HEALTH CONDITIONS CAUSING LIMITATION OF ACTIVITY AMONG WORKING-AGE ADULTS, BY AGE, 2002–2003

This table shows chronic health conditions that may cause limitations of activity among working-age adults. The data show the number of afflicted persons in several age groups as rates per 1,000 persons. Among persons in the 18- to 44-year-old age group, the most frequent conditions causing limitations were arthritis and other musculoskeletal conditions (22.2 per 1,000 persons) and mental illness (12.9 per 1,000 persons). These rates increased for older age groups, with arthritis and other muscoloskeletal conditions reaching 100.7 per 1,000 persons for the 55- to 64-year-old age group. Heart conditions also occurred prominently in older age groups.

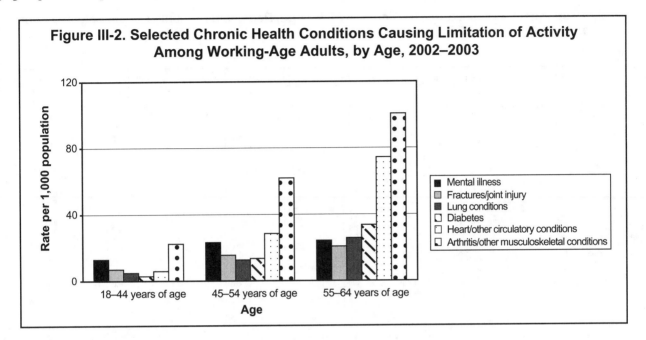

Figure III-2. Selected Chronic Health Conditions Causing Limitation of Activity Among Working-Age Adults, by Age, 2002–2003

Table III-8. Selected Chronic Health Conditions Causing Limitation of Activity Among Working-Age Adults, by Age, 2002–2003

(Number per 1,000 population.)

Type of chronic health conditions	Number of persons with limitations of activity caused by selected chronic health conditions					
	18–44 years		45–54 years		55–64 years	
	Rate per 1,000 population	Standard error	Rate per 1,000 population	Standard error	Rate per 1,000 population	Standard error
Mental illness	12.9	0.5	23.1	1.1	24.1	1.4
Fractures/joint injury	7.0	0.4	15.5	0.9	20.6	1.2
Lung	5.0	0.3	12.6	0.8	25.6	1.3
Diabetes	2.5	0.2	13.4	0.8	33.4	1.5
Heart/other circulatory	5.9	0.3	28.4	1.2	74.3	2.4
Arthritis/other musculoskeletal	22.2	0.7	61.9	1.8	100.7	2.6

Note: Data are for the civilian noninstitutionalized population. Selected chronic health conditions include the four leading causes of activity limitation among adults in each age category. Conditions refer to response categories in the National Health Interview Survey; some conditions include several response categories. "Mental illness" includes depression, anxiety, or other emotional problems. "Heart/other circulatory" includes heart problems, stroke problems, hypertension/high blood pressure, and other circulatory system conditions. "Arthritis/other musculoskeletal" includes arthritis/rheumatism, back or neck problems, and other musculoskeletal system conditions. Persons may report more than one chronic health condition as the cause of their activity limitation.

TABLE III-9. RESPONDENT-ASSESSED HEALTH STATUS BY SEX, AGE, RACE, AND HISPANIC ORIGIN, SELECTED YEARS, 1991–2003

Health status data in this table were obtained by asking respondents to assess their health and the health of family members living in the same household as excellent, very good, good, fair, or poor. In 2003, 9.2 percent of persons had fair or poor health. This rate has held fairly steady over the last five years, but women tended to report fair or poor health more frequently than men.

Minorities (except Asians) reported more health problems than non-Hispanic Whites, and older persons more

Table III-9. Respondent-Assessed Health Status, by Sex, Age, Race, and Hispanic Origin, Selected Years, 1991–2003

(Percent.)

Characteristic	2003	2002	2001	2000	1999	1997	1995 [1]	1991 [1]
PERCENT OF PEOPLE WITH FAIR OR POOR HEALTH								
Total [2, 3]	9.2	9.3	9.2	9.0	8.9	9.2	10.6	10.4
Age								
Under 18 years	1.8	1.9	1.8	1.7	1.6	2.1	2.6	2.6
Under 6 years	1.4	1.6	1.6	1.5	1.4	1.9	2.7	2.7
6–17 years	2.0	2.1	1.9	1.8	1.8	2.1	2.5	2.6
18–44 years	5.6	5.5	5.4	5.1	5.1	5.3	6.6	6.1
18–24 years	3.8	3.6	3.3	3.2	3.4	3.4	4.5	4.8
25–44 years	6.3	6.2	6.0	5.7	5.6	5.9	7.2	6.4
45–54 years	12.1	12.6	11.7	11.9	11.5	11.7	13.4	13.4
55–64 years	18.9	17.9	19.2	17.9	18.5	18.2	21.4	20.7
65 years and over	25.5	26.4	26.6	27.0	26.1	26.7	28.3	29.0
65–74 years	22.3	22.1	23.0	22.6	22.7	23.1	25.6	26.0
75 years and over	29.2	31.4	30.8	32.2	30.2	31.5	32.2	33.6
Sex [2]								
Male	8.8	8.9	9.0	8.8	8.6	8.8	10.1	10.0
Female	9.5	9.6	9.5	9.3	9.2	9.7	11.1	10.8
Race [2, 4]								
White only	8.5	8.6	8.2	8.2	8.0	8.3	9.7	9.6
Black or African American only	14.7	14.1	15.4	14.6	14.6	15.8	17.2	16.8
American Indian and Alaska Native only	16.3	13.1	14.5	17.2	14.7	17.3	18.7	18.3
Asian only	7.4	6.7	8.1	7.4	8.6	7.8	9.3	7.8
Native Hawaiian and Other Pacific Islander only	*	*	*	*	*	...	...	...
Two or more races	14.7	12.6	13.8	16.4	12.9	...	...	...
Black or African American; White	21.4	13.9	*10.1	*14.5	*20 .5	...	...	...
American Indian and Alaska Native; White	18.1	13.5	15.0	18.7	14.5	...	...	...
Hispanic Origin and Race [2, 4]								
Hispanic or Latino	13.9	13.1	12.7	12.9	11.9	13.0	15.1	15.6
Mexican	13.7	13.4	12.5	12.9	12.3	13.1	16.7	17.0
Not Hispanic or Latino	8.7	8.9	8.9	8.7	8.6	8.9	...	...
White only	7.9	8.2	7.9	7.9	7.7	8.0	9.1	9.1
Black or African American only	14.6	14.0	15.5	14.6	14.6	15.8	17.3	16.8
Poverty Status [2, 5]								
Poor	20.4	20.4	20.3	19.7	20.6	20.8	23.7	22.8
Near poor	14.4	14.6	14.5	14.1	14.0	13.9	15.5	14.7
Nonpoor	6.1	6.4	6.4	6.3	6.0	6.1	6.7	6.8
Hispanic Origin and Race and Poverty Status [2, 4, 5]								
Hispanic or Latino								
Poor	20.6	20.9	18.7	18.7	18.3	19.9	22.7	23.6
Near poor	15.5	15.4	14.8	15.4	13.8	13.5	16.9	18.0
Nonpoor	9.8	8.7	8.7	8.5	8.0	8.5	8.7	9.3
Not Hispanic or Latino								
White only								
Poor	19.5	19.1	19.0	18.7	19.4	19.7	22.8	21.9
Near poor	13.9	14.3	13.6	13.4	13.5	13.3	14.8	14.0
Nonpoor	5.6	6.0	5.9	5.8	5.7	5.6	6.2	6.4
Black or African American								
Poor	24.4	24.5	24.9	23.8	25.9	25.3	27.7	25.8
Near poor	18.6	17.4	19.6	18.2	17.5	19.2	19.3	17.0
Nonpoor	9.1	8.8	9.9	9.7	8.3	9.7	9.9	10.9

[1]Data prior to 1997 are not strictly comparable with data for later years due to the 1997 questionnaire redesign.
[2]Estimates are age adjusted to the year 2000 standard population using six age groups: under 18 years, 18–44 years, 45–54 years, 55–64 years, 65–74 years, and 75 years and over.
[3]Includes all other races not shown separately and unknown poverty status.
[4]The race groups, White, Black, American Indian and Alaska Native (AI/AN), Asian, Native Hawaiian and Other Pacific Islander, and two or more races, include persons of Hispanic and non-Hispanic origin. Persons of Hispanic origin may be of any race.
[5]Poor persons are defined as having a total income below the poverty threshold. Near poor persons have incomes of 100 percent to less than 200 percent of the poverty threshold. Nonpoor persons have incomes of 200 percent or more than the poverty threshold. Missing family income data were imputed for 16–18 percent of persons in 1991 and 1995. Starting with *Health, United States, 2004,* a new methodology for imputing family income was used for data years 1997 and beyond. Missing family income data were imputed for 25–29 percent of persons in 1997–1998 and 32–33 percent in 1999–2002.
* = Figure does not meet standards of reliability or precision.
... = Not available.

frequently fell into the category of fair or poor health than younger adults. As many as 29 percent of persons age 75 years or over reported fair or poor health, in comparison to 3.8 percent of those age 18 to 24 years.

Poverty status was a factor related to health, as 20 percent of those living below the poverty level reported fair or poor health, compared to only 6 percent of those with family incomes of more than twice the poverty threshold. Persons living in the South were more likely to report fair or poor health than respondents in other regions, and persons living in urban areas were less likely to report fair or poor health than those in rural areas.

TABLE III-10. SERIOUS PSYCHOLOGICAL DISTRESS AMONG PERSONS 18 YEARS OF AGE AND OVER, ACCORDING TO SELECTED CHARACTERISTICS, SELECTED ANNUAL AVERAGES, 1997–2003

From 2002–2003, 3 percent of the civilian noninstitutional population experienced serious psychological distress. About 4.2 percent of persons age 45 to 54 years experienced serious psychological distress, more than in any other age group. Persons living below the poverty line were more than four times as likely as nonpoor persons—those with incomes greater than 200 percent of the poverty threshold—to experience serious psychological distress (8.7 percent compared with 1.8 percent).

Table III-9. Respondent-Assessed Health Status, by Sex, Age, Race, and Hispanic Origin, Selected Years, 1991–2003—*Continued*

(Percent.)

Characteristic	2003	2002	2001	2000	1999	1997	1995 [1]	1991 [1]
Geographic Region [2]								
Northeast	8.2	8.1	7.4	7.6	7.5	8.0	9.1	8.3
Midwest	8.3	8.3	8.8	8.0	8.0	8.1	9.7	9.1
South	10.7	10.9	10.8	10.7	10.5	10.8	12.3	13.1
West	8.4	8.7	8.6	8.8	8.7	8.8	10.1	9.7
Location of Residence [2]								
Within MSA [6]	8.6	8.7	8.7	8.5	8.3	8.7	10.1	9.9
Outside MSA [6]	11.5	11.7	11.0	11.1	11.1	11.1	12.6	11.9

[1]Data prior to 1997 are not strictly comparable with data for later years due to the 1997 questionnaire redesign.
[2]Estimates are age adjusted to the year 2000 standard population using six age groups: under 18 years, 18–44 years, 45–54 years, 55–64 years, 65–74 years, and 75 years and over.
[6]MSA = Metropolitan Statistical Area.

Table III-10. Serious Psychological Distress[1] Among Persons 18 Years of Age and Over, According to Selected Characteristics, Selected Annual Averages, 1997–2003

(Percent.)

Characteristic	2002–2003	2000–2001	1997–1998
PERCENT OF PEOPLE WITH SERIOUS PSYCHOLOGICAL DISTRESS			
Total, Age-Adjusted [2,3]	3.1	3.2	3.2
Total, Crude	3.1	3.2	3.2
Age			
18–44 years	2.9	3.1	2.9
18–24 years	2.8	2.7	2.7
25–44 years	2.9	3.2	3.0
45–64 years	4.0	3.7	3.7
45–54 years	4.2	3.7	3.9
55–64 years	3.6	3.8	3.4
65 years and over	2.3	2.7	3.1
65–74 years	2.3	2.8	2.5
75 years and over	2.3	2.5	3.8
Sex [2]			
Male	2.3	2.4	2.5
Female	3.9	3.9	3.8
Race [2,4]			
White only	3.0	3.1	3.1
Black or African American only	3.4	3.5	4.0
American Indian and Alaska Native only	*7.1	*9.3	7.8
Asian only	*1.9	*	2.0
Native Hawaiian and Other Pacific Islander only	*	*	...
Two or more races	7.3	5.2	...
Hispanic Origin and Race [2,4]			
Hispanic or Latino	3.9	4.2	5.0
Mexican	3.7	4.0	5.2
Not Hispanic or Latino	3.1	3.1	3.0
White only	3.0	3.1	2.9
Black or African American only	3.2	3.5	3.9
Poverty Status [2,5]			
Poor	8.7	8.3	9.1
Near poor	5.4	5.3	5.0
Nonpoor	1.8	2.0	1.8
Hispanic Origin and Race and Poverty Status [2,4,5]			
Hispanic or Latino			
Poor	7.4	7.2	8.6
Near poor	3.8	4.4	5.4
Nonpoor	2.4	2.8	2.9
Not Hispanic or Latino			
White only			
Poor	10.1	9.4	9.6
Near poor	6.4	6.1	5.2
Nonpoor	1.7	2.0	1.8
Black or African American			
Poor	7.3	7.3	8.7
Near poor	*4.0	4.9	4.3
Nonpoor	*1.3	*1.6	1.6
Geographic Region [2]			
Northeast	3.0	3.1	2.7
Midwest	2.7	3.0	2.6
South	3.5	3.4	3.8
West	3.0	3.2	3.3
Location of Residence [2]			
Within MSA [6]	2.9	3.1	3.0
Outside MSA [6]	3.9	3.5	3.9

[1]Serious psychological distress is measured by a six-question scale that asks respondents how often they experience each of the six symptoms of psychological distress.
[2]Estimates are age adjusted to the year 2000 standard population using six age groups: under 18 years, 18–44 years, 45–54 years, 55–64 years, 65–74 years, and 75 years and over.
[3]Includes all other races not shown separately and unknown poverty status.
[4]The race groups, White, Black, American Indian and Alaska Native (AI/AN), Asian, Native Hawaiian and Other Pacific Islander, and two or more races, include persons of Hispanic and non-Hispanic origin. Persons of Hispanic origin may be of any race.
[5]Poor persons are defined as having a total income below the poverty threshold. Near poor persons have incomes of 100 percent to less than 200 percent of the poverty threshold. Nonpoor persons have incomes of 200 percent or more than the poverty threshold. Missing family income data were imputed for 16–18 percent of persons in 1991 and 1995. Starting with *Health, United States, 2004*, a new methodology for imputing family income was used for data years 1997 and beyond. Missing family income data were imputed for 25–29 percent of persons in 1997–1998 and 32–33 percent in 1999–2002.
[6]MSA = Metropolitan Statistical Area.
* = Figure does not meet standards of reliability or precision.
... = Not available.

TABLE III-11. RESPIRATORY CONDITIONS AMONG ADULTS 18 YEARS OF AGE AND OVER, ACCORDING TO SELECTED CHARACTERISTICS, SELECTED YEARS, 1997–2003

During the 12 months prior to the 2003 interview, 14 percent of the adult population was diagnosed by a doctor with sinusitis, 8.6 percent was diagnosed with hay fever, and 3.3 percent experienced an asthma attack. These percentages were somewhat lower than those in 2002 and 1997. For each of these diseases, the occurrence rates were greater for females than for males. For asthma attacks and hay fever, the incidence rate tended to decline with age, while sinusitis showed increases with age.

Table III-11. Respiratory Conditions Among Adults 18 Years of Age and Over, According to Selected Characteristics, Selected Years, 1997–2003

(Percent.)

Characteristic	Asthma attack [1]			Sinusitis [2]			Hay Fever [2]		
	2003	2002	1997	2003	2002	1997	2003	2002	1997
Total, age-adjusted [3,4]	3.3	3.7	3.7	13.9	14.1	16.3	8.6	8.8	9.2
Total, crude [4]	3.3	3.7	3.7	14.0	14.2	16.3	8.6	8.8	9.3
Age									
18–44 years	3.4	4.0	4.0	11.9	12.3	15.3	8.5	8.4	9.9
18–24 years	3.5	4.6	4.8	8.3	8.2	11.0	5.1	6.2	8.1
25–44 years	3.4	3.8	3.8	13.2	13.7	16.6	9.7	9.2	10.5
45–64 years	3.7	3.7	3.6	17.3	17.8	19.3	9.8	10.8	9.7
45–54 years	3.7	3.9	4.1	16.9	17.4	19.7	10.4	11.7	10.4
55–64 years	3.7	3.4	2.9	17.7	18.4	18.5	9.0	9.6	8.7
65 years and over	2.3	3.0	2.7	13.9	13.2	14.5	6.6	6.1	6.3
65–74 years	2.8	3.4	3.1	15.4	14.2	15.6	7.6	7.0	7.2
75 years and over	1.7	2.4	2.2	12.2	12.0	13.2	5.3	5.0	5.2
Sex [3]									
Male	2.0	2.3	2.6	10.0	10.3	11.5	7.6	7.9	8.5
Female	4.5	5.0	4.7	17.5	17.6	20.8	9.5	9.6	10.0
Sex and Age									
Male									
18–44 years	2.3	2.5	2.7	8.4	8.9	10.8	7.5	7.7	9.0
45–54 years	2.0	2.1	2.7	12.3	12.3	13.4	9.8	10.7	9.7
55–64 years	*1.8	2.4	1.9	12.5	13.3	12.9	7.7	7.7	8.2
65–74 years	*1.6	*2.3	2.8	11.1	11.3	11.8	6.7	7.1	6.5
75 years and over	*	*1.7	*2.0	10.0	9.6	9.4	4.4	4.3	4.4
Female									
18–44 years	4.5	5.4	5.3	15.4	15.6	19.7	9.5	9.2	10.8
45–54 years	5.4	5.5	5.4	21.3	22.3	25.8	11.0	12.6	11.1
55–64 years	5.4	4.4	3.9	22.6	23.1	23.6	10.3	11.3	9.1
65–74 years	3.7	4.4	3.4	18.9	16.7	18.6	8.4	7.0	7.7
75 years and over	2.3	2.9	2.3	13.5	13.5	15.6	5.9	5.5	5.7
Race [3,5]									
White only	3.3	3.7	3.7	14.1	14.5	16.6	8.9	9.1	9.4
Black or African American only	3.7	4.3	3.9	14.3	14.6	16.8	6.7	7.0	8.7
American Indian and Alaska Native only	*	*	*6.3	15.4	*8.3	18.3	*9.5	*	*12.0
Asian only	*	*2.5	*2.2	5.5	7.1	9.9	6.5	8.4	10.8
Native Hawaiian and Other Pacific Islander only	*	*	. . .	*	*	. . .	*	*	. . .
Two or more races	*5.5	9.3	. . .	14.5	19.2	. . .	12.0	8.8	. . .
Hispanic Origin and Race [3,5]									
Hispanic or Latino	2.8	2.3	2.8	8.5	8.6	10.0	6.2	6.8	6.3
Mexican	1.9	1.6	1.7	7.8	7.8	9.1	5.6	6.2	5.6
Not Hispanic or Latino	3.4	3.9	3.8	14.7	14.9	17.0	9.0	9.1	9.6
White only	3.4	3.9	3.9	15.2	15.4	17.4	9.5	9.6	9.7
Black or African American only	3.6	4.2	3.9	14.4	14.4	16.9	6.8	6.9	8.8
Education [6,7]									
25 years and over									
No high school diploma or GED	3.8	3.5	4.4	11.6	12.5	15.9	6.3	6.3	7.8
High school diploma or GED	3.0	3.4	3.2	13.1	14.6	16.5	6.6	8.1	7.9
Some college or more	3.2	3.7	3.4	16.5	15.8	17.9	11.3	10.5	10.9
Poverty Status [8]									
Poor	5.3	5.5	5.9	12.8	14.0	16.1	6.5	7.9	8.7
Near poor	4.1	3.9	4.4	13.5	14.7	15.5	8.2	7.7	8.6
Nonpoor	2.9	3.4	3.1	14.1	14.0	16.7	9.1	9.2	9.6

[1] Only respondents who had ever been told by a doctor or other health professional that they had asthma were asked, "During the past 12 months, have you had an episode of asthma or an asthma attack?"

[2] Respondents were asked in two separate questions, "During the past 12 months, have you been told by a doctor or other health professional that you had sinusitis or hay fever?"

[3] Estimates are age adjusted to the year 2000 standard population using five age groups: 18–44 years, 45–54 years, 55–64 years, 65–74 years, and 75 years and over. Age-adjusted estimates in this table may differ from other age-adjusted estimates based on the same data and presented elsewhere if different age groups are used in the adjustment procedure.

[4] Includes all other races not shown separately.

[5] The race groups, White, Black, American Indian and Alaska Native, Asian, Native Hawaiian and Other Pacific Islander, and two or more races, include persons of Hispanic and non-Hispanic origin. Persons of Hispanic origin may be of any race.

[6] Estimates are for persons 25 years of age and over and are age adjusted to the year 2000 standard population using five age groups: 25–44 years, 45–54 years, 55–64 years, 65–74 years, and 75 years and over.

[7] GED stands for General Educational Development high school equivalency diploma.

[8] Poor persons are defined as having a total income below the poverty threshold. Near poor persons have incomes of 100 percent to less than 200 percent of the poverty threshold. Nonpoor persons have incomes of 200 percent or more than the poverty threshold.

* = Figure does not meet standards of reliability or precision.

. . . = Not available.

Table III-11. Respiratory Conditions Among Adults 18 Years of Age and Over, According to Selected Characteristics, Selected Years, 1997–2003—Continued

(Percent.)

Characteristic	Asthma attack [1]			Sinusitis [2]			Hay Fever [2]		
	2003	2002	1997	2003	2002	1997	2003	2002	1997
Hispanic Origin and Race and Poverty Status [3, 5, 8]									
Hispanic or Latino	3.5	3.7	3.3	8.0	8.4	8.1	5.3	6.9	5.4
Poor	*2.7	*2.0	3.0	7.9	7.9	8.6	6.8	7.4	6.4
Near poor	2.7	1.9	2.4	9.1	9.2	11.5	6.4	6.6	6.9
Nonpoor									
Not Hispanic or Latino									
White only	6.2	6.4	7.2	14.5	16.2	18.4	7.6	9.1	9.7
Poor	4.4	4.7	4.6	15.4	16.8	17.0	9.0	8.5	9.4
Near poor	3.0	3.5	3.4	15.2	15.0	17.4	9.8	9.9	9.9
Nonpoor									
Black or African American only	5.9	5.6	6.0	14.5	15.8	18.9	6.0	7.3	9.2
Poor	4.9	4.2	5.4	14.3	17.4	16.1	7.9	6.2	8.8
Near poor	2.3	3.6	2.2	14.3	12.6	16.5	6.4	6.9	8.8
Nonpoor									
Geographic Region [3]									
Northeast	3.5	4.0	3.4	13.2	13.4	15.0	9.3	9.4	9.2
Midwest	3.5	4.0	3.7	14.1	13.0	15.7	8.0	7.7	8.6
South	3.0	3.3	3.7	16.1	16.6	19.6	7.4	7.7	8.7
West	3.4	4.0	3.9	10.3	11.3	12.6	10.8	11.5	11.1
Location of Residence [3]									
Within MSA [9]	3.3	3.6	3.7	13.4	13.6	15.8	8.6	8.8	9.3
Outside MSA [9]	3.3	4.1	3.5	15.7	15.9	18.4	8.6	8.5	9.0

[1]Only respondents who had ever been told by a doctor or other health professional that they had asthma were asked, "During the past 12 months, have you had an episode of asthma or an asthma attack?"

[2]Respondents were asked in two separate questions, "During the past 12 months, have you been told by a doctor or other health professional that you had sinusitis or hay fever?"

[3]Estimates are age adjusted to the year 2000 standard population using five age groups: 18–44 years, 45–54 years, 55–64 years, 65–74 years, and 75 years and over. Age-adjusted estimates in this table may differ from other age-adjusted estimates based on the same data and presented elsewhere if different age groups are used in the adjustment procedure.

[5]The race groups, White, Black, American Indian and Alaska Native, Asian, Native Hawaiian and Other Pacific Islander, and two or more races, include persons of Hispanic and non-Hispanic origin. Persons of Hispanic origin may be of any race.

[8]Poor persons are defined as having a total income below the poverty threshold. Near poor persons have incomes of 100 percent to less than 200 percent of the poverty threshold. Nonpoor persons have incomes of 200 percent or more than the poverty threshold.

[9]MSA = Metropolitan Statistical Area.

* = Figure does not meet standards of reliability or precision.

TABLE III-12. SEVERE HEADACHE OR MIGRAINE, LOW BACK PAIN, AND NECK PAIN AMONG ADULTS 18 YEARS OF AGE AND OVER, ACCORDING TO SELECTED CHARACTERISTICS, SELECTED YEARS, 1997–2003

During the three months prior to the 2003 interview, 15 percent of the adult population in the United States experienced a migraine or a severe headache, 27 percent experienced low back pain, and 15 percent suffered neck pain. Respondents, who may be represented in more than one category, were instructed to report only pain lasting a whole day or longer.

Table III-12. Severe Headache or Migraine, Low Back Pain, and Neck Pain Among Adults 18 Years of Age and Over, According to Selected Characteristics, Selected Years, 1997–2003

(Percent.)

Characteristic	Severe headache or migraine [1]			Low back pain [1]			Neck pain [1]		
	2003	2002	1997	2003	2002	1997	2003	2002	1997
Percent of Adults with Pain in the Past 3 Months									
Total, age-adjusted [2,3]	15.1	15.0	15.8	27.4	26.4	28.2	14.7	13.8	14.7
Total, crude [3]	15.2	15.1	16.0	27.5	26.4	28.1	14.8	13.8	14.6
Age									
18–44 years	17.8	17.6	18.7	24.2	23.7	26.1	12.5	11.9	13.3
18–24 years	16.8	17.3	18.7	19.6	20.8	21.9	9.1	7.7	9.8
25–44 years	18.1	17.6	18.7	25.8	24.6	27.3	13.7	13.3	14.3
45–64 years	15.1	15.2	15.8	31.5	29.8	31.3	18.2	16.9	17.0
45–54 years	16.5	17.0	17.8	30.2	29.2	31.3	17.9	17.2	17.3
55–64 years	13.1	12.5	12.7	33.4	30.8	31.2	18.5	16.5	16.6
65 years and over	6.9	6.6	7.0	29.9	28.8	29.5	15.1	14.1	15.0
65–74 years	7.9	7.9	8.2	30.8	28.9	30.2	15.6	14.1	15.0
75 years and over	5.7	5.2	5.4	28.9	28.8	28.6	14.5	14.0	15.0
Sex [2]									
Male	9.2	9.2	9.9	25.1	24.3	26.5	12.0	11.7	12.6
Female	20.7	20.6	21.4	29.4	28.3	29.6	17.1	15.7	16.6
Sex and Age									
Male									
18–44 years	10.8	10.7	11.9	22.4	22.1	24.8	10.3	10.4	11.6
45–54 years	9.7	10.3	10.3	29.3	27.6	29.4	14.7	13.8	13.9
55–64 years	8.5	8.4	8.8	30.5	27.9	30.7	15.2	12.7	14.6
65–74 years	5.8	4.1	5.0	25.6	25.9	29.0	12.5	13.2	13.6
75 years and over	3.2	3.6	*2.4	25.1	23.8	22.5	12.6	13.0	12.6
Female									
18–44 years	24.6	24.3	25.4	26.0	25.2	27.3	14.7	13.4	14.9
45–54 years	22.9	23.5	24.9	31.1	30.7	33.1	21.0	20.4	20.6
55–64 years	17.5	16.3	16.3	36.1	33.4	31.7	21.6	20.0	18.4
65–74 years	9.6	11.0	10.7	35.0	31.3	31.1	18.2	14.9	16.1
75 years and over	7.4	6.1	7.4	31.4	31.9	32.4	15.8	14.7	16.5
Race [2,4]									
White only	15.1	15.2	15.9	27.9	26.9	28.7	15.2	14.1	15.1
Black or African American only	15.2	14.9	16.7	25.0	24.0	26.9	12.1	11.7	13.3
American Indian and Alaska Native only	28.6	24.8	18.9	32.2	34.3	33.3	17.4	*18.2	16.2
Asian only	11.9	8.4	11.7	19.7	19.2	21.0	9.1	8.1	9.2
Native Hawaiian and Other Pacific Islander only	*	*	. . .	*	*	. . .	*	*	. . .
Two or more races	23.2	27.0	. . .	34.9	34.0	. . .	20.5	22.3	. . .
Hispanic Origin and Race [2,4]									
Hispanic or Latino	15.9	13.5	15.5	26.5	24.2	26.4	14.6	13.5	13.9
Mexican	15.3	12.5	14.6	24.6	23.2	25.2	12.5	12.3	12.9
Not Hispanic or Latino	15.2	15.4	15.9	27.6	26.7	28.4	14.9	13.9	14.9
White only	15.3	15.6	16.1	28.4	27.4	29.1	15.6	14.4	15.4
Black or African American only	15.2	14.9	16.8	24.9	23.9	26.9	12.0	11.6	13.3
Education [5,6]									
25 years and over									
No high school diploma or GED	17.7	17.9	19.2	31.6	31.6	33.6	17.0	16.4	16.5
High school diploma or GED	15.3	15.9	16.0	29.6	28.6	30.2	14.8	15.1	15.5
Some college or more	13.8	13.2	13.8	27.3	25.6	26.9	15.3	14.0	14.6
Poverty Status [7]									
Poor	21.0	21.3	23.3	33.2	31.3	35.4	17.9	17.0	18.6
Near poor	18.7	17.6	18.9	30.6	30.0	30.8	16.3	15.9	16.1
Nonpoor	13.3	13.5	13.8	25.8	24.9	26.3	13.8	12.9	13.8

[1]In three separate questions, respondents were asked, "During the past 3 months, did you have a severe headache or migraine? Low back pain? Neck pain?" Respondents were instructed to report pain that had lasted a whole day or more and, conversely, not to report fleeting or minor aches or pains. Persons may be represented in more than one column.

[2]Estimates are age adjusted to the year 2000 standard population using five age groups: 18–44 years, 45–54 years, 55–64 years, 65–74 years, and 75 years and over. Age-adjusted estimates in this table may differ from other age-adjusted estimates based on the same data and presented elsewhere if different age groups are used in the adjustment procedure.

[3]Includes all other races not shown separately.

[4]The race groups, White, Black, American Indian and Alaska Native, Asian, Native Hawaiian and Other Pacific Islander, and two or more races, include persons of Hispanic and non-Hispanic origin. Persons of Hispanic origin may be of any race.

[5]Estimates are for persons 25 years of age and over and are age adjusted to the year 2000 standard population using five age groups: 25–44 years, 45–54 years, 55–64 years, 65–74 years, and 75 years and over.

[6]GED stands for General Educational Development high school equivalency diploma.

[7]Poor persons are defined as having a total income below the poverty threshold. Near poor persons have incomes of 100 percent to less than 200 percent of the poverty threshold. Nonpoor persons have incomes of 200 percent or more than the poverty threshold.

* = Figure does not meet standards of reliability or precision.

. . . = Not available.

Women were twice as likely as men to have experienced a recent migraine (21 percent versus 9 percent), and women also reported other pains more frequently. In contrast to many other diseases, the frequency of migraines was inversely related to age. The incidence of migraines declined from 18 percent in the 18- to 44-year-old age group to 6 percent for those age 75 years and over. Age associated declines in pain were not reported for low back or neck pain; on the contrary, there was some increase in occurrence with age in these categories. Among racial groups, American Indians or Alaska Natives reported the most frequent incidences of these types of pains.

Table III-12. Severe Headache or Migraine, Low Back Pain, and Neck Pain Among Adults 18 Years of Age and Over, According to Selected Characteristics, Selected Years, 1997–2003—*Continued*

(Percent.)

Characteristic	Severe headache or migraine [1]			Low back pain [1]			Neck pain [1]		
	2003	2002	1997	2003	2002	1997	2003	2002	1997
Hispanic Origin and Race and Poverty Status [2, 4, 7]									
Hispanic or Latino									
Poor	19.8	19.3	18.9	29.7	28.3	29.5	16.1	18.5	16.4
Near poor	16.4	13.8	15.7	26.6	24.3	26.8	16.9	14.6	12.9
Nonpoor	13.8	11.5	13.4	25.3	22.7	24.3	12.9	11.3	13.3
Not Hispanic or Latino									
White only									
Poor	21.7	23.3	26.2	35.9	33.7	38.9	19.7	17.3	20.5
Near poor	21.0	20.0	20.1	33.0	33.2	33.3	18.0	17.7	18.0
Nonpoor	13.6	14.1	14.1	26.8	25.7	27.1	14.7	13.6	14.4
Black or African American only									
Poor	21.0	20.2	22.7	31.2	30.1	34.5	16.0	14.2	17.9
Near poor	15.9	17.3	17.6	27.6	26.9	27.7	12.7	13.6	14.0
Nonpoor	12.5	11.9	13.4	22.0	20.6	23.1	10.3	10.1	10.9
Geographic Region [2]									
Northeast	14.1	13.9	14.5	27.3	27.4	27.1	14.3	14.0	14.0
Midwest	14.9	15.1	15.6	29.0	27.6	28.7	15.2	13.4	15.3
South	15.6	15.4	17.1	25.1	24.5	27.5	13.5	13.2	13.9
West	15.6	15.2	15.3	29.5	27.6	30.0	16.5	15.2	16.1
Location of Residence [2]									
Within MSA [8]	14.6	14.2	15.2	26.5	25.7	27.0	14.5	13.2	14.2
Outside MSA [8]	17.4	18.1	18.1	30.7	29.2	32.5	15.2	15.9	16.4

[1]In three separate questions, respondents were asked, "During the past 3 months, did you have a severe headache or migraine? Low back pain? Neck pain?" Respondents were instructed to report pain that had lasted a whole day or more and, conversely, not to report fleeting or minor aches or pains. Persons may be represented in more than one column.
[2]Estimates are age adjusted to the year 2000 standard population using five age groups: 18–44 years, 45–54 years, 55–64 years, 65–74 years, and 75 years and over. Age-adjusted estimates in this table may differ from other age-adjusted estimates based on the same data and presented elsewhere if different age groups are used in the adjustment procedure.
[4]The race groups, White, Black, American Indian and Alaska Native, Asian, Native Hawaiian and Other Pacific Islander, and two or more races, include persons of Hispanic and non-Hispanic origin. Persons of Hispanic origin may be of any race.
[7]Poor persons are defined as having a total income below the poverty threshold. Near poor persons have incomes of 100 percent to less than 200 percent of the poverty threshold. Nonpoor persons have incomes of 200 percent or more than the poverty threshold.
[8]MSA = Metropolitan Statistical Area.

TABLE III-13. VISION AND HEARING LIMITATIONS AMONG ADULTS 18 YEARS OF AGE AND OVER, ACCORDING TO SELECTED CHARACTERISTICS, SELECTED YEARS, 1997–2003

In 2003, almost 9 percent of the adult population experienced vision trouble, which is defined as having trouble seeing even with glasses or contact lenses. Significant hearing trouble (or deafness) was reported by 3 percent of adults. These afflictions tended to increase with age.

Table III-13. Vision and Hearing Limitations Among Adults 18 Years of Age and Over, According to Selected Characteristics, Selected Years, 1997–2003

(Percent.)

Characteristic	Any trouble seeing even with eye glasses or contacts [1]				A lot of trouble hearing or deaf [2]			
	2003	2002	2000	1997	2003	2002	2000	1997
Total, age-adjusted [3,4]	8.8	9.3	9.0	10.0	3.1	3.2	3.2	3.2
Total, crude [4]	8.7	9.3	8.9	9.8	3.0	3.1	3.1	3.1
Age								
18–44 years	5.2	5.6	5.3	6.2	0.9	0.9	0.9	1.0
18–24 years	5.1	4.4	4.2	5.4	*	*	*0.7	*0.5
25–44 years	5.2	6.0	5.7	6.5	1.0	1.1	1.0	1.2
45–64 years	10.6	11.0	10.7	12.0	2.8	2.8	3.0	3.1
45–54 years	10.5	11.5	10.9	12.2	1.9	1.9	2.3	2.6
55–64 years	10.7	10.3	10.5	11.6	4.1	4.2	4.0	3.9
65 years and over	16.6	17.6	17.4	18.1	10.5	11.1	10.5	9.8
65–74 years	13.1	14.5	13.6	14.2	6.7	7.2	7.4	6.6
75 years and over	20.6	21.1	21.9	23.1	14.9	15.6	14.3	14.1
Sex [3]								
Male	7.3	8.1	7.9	8.8	4.0	4.2	4.3	4.2
Female	10.1	10.4	10.1	11.1	2.3	2.4	2.3	2.4
Sex and Age								
Male								
18–44 years	4.1	4.8	4.4	5.3	1.1	1.0	1.1	1.2
45–54 years	8.6	10.1	8.8	10.1	2.7	2.2	2.9	3.6
55–64 years	8.6	8.7	9.5	10.5	5.4	5.8	6.2	5.4
65–74 years	11.8	13.3	12.8	13.2	10.2	10.8	10.8	9.4
75 years and over	18.1	18.6	20.7	21.4	17.8	19.7	18.0	17.7
Female								
18–44 years	6.2	6.5	6.2	7.1	0.7	0.7	0.8	0.9
45–54 years	12.3	12.9	12.8	14.2	1.2	1.5	1.8	1.7
55–64 years	12.5	11.9	11.5	12.6	2.8	2.7	1.9	2.6
65–74 years	14.1	15.5	14.4	15.0	3.8	4.1	4.5	4.4
75 years and over	22.3	22.6	22.7	24.2	12.9	13.0	12.1	11.7
Race [3,5]								
White only	8.5	9.0	8.8	9.7	3.3	3.3	3.4	3.4
Black or African American only	10.8	11.7	10.6	12.8	1.7	1.6	1.6	2.0
American Indian and Alaska Native only	18.9	*11.1	16.6	19.2	*	*10.1	*	14.1
Asian only	6.1	7.2	6.3	6.2	*	*2.3	*2.4	*
Native Hawaiian and Other Pacific Islander only	*	*	*	...	*	*	*	...
Two or more races	11.6	14.9	16.2	...	*	*6.3	*5.7	...
Hispanic Origin and Race [3,5]								
Hispanic or Latino	9.1	9.0	9.7	10.0	2.0	2.0	2.3	1.5
Mexican	9.0	8.6	8.3	10.2	2.6	3.0	3.0	1.8
Not Hispanic or Latino	8.8	9.4	9.1	10.0	3.2	3.3	3.3	3.3
White only	8.6	9.1	8.9	9.8	3.4	3.5	3.5	3.5
Black or African American only	10.7	11.8	10.6	12.8	1.8	1.6	1.6	2.0
Education [6,7]								
25 years and over								
No high school diploma or GED	12.6	14.4	12.2	15.0	4.9	4.6	4.6	4.8
High school diploma or GED	9.3	10.3	9.5	10.6	3.5	3.9	3.9	3.7
Some college or more	8.1	8.7	8.9	8.9	2.8	3.3	2.8	2.9
Poverty Status [8]								
Poor	13.7	14.5	12.9	17.0	3.9	4.4	3.7	4.5
Near poor	11.6	12.0	11.6	12.9	3.6	3.6	4.2	3.6
Nonpoor	7.3	8.0	7.8	8.2	2.8	3.0	2.8	3.0

[1] Respondents were asked, "Do you have any trouble seeing, even when wearing glasses or contact lenses?"

[2] Respondents were asked, "Which statement best describes your hearing without a hearing aid: good, a little trouble, a lot of trouble, or deaf?" For this table, "a lot of trouble" and "deaf" are combined into one category.

[3] Estimates are age adjusted to the year 2000 standard population using five age groups: 18–44 years, 45–54 years, 55–64 years, 65–74 years, and 75 years and over. Age-adjusted estimates in this table may differ from other age-adjusted estimates based on the same data and presented elsewhere if different age groups are used in the adjustment procedure.

[4] Includes all other races not shown separately.

[5] The race groups, White, Black, American Indian and Alaska Native, Asian, Native Hawaiian and Other Pacific Islander, and two or more races, include persons of Hispanic and non-Hispanic origin. Persons of Hispanic origin may be of any race.

[6] Estimates are for persons 25 years of age and over and are age adjusted to the year 2000 standard population using five age groups: 25–44 years, 45–54 years, 55–64 years, 65–74 years, and 75 years and over.

[7] GED stands for General Educational Development high school equivalency diploma.

[8] Poor persons are defined as having a total income below the poverty threshold. Near poor persons have incomes of 100 percent to less than 200 percent of the poverty threshold. Nonpoor persons have incomes of 200 percent or more than the poverty threshold.

* = Figure does not meet standards of reliability or precision.

. . . = Not available.

Vision trouble affected 21 percent of people age 75 years and over, and hearing problems were experienced by almost 15 percent of that same age group.

Asians stood out as having relatively few vision or hearing impairments. Poor persons and those without a high school degree tended to have an above-average number of impairments.

Table III-13. Vision and Hearing Limitations Among Adults 18 Years of Age and Over, According to Selected Characteristics, Selected Years, 1997–2003—*Continued*

(Percent.)

Characteristic	Any trouble seeing even with eye glasses or contacts [1]				A lot of trouble hearing or deaf [2]			
	2003	2002	2000	1997	2003	2002	2000	1997
Hispanic Origin and Race and Poverty Status [3,5,8]								
Hispanic or Latino								
Poor	12.4	12.9	11.0	12.8	*3.4	*2.3	3.3	*1.9
Near poor	10.3	9.4	9.4	11.2	*1.6	*1.7	*2.3	*1.5
Nonpoor	6.7	7.2	9.7	7.8	*1.4	*1.9	*1.7	*1.2
Not Hispanic or Latino								
White only								
Poor	14.3	14.7	13.1	17.9	4.7	5.2	4.5	5.8
Near poor	11.8	12.7	12.0	13.1	4.2	4.5	5.0	4.3
Nonpoor	7.3	7.9	7.8	8.2	3.1	3.1	3.0	3.2
Black or African American only								
Poor	14.2	16.6	13.6	17.9	*2.1	*2.3	*1.6	3.3
Near poor	13.0	14.6	12.9	16.0	*2.3	*	*2.0	*2.0
Nonpoor	8.5	9.1	8.1	8.5	*	*1.6	*	*
Geographic Region [3]								
Northeast	7.5	7.8	7.4	8.6	2.9	2.7	2.4	2.2
Midwest	9.3	9.3	9.6	9.5	3.3	3.1	3.5	3.5
South	9.4	9.9	9.2	11.4	3.0	3.3	3.3	3.5
West	8.1	9.7	9.9	9.7	3.2	3.8	3.5	3.4
Location of Residence [3]								
Within MSA [9]	8.2	8.7	8.5	9.5	2.7	3.0	3.0	2.9
Outside MSA [9]	10.7	11.5	11.1	12.0	4.4	3.8	3.9	4.5

[1]Respondents were asked, "Do you have any trouble seeing, even when wearing glasses or contact lenses?"
[2]Respondents were asked, "Which statement best describes your hearing without a hearing aid: good, a little trouble, a lot of trouble, or deaf?" For this table, "a lot of trouble" and "deaf" are combined into one category.
[3]Estimates are age adjusted to the year 2000 standard population using five age groups: 18–44 years, 45–54 years, 55–64 years, 65–74 years, and 75 years and over. Age-adjusted estimates in this table may differ from other age-adjusted estimates based on the same data and presented elsewhere if different age groups are used in the adjustment procedure.
[5]The race groups, White, Black, American Indian and Alaska Native, Asian, Native Hawaiian and Other Pacific Islander, and two or more races, include persons of Hispanic and non-Hispanic origin. Persons of Hispanic origin may be of any race.
[8]Poor persons are defined as having a total income below the poverty threshold. Near poor persons have incomes of 100 percent to less than 200 percent of the poverty threshold. Nonpoor persons have incomes of 200 percent or more than the poverty threshold.
[9]MSA = Metropolitan Statistical Area.
* = Figure does not meet standards of reliability or precision.

TABLE III-14. SUICIDAL IDEATION, SUICIDE ATTEMPTS, AND INJURIOUS SUICIDE ATTEMPTS AMONG STUDENTS IN GRADES 9–12, BY SEX, GRADE LEVEL, RACE, AND HISPANIC ORIGIN, SELECTED YEARS, 1991–2003

(Data are based on a national sample of high school students.)

The rate of students who seriously considered suicide experienced a gradual decline, dropping from 24 percent in 1993 to 17 percent in 2003. For girls, the frequency of suicidal ideation was considerably higher than that for boys. Suicide was attempted by 8.5 percent of this population—about half the rate of suicidal ideation—with girls showing a higher rate of attempts (11.5 percent) than boys (5.4 percent). The percentage of students requiring medical attention due to a suicide attempt was much smaller, in the area of 3 percent, with girls again experiencing a higher rate than boys. Nevertheless, mortality data in Table 46 from *Health, United States, 2005* shows that adolescent boys (15–19 years of age) were five times more likely to die from suicide than adolescent girls, partly reflecting their choice of more lethal methods, such as firearms.

TABLE III-15. HYPERTENSION (ELEVATED BLOOD PRESSURE) AMONG PERSONS 20 YEARS OF AGE AND OVER, ACCORDING TO SEX, AGE, RACE, HISPANIC ORIGIN, AND POVERTY STATUS, 1988–1994 AND 1999–2002

From 1999–2002, based on age-adjusted figures, 25.6 percent of persons age 20 to 74 years had hypertension. The classification of hypertension is based on either elevated blood pressure (systolic pressure of at least 140 mmHg or diastolic pressure of at least 90 mmHg) or the need for anti-hypertensive medication. The data are based on a physical examination of a sample of the civilian population.

When blood pressure was measured, regardless of whether anti-hypertensive medication was taken, 16.4 percent of the population were found to have hypertension. The frequency of hypertension has increased slightly since the 1988–1994 period, perhaps associated with the population's general tendency to gain weight. From 1988–1994, 21.7 percent of the population (3.9 percentage points less) experienced hypertension. Among races, non-Hispanic Blacks were particularly afflicted with hypertension; from 1999–2002, 36.9 percent of Black males and 39.5 percent of Black females had hypertension. The frequency of hypertension tends to increase with age; less than 20 percent of those under age 45 years had hypertension. This proportion rose to 60 percent of males age 65–74 years. For women age 75 years and over, hypertension was found in 83 percent of the population.

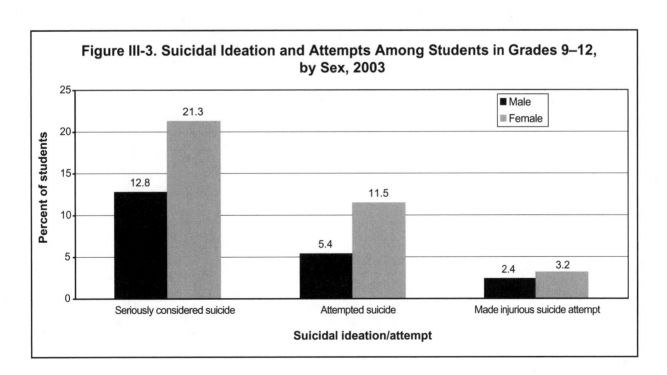

Figure III-3. Suicidal Ideation and Attempts Among Students in Grades 9–12, by Sex, 2003

Table III-14. Suicidal Ideation, Suicide Attempts, and Injurious Suicide Attempts Among Students in Grades 9–12, by Sex, Grade Level, Race, and Hispanic Origin, Selected Years, 1991–2003

(Percent.)

Sex, grade level, race, and Hispanic origin	2003	2001	1999	1997	1995	1993	1991
PERCENT OF STUDENTS WHO SERIOUSLY CONSIDERED SUICIDE [1]							
Total	16.9	19.0	19.3	20.5	24.1	24.1	29.0
Male							
Total	12.8	14.2	13.7	15.1	18.3	18.8	20.8
9th grade	11.9	14.7	11.9	16.1	18.2	17.7	17.6
10th grade	13.2	13.8	13.7	14.5	16.7	18.0	19.5
11th grade	12.9	14.1	13.7	16.6	21.7	20.6	25.3
12th grade	13.2	13.7	15.6	13.5	16.3	18.3	20.7
Not Hispanic or Latino							
White	12.0	14.9	12.5	14.4	19.1	19.1	21.7
Black or African American	10.3	9.2	11.7	10.6	16.7	15.4	13.3
Hispanic or Latino	12.9	12.2	13.6	17.1	15.7	17.9	18.0
Female							
Total	21.3	23.6	24.9	27.1	30.4	29.6	37.2
9th grade	22.2	26.2	24.4	28.9	34.4	30.9	40.3
10th grade	23.8	24.1	30.1	30.0	32.8	31.6	39.7
11th grade	20.0	23.6	23.0	26.2	31.1	28.9	38.4
12th grade	18.0	18.9	21.2	23.6	23.9	27.3	30.7
Not Hispanic or Latino							
White	21.2	24.2	23.2	26.1	31.6	29.7	38.6
Black or African American	14.7	17.2	18.8	22.0	22.2	24.5	29.4
Hispanic or Latino	23.4	26.5	26.1	30.3	34.1	34.1	34.6
PERCENT OF STUDENTS WHO ATTEMPTED SUICIDE [1]							
Total	8.5	8.8	8.3	7.7	8.7	8.6	7.3
Male							
Total	5.4	6.2	5.7	4.5	5.6	5.0	3.9
9th grade	5.8	8.2	6.1	6.3	6.8	5.8	4.5
10th grade	5.5	6.7	6.2	3.8	5.4	5.9	3.3
11th grade	4.6	4.9	4.8	4.4	5.8	3.4	4.1
12th grade	5.2	4.4	5.4	3.7	4.7	4.5	3.8
Not Hispanic or Latino							
White	3.7	5.3	4.5	3.2	5.2	4.4	3.3
Black or African American	7.7	7.5	7.1	5.6	7.0	5.4	3.3
Hispanic or Latino	6.1	8.0	6.6	7.2	5.8	7.4	3.7
Female							
Total	11.5	11.2	10.9	11.6	11.9	12.5	10.7
9th grade	14.7	13.2	14.0	15.1	14.9	14.4	13.8
10th grade	12.7	12.2	14.8	14.3	15.1	13.1	12.2
11th grade	10.0	11.5	7.5	11.3	11.4	13.6	8.7
12th grade	6.9	6.5	5.8	6.2	6.6	9.1	7.8
Not Hispanic or Latino							
White	10.3	10.3	9.0	10.3	10.4	11.3	10.4
Black or African American	9.0	9.8	7.5	9.0	10.8	11.2	9.4
Hispanic or Latino	15.0	15.9	18.9	14.9	21.0	19.7	11.6
PERCENT OF STUDENTS WITH AN INJURIOUS SUICIDE ATTEMPT [1,2]							
Total	2.9	2.6	2.6	2.6	2.8	2.7	1.7
Male							
Total	2.4	2.1	2.1	2.0	2.2	1.6	1.0
9th grade	3.1	2.6	2.6	3.2	2.3	2.1	1.0
10th grade	2.1	2.5	1.8	1.4	2.4	1.3	0.5
11th grade	2.0	1.6	2.1	2.6	2.0	1.1	1.5
12th grade	1.8	1.5	1.7	1.0	2.2	1.5	0.9
Not Hispanic or Latino							
White	1.1	1.7	1.6	1.5	2.1	1.4	1.0
Black or African American	5.2	3.6	3.4	1.8	2.8	2.0	0.4
Hispanic or Latino	4.2	2.5	1.4	2.1	2.9	2.0	0.5
Female							
Total	3.2	3.1	3.1	3.3	3.4	3.8	2.5
9th grade	3.9	3.8	3.8	5.0	6.3	3.5	2.8
10th grade	3.2	3.6	4.0	3.7	3.8	5.1	2.6
11th grade	2.9	2.8	2.8	2.8	2.9	3.9	2.1
12th grade	2.2	1.7	1.3	2.0	1.3	2.9	2.4
Not Hispanic or Latino							
White	2.4	2.9	2.3	2.6	2.9	3.6	2.3
Black or African American	2.2	3.1	2.4	3.0	3.6	4.0	2.9
Hispanic or Latino	5.7	4.2	4.6	3.8	6.6	5.5	2.7

Note: Only youth attending school participated in the survey.

[1] Response is for the 12 months preceding the survey.
[2] A suicide attempt that required medical attention.

Table III-15. Hypertension (Elevated Blood Pressure) Among Persons 20 Years of Age and Over, According to Sex, Age, Race, Hispanic Origin, and Poverty Status, 1988–1994 and 1999–2002

(Percent.)

Sex, age, race, Hispanic origin, and poverty status	Elevated blood pressure or taking antihypertensive medication [1,2]		Elevated blood pressure [1]	
	1999–2002	1988–1994	1999–2002	1988–1994
20–74 Years, Age-Adjusted [3]				
Both sexes [4,5]	25.6	21.7	16.4	15.4
Male	25.2	23.4	16.3	18.2
Female	25.7	20.0	16.1	12.6
Not Hispanic or Latino				
White only, male	24.0	22.6	14.8	17.3
White only, female [4]	23.3	18.4	14.1	11.2
Black or African American only, male	36.9	34.3	25.6	27.9
Black or African American only, female [4]	39.5	35.0	25.7	23.5
Mexican male [6]	22.6	23.4	18.2	19.1
Mexican female [4,6]	23.4	21.0	17.2	16.5
Poverty Status [7]				
Poor	29.0	27.5	19.3	19.0
Near poor	29.3	22.6	19.5	15.8
Nonpoor	24.1	20.4	14.9	14.6
20 Years and Over, Age-Adjusted [3]				
Both sexes [4,5]	30.0	25.5	19.9	18.5
Male	28.8	26.4	19.1	20.6
Female [4]	30.6	24.4	20.2	16.4
Not Hispanic or Latino				
White only, male	27.6	25.6	17.6	19.7
White only, female [4]	28.5	23.0	18.5	15.1
Black or African American only, male	40.6	37.5	28.2	30.3
Black or African American only, female [4]	43.5	38.3	28.9	26.4
Mexican male [4]	26.8	26.9	21.5	22.2
Mexican female [4,6]	27.9	25.0	21.2	20.4
Poverty Status [7]				
Poor	33.9	31.7	23.3	22.5
Near poor	33.5	26.6	23.0	19.3
Nonpoor	28.2	23.9	18.2	17.5
20 Years and Over, Crude				
Both sexes [4,5]	30.2	24.1	19.9	17.6
Male	27.6	23.8	18.2	18.7
Female [4]	32.7	24.4	21.6	16.5
Not Hispanic or Latino				
White only, male	28.3	24.3	17.8	18.7
White only, female	32.9	24.6	21.6	16.4
Black or African American only, male	35.9	31.1	25.2	25.5
Black or African American only, female [4]	42.1	32.5	27.3	22.2
Mexican male [4]	16.5	16.4	14.1	13.9
Mexican female [4,6]	18.8	15.9	13.8	12.7
Poverty Status [7]				
Poor	30.3	25.7	21.1	18.7
Near poor	34.8	26.7	24.1	19.8
Nonpoor	28.2	22.2	17.8	16.2
Male				
20–34 years	*8.1	7.1	*7.3	6.6
35–44 years	17.1	17.1	12.1	15.2
45–54 years	31.0	29.2	20.4	21.9
55–64 years	45.0	40.6	24.8	28.4
65–74 years	59.6	54.4	34.9	39.9
75 years and over	69.0	60.4	50.6	49.7
Female [4]				
20–34 years	*2.7	2.9	*1.4	*2.4
35–44 years	15.1	11.2	8.5	6.4
45–54 years	31.8	23.9	19.1	13.7
55–64 years	53.9	42.6	31.9	27.0
65–74 years	72.7	56.2	53.0	38.2
75 years and over	83.1	73.6	64.4	59.9

[1] Elevated blood pressure is defined as having systolic pressure of at least 140 mmHg or diastolic pressure of at least 90 mmHg. Those with elevated blood pressure may be taking prescribed medicine for high blood pressure.

[2] Respondents were asked, "Are you now taking prescribed medicine for your high blood pressure?"

[3] Age adjusted to the 2000 standard population using five age groups. Age-adjusted estimates may differ from other age-adjusted estimates based on the same data and presented elsewhere if different age groups are used in the adjustment procedure.

[4] Excludes pregnant women.

[5] Includes persons of all races and Hispanic origins, not just those shown separately.

[6] Persons of Mexican origin may be of any race.

[7] Poor persons are defined as having a total income below the poverty threshold. Near poor persons have incomes of 100 percent to less than 200 percent of the poverty threshold. Nonpoor persons have incomes of 200 percent or more than the poverty threshold. Persons with unknown poverty status are excluded.

* = Figure does not meet standards of reliability or precision.

TABLE III-16. SERUM CHOLESTEROL LEVELS AMONG PERSONS 20 YEARS OF AGE AND OVER, ACCORDING TO SEX, AGE, RACE, AND HISPANIC ORIGIN, SELECTED YEARS, 1960–2002

In 1999–2002, based on age-adjusted figures, 17.0 percent of persons from age 20 to 74 years had high cholesterol levels. High cholesterol is defined as equal or above 240mg/dL (or 6.20mmol/L). The data represented a steady reduction in this rate since 1960–1962, when high cholesterol was found in 33.3 percent of this age group. Black men and Mexican women appeared to have lower age-adjusted prevalences of high cholesterol during the 1999–2002 period.

The mean serum cholesterol level for the population age 20 to 74 years was 203mg/dL. The highest level for males occurred between 45 and 54 years of age, and the highest level for females occurred between 65 and 74 years of age.

Table III-16. Serum Cholesterol Levels Among Persons 20 Years of Age and Over, According to Sex, Age, Race, and Hispanic Origin, Selected Years, 1960–2002

(Percent, level.)

Sex, age, race, and Hispanic origin	1999–2002	Standard error	1988–1994	Standard error	1976–1980 [1]	1971–1974	1960–1962
PERCENT OF POPULATION WITH HIGH SERUM CHOLESTEROL [2]							
20–74 Years, Age-Adjusted [3]							
Both sexes [4]	17.0	0.7	19.7	0.6	27.8	28.6	33.3
Male	16.9	0.9	18.8	0.8	26.4	27.9	30.6
Female	17.0	0.8	20.5	0.8	28.8	29.1	35.6
Not Hispanic or Latino							
White only, male	17.0	1.0	18.7	0.9	26.4	. . .	. . .
White only, female	17.4	1.0	20.7	1.0	29.6	. . .	. . .
Black or African American only, male	12.5	1.9	16.4	1.0	25.5	. . .	. . .
Black or African American only, female	16.6	1.2	19.9	0.8	26.3	. . .	. . .
Mexican male [5]	17.6	1.2	18.7	1.5	20.3	. . .	. . .
Mexican female [5]	12.7	1.0	17.7	1.2	20.5	. . .	. . .
20 Years and Over, Age-Adjusted [3]							
Both sexes [4]	17.3	0.7	20.8	0.6	. . .	. . .	. . .
Male	16.4	0.9	19.0	0.7	. . .	. . .	. . .
Female	17.8	0.7	22.0	0.8	. . .	. . .	. . .
Not Hispanic or Latino							
White only, male	16.5	0.9	18.8	0.8	. . .	. . .	. . .
White only, female	18.1	1.0	22.2	1.0	. . .	. . .	. . .
Black or African American only, male	12.4	1.9	16.9	0.9	. . .	. . .	. . .
Black or African American only, female	17.7	1.2	21.4	0.9	. . .	. . .	. . .
Mexican male [5]	17.4	1.2	18.5	1.6	. . .	. . .	. . .
Mexican female [5]	13.8	1.1	18.7	1.3	. . .	. . .	. . .
20 Years and Over, Crude							
Both sexes [4]	17.3	0.7	19.6	0.6	. . .	. . .	. . .
Male	16.6	0.9	17.7	0.7	. . .	. . .	. . .
Female	18.0	0.8	21.3	0.9	. . .	. . .	. . .
Not Hispanic or Latino							
White only, male	16.9	1.0	18.0	0.8	. . .	. . .	. . .
White only, female	19.1	1.1	22.5	1.1	. . .	. . .	. . .
Black or African American only, male	12.2	1.9	14.7	1.0	. . .	. . .	. . .
Black or African American only, female	16.1	1.3	18.2	0.9	. . .	. . .	. . .
Mexican male [5]	15.0	1.2	15.4	1.3	. . .	. . .	. . .
Mexican female [5]	10.7	1.0	14.3	1.1	. . .	. . .	. . .
Male							
20–34 years	9.8	1.1	8.2	0.9	11.9	12.4	15.1
35–44 years	19.8	1.9	19.4	1.6	27.9	31.8	33.9
45–54 years	23.6	2.2	26.6	2.3	36.9	37.5	39.2
55–64 years	19.9	1.9	28.0	2.1	36.8	36.2	41.6
65–74 years	13.7	1.8	21.9	2.2	31.7	34.7	38.0
75 years and over	10.2	1.3	20.4	1.8	. . .	. . .	. . .
Female							
20–34 years	8.9	0.9	7.3	1.0	9.8	10.9	12.4
35–44 years	12.4	1.5	12.3	1.3	20.7	19.3	23.1
45–54 years	21.4	2.1	26.7	2.1	40.5	38.7	46.9
55–64 years	25.6	1.5	40.9	1.9	52.9	53.1	70.1
65–74 years	32.3	2.3	41.3	2.4	51.6	57.7	68.5
75 years and over	26.5	1.8	38.2	2.2	. . .	. . .	. . .

[1] Data for Mexicans are for 1982–1984.
[2] High serum cholesterol is defined as greater than or equal to 240mg/dL (6.20 mmol/L).
[3] Age adjusted to the 2000 standard population using five age groups. Age-adjusted estimates may differ from other age-adjusted estimates based on the same data and presented elsewhere if different age groups are used in the adjustment procedure.
[4] Includes persons of all races and Hispanic origins, not just those shown separately.
[5] Persons of Mexican origin may be of any race.
. . . = Not available.

Table III-16. Serum Cholesterol Levels Among Persons 20 Years of Age and Over, According to Sex, Age, Race, and Hispanic Origin, Selected Years, 1960–2002—*Continued*

(Percent, level.)

Sex, age, race, and Hispanic origin	1999–2002	Standard error	1988–1994	Standard error	1976–1980 [1]	1971–1974	1960–1962
MEAN SERUM CHOLESTEROL LEVEL, MG/DL							
20–74 Years, Age-Adjusted [3]							
Both sexes [4]	203	0.9	205	0.8	215	216	222
Male	203	1.3	204	0.9	213	216	220
Female	202	0.8	205	0.8	216	217	224
Not Hispanic or Latino							
White only, male	202	1.5	204	1.0	213	. . .	. . .
White only, female	204	0.9	206	1.1	216	. . .	. . .
Black or African American only, male	195	2.2	201	1.3	211	. . .	. . .
Black or African American only, female	200	1.6	204	0.6	216	. . .	. . .
Mexican male [5]	205	1.7	206	1.6	209	. . .	. . .
Mexican female [5]	198	1.4	204	1.3	209	. . .	. . .
20 Years and Over, Age-Adjusted [3]							
Both sexes [4]	203	0.8	206	0.7	. . .	. . .	. . .
Male	202	1.3	204	0.9	. . .	. . .	. . .
Female	204	0.7	207	0.8	. . .	. . .	. . .
Not Hispanic or Latino							
White only, male	202	1.5	205	1.0	. . .	. . .	. . .
White only, female	205	0.8	208	1.1	. . .	. . .	. . .
Black or African American only, male	195	2.0	202	1.3	. . .	. . .	. . .
Black or African American only, female	202	1.7	207	0.7	. . .	. . .	. . .
Mexican male [5]	204	1.7	206	1.5	. . .	. . .	. . .
Mexican female [5]	199	1.4	206	1.3	. . .	. . .	. . .
20 Years and Over, Crude							
Both sexes [4]	203	0.9	204	0.8	. . .	. . .	. . .
Male	202	1.2	202	0.9	. . .	. . .	. . .
Female	204	0.9	206	0.9	. . .	. . .	. . .
Not Hispanic or Latino							
White only, male	203	1.5	203	1.0	. . .	. . .	. . .
White only, female	206	1.1	208	1.3	. . .	. . .	. . .
Black or African American only, male	194	2.1	198	1.3	. . .	. . .	. . .
Black or African American only, female	199	1.8	201	0.7	. . .	. . .	. . .
Mexican male [5]	200	2.0	199	1.6	. . .	. . .	. . .
Mexican female [5]	194	1.5	198	1.5	. . .	. . .	. . .
Male							
20–34 years	188	1.6	186	1.2	192	194	198
35–44 years	207	2.4	206	1.6	217	221	227
45–54 years	215	3.0	216	1.8	227	229	231
55–64 years	212	2.4	216	2.2	229	229	233
65–74 years	202	1.7	212	1.9	221	226	230
75 years and over	195	2.8	205	1.9	. . .	. . .	. . .
Female							
20–34 years	185	1.1	184	1.3	189	191	194
35–44 years	198	1.6	195	1.4	207	207	214
45–54 years	211	1.5	217	2.3	232	232	237
55–64 years	221	1.6	235	1.6	249	245	262
65–74 years	224	2.0	233	1.9	246	250	266
75 years and over	217	1.7	229	2.0	. . .	. . .	. . .

[1] Data for Mexicans are for 1982–1984.

[3] Age adjusted to the 2000 standard population using five age groups. Age-adjusted estimates may differ from other age-adjusted estimates based on the same data and presented elsewhere if different age groups are used in the adjustment procedure.

[4] Includes persons of all races and Hispanic origins, not just those shown separately.

[5] Persons of Mexican origin may be of any race.

. . . = Not available.

TABLE III-17. MEAN ENERGY AND MACRONUTRIENT INTAKE AMONG PERSONS 20–74 YEARS OF AGE, ACCORDING TO SEX AND AGE, SELECTED YEARS, 1971–2000

During the 24 hours prior to the interview, males consumed an average of 2,618 kilocalories. They obtained 49 percent of this energy from carbohydrates and 33 percent from fat (of which 11 percent was saturated fat). In contrast, women only consumed 1,877 kilocalories. Women age 60 years and over had a particularly small energy intake of 1,596 kilocalories. Women ate a somewhat larger proportion of carbohydrates than men.

TABLE III-18. LEISURE-TIME PHYSICAL ACTIVITY AMONG ADULTS 18 YEARS OF AGE AND OVER, ACCORDING TO SELECTED CHARACTERISTICS, SELECTED YEARS, 1998–2003

Persons with "regular leisure-time physical activity"— about 33 percent of adults in 2003—were those who exercised vigorously for at least 20 minutes three times a week or those who undertook longer and more frequent moderate activity. The largest percentages occurred among men under 45 years of age. Persons with "some leisure-time physical activity" reported at least one session of physical activity of 10 minutes or more. Thirty percent of adults fell into this category, with representation equally divided among men and women. Almost 38 percent were classified as "inactive." This group had no exercise session lasting 10 minutes or more. Older persons had particularly large percentages of inactivity. Hispanics and non-Hispanic Blacks had more inactive participants than non-Hispanic Whites. However, some of those classified as inactive may be physically active on the job. In addition, physical activity was positively associated with increased levels of educational attainment.

Table III-17. Mean Energy and Macronutrient Intake Among Persons 20–74 Years of Age, According to Sex and Age, Selected Years, 1971–2000

(Number, percent.)

Characteristic	1999–2000	1988–1994	1976–1980	1971–1974
Energy Intake in Kcals				
Male, age-adjusted [1]	2 618	2 666	2 439	2 450
20–39 years	2 828	2 965	2 753	2 784
40–59 years	2 590	2 568	2 315	2 303
60–74 years	2 123	2 105	1 906	1 918
Female, age-adjusted [1]	1 877	1 798	1 522	1 542
20–39 years	2 028	1 958	1 643	1 652
40–59 years	1 828	1 736	1 473	1 510
60–74 years	1 596	1 522	1 322	1 325
Percent Kcals from Carbohydrate				
Male, age-adjusted [1]	49.0	48.2	42.6	42.4
20–39 years	50.0	48.1	43.1	42.2
40–59 years	47.5	47.8	41.5	41.6
60–74 years	49.7	49.7	44.1	44.8
Female, age-adjusted [1]	51.6	50.6	46.0	45.4
20–39 years	52.6	50.6	46.0	45.8
40–59 years	50.9	50.0	45.0	44.4
60–74 years	51.1	52.5	48.6	46.8
Percent Kcals from Total Fat				
Male, age-adjusted [1]	32.8	33.9	36.8	36.9
20–39 years	32.1	34.0	36.2	37.0
40–59 years	33.4	34.2	37.3	36.9
60–74 years	33.0	32.9	36.9	36.4
Female, age-adjusted [1]	32.8	33.4	36.0	36.1
20–39 years	32.3	33.6	36.0	36.3
40–59 years	33.1	34.0	36.5	36.3
60–74 years	33.3	31.6	34.7	34.9
Percent Kcals from Saturated Fat				
Male, age-adjusted [1]	10.9	11.3	13.2	13.5
20–39 years	10.8	11.5	13.1	13.6
40–59 years	11.1	11.3	13.5	13.5
60–74 years	10.7	10.9	13.1	13.3
Female, age-adjusted [1]	11.0	11.2	12.5	13.0
20–39 years	10.9	11.4	12.6	13.0
40–59 years	11.1	11.3	12.7	13.1
60–74 years	10.9	10.4	11.8	12.4

Note: Estimates of energy intake include kilocalories (kcals) from all foods and beverages, including alcoholic beverages, consumed during the preceding 24 hours.

[1] Age adjusted to the 2000 standard population using three age groups, 20–39 years, 40–59 years, and 60–74 years.

Table III-18. Leisure-Time Physical Activity Among Adults 18 Years of Age and Over, According to Selected Characteristics, Selected Years, 1998–2003

(Percent.)

Characteristic	Inactive [1]			Some leisure-time activity [1]			Regular leisure-time activity [1]		
	2003	2002	1998	2003	2002	1998	2003	2002	1998
Total, age-adjusted [2,3]	37.6	38.2	40.5	29.5	30.1	30.0	32.8	31.7	29.5
Total, crude [3]	37.6	38.1	40.2	29.6	30.1	30.0	32.8	31.7	29.8
Age									
18–44 years	32.9	33.1	35.2	30.3	31.0	31.4	36.8	35.9	33.5
18–24 years	29.6	32.9	32.8	28.2	28.3	30.1	42.3	38.8	37.1
25–44 years	34.0	33.2	35.9	31.0	31.9	31.8	34.9	34.9	32.4
45–64 years	38.2	38.4	41.2	30.5	31.5	30.6	31.3	30.1	28.2
45–54 years	36.5	37.5	38.9	30.8	31.2	31.4	32.8	31.3	29.8
55–64 years	40.8	39.7	44.9	30.1	32.0	29.3	29.2	28.3	25.8
65 years and over	51.4	53.6	55.4	25.3	24.8	24.7	23.3	21.6	19.9
65–74 years	45.8	46.9	49.1	25.8	27.1	26.5	28.4	26.0	24.4
75 years and over	57.5	61.3	63.3	24.8	22.2	22.4	17.7	16.6	14.3
Sex [2]									
Male	35.4	36.1	37.8	29.2	28.8	28.7	35.4	35.1	33.5
Female	39.5	40.1	42.9	29.9	31.3	31.1	30.6	28.7	26.0
Sex and Age									
Male									
18–44 years	30.9	30.6	32.0	29.5	29.7	30.7	39.6	39.7	37.2
45–54 years	36.4	37.5	37.7	30.5	29.8	29.6	33.2	32.8	32.6
55–64 years	39.5	39.1	44.5	29.7	30.9	26.9	30.8	30.0	28.6
65–74 years	43.0	44.3	45.3	24.9	26.1	23.6	32.1	29.6	31.1
75 years and over	48.1	55.6	57.4	28.9	21.0	21.6	23.0	23.5	20.9
Female									
18–44 years	34.9	35.6	38.2	31.1	32.3	32.0	34.0	32.1	29.8
45–54 years	36.5	37.5	39.9	31.1	32.6	33.0	32.4	29.9	27.1
55–64 years	41.9	40.2	45.2	30.4	33.0	31.5	27.6	26.8	23.3
65–74 years	48.0	49.0	52.2	26.6	27.9	28.7	25.4	23.1	19.0
75 years and over	63.7	64.8	67.0	22.0	22.9	22.9	14.3	12.3	10.1
Race [2,4]									
White only	36.3	36.5	38.8	29.8	30.4	30.5	33.9	33.1	30.7
Black or African American only	48.5	48.5	52.2	26.1	27.1	25.2	25.5	24.4	22.6
American Indian and Alaska Native only	54.7	45.4	49.2	20.0	28.9	19.0	25.2	25.7	31.8
Asian only	35.9	39.0	39.4	31.1	33.1	35.2	33.1	27.9	25.4
Native Hawaiian and Other Pacific Islander only	*	*	. . .	*	*	. . .	*	*	. . .
Two or more races	33.3	30.6	. . .	34.1	32.5	. . .	32.6	36.9	. . .
Hispanic Origin and Race [2,4]									
Hispanic or Latino	51.9	53.9	55.5	23.6	23.5	23.4	24.4	22.7	21.1
Mexican	52.0	54.9	56.7	23.7	23.1	23.9	24.3	22.0	19.4
Not Hispanic or Latino	35.5	36.0	38.8	30.3	30.9	30.7	34.2	33.1	30.5
White only	33.4	33.9	36.7	30.9	31.5	31.3	35.8	34.6	32.0
Black or African American only	48.5	48.6	52.2	26.0	26.9	25.1	25.5	24.6	22.6
Education [5,6]									
25 years and over									
No high school diploma or GED	61.2	63.2	64.8	20.6	19.5	19.4	18.1	17.2	15.8
High school diploma or GED	45.5	45.4	47.6	27.5	28.5	28.7	27.0	26.2	23.7
Some college or more	28.1	28.1	30.2	33.8	34.7	34.3	38.2	37.1	35.5
Poverty Status [7]									
Poor	55.1	56.5	59.4	22.0	22.5	20.5	22.9	21.0	20.1
Near poor	50.5	50.5	52.2	24.8	25.8	26.2	24.7	23.7	21.6
Nonpoor	31.4	32.3	34.7	32.0	32.3	32.4	36.7	35.4	33.0

[1]Respondents were asked about the frequency and duration of vigorous and light/moderate physical activity during leisure time. Adults classified as inactive reported no sessions of light/moderate or vigorous leisure-time activity of at least 10 minutes duration; adults classified with some leisure-time activity reported at least one session of light/moderate or vigorous physical activity of at least 10 minutes duration but did not meet the definition for regular leisure-time activity; adults classified with regular leisure-time activity reported three or more sessions per week of vigorous activity lasting at least 20 minutes or five or more sessions per week of light/moderate activity lasting at least 30 minutes in duration.

[2]Estimates are age adjusted to the year 2000 standard population using five age groups: 18–44 years, 45–54 years, 55–64 years, 65–74 years, and 75 years and over. Age-adjusted estimates in this table may differ from other age-adjusted estimates based on the same data and presented elsewhere if different age groups are used in the adjustment procedure.

[3]Includes all other races not shown separately.

[4]The race groups, White, Black, American Indian and Alaska Native, Asian, Native Hawaiian and Other Pacific Islander, and two or more races, include persons of Hispanic and non-Hispanic origin. Persons of Hispanic origin may be of any race.

[5]Estimates are for persons 25 years of age and over and are age adjusted to the year 2000 standard population using five age groups: 25–44 years, 45–54 years, 55–64 years, 65–74 years, and 75 years and over.

[6]GED stands for General Educational Development high school equivalency diploma.

[7]Poor persons are defined as having a total income below the poverty threshold. Near poor persons have incomes of 100 percent to less than 200 percent of the poverty threshold. Nonpoor persons have incomes of 200 percent or more than the poverty threshold.

* = Figure does not meet standards of reliability or precision.

. . . = Not available.

Table III-18. Leisure-Time Physical Activity Among Adults 18 Years of Age and Over, According to Selected Characteristics, Selected Years, 1998–2003—Continued

(Percent.)

Characteristic	Inactive [1]			Some leisure-time activity [1]			Regular leisure-time activity [1]		
	2003	2002	1998	2003	2002	1998	2003	2002	1998
Hispanic Origin and Race and Poverty Status [2, 4, 7]									
Hispanic or Latino									
Poor	64.2	65.5	68.6	19.1	19.0	18.0	16.7	15.5	13.4
Near poor	58.8	61.0	60.8	21.0	20.5	21.2	20.3	18.5	18.0
Nonpoor	41.8	45.5	45.6	27.3	26.3	27.6	30.9	28.1	26.8
Not Hispanic or Latino									
White only									
Poor	49.3	49.8	53.7	22.6	25.1	22.5	28.0	25.1	23.8
Near poor	45.7	46.4	49.0	27.4	27.5	27.6	27.0	26.1	23.4
Nonpoor	29.2	29.8	32.7	32.4	32.9	32.9	38.3	37.3	34.4
Black or African American only									
Poor	61.3	64.6	64.3	20.9	18.5	17.4	17.8	16.8	18.3
Near poor	55.3	52.8	55.6	22.9	25.4	24.4	21.8	21.8	19.9
Nonpoor	40.7	40.6	46.0	29.1	30.8	28.7	30.2	28.6	25.3
Geographic Region [2]									
Northeast	34.4	35.0	39.4	29.2	31.5	31.3	36.4	33.5	29.4
Midwest	34.7	35.5	37.3	32.2	32.7	31.7	33.1	31.8	31.0
South	42.6	42.5	46.9	27.7	28.2	27.1	29.7	29.2	26.0
West	34.9	36.5	33.9	29.9	29.0	31.6	35.2	34.5	34.6
Location of Residence [2]									
Within MSA [8]	36.4	36.9	39.3	29.9	30.7	30.6	33.7	32.4	30.0
Outside MSA [8]	42.4	43.5	44.7	28.1	27.7	27.5	29.5	28.9	27.8

[1]Respondents were asked about the frequency and duration of vigorous and light/moderate physical activity during leisure time. Adults classified as inactive reported no sessions of light/moderate or vigorous leisure-time activity of at least 10 minutes duration; adults classified with some leisure-time activity reported at least one session of light/moderate or vigorous physical activity of at least 10 minutes duration but did not meet the definition for regular leisure-time activity; adults classified with regular leisure-time activity reported three or more sessions per week of vigorous activity lasting at least 20 minutes or five or more sessions per week of light/moderate activity lasting at least 30 minutes in duration.

[2]Estimates are age adjusted to the year 2000 standard population using five age groups: 18–44 years, 45–54 years, 55–64 years, 65–74 years, and 75 years and over. Age-adjusted estimates in this table may differ from other age-adjusted estimates based on the same data and presented elsewhere if different age groups are used in the adjustment procedure.

[4]The race groups, White, Black, American Indian and Alaska Native, Asian, Native Hawaiian and Other Pacific Islander, and two or more races, include persons of Hispanic and non-Hispanic origin. Persons of Hispanic origin may be of any race.

[7]Poor persons are defined as having a total income below the poverty threshold. Near poor persons have incomes of 100 percent to less than 200 percent of the poverty threshold. Nonpoor persons have incomes of 200 percent or more than the poverty threshold.

[8]MSA = Metropolitan Statistical Area.

TABLE III-19. OVERWEIGHT, OBESITY, AND HEALTHY WEIGHT AMONG PERSONS 20 YEARS OF AGE AND OVER, ACCORDING TO SEX, AGE, RACE, AND HISPANIC ORIGIN, SELECTED YEARS, 1960–2002

Adults are shown in three partly overlapping categories: healthy weight with a body mass index (BMI) over 18.5, but less than 25; overweight with BMI of 25 or above; and obese with BMI of 30 or above. BMI is a measure that adjusts body weight for height; weight in kilograms is divided by height in meters squared.

From 1999–2002, 65 percent of the population age 20 to 74 years was classified as overweight. Almost half of these, 31 percent, were reported to be obese (age-adjusted). The percentage of obese persons doubled in size between the 1976–1980 period and the 1999–2002 period. Especially high obesity rates were reported for non-Hispanic Black women (excluding pregnant women) and, to a lesser extent, for Mexican women. (The table does not provide global figures for Hispanics.)

For the population age 20 to 74 years, 33 percent were of healthy weight in 1999–2002, down from 51 percent in 1960–1962 (age-adjusted). Non-Hispanic White females and non-Hispanic Black males had higher than average percentages with healthy weight, while only 21 percent of non-Hispanic Black females reportedly had healthy weights. By age, the largest participation in the healthy weight group occurred between age 20 and 34 years, and the smallest was reported between age 65 and 74 years.

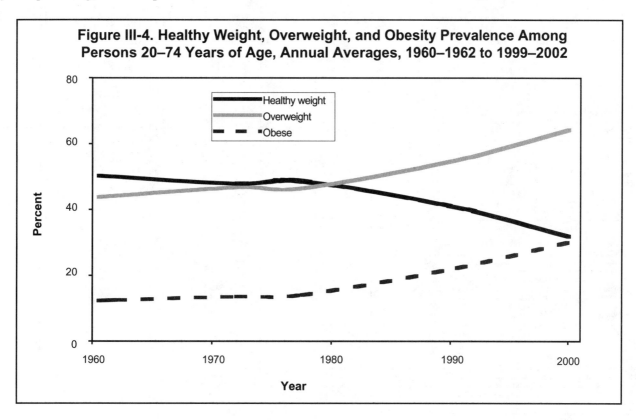

Figure III-4. Healthy Weight, Overweight, and Obesity Prevalence Among Persons 20–74 Years of Age, Annual Averages, 1960–1962 to 1999–2002

Table III-19. Overweight, Obesity, and Healthy Weight Among Persons 20 Years of Age and Over, According to Sex, Age, Race, and Hispanic Origin, Selected Years, 1960–2002

(Percent.)

Sex, age, race, and Hispanic origin	1999–2002	Standard error	1988–1994	Standard error	1976–1980 [1]	1971–1974	1960–1962
PERCENT OF POPULATION OVERWEIGHT [2]							
20–74 Years, Age-Adjusted [3]							
Both sexes [4,5]	65.2	0.8	56.0	0.9	47.4	47.7	44.8
Male	68.8	1.0	61.0	1.0	52.9	54.7	49.5
Female [4]	61.7	1.2	51.2	1.1	42.0	41.1	40.2
Not Hispanic or Latino							
White only, male	69.5	1.3	61.6	1.2	53.8	. . .	. . .
White only, female [4]	57.0	1.7	47.2	1.4	38.7	. . .	. . .
Black or African American only, male	62.0	1.8	58.2	1.2	51.3	. . .	. . .
Black or African American only, female [4]	77.5	1.4	68.5	1.4	62.6	. . .	. . .
Mexican male [6]	74.1	1.7	69.4	1.1	61.6	. . .	. . .
Mexican female [4,6]	71.4	2.0	69.6	1.7	61.7	. . .	. . .
Poverty Status [7]							
Poor	65.2	1.7	59.8	1.8	50.0	49.3	. . .
Near poor	68.0	1.7	58.2	1.5	49.0	50.9	. . .
Nonpoor	64.9	1.0	54.5	1.1	46.6	46.7	. . .
20 Years and Over, Age-Adjusted [3]							
Both sexes [4,5]	65.1	0.8	56.0	0.8	. . .	. . .	. . .
Male	68.8	0.9	60.9	1.0	. . .	. . .	. . .
Female [4]	61.6	1.2	51.4	1.0	. . .	. . .	. . .
Not Hispanic or Latino							
White only, male	69.4	1.2	61.6	1.2	. . .	. . .	. . .
White only, female [4]	57.2	1.7	47.5	1.3	. . .	. . .	. . .
Black or African American only, male	62.6	1.7	57.8	1.2	. . .	. . .	. . .
Black or African American only, female [4]	77.1	1.5	68.2	1.3	. . .	. . .	. . .
Mexican male [6]	73.2	1.8	68.9	1.1	. . .	. . .	. . .
Mexican female [4,6]	71.2	2.0	68.9	1.6	. . .	. . .	. . .
Poverty Status [7]							
Poor	64.6	1.5	59.6	1.7	. . .	. . .	. . .
Near poor	67.3	1.6	58.0	1.4	. . .	. . .	. . .
Nonpoor	65.1	0.9	54.8	1.0	. . .	. . .	. . .
20 Years and Over, Crude							
Both sexes [4,5]	65.2	0.8	54.9	0.8	. . .	. . .	. . .
Male	68.6	0.9	59.4	1.0	. . .	. . .	. . .
Female [4]	62.0	1.2	50.7	1.0	. . .	. . .	. . .
Not Hispanic or Latino							
White only, male	69.9	1.2	60.6	1.2	. . .	. . .	. . .
White only, female [4]	58.2	1.8	47.4	1.2	. . .	. . .	. . .
Black or African American only, male	61.7	1.7	56.7	1.2	. . .	. . .	. . .
Black or African American only, female [4]	76.8	1.5	66.0	1.4	. . .	. . .	. . .
Mexican male [6]	70.1	2.2	63.9	1.5	. . .	. . .	. . .
Mexican female [4,6]	69.3	2.3	65.9	1.4	. . .	. . .	. . .
Poverty Status [7]							
Poor	62.5	1.6	56.8	1.6	. . .	. . .	. . .
Near poor	66.2	1.5	55.7	1.5	. . .	. . .	. . .
Nonpoor	65.8	1.0	54.2	1.0	. . .	. . .	. . .
Male [4]							
20–34 years	57.4	1.5	47.5	1.4	41.2	42.8	42.7
35–44 years	70.5	1.8	65.5	1.7	57.2	63.2	53.5
45–54 years	75.7	2.1	66.1	2.1	60.2	59.7	53.9
55–64 years	75.4	2.2	70.5	2.1	60.2	58.5	52.2
65–74 years	76.2	1.8	68.5	2.1	54.2	54.6	47.8
75 years and over	67.4	2.3	56.5	2.0	. . .	. . .	. . .
Female [4]							
20–34 years	52.8	2.1	37.0	1.4	27.9	25.8	21.2
35–44 years	60.6	2.4	49.6	2.4	40.7	40.5	37.2
45–54 years	65.1	2.2	60.3	2.5	48.7	49.0	49.3
55–64 years	72.2	2.4	66.3	1.6	53.7	54.5	59.9
65–74 years	70.9	3.1	60.3	1.8	59.5	55.9	60.9
75 years and over	59.9	3.3	52.3	1.5	. . .	. . .	. . .

Note: Percents do not sum to 100 because the percent of persons with BMI less than 18.5 is not shown, and the percent of persons with obesity is a subset of the percent that is overweight.

[1] Data for Mexicans are for 1982–1984.
[2] Body mass index (BMI) greater than or equal to 25 kilograms/meter squared.
[3] Age adjusted to the 2000 standard population using five age groups. Age-adjusted estimates may differ from other age-adjusted estimates based on the same data and presented elsewhere if different age groups are used in the adjustment procedure.
[4] Excludes pregnant women.
[5] Includes persons of all races and Hispanic origins, not just those shown separately.
[6] Persons of Mexican origin may be of any race.
[7] Poor persons are defined as having a total income below the poverty threshold. Near poor persons have incomes of 100 percent to less than 200 percent of the poverty threshold. Nonpoor persons have incomes of 200 percent or greater than the poverty threshold. Persons with unknown poverty status are excluded.
. . . = Not available.

Table III-19. Overweight, Obesity, and Healthy Weight Among Persons 20 Years of Age and Over, According to Sex, Age, Race, and Hispanic Origin, Selected Years, 1960–2002—*Continued*

(Percent.)

Sex, age, race, and Hispanic origin	1999–2002	Standard error	1988–1994	Standard error	1976–1980 [1]	1971–1974	1960–1962
PERCENT OF POPULATION OBESE [8]							
20–74 Years, Age-Adjusted [3]							
Both sexes [4], [5]	31.1	1.0	23.3	0.7	15.1	14.6	13.3
Male	28.1	0.9	20.6	0.7	12.8	12.2	10.7
Female [4]	34.0	1.2	26.0	1.0	17.1	16.8	15.7
Not Hispanic or Latino							
White only, male	28.7	1.1	20.7	0.9	12.4	. . .	. . .
White only, female [4]	31.3	1.4	23.3	1.2	15.4	. . .	. . .
Black or African American only, male	27.9	1.3	21.3	1.0	16.5	. . .	. . .
Black or African American only, female [4]	49.6	1.8	39.1	1.4	31.0	. . .	. . .
Mexican male [6]	29.0	1.5	24.4	1.1	15.7	. . .	. . .
Mexican female [4], [6]	38.9	2.6	36.1	1.4	26.6	. . .	. . .
Poverty Status [7]							
Poor	36.0	2.1	29.2	1.5	21.9	20.7	. . .
Near poor	35.4	1.8	26.6	1.5	18.7	18.4	. . .
Nonpoor	29.2	1.2	21.4	0.9	12.9	12.4	. . .
20 Years and Over, Age-Adjusted [3]							
Both sexes [4], [5]	30.4	0.9	22.9	0.7	. . .	. . .	. . .
Male	27.5	0.9	20.2	0.7	. . .	. . .	. . .
Female [4]	33.2	1.2	25.5	0.9	. . .	. . .	. . .
Not Hispanic or Latino							
White only, male	28.0	1.0	20.3	0.8	. . .	. . .	. . .
White only, female [4]	30.7	1.3	22.9	1.1	. . .	. . .	. . .
Black or African American only, male	27.8	1.4	20.9	1.0	. . .	. . .	. . .
Black or African American only, female [4]	48.8	2.0	38.3	1.4	. . .	. . .	. . .
Mexican male [6]	27.8	1.5	23.8	1.0	. . .	. . .	. . .
Mexican female [4], [6]	38.0	2.6	35.2	1.4	. . .	. . .	. . .
Poverty Status [7]							
Poor	34.7	2.0	28.1	1.4	. . .	. . .	. . .
Near poor	34.1	1.6	26.1	1.4	. . .	. . .	. . .
Nonpoor	28.7	0.2	21.1	0.8	. . .	. . .	. . .
20 Years and Over, Crude							
Both sexes [4], [5]	30.5	0.9	22.3	0.6	. . .	. . .	. . .
Male	27.5	0.9	19.5	0.7	. . .	. . .	. . .
Female [4]	33.4	1.2	25.0	0.9	. . .	. . .	. . .
Not Hispanic or Latino							
White only, male	28.4	1.0	19.9	0.8	. . .	. . .	. . .
White only, female [4]	31.3	1.3	22.7	1.1	. . .	. . .	. . .
Black or African American only, male	27.5	1.3	20.7	1.0	. . .	. . .	. . .
Black or African American only, female [4]	48.8	2.0	36.7	1.4	. . .	. . .	. . .
Mexican male [6]	26.0	1.8	20.6	1.2	. . .	. . .	. . .
Mexican female [4], [6]	37.0	2.9	33.3	1.3	. . .	. . .	. . .
Poverty Status [7]							
Poor	33.0	1.6	25.9	1.3	. . .	. . .	. . .
Near poor	32.8	1.5	24.3	1.3	. . .	. . .	. . .
Nonpoor	29.3	1.2	20.9	0.8	. . .	. . .	. . .
Male							
20–34 years	21.7	1.2	14.1	1.0	8.9	9.7	9.2
35–44 years	28.5	1.8	21.5	1.2	13.5	13.5	12.1
45–54 years	30.6	1.8	23.2	1.7	16.7	13.7	12.5
55–64 years	35.5	2.4	27.2	2.2	14.1	14.1	9.2
65–74 years	31.9	2.3	24.1	1.8	13.2	10.9	10.4
75 years and over	18.0	2.2	13.2	2.1	. . .	. . .	. . .
Female [4]							
20–34 years	28.4	1.8	18.5	1.1	11.0	9.7	7.2
35–44 years	32.1	1.9	25.5	2.1	17.8	17.7	14.7
45–54 years	36.9	2.4	32.4	1.9	19.6	18.9	20.3
55–64 years	42.1	3.0	33.7	1.8	22.9	24.1	24.4
65–74 years	39.3	3.2	26.9	1.5	21.5	22.0	23.2
75 years and over	23.6	2.2	19.2	1.3	. . .	. . .	. . .

Note: Percents do not sum to 100 because the percent of persons with BMI less than 18.5 is not shown, and the percent of persons with obesity is a subset of the percent that is overweight.

[1] Data for Mexicans are for 1982–1984.
[3] Age adjusted to the 2000 standard population using five age groups. Age-adjusted estimates may differ from other age-adjusted estimates based on the same data and presented elsewhere if different age groups are used in the adjustment procedure.
[4] Excludes pregnant women.
[5] Includes persons of all races and Hispanic origins, not just those shown separately.
[6] Persons of Mexican origin may be of any race.
[7] Poor persons are defined as having a total income below the poverty threshold. Near poor persons have incomes of 100 percent to less than 200 percent of the poverty threshold. Nonpoor persons have incomes of 200 percent or greater than the poverty threshold. Persons with unknown poverty status are excluded.
[8] Body mass index (BMI) of 30 or more kilograms/meter squared.
. . . = Not available.

Table III-19. Overweight, Obesity, and Healthy Weight Among Persons 20 Years of Age and Over, According to Sex, Age, Race, and Hispanic Origin, Selected Years, 1960–2002—*Continued*

(Percent.)

Sex, age, race, and Hispanic origin	1999–2002	Standard error	1988–1994	Standard error	1976–1980 [1]	1971–1974	1960–1962
PERCENT OF POPULATION WITH A HEALTHY WEIGHT [9]							
20–74 Years, Age-Adjusted [3]							
Both sexes [4],[5]	32.9	0.8	41.7	0.9	49.6	48.8	51.2
Male	30.2	1.0	37.9	1.0	45.4	43.0	48.3
Female [4]	35.6	1.2	45.3	1.1	53.7	54.3	54.1
Not Hispanic or Latino							
White only, male	29.5	1.3	37.4	1.2	45.3	. . .	. . .
White only, female [4]	39.7	1.7	49.2	1.4	56.7	. . .	. . .
Black or African American only, male	35.5	1.7	40.0	1.2	46.6	. . .	. . .
Black or African American only, female [4]	21.3	1.3	28.9	1.2	35.0	. . .	. . .
Mexican male [6]	25.6	1.7	29.8	1.1	37.1	. . .	. . .
Mexican female [4],[6]	27.5	1.9	29.0	1.7	36.4	. . .	. . .
Poverty Status [7]							
Poor	32.4	1.7	37.3	1.8	45.1	45.8	. . .
Near poor	29.7	1.5	39.2	1.5	47.6	45.1	. . .
Nonpoor	33.5	1.0	43.4	1.1	51.0	50.2	. . .
20 Years and Over, Age-Adjusted [3]							
Both sexes [4],[5]	33.0	0.8	41.6	0.8	. . .	. . .	. . .
Male	30.2	0.9	37.9	1.0	. . .	. . .	. . .
Female [4]	35.7	1.2	45.0	1.0	. . .	. . .	. . .
Not Hispanic or Latino							
White only, male	29.6	1.2	37.3	1.1	. . .	. . .	. . .
White only, female [4]	39.5	1.6	48.7	1.3	. . .	. . .	. . .
Black or African American only, male	34.7	1.8	40.1	1.2	. . .	. . .	. . .
Black or African American only, female [4]	21.7	1.4	29.2	1.2	. . .	. . .	. . .
Mexican male [6]	26.5	1.8	30.2	1.0	. . .	. . .	. . .
Mexican female [4],[6]	27.5	1.9	29.7	1.6	. . .	. . .	. . .
Poverty Status [7]							
Poor	32.7	1.7	37.5	1.6	. . .	. . .	. . .
Near poor	30.5	1.5	39.3	1.4	. . .	. . .	. . .
Nonpoor	33.4	0.9	43.1	1.0	. . .	. . .	. . .
20 Years and Over, Crude							
Both sexes [4],[5]	32.9	0.8	42.6	0.8	. . .	. . .	. . .
Male	30.4	0.9	39.4	1.0	. . .	. . .	. . .
Female [4]	35.4	1.2	45.7	1.0	. . .	. . .	. . .
Not Hispanic or Latino							
White only, male	29.2	1.2	38.2	1.2	. . .	. . .	. . .
White only, female [4]	38.7	1.7	48.8	1.2	. . .	. . .	. . .
Black or African American only, male	35.9	1.8	41.5	1.2	. . .	. . .	. . .
Black or African American only, female [4]	21.9	1.4	31.2	1.3	. . .	. . .	. . .
Mexican male [6]	29.4	2.3	35.2	1.5	. . .	. . .	. . .
Mexican female [4],[6]	29.4	2.2	32.4	1.5	. . .	. . .	. . .
Poverty Status [7]							
Poor	34.5	1.7	39.8	1.5	. . .	. . .	. . .
Near poor	31.5	1.4	41.5	1.5	. . .	. . .	. . .
Nonpoor	32.8	1.0	43.6	1.0	. . .	. . .	. . .
Male							
20–34 years	40.3	1.6	51.1	1.5	57.1	54.7	55.3
35–44 years	29.0	1.8	33.4	1.7	41.3	35.2	45.2
45–54 years	24.0	2.1	33.6	2.0	38.7	38.5	44.8
55–64 years	23.8	2.0	28.6	2.1	38.7	38.3	44.9
65–74 years	22.8	1.8	30.1	2.2	42.3	42.1	46.2
75 years and over	32.0	2.2	40.9	1.9	. . .	. . .	. . .
Female [4]							
20–34 years	42.6	1.9	57.9	1.3	65.0	65.8	67.6
35–44 years	37.1	2.3	47.1	2.5	55.6	56.7	58.4
45–54 years	33.1	2.1	37.2	2.3	48.7	49.3	47.6
55–64 years	27.6	2.4	31.5	1.5	43.5	41.1	38.1
65–74 years	26.4	3.2	37.0	2.0	37.8	40.6	36.4
75 years and over	36.9	3.3	43.0	1.6	. . .	. . .	. . .

Note: Percents do not sum to 100 because the percent of persons with BMI less than 18.5 is not shown, and the percent of persons with obesity is a subset of the percent that is overweight.

[1] Data for Mexicans are for 1982–1984.
[3] Age adjusted to the 2000 standard population using five age groups. Age-adjusted estimates may differ from other age-adjusted estimates based on the same data and presented elsewhere if different age groups are used in the adjustment procedure.
[4] Excludes pregnant women.
[5] Includes persons of all races and Hispanic origins, not just those shown separately.
[6] Persons of Mexican origin may be of any race.
[7] Poor persons are defined as having a total income below the poverty threshold. Near poor persons have incomes of 100 percent to less than 200 percent of the poverty threshold. Nonpoor persons have incomes of 200 percent or greater than the poverty threshold. Persons with unknown poverty status are excluded.
[9] Body mass index (BMI) of 18.5 to less than 25 kilograms/meter squared.
. . . = Not available.

TABLE III–20. OVERWEIGHT CHILDREN AND ADOLES-CENTS 6–19 YEARS OF AGE, ACCORDING TO SEX, AGE, RACE, HISPANIC ORIGIN, AND POVERTY STATUS, SELECTED YEARS, 1963–2002

In this table, "overweight" is defined as having a body mass index (BMI) at or above the sex- and age-specific 95th percentile. BMI cut off-points come from the 2000 CDC Growth Charts (*Vital and Health Statistics* #314,

National Center for Health Statistics, 2000).

In the 6- to 11-year-old age group, 16 percent of children were classified as overweight from 1999–2002; in the 12- to 19 year-old age group, 16 percent also fell into this classification. These proportions represented sizeable increases over the last three and a half decades. Mexican boys and non-Hispanic Black girls were more likely than average to be overweight.

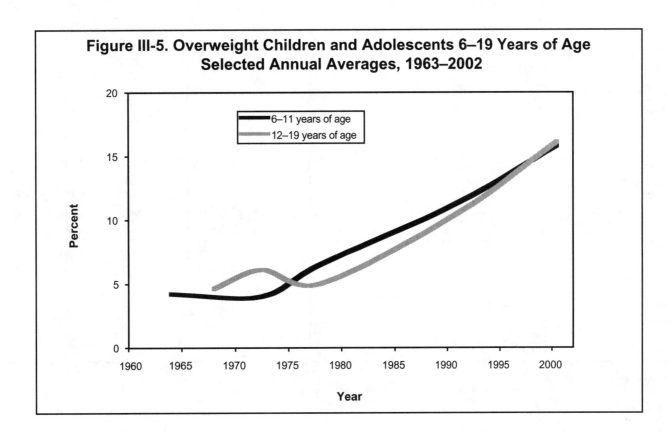

Table III-20. Overweight Children and Adolescents 6–19 Years of Age, According to Sex, Age, Race, Hispanic Origin, and Poverty Status, Selected Years, 1963–2002

(Percent.)

Sex, age, race, and Hispanic origin	1999–2002	1988–1994	1976–1980 [1]	1971–1974	1963–1966 and 1966–1970 [2]
PERCENT OF POPULATION OVERWEIGHT [3]					
6–11 Years of Age					
Both sexes [4]	15.8	11.3	6.5	4.0	4.2
Boys	16.9	11.6	6.6	*4.3	4.0
Not Hispanic or Latino					
White only	14.0	10.7	6.1	...	...
Black or African American only	17.0	12.3	6.8	...	...
Mexican [5]	26.5	17.5	13.3	...	...
Girls [6]	14.7	11.0	6.4	*3.6	4.5
Not Hispanic or Latino					
White only	13.1	*9.8	5.2	...	...
Black or African American only	22.8	17.0	11.2	...	...
Mexican [5]	17.1	15.3	9.8	...	...
Poverty Status [7]					
Poor	19.1	11.4	...	...	...
Near poor	16.4	11.1	...	...	...
Nonpoor	14.3	11.1	...	...	...
12–19 Years of Age					
Both sexes	16.1	10.5	5.0	6.1	4.6
Boys	16.7	11.3	4.8	6.1	4.5
Not Hispanic or Latino					
White only	14.6	11.6	3.8	...	...
Black or African American only	18.7	10.7	6.1	...	...
Mexican [5]	24.7	14.1	7.7	...	...
Girls [6]	15.4	9.7	5.3	6.2	4.7
Not Hispanic or Latino					
White only	12.7	8.9	4.6	...	...
Black or African American only	23.6	16.3	10.7	...	...
Mexican [5]	19.9	*13.4	8.8	...	...
Poverty Status [7]					
Poor	19.9	15.8	...	...	...
Near poor	15.2	11.2	...	...	...
Nonpoor	14.9	7.9	...	...	...

[1] Data for Mexicans are for 1982–1984.

[2] Data for 1963–1965 are for children 6–11 years of age; data for 1966–1970 are for adolescents 12–17 years of age, not 12–19 years.

[3] Overweight is defined as body mass index (BMI) at or above the sex and age-specific 95th percentile BMI cutoff points from the 2000 CDC Growth Charts.

[4] Includes persons of all races and Hispanic origins, not just those shown separately.

[5] Persons of Mexican origin may be of any race.

[6] Excludes pregnant women.

[7] Poverty status is based on family income and family size. Poor persons are defined as having a total income below the poverty threshold. Near poor persons have incomes of 100 percent to less than 200 percent of the poverty threshold. Nonpoor persons have incomes of 200 percent or more than the poverty threshold. Persons with unknown poverty status are excluded.

* = Figure does not meet standards of reliability or precision.

. . . = Not available.

USE OF ADDICTIVE SUBSTANCES

TABLE III-21. CURRENT CIGARETTE SMOKING BY PERSONS 18 YEARS OF AGE AND OVER, ACCORDING TO SEX, RACE, AND AGE, SELECTED YEARS, 1965–2003

One of health care's big successes in recent decades has been the pronounced decline in smoking. In 1965, 41.9 percent of persons 18 years of age and over were current cigarette smokers; by 2003, this percentage had dropped to 21.54 percent. In a large interview survey, persons who smoked 100 cigarettes in their lifetime and who now smoke every day or some days were defined as current smokers. Current smokers included 23.7 percent of all males and 19.4 percent of all females. Only 17.9 percent of Black females were current smokers.

Among the age and sex groups, 25- to 34-year-old males were the most frequent smokers in 2003; for older males, rates remained fairly steady until declining sharply after age 64. Smoking rates for females also reflected these patterns.

Table III-21. Current Cigarette Smoking by Persons [1] 18 Years of Age and Over, According to Sex, Race, and Age, Selected Years, 1965–2003

(Percent of persons who are current cigarette smokers.)

Sex, race, and age	2003	2002	2001	2000	1999	1998	1995[2]	1990[2]	1985[2]	1979[2]	1974[2]	1965[2]
18 Years and Over, Age-Adjusted [3]												
All persons	21.5	22.3	22.6	23.1	23.3	24.0	24.6	25.3	29.9	33.3	37.0	41.9
Male	23.7	24.6	24.6	25.2	25.2	25.9	26.5	28.0	32.2	37.0	42.8	51.2
Female	19.4	20.0	20.7	21.1	21.6	22.1	22.7	22.9	27.9	30.1	32.2	33.7
White male [4]	23.8	24.9	24.8	25.4	25.0	26.0	26.2	27.6	31.3	36.4	41.7	50.4
Black or African American male [4]	25.3	26.6	27.5	25.7	28.4	29.0	29.4	32.8	40.2	43.9	53.6	58.8
White female [4]	20.1	21.0	22.0	22.0	22.5	23.0	23.4	23.5	27.9	30.3	32.0	33.9
Black or African American female [4]	17.9	18.3	18.0	20.7	20.5	21.1	23.5	20.8	30.9	30.5	35.6	31.8
18 Years and Over, Crude												
All persons	21.6	22.4	22.7	23.2	23.5	24.1	24.7	25.5	30.1	33.5	37.1	42.4
Male	24.1	25.1	25.1	25.6	25.7	26.4	27.0	28.4	32.6	37.5	43.1	51.9
Female	19.2	19.8	20.6	20.9	21.5	22.0	22.6	22.8	27.9	29.9	32.1	33.9
White male [4]	24.0	25.0	25.0	25.7	25.3	26.3	26.6	28.0	31.7	36.8	41.9	51.1
Black or African American male [4]	25.7	27.0	27.6	26.2	28.6	29.0	28.5	32.5	39.9	44.1	54.3	60.4
White female [4]	19.7	20.6	21.5	21.4	22.1	22.6	23.1	23.4	27.7	30.1	31.7	34.0
Black or African American female [4]	18.1	18.5	18.1	20.8	20.6	21.1	23.5	21.2	31.0	31.1	36.4	33.7
All Males												
18–24 years	26.3	32.1	30.2	28.1	29.5	31.3	27.8	26.6	28.0	35.0	42.1	54.1
25–34 years	28.7	27.2	26.9	28.9	29.1	28.5	29.5	31.6	38.2	43.9	50.5	60.7
35–44 years	28.1	29.7	27.3	30.2	30.0	30.2	31.5	34.5	37.6	41.8	51.0	58.2
45–64 years	23.9	24.5	26.4	26.4	25.8	27.7	27.1	29.3	33.4	39.3	42.6	51.9
65 years and over	10.1	10.1	11.5	10.2	10.5	10.4	14.9	14.6	19.6	20.9	24.8	28.5
White Males [4]												
18–24 years	27.7	34.3	32.3	30.4	30.5	34.1	28.4	27.4	28.4	34.3	40.8	53.0
25–34 years	28.8	27.7	28.7	29.7	30.8	29.2	29.9	31.6	37.3	43.6	49.5	60.1
35–44 years	28.8	29.7	27.8	30.6	29.5	29.6	31.2	33.5	36.6	41.3	50.1	57.3
45–64 years	23.3	24.4	25.1	25.8	24.5	27.0	26.3	28.7	32.1	38.3	41.2	51.3
65 years and over	9.6	9.3	10.7	9.8	10.0	10.0	14.1	13.7	18.9	20.5	24.3	27.7
Black or African American Males [4]												
18–24 years	18.6	22.7	21.6	20.9	23.6	19.7	*14.6	21.3	27.2	40.2	54.9	62.8
25–34 years	31.0	28.9	23.8	23.2	22.7	25.2	25.1	33.8	45.6	47.5	58.5	68.4
35–44 years	23.6	28.3	29.9	30.7	34.8	36.1	36.3	42.0	45.0	48.6	61.5	67.3
45–64 years	30.1	29.8	34.3	32.2	35.7	37.3	33.9	36.7	46.1	50.0	57.8	57.9
65 years and over	18.0	19.4	21.1	14.2	17.3	16.3	28.5	21.5	27.7	26.2	29.7	36.4
All Females												
18–24 years	21.5	24.5	23.2	24.9	26.3	24.5	21.8	22.5	30.4	33.8	34.1	38.1
25–34 years	21.3	21.3	22.7	22.3	23.5	24.6	26.4	28.2	32.0	33.7	38.8	43.7
35–44 years	24.2	23.7	25.7	26.2	26.5	26.5	27.1	24.8	31.5	37.0	39.8	43.7
45–64 years	20.2	21.1	21.4	21.7	21.0	22.5	24.0	24.8	29.9	30.7	33.4	32.0
65 years and over	8.3	8.6	9.1	9.3	10.7	11.2	11.5	11.5	13.5	13.2	12.0	9.6
White Females [4]												
18–24 years	23.6	26.7	27.1	28.5	29.6	28.1	24.9	25.4	31.8	34.5	34.0	38.4
25–34 years	22.5	23.8	25.2	24.9	25.5	26.9	27.3	28.5	32.0	34.1	38.6	43.4
35–44 years	25.2	24.4	26.9	26.6	26.9	26.6	27.0	25.0	31.0	37.2	39.3	43.9
45–64 years	20.1	21.5	21.6	21.4	21.2	22.5	24.3	25.4	29.7	30.6	33.0	32.7
65 years and over	8.4	8.5	9.4	9.1	10.5	11.2	11.7	11.5	13.3	13.8	12.3	9.8
Black or African American Females [4]												
18–24 years	10.8	17.1	10.0	14.2	14.8	*8.1	*8.8	10.0	23.7	31.8	35.6	37.1
25–34 years	17.0	13.9	16.8	15.5	18.2	21.5	26.7	29.1	36.2	35.2	42.2	47.8
35–44 years	23.2	24.0	24.0	30.2	28.8	30.0	31.9	25.5	40.2	37.7	46.4	42.8
45–64 years	23.3	22.2	22.6	25.6	22.3	25.4	27.5	22.6	33.4	34.2	38.9	25.7
65 years and over	8.0	9.4	9.3	10.2	13.5	11.5	13.3	11.1	14.5	*8.5	*8.9	7.1

[1]Beginning in 1993, current cigarette smokers reported ever smoking 100 cigarettes in their lifetime and currently smoking every day or some days.
[2]Data prior to 1997 are not strictly comparable with data for later years due to the 1997 questionnaire redesign.
[3]Estimates are age adjusted to the year 2000 standard population using five age groups: 18–24 years, 25–34 years, 35–44 years, 45–64 years, and 65 years and over.
[4]The race groups, White, Black, American Indian and Alaska Native (AI/AN), Asian, Native Hawaiian and Other Pacific Islander, and two or more races, include persons of Hispanic and non-Hispanic origin. Persons of Hispanic origin may be of any race.
* = Figure does not meet standards of reliability or precision.

TABLE III-22. CURRENT CIGARETTE SMOKING BY PERSONS 25 YEARS OF AGE AND OVER, ACCORDING TO SEX, RACE, AND EDUCATION, SELECTED YEARS, 1974–2003

For both sexes, and for Blacks as well as Whites, the frequency of smoking declined as educational attainment levels increased. Current smokers made up 29.7 percent of all persons 25 years and over without a high school diploma in 2003, but made up only 10.2 percent of those with a bachelor's degree or more. Rates for other levels of educational attainment fell between these percentages. Among Black males, the contrast between educational

attainment levels was even greater: 37.4 percent of those without a high school diploma were smokers, while only about 10.3 percent of those with a college degree smoked.

The rankings according to educational attainment have remained steady since 1974, but the rates of decline in smoking have differed. For instance, 14.0 percent of persons without a high school degree "dropped" smoking between 1974 and 2001, lowering the overall rate from 43.7 percent to 29.7 percent, while a larger drop (17.0 percent) occurred for those with college degrees.

Table III-22. Current Cigarette Smoking by Persons[1] 25 Years of Age and Over, According to Sex, Race, and Education, Selected Years, 1974–2003

(Percent of people who are current cigarette smokers.)

Sex, race, and education	2003	2002	2001	2000	1999	1998	1995[2]	1990[2]	1985[2]	1979[2]	1974[2]
25 YEARS AND OVER, AGE-ADJUSTED[3]											
All Persons[4]	21.1	21.4	22.0	22.6	22.7	23.4	24.5	25.4	30.0	33.1	36.9
No high school diploma or GED	29.7	30.5	30.5	31.6	32.2	34.4	35.6	36.7	40.8	40.7	43.7
High school diploma or GED	27.8	27.9	28.1	29.2	28.0	28.9	29.1	29.1	32.0	33.6	36.2
Some college, no bachelor's degree	21.1	21.5	22.2	21.7	23.3	23.5	22.6	23.4	29.5	33.2	35.9
Bachelor's degree or higher	10.2	10.0	10.8	10.9	11.1	10.9	13.6	13.9	18.5	22.6	27.2
All Males[4]	23.3	23.5	23.8	24.7	24.5	25.1	26.4	28.2	32.8	37.3	42.9
No high school diploma or GED	34.4	34.0	34.2	36.0	36.2	37.5	39.7	42.0	45.7	47.6	52.3
High school diploma or GED	29.9	31.0	30.2	32.1	30.4	32.0	32.7	33.1	35.5	38.9	42.4
Some college, no bachelor's degree	22.7	23.2	24.3	23.3	24.8	25.4	23.7	25.9	32.9	36.5	41.8
Bachelor's degree or higher	11.2	11.0	11.2	11.6	11.8	11.0	13.8	14.5	19.6	22.7	28.3
White Males[4, 5]	23.2	23.5	23.7	24.7	24.2	24.8	25.9	27.6	31.7	36.7	41.9
No high school diploma or GED	33.6	35.6	34.8	38.2	36.3	37.4	38.7	41.8	45.0	47.6	51.5
High school diploma or GED	29.6	31.0	30.3	32.4	30.5	32.2	32.9	32.9	34.8	38.5	42.0
Some college, no bachelor's degree	23.3	23.2	24.5	23.5	24.7	25.2	23.3	25.4	32.2	36.4	41.6
Bachelor's degree or higher	11.2	11.1	11.2	11.3	11.8	10.9	13.4	14.4	19.1	22.5	27.8
Black or African American Males[4, 5]	26.3	27.2	28.4	26.4	29.1	30.4	31.6	34.5	42.1	44.4	53.4
No high school diploma or GED	37.4	37.2	37.9	38.2	43.8	42.9	41.9	41.6	50.5	49.7	58.1
High school diploma or GED	33.4	31.3	33.4	29.0	32.5	32.8	36.6	37.4	41.8	48.6	*50.7
Some college, no bachelor's degree	19.5	25.6	24.1	19.9	23.4	28.4	26.4	28.1	41.8	39.2	*45.3
Bachelor's degree or higher	*10.3	*10.8	11.3	14.6	11.3	*15.3	*17.3	*20.8	*32.0	*36.8	*41.4
All Females[4]	19.1	19.3	20.4	20.5	20.9	21.7	22.9	22.9	27.5	29.5	32.0
No high school diploma or GED	24.9	26.9	26.9	27.1	28.2	31.3	31.7	31.8	36.5	34.8	36.6
High school diploma or GED	25.8	25.2	26.4	26.6	25.9	26.2	26.4	26.1	29.5	29.8	32.2
Some college, no bachelor's degree	19.7	20.0	20.4	20.4	21.9	21.8	21.6	21.0	26.3	30.0	30.1
Bachelor's degree or higher	9.3	9.0	10.5	10.1	10.4	10.7	13.3	13.3	17.1	22.5	25.9
White Females[4, 5]	19.6	20.2	21.3	21.0	21.4	22.3	23.1	23.3	27.3	29.7	31.7
No high school diploma or GED	25.0	29.0	29.2	28.4	29.5	33.0	32.4	33.4	36.7	35.8	36.8
High school diploma or GED	26.8	26.8	28.3	27.8	27.2	27.1	26.8	26.5	29.4	29.9	31.9
Some college, no bachelor's degree	20.6	20.5	21.3	21.1	22.3	22.2	22.2	21.2	26.7	30.7	30.4
Bachelor's degree or higher	9.4	9.6	10.9	10.2	10.5	11.5	13.5	13.4	16.5	21.9	25.5
Black or African American Females[4, 5]	18.9	18.4	19.1	21.6	21.4	23.0	25.7	22.4	32.0	30.3	35.6
No high school diploma or GED	26.9	27.1	26.3	31.1	30.1	32.8	32.3	26.3	39.4	31.6	36.1
High school diploma or GED	23.3	19.5	21.3	25.4	22.4	24.3	27.8	24.1	32.1	32.6	40.9
Some college, no bachelor's degree	17.0	20.7	17.4	20.4	22.3	21.7	20.8	22.7	23.9	*28.9	32.3
Bachelor's degree or higher	11.4	*7.7	11.6	10.8	13.4	9.0	17.3	17.0	26.6	*43.3	*36.3

[1]Beginning in 1993, current cigarette smokers reported ever smoking 100 cigarettes in their lifetime and currently smoking every day or some days.

[2]Data prior to 1997 are not strictly comparable with data for later years due to the 1997 questionnaire redesign.

[3]Estimates are age adjusted to the year 2000 standard population using four age groups: 25–34 years, 35–44 years, 45–64 years, and 65 years and over.

[4]Includes unknown education. Education quantities shown apply to 1997 and subsequent years. GED stands for General Educational Development high school equivalency diploma. From 1974–1995, the following categories based on the number of years of school completed were used: less than 12 years, 12 years, 13–15 years, and 16 years or more.

[5]The race groups, White and Black, include persons of Hispanic and non-Hispanic origin. Starting with data year 1999, race-specific estimates are tabulated according to the 1997 Standards for Federal Data on Race and Ethnicity and are not strictly comparable with estimates for earlier years. The single race categories shown in the table conform to the 1997 standards. Starting with data year 1999, race-specific estimates are for persons who reported only one racial group. Prior to data year 1999, data were tabulated according to the 1977 standards. Estimates for single race categories prior to 1999 included persons who reported one race or, if they reported more than one race, identified one race as best representing their race.

* = Figure does not meet standards of reliability or precision.

TABLE III-23. CURRENT CIGARETTE SMOKING BY ADULTS, ACCORDING TO SEX, RACE, HISPANIC ORIGIN, AGE, AND EDUCATION, SELECTED ANNUAL AVERAGES, 1990–2003

This table, with its detail on race, indicates that American Indians or Alaskan Natives—including women—have been the most frequent smokers, and Asians have been the group that smoked the least. In between, Black men (but not Black women) tended to smoke somewhat more than Whites, and Hispanics tended to smoke less than non-Hispanics. Women of Mexican origin had a low smoking rate of 9.6 percent. It should be noted that persons who reported belonging to more than one race, a classification system first used with the 2000 census, are indicated as having an especially high frequency of smoking.

Table III-23. Current Cigarette Smoking by Adults, [1] According to Sex, Race, Hispanic Origin, Age, and Education, Selected Annual Averages, 1990–2003

(Percent of persons who are current cigarette smokers.)

Characteristic	Male			Female		
	2001–2003	1995–1998[2]	1990–1992[2]	2001–2003	1995–1998[2]	1990–1992[2]
18 Years and Over, Age-Adjusted [3]						
All persons [4]	24.3	26.5	27.9	20.0	22.1	23.7
Race [5]						
White only	24.5	26.4	27.4	21.0	22.9	24.3
Black or African American only	26.5	30.7	33.9	18.0	21.8	23.1
American Indian and Alaska Native only	32.8	40.5	34.2	31.0	28.9	36.7
Asian only	17.4	18.1	24.8	6.3	11.0	6.3
Native Hawaiian and Other Pacific Islander only	*	...	...	*	...	...
Two or more races	32.3	...	...	30.9	...	...
American Indian and Alaska Native; White	39.3	...	...	38.0	...	...
Hispanic Origin and Race [5]						
Hispanic or Latino	21.1	24.4	25.7	10.9	13.7	15.8
Mexican	21.3	24.5	26.2	9.6	12.0	14.8
Not Hispanic or Latino	24.9	26.9	28.1	21.4	23.1	24.4
White only	25.2	26.9	27.7	22.7	24.1	25.2
Black or African American only	26.5	30.7	33.9	18.1	21.9	23.2
18 Years and Over, Crude						
All persons	24.8	27.0	28.4	19.9	22.0	23.6
Race [5]						
White only	24.7	26.8	27.8	20.6	22.6	24.1
Black or African American only	26.8	30.6	33.2	18.2	21.8	23.3
American Indian and Alaska Native only	35.0	39.2	35.5	33.0	31.2	37.3
Asian only	18.4	20.0	24.9	6.5	11.2	6.3
Native Hawaiian and Other Pacific Islander only	*	...	...	*	...	...
Two or more races	33.4	...	...	31.5	...	...
American Indian and Alaska Native; White	39.9	...	...	37.9	...	...
Hispanic Origin, Race, and Age [5]						
Hispanic or Latino	22.2	25.5	26.5	11.0	13.8	16.6
Mexican	22.3	25.2	27.1	9.4	11.6	15.0
Not Hispanic or Latino	25.1	27.2	28.5	21.0	22.9	24.2
White only	25.0	27.0	28.0	21.8	23.5	24.8
Black or African American only	26.8	30.6	33.3	18.3	21.9	23.3
18–24 years						
Hispanic or Latino	23.1	26.5	19.3	9.8	12.0	12.8
Not Hispanic or Latino						
White only	33.2	35.5	28.9	28.8	31.6	28.7
Black or African American only	20.9	21.3	17.7	12.9	9.8	10.8
25–34 years						
Hispanic or Latino	21.9	25.9	29.9	10.3	12.6	19.2
Not Hispanic or Latino						
White only	30.1	30.5	32.7	26.9	28.5	30.9
Black or African American only	27.4	28.5	34.6	15.8	22.0	29.2
35–44 years						
Hispanic or Latino	24.8	26.2	32.1	12.8	17.6	19.9
Not Hispanic or Latino						
White only	29.3	31.5	32.3	27.5	28.1	27.3
Black or African American only	27.3	34.7	44.1	23.7	30.3	31.3
45–64 years						
Hispanic or Latino	22.1	26.8	26.6	13.4	14.7	17.1
Not Hispanic or Latino						
White only	24.4	26.8	28.4	21.8	22.3	26.1
Black or African American only	31.7	38.8	38.0	22.9	26.9	26.1
65 years and over						
Hispanic or Latino	12.2	14.7	16.1	5.4	9.4	6.6
Not Hispanic or Latino						
White only	9.7	10.6	14.2	8.9	11.6	12.3
Black or African American only	19.5	20.9	25.2	9.0	11.2	10.7

[1]Beginning in 1993, current cigarette smokers reported ever smoking 100 cigarettes in their lifetime and currently smoking every day or some days.

[2]Data prior to 1997 are not strictly comparable with data for later years due to the 1997 questionnaire redesign.

[3]Estimates are age adjusted to the year 2000 standard population using five age groups: 18–24 years, 25–34 years, 35–44 years, 45–64 years, and 65 years and over.

[4]Includes all other races not shown separately.

[5]The race groups, White, Black, American Indian and Alaska Native (AI/AN), Asian, Native Hawaiian and Other Pacific Islander, and two or more races, include persons of Hispanic and non-Hispanic origin. Persons of Hispanic origin may be of any race.

* = Figure does not meet standards of reliability or precision.

. . . = Not available.

By age group, the data confirm large declines in smoking among persons age 65 years and older. These declines affected both to men and women, and Hispanics as well as non-Hispanics.

The general decline in smoking with increased educational attainment was not in evidence for Hispanics; their rate of smoking was usually lower, even with less education.

Table III-23.   Current Cigarette Smoking by Adults, [1] According to Sex, Race, Hispanic Origin, Age, and Education, Selected Annual Averages, 1990–2003—*Continued*

(Percent of persons who are current cigarette smokers.)

Characteristic	Male			Female		
	2001–2003	1995–1998 [2]	1990–1992 [2]	2001–2003	1995–1998 [2]	1990–1992 [2]
Education, Hispanic Origin, and Race [5, 6]						
25 Years and Over, Age-Adjusted [7]						
No High School Diploma or GED						
Hispanic or Latino	23.6	27.6	30.2	10.5	13.3	15.8
Not Hispanic or Latino						
White only	43.6	43.9	46.1	41.1	40.7	40.4
Black or African American only	37.9	44.6	45.4	26.9	30.0	31.3
High School Diploma or GED						
Hispanic or Latino	21.2	26.7	29.6	12.1	16.4	18.4
Not Hispanic or Latino						
White only	31.5	32.8	32.9	29.3	28.8	28.4
Black or African American only	32.7	35.7	38.2	21.5	26.6	25.4
Some College or More						
Hispanic or Latino	16.0	16.6	20.4	10.7	13.5	14.3
Not Hispanic or Latino						
White only	17.3	18.3	19.3	15.9	17.2	18.1
Black or African American only	18.7	23.3	25.6	15.4	18.9	22.8

[1]Beginning in 1993, current cigarette smokers reported ever smoking 100 cigarettes in their lifetime and currently smoking every day or some days.

[2]Data prior to 1997 are not strictly comparable with data for later years due to the 1997 questionnaire redesign.

[5]The race groups, White, Black, American Indian and Alaska Native (AI/AN), Asian, Native Hawaiian and Other Pacific Islander, and two or more races, include persons of Hispanic and non-Hispanic origin. Persons of Hispanic origin may be of any race.

[6]Education categories shown are for 1997 and subsequent years. GED stands for General Educational Development high school equivalency diploma. In years prior to 1997, the following categories based on number of years of school completed were used: less than 12 years, 12 years, and 13 years or more.

[7]Estimates are age adjusted to the year 2000 standard population using four age groups: 25–34 years, 35–44 years, 45–64 years, and 65 years and over.

TABLE III-24. USE OF SELECTED SUBSTANCES IN THE PAST MONTH BY PERSONS 12 YEARS OF AGE AND OVER, BY AGE, SEX, RACE, AND HISPANIC ORIGIN, 2002–2003

Based on personal interviews in 2003, 6.2 percent of persons 12 years of age and over used marijuana at least once during the 30 days before the interview. The most frequent use, 17 percent, was for persons in the 18- to 25-year-old age group. Persons age 16 to 17 years old reported a percentage that was nearly as high. Percentages rapidly tapered off at earlier and later ages. The use of other illicit drugs (including cocaine, heroin, hallucinogens, inhalants, and nonmedical use of psychoactive medications) followed similar patterns, with about 20 percent of 16–19 year olds reporting their usage.

About half of the population age 12 years and over reported having at least one drink of alcohol during the month prior to the interview. The highest percentage of use, 61.4 percent, was among persons age 18–25 years. Binge alcohol use was as high as 41.6 percent for this same age group. For all age groups combined, males tended to indulge in "binges" about twice as often as females. The definition of a binge is drinking at least 5 drinks on the same occasion during at least 1 of the past 30 days. If the respondent "binged" on 5 or more days during the month, he or she was additionally reported as being in the "heavy alcohol use" category. Among the population age 11 years and over, 6.8 percent were heavy alcohol users in 2003. American Indians or Alaska Natives and Native Hawaiians and Other Pacific Islanders were the most frequent heavy alcohol users, with rates of about 10 percent for each population group.

Cigarette use, according to household surveys, declined from 26.0 percent in 2002 to 25.4 percent in 2003 among persons age 12 years and over. Respondents who had smoked one cigarette or more in the past 30 days were counted as cigarette users. Smoking was most frequent in the 18- to 25-year-old age group, in which 40.2 percent used cigarettes. Overall, men had a 5 percentage point lead over women in cigarette use in 2003, but the trend was reversed for the very young (those between 12 and 17 years old): 12.5 percent of females in this age group used cigarettes, compared to 11.9 percent of males.

Table III-24. Use of Selected Substances in the Past Month by Persons 12 Years of Age and Over, by Age, Sex, Race, and Hispanic Origin, 2002–2003

(Percent of persons who have specified substance abuse.)

Age, sex, race, and Hispanic origin	Any illicit drug [1]		Marijuana		Nonmedical use of any psychotherapeutic drug [2]	
	2003	2002	2003	2002	2003	2002
12 years and over	8.2	8.3	6.2	6.2	2.7	2.6
Age						
12–13 years	3.8	4.2	1.0	1.4	1.8	1.7
14–15 years	10.9	11.2	7.2	7.6	4.1	4.0
16–17 years	19.2	19.8	15.6	15.7	6.1	6.2
18–25 years	20.3	20.2	17.0	17.3	6.0	5.4
26–34 years	10.7	10.5	8.4	7.7	3.4	3.6
35 years and over	4.4	4.6	3.0	3.1	1.5	1.6
Sex						
Male	10.0	10.3	8.1	8.1	2.7	2.7
Female	6.5	6.4	4.4	4.4	2.6	2.6
Age and Sex						
12–17 years	11.2	11.6	7.9	8.2	4.0	4.0
Male	11.4	12.3	8.6	9.1	3.7	3.6
Female	11.1	10.9	7.2	7.2	4.2	4.3
Hispanic Origin [3] and Race						
Not Hispanic or Latino						
White only	8.3	8.5	6.4	6.5	2.8	2.8
Black or African American only	8.7	9.7	6.7	7.4	1.8	2.0
American Indian and Alaska Native only	12.1	10.1	10.3	6.7	4.8	3.2
Native Hawaiian and Other Pacific Islander only	11.1	7.9	7.3	4.4	3.2	3.8
Asian only	3.8	3.5	1.9	1.8	1.7	0.7
Two or more races	12.0	11.4	9.3	9.0	2.4	3.5
Hispanic or Latino	8.0	7.2	4.9	4.3	3.0	2.9

Age, sex, race, and Hispanic origin	Alcohol use		Binge alcohol use [4]		Heavy alcohol use [5]	
	2003	2002	2003	2002	2003	2002
12 years and over	50.1	51.0	22.6	22.9	6.8	6.7
Age						
12–13 years	4.5	4.3	1.6	1.8	0.1	0.3
14–15 years	17.0	16.6	9.4	9.2	2.2	1.9
16–17 years	31.8	32.6	21.2	21.4	5.5	5.6
18–25 years	61.4	60.5	41.6	40.9	15.1	14.9
26–34 years	60.2	61.4	32.9	33.1	9.4	9.0
35 years and over	50.7	52.1	18.1	18.6	5.1	5.2
Sex						
Male	57.3	57.4	30.9	31.2	10.4	10.8
Female	43.2	44.9	14.8	15.1	3.4	3.0
Age and Sex						
12–17 years	17.7	17.6	10.6	10.7	2.6	2.5
Male	17.1	17.4	11.1	11.4	2.9	3.1
Female	18.3	17.9	10.1	9.9	2.3	1.9
Hispanic Origin [3] and Race						
Not Hispanic or Latino						
White only	54.4	55.0	23.6	23.4	7.7	7.5
Black or African American only	37.9	39.9	19.0	21.0	4.5	4.4
American Indian and Alaska Native only	42.0	44.7	29.6	27.9	10.0	8.7
Native Hawaiian and Other Pacific Islander only	43.3	*	29.8	25.2	10.4	8.3
Asian only	39.8	37.1	11.0	12.4	2.3	2.6
Two or more races	44.4	49.9	21.8	19.8	6.1	7.5
Hispanic or Latino	41.5	42.8	24.2	24.8	5.2	5.9

Note: Due to methodological differences among the National Survey on Drug Use & Health (formerly called NHSDA), Monitoring the Future Study (MTF), and the Youth Risk Behavior Survey (YRBS), rates of substance use measured by these surveys are not directly comparable.

[1] Any illicit drug includes marijuana/hashish, cocaine (including crack), heroin, hallucinogens (including LSD and PCP), inhalants, or any prescription-type psychotherapeutic drug used nonmedically.
[2] Psychotherapeutic drugs include prescription-type pain relievers, tranquilizers, stimulants, or sedatives; does not include over-the-counter drugs.
[3] May be of any race.
[4] Binge alcohol use is defined as drinking 5 or more drinks on the same occasion on at least 1 day in the past 30 days. Occasion is defined as at the same time or within a couple of hours of each other.
[5] Heavy alcohol use is defined as drinking 5 or more drinks on the same occasion on each of 5 or more days in the past 30 days; all heavy alcohol users are also "binge" alcohol users.
* = Figure does not meet standards of reliability or precision.

Table III-24. Use of Selected Substances in the Past Month by Persons 12 Years of Age and Over, by Age, Sex, Race, and Hispanic Origin, 2002–2003—*Continued*

(Percent of persons who have specified substance abuse.)

Age, sex, race, and Hispanic origin	Any tobacco [6]		Cigarettes		Cigars	
	2003	2002	2003	2002	2003	2002
12 years and over	29.8	30.4	25.4	26.0	5.4	5.4
Age						
12–13 years	3.2	3.8	2.5	3.2	0.8	0.7
14–15 years	13.3	13.4	11.0	11.2	3.9	3.8
16–17 years	27.0	29.0	23.2	24.9	8.8	9.3
18–25 years	44.8	45.3	40.2	40.8	11.4	11.0
26–34 years	38.8	38.2	33.4	32.7	6.9	6.6
35 years and over	27.0	27.9	22.6	23.4	3.9	4.1
Sex						
Male	35.9	37.0	28.1	28.7	9.0	9.4
Female	24.0	24.3	23.0	23.4	2.0	1.7
Age and Sex						
12–17 years	14.4	15.2	12.2	13.0	4.5	4.5
Male	15.6	16.0	11.9	12.3	6.2	6.2
Female	13.3	14.4	12.5	13.6	2.7	2.7
Hispanic Origin [3] and Race						
Not Hispanic or Latino						
White only	31.6	32.0	26.6	26.9	5.4	5.5
Black or African American only	30.0	28.8	25.9	25.3	7.2	6.8
American Indian and Alaska Native only	41.8	44.3	36.1	37.1	8.3	5.2
Native Hawaiian and Other Pacific Islander only	37.0	28.8	33.1	*	8.0	4.1
Asian only	13.8	18.6	12.6	17.7	1.8	1.1
Two or more races	34.4	38.1	30.7	35.0	6.2	5.5
Hispanic or Latino	23.7	25.2	21.4	23.0	4.9	5.0

Note: Due to methodological differences among the National Survey on Drug Use & Health (formerly called NHSDA), Monitoring the Future Study (MTF), and the Youth Risk Behavior Survey (YRBS), rates of substance use measured by these surveys are not directly comparable.

[3] May be of any race.
[6] Any tobacco product includes cigarettes, smokeless tobacco (chewing tobacco or snuff), cigars, or pipe tobacco.
* = Figure does not meet standards of reliability or precision.

TABLE III-25. USE OF SELECTED SUBSTANCES BY HIGH SCHOOL SENIORS, TENTH GRADERS, AND EIGHTH GRADERS, ACCORDING TO SEX AND RACE, SELECTED YEARS, 1980–2004

This survey presents separate data concerning the use of cigarettes, marijuana, cocaine, inhalants, ecstasy, and alcohol by 8th graders, 10th graders, and high school seniors. Cigarettes were used at least once during the past month by 9 percent of 8th graders; this rate increased to 25 percent for high school seniors. Marijuana usage was reported at 6 percent for 8th graders and 20 percent for seniors. Alcohol use was substantially more prevalent, ranging from 19 percent for 8th graders to 48 percent for seniors. Binge drinking was indulged in by 29 percent of seniors. Other substances were used much less frequently. Inhalants were used by 4.5 percent of 8th graders, but only by 1.5 percent of seniors. Cocaine had its greatest use among male high school seniors (2.9 percent), but only 1.7 percent of female seniors reported using the drug.

TABLE III-26. COCAINE-RELATED EMERGENCY DEPARTMENT EPISODES, ACCORDING TO AGE, SEX, RACE, AND HISPANIC ORIGIN, SELECTED YEARS, 1990–2002

In 2002, there were almost 200,000 cocaine-related episodes in hospital emergency departments, which is equivalent to 79 cases per 100,000 persons. These cases may have represented drug overdose, unexpected drug reactions, chronic abuse, detoxification, or other drug-related reasons. Such episodes have been increasing since 1990. Occurrences were about twice as frequent for men as for women, with the highest rate occurring in the 26- to 34-year-old age bracket. Blacks had a proportionately high incidence of cocaine-related ER episodes, especially among men and women age 35 years and over.

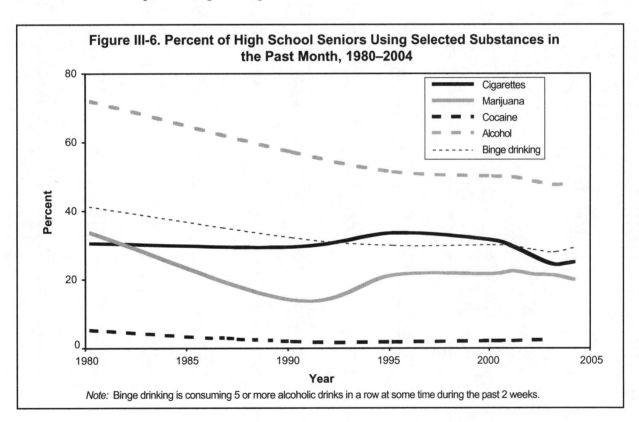

Figure III-6. Percent of High School Seniors Using Selected Substances in the Past Month, 1980–2004

Note: Binge drinking is consuming 5 or more alcoholic drinks in a row at some time during the past 2 weeks.

Table III-25. Use of Selected Substances by High School Seniors, Tenth Graders, and Eighth Graders, According to Sex and Race, Selected Years, 1980–2004

(Percent using substance in the past month.)

Substance, sex, race, and grade in school	Percent using in the last month								
	2004	2003	2002	2001	2000	1995	1991	1990	1980
Cigarettes									
All seniors	25.0	24.4	26.7	29.5	31.4	33.5	28.3	29.4	30.5
Male	25.3	26.2	27.4	29.7	32.8	34.5	29.0	29.1	26.8
Female	24.1	22.1	25.5	28.7	29.7	32.0	27.5	29.2	33.4
White	28.2	28.2	30.9	34.1	36.6	37.3	31.8	32.5	31.0
Black or African American	11.3	9.0	11.3	12.9	13.6	15.0	9.4	12.0	25.2
All 10th graders	16.0	16.7	17.7	21.3	23.9	27.9	20.8	...	...
Male	16.2	16.2	16.7	20.9	23.8	27.7	20.8	...	...
Female	15.7	17.0	18.6	21.5	23.6	27.9	20.7	...	...
White	18.1	19.3	20.8	24.0	27.3	31.2	23.9	...	...
Black or African American	9.6	8.8	9.1	10.9	11.3	12.2	6.4	...	...
All 8th graders	9.2	10.2	10.7	12.2	14.6	19.1	14.3	...	...
Male	8.3	9.6	11.0	12.2	14.3	18.8	15.5	...	...
Female	9.9	10.6	10.4	12.0	14.7	19.0	13.1	...	...
White	9.4	10.6	11.1	12.8	16.4	21.7	15.0	...	...
Black or African American	7.5	6.4	7.3	8.0	8.4	8.2	5.3	...	...
Marijuana									
All seniors	19.9	21.2	21.5	22.4	21.6	21.2	13.8	14.0	33.7
Male	23.0	24.7	25.3	25.6	24.7	24.6	16.1	16.1	37.8
Female	16.6	17.3	17.4	19.1	18.3	17.2	11.2	11.5	29.1
White	21.5	22.8	22.8	23.9	22.0	21.5	15.0	15.6	34.2
Black or African American	14.2	16.1	16.4	16.5	17.5	17.8	6.5	5.2	26.5
All 10th graders	15.9	17.0	17.8	19.8	19.7	17.2	8.7	...	...
Male	17.4	19.0	19.3	22.7	23.3	19.2	10.1	...	...
Female	14.2	15.0	16.4	16.8	16.2	15.0	7.3	...	...
White	15.8	17.4	19.1	20.4	20.1	17.7	9.4	...	...
Black or African American	17.2	15.6	14.4	16.5	17.0	15.1	3.8	...	...
All 8th graders	6.4	7.5	8.3	9.2	9.1	9.1	3.2	...	...
Male	6.3	8.5	9.5	11.0	10.2	9.8	3.8	...	...
Female	6.3	6.4	7.1	7.3	7.8	8.2	2.6	...	...
White	5.5	7.0	7.9	8.6	8.3	9.0	3.0	...	...
Black or African American	8.1	7.4	7.1	7.7	8.5	7.0	2.1	...	...
Cocaine									
All seniors	2.3	2.1	2.3	2.1	2.1	1.8	1.4	1.9	5.2
Male	2.9	2.6	2.7	2.5	2.7	2.2	1.7	2.3	6.0
Female	1.7	1.4	1.8	1.6	1.6	1.3	0.9	1.3	4.3
White	2.5	2.1	2.8	2.3	2.2	1.7	1.3	1.8	5.4
Black or African American	0.9	1.0	0.2	0.6	1.0	0.4	0.8	0.5	2.0
All 10th graders	1.7	1.3	1.6	1.3	1.8	1.7	0.7	...	...
Male	1.9	1.3	1.8	1.5	2.1	1.8	0.7	...	...
Female	1.4	1.3	1.4	1.2	1.4	1.5	0.6	...	...
White	1.7	1.4	1.7	1.2	1.7	1.7	0.6	...	...
Black or African American	0.4	0.5	0.4	0.3	0.4	0.4	0.2	...	...
All 8th graders	0.9	0.9	1.1	1.2	1.2	1.2	0.5	...	...
Male	0.8	1.0	1.1	1.1	1.3	1.1	0.7	...	...
Female	1.0	0.8	1.1	1.2	1.1	1.2	0.4	...	...
White	0.8	0.8	1.0	1.1	1.1	1.0	0.4	...	...
Black or African American	0.8	0.5	0.5	0.4	0.5	0.4	0.4	...	...
Inhalants									
All seniors	1.5	1.5	1.5	1.7	2.2	3.2	2.4	2.7	1.4
Male	1.7	2.0	2.2	2.3	2.9	3.9	3.3	3.5	1.8
Female	1.3	1.1	0.8	1.1	1.7	2.5	1.6	2.0	1.0
White	1.6	1.7	1.3	1.8	2.1	3.7	2.4	3.0	1.4
Black or African American	1.0	0.7	1.2	1.3	2.1	1.1	1.5	1.5	1.0
All 10th graders	2.4	2.2	2.4	2.5	2.6	3.5	2.7	...	...
Male	2.4	2.3	2.3	2.5	3.0	3.8	2.9	...	...
Female	2.3	2.2	2.4	2.4	2.2	3.2	2.6	...	...
White	2.6	2.6	2.6	2.5	2.8	3.9	2.9	...	...
Black or African American	1.4	0.5	1.5	0.9	1.5	1.2	2.0	...	...
All 8th graders	4.5	4.1	3.8	4.0	4.5	6.1	4.4	...	...
Male	4.0	3.4	3.5	3.6	4.1	5.6	4.1	...	...
Female	5.1	4.7	3.9	4.3	4.8	6.6	4.7	...	...
White	4.4	4.3	3.9	4.1	4.5	7.0	4.5	...	...
Black or African American	3.8	2.3	2.7	2.6	2.3	2.3	2.3	...	...
MDMA (Ecstasy)									
All seniors	1.2	1.3	2.4	2.8	3.6	...	...	...	...
Male	1.6	1.3	2.6	3.7	4.1	...	...	...	...
Female	0.9	1.2	2.1	2.0	3.1	...	...	...	...
White	1.2	1.3	2.5	2.8	3.9	...	...	...	...
Black or African American	1.1	0.6	0.5	0.9	1.9	...	...	...	...
All 10th graders	0.8	1.1	1.8	2.6	2.6	...	...	...	...
Male	1.0	1.2	1.6	3.5	2.5	...	...	...	...
Female	0.6	1.1	1.8	1.6	2.5	...	...	...	...
White	0.9	1.2	2.3	2.6	2.5	...	...	...	...
Black or African American	0.1	0.7	0.5	1.0	1.8	...	...	...	...
All 8th graders	0.8	0.7	1.4	1.8	1.4	...	...	...	...
Male	0.7	0.7	1.5	1.9	1.6	...	...	...	...
Female	0.9	0.7	1.3	1.8	1.2	...	...	...	...
White	0.6	0.7	1.0	2.0	1.4	...	...	...	...
Black or African American	1.2	0.4	0.6	1.1	0.8	...	...	...	...

. . . = Not available.

Table III-25.   Use of Selected Substances by High School Seniors, Tenth Graders, and Eighth Graders, According to Sex and Race, Selected Years, 1980–2004—*Continued*

(Percent using substance in the past month.)

Substance, sex, race, and grade in school	Percent using in the last month								
	2004	2003	2002	2001	2000	1995	1991	1990	1980
Alcohol [1]									
All seniors	48.0	47.5	48.6	49.8	50.0	51.3	54.0	57.1	72.0
Male	51.1	51.7	52.3	54.7	54.0	55.7	58.4	61.3	77.4
Female	45.1	43.8	45.1	45.1	46.1	47.0	49.0	52.3	66.8
White	52.5	52.0	52.7	55.3	55.3	54.8	57.7	62.2	75.8
Black or African American	29.2	29.2	30.7	29.6	29.3	37.4	34.4	32.9	47.7
All 10th graders	35.2	35.4	35.4	39.0	41.0	38.8	42.8	...	...
Male	36.3	35.3	35.3	41.1	43.3	39.7	45.5	...	...
Female	34.0	35.3	35.7	36.8	38.6	37.8	40.3	...	...
White	37.3	38.4	39.0	41.0	44.3	41.3	45.7	...	...
Black or African American	25.4	24.0	23.2	26.0	24.7	24.9	30.2	...	...
All 8th graders	18.6	19.7	19.6	21.5	22.4	24.6	25.1	...	...
Male	17.9	19.4	19.1	22.3	22.5	25.0	26.3	...	...
Female	19.0	19.8	20.0	20.6	22.0	24.0	23.8	...	...
White	18.6	19.9	20.4	22.5	23.9	25.4	26.0	...	...
Black or African American	16.0	16.5	14.7	14.9	15.1	17.3	17.8	...	...
Binge Drinking [2]									
All seniors	29.2	27.9	28.6	29.7	30.0	29.8	29.8	32.2	41.2
Male	34.3	34.2	34.2	36.0	36.7	36.9	37.8	39.1	52.1
Female	24.2	22.1	23.0	23.7	23.5	23.0	21.2	24.4	30.5
White	33.1	31.9	32.9	34.5	34.4	32.9	32.9	36.2	44.6
Black or African American	11.7	11.1	10.4	12.6	11.0	15.5	11.8	11.6	17.0
All 10th graders	22.0	22.2	22.4	24.9	26.2	24.0	22.9	...	...
Male	23.8	23.2	23.8	28.6	29.8	26.4	26.4	...	...
Female	20.2	21.2	21.0	21.4	22.5	21.5	19.5	...	...
White	23.7	24.3	24.6	26.4	28.5	25.7	24.4	...	...
Black or African American	11.5	11.7	12.4	12.3	12.9	12.3	14.4	...	...
All 8th graders	11.4	11.9	12.4	13.2	14.1	14.5	12.9	...	...
Male	10.8	12.2	12.5	13.7	14.4	15.1	14.3	...	...
Female	11.8	11.6	12.1	12.4	13.6	13.9	11.4	...	...
White	11.2	11.4	12.3	13.1	14.6	14.5	12.6	...	...
Black or African American	8.6	10.9	9.9	8.8	9.3	10.0	9.9	...	...

[1] In 1993, the alcohol question was changed to indicate that a "drink" meant "more than a few sips."
[2] Five or more alcoholic drinks in a row at least once in the prior two-week period.
. . . = Not available.

Table III-26. Cocaine-Related Emergency Department Episodes, According to Age, Sex, Race, and Hispanic Origin, Selected Years, 1990–2002

(Number, rate per 100,000 population.)

Age, sex, race, and Hispanic origin	2002	2001	2000	1999	1998	1997	1995	1991	1990
NUMBER									
All Races, Both Sexes [1]									
All ages [2]	199 198	193 034	174 881	168 751	172 011	161 083	135 711	101 189	80 355
6–17 years	3 502	3 514	4 402	3 299	4 362	3 642	2 051	2 210	1 877
18–25 years	30 808	28 666	25 753	25 264	24 507	25 218	21 110	21 766	19 614
26–34 years	52 743	53 693	51 007	54 058	59 008	57 143	54 881	46 137	35 639
35 years and over	111 937	106 810	93 357	85 869	83 730	74 600	57 341	30 582	23 054
Male									
Not Hispanic or Latino									
White									
All ages [2]	49 305	43 387	36 508	35 378	32 767	32 778	25 634	19 385	15 512
6–17 years	903	935	897	666	1 302	898	493	486	527
18–25 years	10 138	9 726	7 294	7 367	6 069	6 644	5 459	5 284	3 810
26–34 years	15 881	12 282	11 143	11 421	11 302	11 697	10 426	8 777	6 724
35 years and over	22 360	20 424	17 148	15 893	14 075	13 464	9 226	4 747	4 432
Black or African American									
All ages [2]	52 463	53 282	49 612	49 944	55 562	54 257	48 872	36 597	27 745
6–17 years	104	91	305	404	236	388	304	244	241
18–25 years	3 628	3 756	3 836	4 066	4 153	4 725	4 735	5 743	5 104
26–34 years	10 432	11 924	11 608	13 433	17 578	18 052	18 756	16 232	12 160
35 years and over	38 230	37 437	33 758	31 978	33 511	30 850	25 016	14 110	10 202
Hispanic or Latino [3]									
All ages [2]	15 881	18 293	16 774	15 111	14 844	11 540	7 886	6 571	4 821
6–17 years	542	485	612	899	725	402	181	201	144
18–25 years	3 369	4 108	4 268	4 027	3 871	3 467	1 892	1 831	1 774
26–34 years	4 900	6 080	5 510	4 582	4 694	3 575	2 901	2 723	1 758
35 years and over	7 051	7 615	6 375	5 540	5 536	4 077	2 907	1 801	1 125
Female									
Not Hispanic or Latino									
White									
All ages [2]	29 736	27 365	22 419	20 884	19 687	17 593	13 566	9 541	8 331
6–17 years	1 012	838	1 208	837	1 125	1 021	495	529	486
18–25 years	7 306	5 675	4 259	4 348	4 368	3 742	2 962	2 765	2 663
26–34 years	8 509	8 936	7 471	8 022	6 621	6 771	5 976	4 427	3 636
35 years and over	12 902	11 801	9 414	7 667	7 504	6 043	4 126	1 808	1 539
Black or African American									
All ages [2]	27 089	26 257	25 480	27 625	28 361	27 298	24 138	19 149	14 833
6–17 years	82	175	99	125	80	100	153	210	177
18–25 years	2 114	1 824	1 947	2 012	2 245	3 407	3 307	3 892	3 820
26–34 years	6 018	6 927	7 962	9 994	11 312	11 004	10 831	9 481	7 418
35 years and over	18 843	17 305	15 453	15 473	14 687	12 752	9 822	5 512	3 369
Hispanic or Latino [3]									
All ages [2]	7 841	6 491	6 598	5 224	6 238	5 063	3 515	2 356	1 719
6–17 years	*	*	*	146	*	*	128	183	64
18–25 years	*	1 112	*	1 167	*	*	901	616	634
26–34 years	2 511	2 409	1 967	2 091	2 278	1 698	1 280	1 044	663
35 years and over	3 028	2 419	2 029	1 811	1 821	1 402	1 203	513	357
RATE									
Both Sexes									
6 years and over, age-adjusted [4]	79.0	77.6	70.8	69.2	70.7	66.4	56.2	41.0	...
6 years and over, crude [5]	77.6	76.1	70.7	69.4	71.5	67.7	58.3	45.2	...
6–11 years	*	*	*	*	*	*	*	*	...
12–17 years	14.2	14.5	18.8	14.0	18.8	16.0	9.3	10.6	...
18–25 years	90.7	85.5	88.9	89.5	88.2	91.8	76.2	76.9	...
26–34 years	171.1	176.4	154.6	161.9	173.1	164.5	153.7	120.5	...
35 years and over	79.0	76.2	67.7	63.7	63.2	57.4	46.0	26.5	...
Male									
6 years and over, age-adjusted [4]	105.5	104.5	95.7	93.4	96.4	91.2	77.5	56.2	...
6 years and over, crude [5]	102.6	101.8	94.8	93.0	96.7	92.2	79.9	61.6	...
6–11 years	*	*	*	*	*	*	*	*	...
12–17 years	13.8	14.3	16.7	17.4	20.7	15.3	10.5	9.5	...
18–25 years	109.9	112.8	118.5	120.5	115.2	116.1	98.1	102.7	...
26–34 years	221.8	220.8	193.8	195.5	219.7	211.3	196.2	152.8	...
35 years and over	110.2	108.0	97.1	92.0	92.2	85.6	69.2	40.7	...
Female									
6 years and over, age-adjusted [4]	53.6	51.4	46.3	46.0	46.1	42.6	35.5	26.5	...
6 years and over, crude [5]	52.9	50.4	46.4	46.4	46.7	43.5	37.0	29.1	...
6–11 years	*	*	*	*	*	*	*	*	...
12–17 years	14.6	14.5	20.9	10.2	16.7	16.6	7.8	11.0	...
18–25 years	70.9	55.6	58.2	57.7	61.7	66.4	54.1	53.0	...
26–34 years	118.4	130.0	112.9	127.3	125.0	117.0	108.6	86.1	...
35 years and over	50.1	46.6	40.1	37.9	36.6	31.3	24.8	13.6	...

[1] Includes other races and unknown race, Hispanic origin, and/or sex.
[2] Includes unknown age.
[3] May be of any race.
[4] Age adjusted to the year 2000 standard population using five age groups.
[5] Includes unknown age and sex.
* = Figure does not meet standards of reliability or precision.
. . . = Not available.

TABLE III-27. ALCOHOL CONSUMPTION BY PERSONS 18 YEARS OF AGE AND OVER, ACCORDING TO SELECTED CHARACTERISTICS, SELECTED YEARS, 1997–2003

Respondents age 18 years and over were divided into several categories (age-adjusted): lifetime abstainers (31.3 percent in 2003); former drinkers, who had gone without a drink for a year (13.6 percent in 2003); current infrequent drinkers, who had fewer than 12 drinks in the past year (15.9 percent in 2003); and current regular drinkers, who had at least 12 drinks in the past year (39.0 percent in 2003).

The table also categorizes drinkers in a number of additional ways. One panel classifies current drinkers according to the frequency of drinking. Almost 80 percent of drinkers were light drinkers who consumed 3 or fewer drinks per week. Moderate drinkers, representing nearly 14 percent of current drinkers, consumed between 3 and 14 drinks per week for men, and between 3 and 7 drinks per week for women. (The distinction between the sexes is based on dietary guidelines from the Department of Agriculture.) Heavy drinkers (some 7 percent of current drinkers) were those who exceeded the limits of moderate drinking for their genders.

Drinking, like smoking, became much less frequent at age 65 and over, with gradual reductions beginning at age 55. Binge drinking (five or more drinks in one day) was somewhat more frequent in the Midwest than in other regions of the country. The South had considerably fewer drinkers than other regions.

Table III-27. Alcohol Consumption by Persons 18 Years of Age and Over, According to Selected Characteristics, Selected Years, 1997–2003

(Percent.)

Characteristic	Both sexes			Male			Female		
	2003	2002	1997	2003	2002	1997	2003	2002	1997
DRINKING STATUS PERCENT DISTRIBUTION [1]									
18 Years and Over, Age-Adjusted [2]									
All	100.0	100.0	100.0	100.0	100.0	100.0	100.0	100.0	100.0
Lifetime abstainer	24.9	22.3	21.4	17.8	14.8	14.1	31.3	28.8	27.8
Former drinker	14.3	15.3	15.8	15.2	15.8	16.4	13.6	14.9	15.4
Infrequent	7.7	8.4	9.0	7.1	7.4	7.8	8.4	9.3	10.2
Regular	6.5	6.8	6.8	8.0	8.3	8.6	5.2	5.5	5.3
Current drinker	60.8	62.5	62.8	67.1	69.4	69.5	55.2	56.3	56.8
Infrequent	12.9	13.3	13.9	9.8	9.8	10.2	15.9	16.6	17.4
Regular	47.4	48.7	48.5	56.7	58.9	58.7	39.0	39.3	39.2
18 Years and Over, Crude									
All	100.0	100.0	100.0	100.0	100.0	100.0	100.0	100.0	100.0
Lifetime abstainer	24.8	22.2	21.3	17.7	14.8	14.1	31.4	28.9	27.8
Former drinker	14.3	15.2	15.6	14.9	15.3	15.7	13.7	15.1	15.5
Infrequent	7.8	8.4	8.9	7.0	7.2	7.5	8.5	9.4	10.2
Regular	6.5	6.8	6.7	7.9	8.0	8.2	5.2	5.6	5.3
Current drinker	60.9	62.6	63.1	67.4	69.9	70.2	54.9	56.0	56.7
Infrequent	13.0	13.3	14.0	9.8	9.8	10.2	15.9	16.6	17.4
Regular	47.5	48.8	48.8	57.1	59.4	59.4	38.7	39.1	39.1
PERCENT CURRENT DRINKERS AMONG ALL PERSONS									
All Persons									
18–44 years	66.4	68.8	68.5	72.3	75.6	73.8	60.7	62.3	63.3
18–24 years	59.5	63.7	61.3	64.6	70.5	65.5	54.5	56.8	57.0
25–44 years	68.7	70.6	70.6	74.9	77.4	76.3	62.8	64.1	65.2
45–64 years	60.4	62.5	62.7	65.7	67.7	69.8	55.4	57.7	55.9
45–54 years	63.8	65.6	66.5	68.0	70.5	73.0	59.9	60.9	60.3
55–64 years	55.5	57.9	56.7	62.4	63.3	64.8	49.0	53.0	49.2
65 years and over	42.4	40.8	42.8	51.1	51.1	52.0	36.0	33.1	36.0
65–74 years	46.5	44.9	47.9	53.7	55.6	56.1	40.6	36.0	41.4
75 years and over	37.8	35.9	36.0	47.6	45.0	45.9	31.4	30.0	29.7
Race [3]									
White only	63.3	65.3	65.3	69.1	71.4	71.0	58.0	59.7	60.1
Black or African American only	47.4	46.9	46.7	54.7	56.4	55.5	41.8	39.6	40.0
American Indian and Alaska Native only	46.5	52.0	52.2	47.8	60.2	64.6	45.2	46.8	43.4
Asian only	39.1	47.7	45.7	49.4	58.5	59.8	30.3	35.0	31.6
Native Hawaiian and Other Pacific Islander	*	*	. . .	*	*	. . .	*	*	. . .
Two or more races	54.5	62.4	. . .	62.4	62.8	. . .	48.4	61.9	. . .
Hispanic Origin and Race [3]									
Hispanic or Latino	49.5	50.5	52.9	61.7	64.2	63.9	37.3	37.8	41.9
Mexican	47.5	50.7	52.7	60.9	64.6	66.3	33.4	36.6	38.7
Not Hispanic or Latino	62.1	63.7	63.3	67.4	69.8	69.3	57.4	58.3	58.0
White only	65.7	67.2	66.7	70.3	72.4	71.7	61.6	62.4	62.2
Black or African American only	47.2	46.7	46.7	54.3	55.9	55.7	41.8	39.6	39.8

[1]Drinking status categories are based on self-reported responses to questions about alcohol consumption. Lifetime abstainers had fewer than 12 drinks in their lifetime. Former drinkers had at least 12 drinks in their lifetime and none in the past year. Former infrequent drinkers are former drinkers who had fewer than 12 drinks in any one year. Former regular drinkers are former drinkers who had at least 12 drinks in any one year. Current drinkers had 12 drinks in their lifetime and at least one drink in the past year. Current infrequent drinkers are current drinkers who had fewer than 12 drinks in the past year. Current regular drinkers are current drinkers who had at least 12 drinks in the past year.

[2]Estimates are age adjusted to the year 2000 standard population using four age groups: 18–24 years, 25–44 years, 45–64 years, and 65 years and over.

[3]The race groups, White, Black, American Indian and Alaska Native (AI/AN), Asian, Native Hawaiian and Other Pacific Islander, and two or more races, include persons of Hispanic and non-Hispanic origin. Persons of Hispanic origin may be of any race.

* = Figure does not meet standards of reliability or precision.

. . . = Not available.

Table III-27. Alcohol Consumption by Persons 18 Years of Age and Over, According to Selected Characteristics, Selected Years, 1997–2003—*Continued*

(Percent.)

Characteristic	Both sexes			Male			Female		
	2003	2002	1997	2003	2002	1997	2003	2002	1997
Geographic Region									
Northeast	67.8	69.3	67.9	73.7	74.7	73.4	62.9	64.8	63.3
Midwest	64.5	66.4	65.7	68.8	73.4	71.6	60.7	60.1	60.3
South	54.3	55.7	55.5	61.7	63.5	63.0	47.6	48.6	48.7
West	60.4	62.3	64.4	67.0	68.8	71.2	54.1	56.1	58.1
Location of Residence									
Within MSA [4]	62.3	63.7	63.9	68.2	70.4	70.1	57.0	57.6	58.5
Outside MSA [4]	53.8	56.6	56.5	61.5	64.0	64.6	47.1	50.0	48.8
PERCENT DISTRIBUTION OF CURRENT DRINKERS									
Level of Alcohol Consumption in Past Year [5]									
18 Years and Over, Age-Adjusted [2]									
All drinking levels	100.0	100.0	100.0	100.0	100.0	100.0	100.0	100.0	100.0
Light	68.4	68.5	69.6	58.9	58.8	59.5	78.9	79.6	81.0
Moderate	23.7	23.4	22.5	32.8	32.7	31.8	13.7	12.8	12.0
Heavier	7.9	8.1	7.9	8.3	8.5	8.7	7.4	7.6	7.0
18 Years and Over, Crude									
All drinking levels	100.0	100.0	100.0	100.0	100.0	100.0	100.0	100.0	100.0
Light	68.6	68.7	69.8	59.1	58.9	59.6	79.2	79.9	81.4
Moderate	23.5	23.2	22.3	32.5	32.6	31.7	13.5	12.5	11.7
Heavier	7.9	8.1	7.9	8.4	8.5	8.8	7.3	7.5	6.9
NUMBER OF DAYS IN PAST YEAR WITH 5 OR MORE DRINKS, PERCENT DISTRIBUTION OF CURRENT DRINKERS									
18 Years and Over, Crude									
All current drinkers	100.0	100.0	100.0	100.0	100.0	100.0	100.0	100.0	100.0
No days	68.1	67.7	65.8	58.1	57.6	54.5	79.1	79.1	78.5
At least 1 day	31.9	32.3	34.2	41.9	42.4	45.5	20.9	20.9	21.5
1–11 days	17.0	16.8	18.5	19.5	19.7	22.0	14.2	13.5	14.6
12 or more days	14.9	15.5	15.6	22.4	22.8	23.5	6.7	7.4	6.9
PERCENT ADULT CURRENT DRINKERS WHO DRANK 5 OR MORE DRINKS ON AT LEAST 1 DAY									
All Persons									
18 years and over, age-adjusted	30.8	31.0	32.4	40.3	40.7	43.4	20.3	20.0	20.2
18 years and over, crude	31.9	32.3	34.2	41.9	42.4	45.5	20.9	20.9	21.5
18–44 years	41.1	42.0	42.5	52.1	53.1	54.8	28.7	29.1	28.7
18–24 years	51.2	53.5	51.6	59.3	63.1	61.5	41.9	41.7	40.2
25–44 years	38.2	38.5	40.2	50.0	50.0	53.0	24.9	25.4	25.8
45–64 years	23.9	22.3	25.3	33.5	31.9	36.1	13.2	12.0	12.8
45–54 years	26.3	25.5	28.5	37.0	35.9	40.2	14.9	14.3	15.2
55–64 years	19.8	16.9	19.5	28.0	25.1	28.8	10.2	8.2	8.3
65 years and over	8.4	9.2	11.2	12.5	14.0	17.8	4.2	3.7	4.3
65–74 years	10.8	12.4	13.8	16.1	17.9	21.6	5.0	5.5	5.4
75 years and over	5.2	4.5	6.6	7.3	7.5	10.8	*3.1	*	*2.5
Race [3]									
White only	31.9	31.8	33.3	41.3	41.8	44.4	21.4	20.7	20.9
Black or African American only	21.6	22.7	23.9	31.0	29.2	32.0	12.2	15.3	15.0
American Indian and Alaska Native only	34.1	40.8	54.4	43.8	49.0	70.5	*23.1	38.6	37.6
Asian only	15.3	20.7	25.6	20.3	26.8	30.8	*8.4	*9.6	16.6
Native Hawaiian and Other Pacific Islander	*	*	. . .	*	*	. . .	*	*	. . .
Hispanic Origin and Race [3]									
Hispanic or Latino	30.2	34.3	37.0	39.1	45.0	46.6	15.4	17.5	22.4
Mexican	34.2	39.4	39.1	43.0	50.7	50.2	18.2	19.6	20.3
Not Hispanic or Latino	30.6	30.3	31.9	40.1	39.7	42.8	20.6	20.0	20.0
White only	32.3	31.8	33.2	41.9	41.8	44.5	22.1	21.0	21.0
Black or African American only	21.2	22.8	23.7	30.5	29.3	32.0	11.9	15.4	14.5
Geographic Area									
Northeast	29.1	29.1	31.4	37.2	39.2	43.3	21.0	18.9	19.0
Midwest	33.9	33.8	33.7	44.6	43.5	44.6	22.5	22.9	21.6
South	28.2	28.5	30.9	36.9	37.3	40.6	17.9	17.8	19.3
West	31.5	31.7	33.5	41.7	41.9	44.7	19.6	19.8	20.7
Location of Residence									
Within MSA [4]	29.9	30.4	31.7	39.0	39.7	42.4	19.8	19.8	19.9
Outside MSA [4]	33.2	31.7	34.9	43.7	42.0	45.7	21.2	19.9	21.2

[2]Estimates are age adjusted to the year 2000 standard population using four age groups: 18–24 years, 25–44 years, 45–64 years, and 65 years and over.

[3]The race groups, White, Black, American Indian and Alaska Native (AI/AN), Asian, Native Hawaiian and Other Pacific Islander, and two or more races, include persons of Hispanic and non-Hispanic origin. Persons of Hispanic origin may be of any race.

[4]MSA = Metropolitan Statistical Area.

[5]Level of alcohol consumption categories are based on self-reported responses to questions about average alcohol consumption and defined as follows—light drinkers: three drinks or fewer per week; moderate drinkers: more than three drinks and up to fourteen drinks per week for men and more than three drinks and up to seven drinks per week for women; heavier drinkers: more than fourteen drinks per week for men and more than seven drinks per week for women.

* = Figure does not meet standards of reliability or precision.

. . . = Not available.

AMBULATORY CARE

TABLE III-28. HEALTH CARE VISITS TO DOCTORS' OFFICES, EMERGENCY DEPARTMENTS, AND HOME VISITS WITHIN THE PAST 12 MONTHS, ACCORDING TO SELECTED CHARACTERISTICS, SELECTED YEARS, 1997–2003

The number of health care visits by patients during a 12-month period ending in 2003 differed widely, but the most frequent rate was 1 to 3 visits. However, persons 65 years old and over had a rate of 4 to 9 visits. About 16 percent of all persons reported having no visits during the year. This rate dropped to 5 percent for persons 75 years old and over. Only 5.5 percent of children under 6 years of age had no health care visits.

The frequency of health care visits was not substantially different between Blacks and Whites, but Asians and Hispanics tended to have a lower number of visits. Hispanics were the group most likely to have had no health care visits during the last 12 months.

Persons in poverty generally had fewer health care visits. However, for the highest category (10 visits or more), poor respondents showed a somewhat higher frequency than nonpoor respondents. This could reflect more ailments or more insurance coverage under Medicaid.

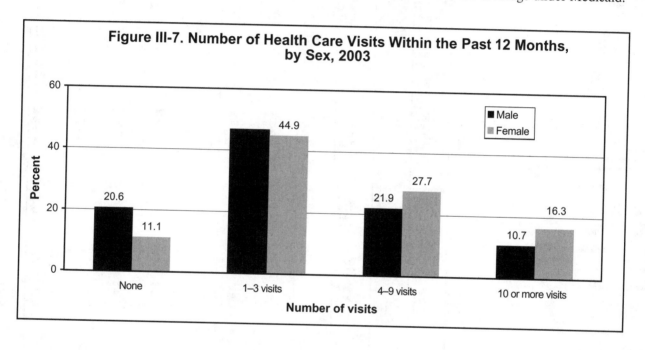

Figure III-7. Number of Health Care Visits Within the Past 12 Months, by Sex, 2003

Table III-28. Health Care Visits to Doctors' Offices, Emergency Departments, and Home Visits Within the Past 12 Months, According to Selected Characteristics, Selected Years, 1997–2003

(Percent.)

Characteristic	Number of health care visits											
	None			1–3 visits			4–9 visits			10 or more visits		
	2003	2002	1997	2003	2002	1997	2003	2002	1997	2003	2002	1997
All persons [1,2]	15.8	15.9	16.5	45.8	45.5	46.2	24.8	25.2	23.6	13.6	13.4	13.7
Age												
Under 18 years	11.3	10.6	11.8	54.5	55.1	54.1	26.7	27.1	25.2	7.5	7.2	8.9
Under 6 years	5.5	5.6	5.0	46.0	47.0	44.9	39.0	37.1	37.0	9.4	10.4	13.0
6–17 years	14.0	13.0	15.3	58.7	59.0	58.7	20.8	22.3	19.3	6.6	5.7	6.8
18–44 years	22.4	22.6	21.7	46.7	45.7	46.7	19.1	19.4	19.0	11.8	12.4	12.6
18–24 years	23.6	24.8	22.0	47.2	45.6	46.8	18.2	18.7	20.0	11.0	10.8	11.2
25–44 years	22.0	21.8	21.6	46.6	45.7	46.7	19.4	19.6	18.7	12.0	12.9	13.0
45–64 years	14.7	14.8	16.9	42.2	41.9	42.9	26.6	26.9	24.7	16.5	16.4	15.5
45–54 years	16.9	17.0	17.9	44.2	43.3	43.9	24.5	25.4	23.4	14.3	14.3	14.8
55–64 years	11.4	11.5	15.3	39.2	39.7	41.3	29.8	29.0	26.7	19.6	19.7	16.7
65 years and over	6.3	8.2	8.9	31.5	31.3	34.7	35.8	36.4	32.5	26.4	24.1	23.8
65–74 years	7.1	9.1	9.8	34.0	33.7	36.9	35.7	36.8	31.6	23.3	20.5	21.6
75 years and over	5.4	7.3	7.7	28.6	28.6	31.8	36.0	35.8	33.8	30.0	28.3	26.6
Sex [2]												
Male	20.6	20.6	21.3	46.8	46.5	47.1	21.9	22.2	20.6	10.7	10.7	11.0
Female	11.1	11.4	11.8	44.9	44.5	45.4	27.7	28.0	26.5	16.3	16.1	16.3
Race [2,3]												
White only	15.7	15.6	16.0	45.6	45.1	46.1	25.1	25.4	23.9	13.6	13.8	14.0
Black or African American only	14.7	15.3	16.8	45.8	45.8	46.1	25.2	26.0	23.2	14.3	13.0	13.9
American Indian and Alaska Native only	23.3	18.1	17.1	41.4	43.7	38.0	20.6	21.7	24.2	14.7	16.6	20.7
Asian only	22.6	21.2	22.8	47.8	49.7	49.1	20.7	20.3	19.7	8.9	8.8	8.3
Native Hawaiian and Other Pacific Islander only	*	*	. . .	*	*	. . .	*	*	. . .	*	*	. . .
Two or more races	11.1	13.5	. . .	44.9	43.7	. . .	23.0	27.3	. . .	21.0	15.4	. . .
Hispanic Origin and Race [2,3]												
Hispanic or Latino	25.3	25.7	24.9	42.9	41.5	42.3	20.3	21.1	20.3	11.5	11.7	12.5
Mexican	27.8	28.8	28.9	42.5	40.5	40.8	18.8	19.3	18.5	11.0	11.5	11.8
Not Hispanic or Latino	14.1	14.5	15.4	46.3	46.0	46.7	25.6	25.8	24.0	14.0	13.7	13.9
White only	13.5	14.0	14.7	46.2	45.8	46.6	26.1	26.1	24.4	14.2	14.2	14.3
Black or African American only	14.6	15.3	16.9	45.9	45.7	46.1	25.3	26.0	23.1	14.2	13.1	13.8
Respondent-Assessed Health Status [2]												
Fair or poor	8.7	10.1	7.8	23.2	22.2	23.3	28.8	29.4	29.0	39.3	38.3	39.9
Good to excellent	16.4	16.6	17.2	48.1	47.7	48.4	24.5	24.9	23.3	10.9	10.8	11.1
Poverty Status [2,4]												
Poor	20.9	19.9	20.6	37.8	38.3	37.8	23.7	23.9	22.7	17.6	17.9	18.9
Near poor	19.8	20.0	20.1	41.5	41.2	43.3	23.6	23.8	21.7	15.1	15.0	14.9
Nonpoor	13.7	14.2	14.5	48.4	47.6	48.7	25.4	25.7	24.2	12.6	12.4	12.6
Hispanic Origin, Race and Poverty Status [2,3,4]												
Hispanic or Latino												
Poor	29.9	30.0	30.2	37.0	35.4	34.8	18.5	18.9	19.9	14.6	15.7	15.0
Near poor	28.6	30.2	28.7	40.2	37.8	39.7	20.6	19.9	20.4	10.5	12.2	11.2
Nonpoor	20.7	21.1	18.9	47.7	46.8	48.8	21.2	22.3	20.4	10.3	9.8	11.9
Not Hispanic or Latino White only												
Poor	17.0	16.1	17.0	37.5	38.4	38.3	25.9	25.6	23.9	19.5	19.9	20.9
Near poor	16.6	16.7	17.3	41.0	41.3	44.1	24.9	25.0	22.2	17.4	17.0	16.3
Nonpoor	12.5	13.3	13.8	48.1	47.3	48.2	26.3	26.4	24.9	13.1	13.1	13.1
Not Hispanic or Latino Black or African American only												
Poor	15.7	17.3	17.4	38.1	39.7	38.5	26.5	25.9	23.4	19.6	17.1	20.7
Near poor	15.4	15.6	18.8	44.2	43.4	43.7	25.9	26.9	22.9	14.5	14.1	14.5
Nonpoor	13.7	14.4	15.6	50.6	49.1	51.7	24.3	25.3	22.7	11.4	11.1	10.0

[1] Includes all other races not shown separately, unknown poverty status, and unknown health insurance status.

[2] Estimates are age adjusted to the year 2000 standard population using six age groups: under 18 years, 18–44 years, 45–54 years, 55–64 years, 65–74 years, and 75 years and over.

[3] The race groups, White, Black, American Indian and Alaska Native (AI/AN), Asian, Native Hawaiian and Other Pacific Islander, and two or more races, include persons of Hispanic and non-Hispanic origin. Persons of Hispanic origin may be of any race.

[4] Poor persons are defined as having a total income below the poverty threshold. Near poor persons have incomes of 100 percent to less than 200 percent of the poverty threshold. Nonpoor persons have incomes of 200 percent or more than the poverty threshold.

* = Figure does not meet standards of reliability or precision.

. . . = Not available.

Table III-28.   Health Care Visits to Doctors' Offices, Emergency Departments, and Home Visits Within the Past 12 Months, According to Selected Characteristics, Selected Years, 1997–2003—*Continued*

(Percent.)

Characteristic	Number of health care visits											
	None			1–3 visits			4–9 visits			10 or more visits		
	2003	2002	1997	2003	2002	1997	2003	2002	1997	2003	2002	1997
Health Insurance Status [4,5]												
Under 65 years of age												
Insured	12.8	13.3	14.3	49.1	48.7	49.0	25.2	25.1	23.6	12.9	12.9	13.1
Private	13.2	13.6	14.7	51.1	50.5	50.6	24.6	24.8	23.1	11.1	11.1	11.6
Medicaid	9.9	9.9	9.8	35.2	34.9	35.5	28.1	27.4	26.5	26.8	27.7	28.2
Uninsured	38.1	36.3	33.7	42.4	42.1	42.8	13.4	14.7	15.3	6.1	6.9	8.2
65 years of age and over												
Medicare HMO	5.4	7.7	8.9	30.6	30.9	35.8	38.9	40.9	33.1	25.2	20.5	22.3
Private	4.8	6.1	7.3	33.5	32.0	35.9	35.9	38.1	34.0	25.8	23.8	22.7
Medicaid	*4.9	9.3	9.3	21.1	15.8	19.2	29.7	34.2	27.9	44.3	40.8	43.7
Medicare fee-for-service only	11.6	14.4	15.5	28.7	33.4	34.0	35.3	30.7	28.1	24.5	21.4	22.4
Poverty Status and Health Insurance Status [4,5]												
Under 65 years of age												
Poor												
Insured	13.0	12.5	14.0	40.8	41.4	39.2	25.9	26.5	25.1	20.4	19.5	21.7
Uninsured	41.8	39.8	37.0	38.4	37.5	39.6	13.5	13.6	14.4	6.3	9.1	8.9
Near poor												
Insured	13.8	14.9	15.8	44.5	44.1	46.2	24.8	24.5	22.3	16.8	16.6	15.8
Uninsured	37.9	38.1	34.8	40.0	39.8	42.0	15.4	16.3	15.1	6.7	5.8	8.1
Nonpoor												
Insured	12.5	13.1	13.8	51.0	50.3	51.0	25.2	25.1	23.6	11.4	11.5	11.7
Uninsured	35.5	32.8	29.7	47.3	46.3	46.0	11.6	14.2	16.3	5.6	6.7	8.0
Geographic Region												
Northeast	10.4	11.0	13.2	47.6	45.5	45.9	27.0	27.7	26.0	15.0	15.7	14.9
Midwest	14.2	14.4	15.9	47.2	47.7	47.7	25.4	25.0	22.8	13.2	13.0	13.6
South	16.5	17.4	17.2	45.1	44.7	46.1	24.8	25.2	23.3	13.6	12.8	13.5
West	21.0	19.9	19.1	44.2	44.2	44.8	22.2	23.0	22.8	12.6	12.9	13.3
Location of Residence												
Within MSA [6]	16.0	15.8	16.2	45.9	45.8	46.4	24.8	25.1	23.7	13.3	13.3	13.7
Outside MSA [6]	15.0	16.3	17.3	45.6	44.1	45.4	24.9	25.6	23.3	14.5	14.0	13.9

[4]Poor persons are defined as having a total income below the poverty threshold. Near poor persons have incomes of 100 percent to less than 200 percent of the poverty threshold. Nonpoor persons have incomes of 200 percent or more than the poverty threshold.

[5]Health insurance categories are mutually exclusive. Persons who reported both Medicaid and private coverage are classified as having private coverage. Persons 65 years of age and over who reported Medicare HMO (health maintenance organization) and some other type of health insurance coverage are classified as having Medicare HMO.

[6]MSA = Metropolitan Statistical Area.

* = Figure does not meet standards of reliability or precision.

TABLE III-29. INFLUENZA AND PNEUMOCOCCAL VACCINATIONS AMONG PERSONS 18 YEARS OF AGE AND OVER, ACCORDING TO SELECTED CHARACTERISTICS, SELECTED YEARS, 1989–2003

In 2003, 29 percent of adults received influenza vaccinations, a rate three times as high as that in 1989 but only slightly higher than that in 2002. The frequency of these vaccinations increased substantially with age, and climbed to 71 percent for persons age 75 years and over. Medicare generally paid for the vaccinations of older persons.

The percentage of adults who had received a pneumococcal vaccinaton at any time was 16.3 percent in 2003. This percentage also rose significantly with advancing age.

Table III-29. Influenza and Pneumococcal Vaccinations Among Persons 18 Years of Age and Over, According to Selected Characteristics, Selected Years, 1989–2003

(Percent.)

Characteristic	Percent receiving influenza vaccination in the past 12 months [1]				Percent ever receiving pneumococcal vaccination [2]			
	2003	2002	1995	1989	2003	2002	1995	1989
Total, age-adjusted [3,4]	29.1	28.2	23.5	9.5	16.3	16.4	11.7	4.6
Total, crude [4]	29.0	28.0	24.4	9.1	16.0	16.0	12.5	4.4
Age								
18–44 years	15.4	14.8	12.3	3.3	5.1	5.3	6.3	2.1
18–24 years	14.9	13.3	11.2	3.2	6.4	5.7	10.3	2.9
25–44 years	15.5	15.3	12.5	3.3	4.7	5.2	5.4	1.8
45–64 years	32.9	30.7	24.5	8.8	14.0	13.4	9.1	3.7
45–54 years	27.7	25.9	21.0	5.6	9.8	8.7	6.9	2.3
55–64 years	40.4	37.9	29.2	12.6	20.0	20.4	12.1	5.2
65 years and over	65.5	65.7	57.0	30.4	55.6	56.0	32.9	14.1
65–74 years	60.5	60.9	54.0	28.0	49.8	50.2	30.3	13.1
75 years and over	71.0	71.3	61.2	34.2	62.1	62.8	36.7	15.7
50 years and over	48.9	47.7	43.0	19.9	33.1	33.3	22.4	9.0
Sex [3]								
Male	27.9	27.1	22.9	9.5	15.9	16.5	13.2	4.7
Female	30.3	29.4	24.2	9.6	16.6	16.3	10.7	4.5
Sex and Age								
Male								
18–44 years	14.3	13.6	12.1	3.2	5.7	5.6	8.9	2.4
45–54 years	25.3	22.9	18.3	4.6	8.6	8.8	7.4	2.2
55–64 years	37.4	35.8	25.7	11.8	18.2	19.0	11.2	4.9
65–74 years	60.4	62.1	54.1	28.3	47.9	49.3	28.9	12.6
75 years and over	73.2	74.1	65.3	37.5	61.2	65.2	39.7	16.3
50 years and over	46.8	45.1	40.9	19.2	30.2	31.5	21.2	8.4
Female								
18–44 years	16.4	16.0	12.3	3.3	4.5	5.0	4.4	1.8
45–54 years	30.1	28.8	23.3	6.5	11.0	8.7	6.4	2.5
55–64 years	43.1	39.9	32.1	13.2	21.6	21.7	12.8	5.4
65–74 years	60.7	59.9	53.9	27.8	51.4	51.0	31.3	13.5
75 years and over	69.6	69.6	59.3	32.3	62.7	61.4	35.3	15.3
50 years and over	50.7	49.8	44.4	20.6	35.4	34.9	23.2	9.4
Race [3,5]								
White only	29.5	28.7	24.0	9.8	16.5	16.8	11.5	4.7
Black or African American only	24.4	23.9	20.5	7.3	14.1	13.1	12.0	3.7
American Indian and Alaska Native only	24.3	29.2	22.6	12.8	16.1	*16.2	20.1	9.4
Asian only	28.9	28.4	23.8	5.7	11.3	11.0	8.7	*
Native Hawaiian and Other Pacific Islander only	*	*	. . .	. . .	*	*	. . .	. . .
Two or more races	34.2	30.8	. . .	. . .	18.7	21.9	. . .	. . .
Hispanic Origin and Race [3,5]								
Hispanic or Latino	21.2	21.4	21.1	8.0	10.0	9.2	9.6	3.6
Mexican	20.8	21.0	22.4	7.3	10.1	9.3	8.9	4.0
Not Hispanic or Latino	30.0	28.9	23.9	9.5	16.8	16.9	11.8	4.6
White only	30.6	29.3	24.3	9.8	17.1	17.3	11.7	4.7
Black or African American only	24.5	24.0	20.5	7.2	14.1	13.2	11.8	3.6
Education [6,7]								
25 years and over								
No high school diploma or GED	24.6	24.8	22.6	9.5	15.7	16.1	12.2	4.6
High school diploma or GED	29.4	29.2	25.0	10.5	17.9	18.6	13.1	5.0
Some college or more	34.4	33.3	26.9	11.9	18.9	19.1	13.3	5.8

[1] Respondents were asked, "During the past 12 months, have you had a flu shot? A flu shot is usually given in the fall and protects against influenza for the flu season."

[2] Respondents were asked, "Have you ever had a pneumonia shot? This shot is usually given only once or twice in a person's lifetime and is different from the flu shot. It is also called the pneumococcal vaccine."

[3] Estimates are age adjusted to the year 2000 standard population using five age groups: 18-44 years, 45-54 years, 55-64 years, 65-74 years, and 75 years and over. Age-adjusted estimates in this table may differ from other age-adjusted estimates based on the same data and presented elsewhere if different age groups are used in the adjustment procedure.

[4] Includes all other races not shown separately.

[5] The race groups, White, Black, American Indian and Alaska Native, Asian, Native Hawaiian and Other Pacific Islander, and two or more races, include persons of Hispanic and non-Hispanic origin. Persons of Hispanic origin may be of any race.

[6] Estimates are for persons 25 years of age and over and are age adjusted to the year 2000 standard population using five age groups: 25-44 years, 45-54 years, 55-64 years, 65-74 years, and 75 years and over.

[7] GED stands for General Educational Development high school equivalency diploma.

* = Figure does not meet standards of reliability or precision.

. . . = Not available.

Table III-29. Influenza and Pneumococcal Vaccinations Among Persons 18 Years of Age and Over, According to Selected Characteristics, Selected Years, 1989–2003—*Continued*

(Percent.)

Characteristic	Percent receiving influenza vaccination in the past 12 months [1]				Percent ever receiving pneumococcal vaccination [2]			
	2003	2002	1995	1989	2003	2002	1995	1989
Poverty Status [3, 8]								
Poor	23.9	24.0	21.1	9.4	15.9	14.7	12.4	5.2
Near poor	25.6	24.5	22.2	9.6	17.9	15.8	12.9	5.0
Nonpoor	30.8	29.8	25.1	10.3	16.1	16.9	11.7	4.7
Hispanic Origin and Race and Poverty Status [3, 5, 8]								
Hispanic or Latino								
Poor	18.4	20.2	19.3	7.3	8.9	8.4	9.2	*3.3
Near poor	18.1	19.7	22.5	10.3	8.1	8.5	11.0	4.3
Nonpoor	24.5	23.3	23.3	9.2	12.1	10.4	8.9	3.8
Not Hispanic or Latino								
White only								
Poor	26.1	23.4	22.7	10.2	18.8	16.4	14.4	6.2
Near poor	26.9	25.6	22.2	9.8	19.8	17.3	13.3	5.0
Nonpoor	31.9	30.8	25.4	10.4	16.5	17.5	11.6	4.8
Black or African American only								
Poor	23.2	26.8	20.2	7.9	14.3	12.9	9.7	4.3
Near poor	25.2	22.5	19.0	6.7	16.3	13.8	11.9	4.2
Nonpoor	24.4	23.7	22.8	8.3	13.3	13.1	13.7	3.2
Geographic Region [3]								
Northeast	29.8	28.0	21.8	8.4	14.9	15.4	9.8	3.3
Midwest	29.6	29.2	23.6	9.3	16.4	16.9	11.0	4.4
South	29.7	27.8	24.6	9.8	17.2	16.1	12.4	5.0
West	26.9	28.1	23.6	10.4	15.9	17.2	13.4	5.6
Location of Residence [3]								
Within MSA [9]	29.0	28.1	23.5	9.5	16.1	16.2	11.7	4.6
Outside MSA [9]	29.6	28.8	26.3	9.3	17.3	17.1	12.6	4.2

[1] Respondents were asked, "During the past 12 months, have you had a flu shot? A flu shot is usually given in the fall and protects against influenza for the flu season."

[2] Respondents were asked, "Have you ever had a pneumonia shot? This shot is usually given only once or twice in a person's lifetime and is different from the flu shot. It is also called the pneumococcal vaccine."

[3] Estimates are age adjusted to the year 2000 standard population using five age groups: 18-44 years, 45-54 years, 55-64 years, 65-74 years, and 75 years and over. Age-adjusted estimates in this table may differ from other age-adjusted estimates based on the same data and presented elsewhere if different age groups are used in the adjustment procedure.

[5] The race groups, White, Black, American Indian and Alaska Native, Asian, Native Hawaiian and Other Pacific Islander, and two or more races, include persons of Hispanic and non-Hispanic origin. Persons of Hispanic origin may be of any race.

[8] Poor persons are defined as having a total income below the poverty threshold. Near poor persons have incomes of 100 percent to less than 200 percent of the poverty threshold. Nonpoor persons have incomes of 200 percent or more than the poverty threshold.

[9] MSA = Metropolitan Statistical Area.

* = Figure does not meet standards of reliability or precision.

TABLE III-30. VACCINATIONS OF CHILDREN 19–35 MONTHS OF AGE FOR SELECTED DISEASES, ACCORDING TO RACE, HISPANIC ORIGIN, POVERTY STATUS, AND RESIDENCE IN METROPOLITAN STATISTICAL AREA (MSA), SELECTED YEARS, 1995–2003

According to a 2003 sample survey, 81 percent of all children 19 to 35 months of age (including 75 percent of Black children) received a combined series of shots (4:3:1:3), which consisted of 4 or more doses of diphtheria and tetanus toxoids and pertussis vaccine (DTP) or variants of these items, 3 or more doses of any polio virus vaccine, 1 or more doses of a measles-containing vaccine (MCV), and 3 or more doses of Haemophilus influenzae type b vaccine (Hib).

Children who did not receive the combined series (4:3:1:3) frequently received vaccinations in other combi-

Table III-30. Vaccinations of Children 19–35 Months of Age for Selected Diseases, According to Race, Hispanic Origin, Poverty Status, and Residence In Metropolitan Statistical Area (MSA), Selected Years, 1995–2003

(Percent.)

Vaccination and year	Race and Hispanic origin								Poverty status		Location of residence		
	Not Hispanic or Latino							Hispanic or Latino [2]	Below poverty	At or above poverty	Inside MSA		Outside MSA
	All	White	Black or African American	American Indian or Alaskan Native	Asian [1]	Native Hawaiian or Pacific Islander [1]	Two or more races				Central city	Remaining areas	
PERCENT													
Combined Series (4:3:1:3) [3]													
2003	81	84	75	77	81	*	81	79	76	83	80	82	81
2002	78	80	71	*	83	*	74	76	72	79	75	80	77
2001	77	79	71	76	77	...	...	77	72	79	75	78	79
2000	76	79	71	69	75	...	...	73	71	78	73	78	79
1999	78	81	74	75	77	...	...	75	73	81	77	79	80
1998	79	82	73	78	79	...	...	75	74	82	77	81	81
1995	74	76	70	69	76	...	...	68	67	77	72	75	75
DTP/DT/DTaP (4 or more doses)													
2003	85	88	80	80	89	*	84	82	80	87	84	86	83
2002	82	84	76	*	88	*	78	79	75	84	79	84	80
2001	82	84	76	77	84	...	...	83	77	84	81	83	82
2000	82	84	76	75	85	...	...	79	76	84	80	83	83
1999	83	86	79	80	87	...	...	80	79	85	82	84	83
1998	84	87	77	83	89	...	...	81	80	86	82	85	85
1995	78	80	74	71	84	...	...	75	71	81	77	79	78
Polio (3 or more doses)													
2003	92	93	89	91	91	90	91	90	89	93	91	92	92
2002	90	91	87	*	92	95	87	90	88	91	89	91	90
2001	89	90	85	88	90	...	...	91	87	90	88	90	91
2000	90	91	87	90	93	...	...	88	87	90	88	90	91
1999	90	90	87	88	90	...	...	89	87	91	89	90	90
1998	91	92	88	85	93	...	...	89	90	92	89	91	93
1995	88	89	84	86	90	...	...	87	85	89	87	88	89
Measels, Mumps, and Rubella													
2003	93	93	92	92	96	*	94	93	92	93	93	93	92
2002	92	93	90	84	95	94	89	91	90	92	90	93	90
2001	91	92	89	94	90	...	...	92	89	92	91	92	91
2000	91	92	88	87	90	...	...	90	89	91	90	91	91
1999	92	92	90	92	93	...	...	90	90	92	91	92	90
1998	92	93	89	91	92	...	...	91	90	93	92	92	93
1995	90	91	87	88	95	...	...	88	86	91	90	90	89
Hib (3 or more doses)													
2003	94	95	92	89	91	*	93	93	91	95	94	94	94
2002	93	94	92	*	95	93	90	92	90	94	92	94	93
2001	93	94	90	91	92	...	...	93	90	94	91	94	93
2000	93	95	93	90	92	...	...	91	90	95	92	94	95
1999	94	95	92	91	90	...	...	92	91	95	92	95	93
1998	93	95	90	90	92	...	...	92	91	95	92	94	94
1995	91	93	88	93	90	...	...	89	88	93	91	92	92
Hepatitis B (3 or more doses)													
2003	92	93	92	90	94	*	93	91	91	93	92	93	93
2002	90	91	88	*	94	94	84	90	88	90	89	91	90
2001	89	90	85	86	90	...	...	90	87	90	88	90	89
2000	90	91	89	91	91	...	...	88	87	91	89	90	92
1999	88	89	87	*	88	...	...	87	87	89	87	89	88
1998	87	88	84	82	89	...	...	86	85	88	85	88	87
1995	68	68	66	52	80	...	...	70	65	69	69	71	59
Varicella [4]													
2003	85	84	85	81	91	*	86	86	84	85	86	86	80
2002	81	79	83	71	87	*	79	82	79	81	81	83	75
2001	76	75	75	69	82	...	...	80	74	77	78	78	68
2000	68	66	67	62	77	...	...	70	64	69	69	70	60
1999	58	56	58	*	64	...	...	61	55	58	59	61	47
1998	43	42	42	28	53	...	...	47	41	44	45	45	34
PCV (3 or more doses) [5]													
2003	68	71	62	60	71	*	66	66	62	71	68	71	61
2002	41	44	34	33	55	*	38	37	33	43	41	45	32

Note: Final estimates from the National Immunization Survey include an adjustment for children with missing immunization provider data. Poverty status is based on family income and family size using Census Bureau poverty thresholds.

[1] Prior to the data year 2002 the category "Asian" included Native Hawaiian and Other Pacific Islander.
[2] May be of any race.
[3] The 4:3:1:3 combined series consists of four or more doses of diphtheria and tetanus toxoids and pertussis vaccine (DTP), diphtheria and tetanus toxoids (DT), or diphtheria and tetanus toxoids and acellular pertussis vaccine (DTaP); three or more doses of any poliovirus vaccine; one or more doses of a measles-containing vaccine (MCV); and three or more doses of Haemophilus influenzae type b vaccine (Hib).
[4] Recommended in 1996. Data collection for varicella began in July 1996.
[5] Pneumococcal conjugate vaccine. Recommended in 2000. Data collection for PCV began in July 2001.
* = Figure does not meet standards of reliability or precision.
. . . = Not available.

nations. For example, 92 percent of all children received 3 doses or more of polio vaccine (including 89 percent of Black children), and 93 percent were immunized for measles, mumps, and rubella (including 92 percent of Black children).

The table also shows differences between children raised above and below the poverty line. Children raised below the poverty line received vaccinations for the combined series at a rate of 7 percentage points less than children raised above the poverty line.

TABLE III-31. VACCINATION COVERAGE AMONG CHILDREN 19–35 MONTHS OF AGE, ACCORDING TO GEOGRAPHIC DIVISION, STATE, AND SELECTED URBAN AREAS, 1995–2003

This table reports the frequency of vaccinations for the combined series (4:3:1:3) among children 19 to 35 months of age. For the United States in 2003, the frequency of vaccination was 81 percent, up from 74 percent in 1995. Among the states and regions, New England had the highest rate of vaccination in 2003, with states in the region posting rates between 87 and 95 percent. States with low coverage rates were Oklahoma and Louisiana (both with rates of 72 percent), and Texas, Wyoming, West Virginia, and the District of Columbia (each with a vaccination coverage rate of 77 percent).

Among urban areas, Boston, Los Angeles, and Santa Clara County (in California), had high rates of vaccination coverage. The immunization rate was low in Newark, New Jersey (74 percent); New Orleans, Louisiana (74 percent); and Detroit, Michigan (71 percent).

Table III-30. Vaccinations of Children 19–35 Months of Age for Selected Diseases, According to Race, Hispanic Origin, Poverty Status and Residence In Metropolitan Statistical Area (MSA), 1995–2003—Continued

(Percent.)

Vaccination and year	Not Hispanic or Latino				Hispanic or Latino [2]	
	White		Black or African American		Below poverty	At or above poverty
	Below poverty	At or above poverty	Below poverty	At or above poverty		
Combined Series (4:3:1:3) [3]						
2003	79	85	70	79	78	81
2002	72	81	68	72	75	76
2001	71	80	69	74	73	79
2000	73	80	69	72	70	74
1999	76	82	72	77	73	78
1998	77	83	72	74	73	79
1995	69	78	70	73	63	72

Note: Final estimates from the National Immunization Survey include an adjustment for children with missing immunization provider data. Poverty status is based on family income and family size using Census Bureau poverty thresholds.

[2]May be of any race.

[3]The 4:3:1:3 combined series consists of four or more doses of diphtheria and tetanus toxoids and pertussis vaccine (DTP), diphtheria and tetanus toxoids (DT), or diphtheria and tetanus toxoids and acellular pertussis vaccine (DTaP), three or more doses of any poliovirus vaccine, one or more doses of a measles-containing vaccine (MCV), and three or more doses of Haemophilus influenzae type b vaccine (Hib).

Table III-31. Vaccination Coverage Among Children 19–35 Months of Age, According to Geographic Division, State, and Selected Urban Areas, 1995–2003

(Percent.)

Geographic division and state	2003	2002	2001	2000	1999	1998	1997	1996	1995
PERCENT OF CHILDREN 19–35 MONTHS OF AGE WITH 4:3:1:3 SERIES [1]									
United States	81	78	77	76	78	79	76	76	74
New England									
Connecticut	95	86	84	85	86	90	86	88	86
Maine	82	83	82	83	83	86	87	86	88
Massachusetts	92	89	81	85	85	87	88	87	81
New Hampshire	88	87	84	83	85	82	85	83	89
Rhode Island	87	86	84	82	87	86	82	84	83
Vermont	90	87	88	83	91	86	87	87	87
Middle Atlantic									
New Jersey	76	80	76	76	81	82	76	75	70
New York	82	81	81	75	81	85	75	80	74
Pennsylvania	87	77	82	78	86	83	79	79	77
East North Central									
Illinois	85	80	76	75	77	78	74	75	78
Indiana	82	78	74	76	74	78	72	70	74
Michigan	83	84	74	75	74	78	75	75	68
Ohio	84	77	75	72	78	78	72	78	71
Wisconsin	83	82	83	80	85	78	81	77	74
West North Central									
Iowa	83	80	79	83	83	82	77	81	83
Kansas	78	73	76	76	79	82	84	72	70
Minnesota	84	79	79	86	85	82	78	84	75
Missouri	84	77	78	78	75	85	79	75	75
Nebraska	82	79	80	79	82	76	74	78	71
North Dakota	83	79	83	81	80	79	80	80	79
South Dakota	83	81	79	78	82	74	77	81	79
South Atlantic									
Delaware	80	81	79	75	78	79	80	81	68
District of Columbia	77	72	74	71	78	71	71	76	69
Florida	83	77	77	74	80	79	74	79	74
Georgia	77	82	80	81	82	80	78	81	77
Maryland	84	81	78	78	79	77	81	79	77
North Carolina	89	87	85	87	82	83	80	78	80
South Carolina	85	80	81	80	81	88	81	85	78
Virginia	85	77	78	74	80	80	72	76	69
West Virginia	77	79	81	76	81	82	81	71	71
East South Central									
Alabama	82	80	83	81	78	82	87	74	73
Kentucky	81	74	79	81	88	82	78	76	81
Mississippi	84	78	84	81	82	84	80	81	79
Tennessee	81	80	84	81	78	82	79	79	74
West South Central									
Arkansas	80	74	74	72	77	73	80	70	73
Louisiana	72	69	69	75	77	78	77	79	77
Oklahoma	72	67	76	71	73	75	70	72	74
Texas	77	71	74	69	72	74	74	71	71
Mountain									
Arizona	79	70	73	72	72	76	71	70	69
Colorado	69	64	75	74	76	76	74	80	75
Idaho	82	73	74	74	69	76	71	65	66
Montana	85	71	82	77	83	82	75	75	71
Nevada	78	78	72	74	73	76	70	67	67
New Mexico	77	67	71	68	73	71	73	78	74
Utah	80	79	74	77	80	76	69	65	65
Wyoming	77	77	81	79	83	80	75	77	71
Pacific									
Alaska	81	78	74	77	80	81	75	72	74
California	80	76	75	75	75	76	74	74	70
Hawaii	83	81	73	75	82	79	77	80	75
Oregon	79	75	73	79	72	76	72	70	71
Washington	80	73	76	77	75	81	79	78	76

Note: Urban areas were chosen because they were at a high risk for under-vaccination. Final estimates from the National Immunization Survey include an adjustment for children with missing immunization provider data.

[1] The 4:3:1:3 combined series consists of four or more doses of diphtheria and tetanus toxoids and pertussis vaccine (DTP), diphtheria and tetanus toxoids (DT), or diphtheria and tetanus toxoids and acellular pertussis vaccine (DTaP); three or more doses of any poliovirus vaccine; one or more doses of a measles-containing vaccine (MCV); and three or more doses of Haemophilus influenzae type b vaccine (Hib).

Table III-31. Vaccination Coverage Among Children 19–35 Months of Age, According to Geographic Division, State, and Selected Urban Areas, 1995–2003—*Continued*

(Percent.)

Geographic division and state	2003	2002	2001	2000	1999	1998	1997	1996	1995
New England									
Boston, Massachusetts	90	80	85	79	84	89	86	85	85
Middle Atlantic									
New York City, New York	77	81	76	68	78	81	72	78	72
Newark, New Jersey	74	60	64	63	67	64	68	64	67
Philadelphia, Pennsylvania	80	74	74	74	81	80	81	74	67
East North Central									
Chicago, Illinois	77	72	69	65	71	64	66	72	70
Cuyahoga County (Cleveland), Ohio	75	74	73	73	74	75	70	79	72
Detroit, Michigan	71	66	63	59	66	70	60	60	54
Franklin County (Columbus), Ohio	83	84	78	77	78	78	73	80	75
Marion County (Indianapolis), Indiana	79	75	72	69	79	78	80	72	77
Milwaukee County (Milwaukee), Wisconsin	81	70	70	69	74	73	72	70	69
South Atlantic									
Baltimore, Maryland	81	75	72	70	72	81	84	80	*
District of Columbia	77	72	74	71	78	71	71	76	67
Duval County (Jacksonville), Florida	81	77	76	79	78	79	69	76	69
Fulton/DeKalb Counties (Atlanta), Georgia	75	79	75	80	83	71	74	76	*
Miami-Dade County (Miami), Florida	83	73	78	78	84	75	75	79	78
East South Central									
Davidson County (Nashville), Tennessee	83	80	82	73	73	80	76	80	72
Jefferson County (Birmingham), Alabama	83	82	87	79	85	85	83	76	86
Shelby County (Memphis), Tennessee	77	73	74	77	75	71	70	70	69
West South Central									
Bexar County (San Antonio), Texas	79	76	73	68	70	79	79	74	76
Dallas County (Dallas), Texas	75	76	67	67	72	71	75	68	70
El Paso County (El Paso), Texas	81	77	69	70	73	78	63	61	72
Houston, Texas	75	64	69	65	63	61	62	62	64
Orleans Parish (New Orleans), Louisiana	74	63	68	70	72	79	69	72	78
Mountain									
Maricopa County (Phoenix), Arizona	80	73	72	71	71	77	70	72	67
Pacific									
King County (Seattle), Washington	83	77	72	75	77	86	81	82	84
Los Angeles County (Los Angeles), California	84	77	73	77	76	76	72	75	68
San Diego County (San Diego), California	81	78	80	76	75	77	76	74	72
Santa Clara County (Santa Clara), California	85	84	77	76	82	84	69	80	76

Note: Urban areas were chosen because they were at a high risk for under-vaccination. Final estimates from the National Immunization Survey include an adjustment for children with missing immunization provider data.

* = Figure does not meet standards of reliability or precision.

TABLE III-32. NO HEALTH CARE VISITS TO AN OFFICE OR CLINIC WITHIN THE PAST 12 MONTHS AMONG CHILDREN UNDER 18 YEARS OF AGE, ACCORDING TO SELECTED CHARACTERISTICS, SELECTED ANNUAL AVERAGES, 1997–2003

Household interviews conducted on a sample basis indicated that, in 2002–2003, 12 percent of all children under 18 years of age had not received medical attention in a doctor's office or at a clinic during the previous 12 months. This percentage was slightly lower than that from 1997–1998 interview period. When medical visits of children under 6 years of age were compared with medical visits of children between 6 and 17 years of age, the younger age group showed a much higher rate of visits. No visits occurred for 6.2 percent of the younger group, while 14.5 percent of older children had no visits.

The percentage rate of no visits was high for both Hispanic children and for poor households. It was especially high for poor Hispanics. Insurance status contributed to considerable differences: an average of 31.8 percent of uninsured children had no medical visits during the 2002–2003 survey period, compared to 9.5 percent of children with insurance. When lack of insurance was combined with poverty status, the percentages of no visits for poor families increased even further: 21.6 percent of children under 6 years old had no visits, and 42.7 percent of children age 6–17 years had no medical visits. The West was the region with the highest percentage of children with no health care visits.

TABLE III-33. NO USUAL SOURCE OF HEALTH CARE AMONG CHILDREN UNDER 18 YEARS OF AGE, ACCORDING TO SELECTED CHARACTERISTICS, SELECTED ANNUAL AVERAGES, 1993–2003

In a household interview, the respondent was asked whether there was a regular place for a sick child in the household to receive medical care, or whether there was a regular place to seek out advice about the child's health. Persons who reported the emergency department of a hospital as their usual source of care were defined as having no usual source of care. The question was phrased slightly differently prior to 1997.

In 2002–2003, some 4.1 percent of children under 6 years old were reported to have no usual source of care, and 6.5 percent of children age 6 to 17 years old also had no usual source of care. These figures were smaller than those in 1993–1994. Hispanics had a greater than average frequency of no usual source of health care.

Medical insurance had a big impact: only 2.0 percent of insured children under 6 years old and 3.6 percent of children age 6 to 17 years lacked a usual source of medical care. For the uninsured, 25.5 percent of children under 6 years old and 30.6 percent of children 6 to 17 years old lacked a usual source of care.

TABLE III-34. EMERGENCY DEPARTMENT VISITS WITHIN THE PAST 12 MONTHS AMONG CHILDREN UNDER 18 YEARS OF AGE, ACCORDING TO SELECTED CHARACTERISTICS, SELECTED YEARS, 1997–2003

In 2002, 20.9 percent of children under 18 years old had one or more visits to the emergency department of a hospital. For children under 6 years old, 26.5 percent paid at least one visit to the ER, while those age 6 to 17 years had a visitation rate of 18.2 percent. Blacks made more frequent visits than Whites, especially among the younger age group.

Poor households made visits to emergency departments more frequently than nonpoor households, partly reflecting the lack of attachment to a physician by some of the poor. Also, many poor households have Medicaid insurance, and data show that Medicaid-covered families made frequent use of emergency departments: 35.1 percent of Medicaid-covered children under 6 years old made at least one visit to the ER; this rate dropped to 24.5 percent for Medicaid-covered children between 6 to 17 years old.

Visits to emergency departments occurred more frequently among residents outside of a metropolitan statistical area (MSA) than among those living within a metropolitan area.

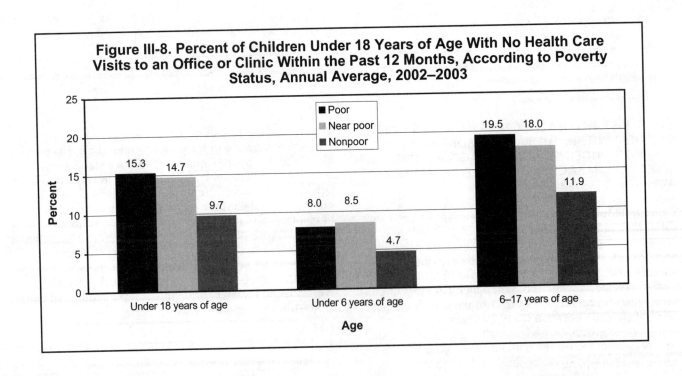

Figure III-8. Percent of Children Under 18 Years of Age With No Health Care Visits to an Office or Clinic Within the Past 12 Months, According to Poverty Status, Annual Average, 2002–2003

Table III-32. No Health Care Visits to an Office or Clinic Within the Past 12 Months Among Children Under 18 Years of Age, According to Selected Characteristics, Selected Annual Averages, 1997–2003

(Percent.)

Characteristic	Under 18 years of age			Under 6 years of age			6–17 years of age		
	2002–2003	2000–2001	1997–1998	2002–2003	2000–2001	1997–1998	2002–2003	2000–2001	1997–1998
PERCENT OF CHILDREN WITHOUT A HEALTH CARE VISIT [1]									
All children [2]	11.8	12.9	12.8	6.2	6.6	5.7	14.5	15.9	16.3
Race [3]									
White only	11.7	12.1	12.2	6.3	6.6	5.5	14.3	14.7	15.5
Black or African American only	11.4	15.0	14.3	6.1	6.3	6.5	13.9	19.0	18.1
American Indian and Alaska Native only	*15.6	22.4	13.8	*	*	*	*18.6	*25.0	*17.6
Asian only	17.1	15.2	16.3	*7.8	*8.8	*5.6	21.9	18.9	22.1
Native Hawaiian and Other Pacific Islander only	*	*	. . .	*	*	. . .	*	*	. . .
Two or more races	8.5	8.5	. . .	*	*	. . .	12.4	13.5	. . .
Hispanic Origin and Race [3]									
Hispanic or Latino	18.6	19.8	19.3	10.1	10.0	9.7	23.5	25.5	25.3
Not Hispanic or Latino	10.3	11.4	11.6	5.3	5.8	4.8	12.6	14.0	14.9
White only	9.7	10.4	10.7	5.0	5.5	4.3	11.8	12.6	13.7
Black or African American only	11.4	14.7	14.5	6.0	6.5	6.5	13.9	18.4	18.3
Poverty Status [4]									
Poor	15.3	18.2	17.6	8.0	9.9	8.1	19.5	22.8	23.6
Near poor	14.7	17.0	16.2	8.5	9.2	7.2	18.0	21.1	20.8
Nonpoor	9.7	9.9	9.9	4.7	4.5	4.1	11.9	12.3	12.6
Hispanic Origin, Race and Poverty Status [3, 4]									
Hispanic or Latino									
Poor	20.6	23.6	23.2	10.5	11.6	11.7	26.9	30.8	31.1
Near poor	21.2	22.6	20.9	11.4	13.4	9.7	26.8	28.0	28.1
Nonpoor	14.6	14.1	13.4	8.3	5.1	7.2	17.8	18.8	16.8
Not Hispanic or Latino									
White only									
Poor	12.4	15.1	14.0	*6.6	*9.6	*5.6	15.7	18.2	19.7
Near poor	12.2	14.1	14.1	7.8	7.5	6.0	14.6	17.4	18.0
Nonpoor	8.7	8.9	9.2	3.9	4.3	3.6	10.7	10.8	11.7
Black or African American only									
Poor	12.6	16.1	15.8	*6.9	*8.2	7.6	15.4	20.1	20.5
Near poor	11.5	16.7	16.4	*6.1	*7.1	*7.7	13.8	21.2	20.4
Nonpoor	10.5	12.3	11.8	*5.3	*4.4	*4.1	12.9	15.5	14.8
Health Insurance Status [5]									
Insured	9.5	10.6	10.4	5.1	5.2	4.5	11.7	13.2	13.4
Private	9.5	10.4	10.4	4.9	4.7	4.3	11.5	12.9	13.1
Medicaid	9.3	11.1	10.1	5.3	6.3	5.0	12.1	14.2	14.4
Uninsured	31.8	30.8	28.8	18.5	18.8	14.6	37.0	35.9	34.9
Poverty Status and Health Insurance Status [4]									
Poor									
Insured	11.2	13.2	13.0	6.1	7.5	6.0	14.3	16.6	17.8
Uninsured	36.8	37.0	34.3	21.6	20.8	18.2	42.7	44.3	41.3
Near poor									
Insured	11.0	13.4	12.6	6.4	6.5	4.9	13.6	17.2	16.7
Uninsured	33.7	31.8	28.2	21.0	21.9	16.0	39.2	36.3	33.7
Nonpoor									
Insured	8.6	9.1	9.0	4.3	4.1	3.8	10.6	11.3	11.4
Uninsured	26.0	23.0	22.7	*12.8	11.8	*7.8	30.5	27.1	28.7
Geographic Region									
Northeast	5.1	6.5	7.0	3.1	4.6	3.1	6.1	7.4	8.9
Midwest	10.5	10.5	12.2	4.8	5.3	5.9	13.3	12.9	15.3
South	13.1	15.2	14.3	7.1	7.4	5.6	16.1	19.0	18.5
West	16.5	17.0	16.3	8.9	8.2	7.9	20.3	21.5	20.7
Location of Residence									
Within MSA [6]	11.4	12.4	12.3	6.0	6.6	5.4	14.1	15.3	15.9
Outside MSA [6]	13.3	14.8	14.6	7.4	6.8	6.9	16.0	18.2	17.9

[1] Respondents were asked how many times a doctor or other health care professional was seen in the past 12 months at a doctor's office, clinic, or some other place. Excluded are visits to emergency rooms, hospitalizations, home visits, and telephone calls. Beginning in 2000, dental visits were also excluded.
[2] Includes all other races not shown separately, unknown poverty status, and unknown health insurance status.
[3] The race groups, White, Black, American Indian and Alaska Native (AI/AN), Asian, Native Hawaiian and Other Pacific Islander, and two or more races, include persons of Hispanic and non-Hispanic origin. Persons of Hispanic origin may be of any race.
[4] Poor persons are defined as having a total income below the poverty threshold. Near poor persons have incomes of 100 percent to less than 200 percent of the poverty threshold. Nonpoor persons have incomes of 200 percent or more than the poverty threshold.
[5] Health insurance categories are mutually exclusive. Persons who reported both Medicaid and private coverage are classified as having private coverage. Starting in 1997, Medicaid includes state-sponsored health plans and the State Children's Health Insurance Program (SCHIP).
[6] MSA = Metropolitan Statistical Area.
* = Figure does not meet standards of reliability or precision.
. . . = Not available.

Table III-33. No Usual Source of Health Care Among Children Under 18 Years of Age, According to Selected Characteristics, Selected Annual Averages, 1993–2003

(Percent.)

Characteristic	Percent of children without a usual source of health care [1]								
	Under 18 years of age			Under 6 years of age			6–17 years of age		
	2002–2003	2000–2001	1993–1994[2]	2002–2003	2000–2001	1993–1994[2]	2002–2003	2000–2001	1993–1994[2]
PERCENT OF CHILDREN WITHOUT A USUAL SOURCE OF HEALTH CARE									
All children [3]	5.7	6.5	7.7	4.1	4.4	5.2	6.5	7.4	9.0
Race [4]									
White only	5.2	5.7	7.0	3.9	4.2	4.7	5.8	6.4	8.3
Black or African American only	6.7	7.4	10.3	3.3	4.0	7.6	8.2	8.9	11.9
American Indian and Alaska Native only	*	*8.8	*9.3	*	*	*	*	*	*8.7
Asian only	10.3	9.9	9.7	*	*7.4	*3.4	13.3	11.3	13.5
Native Hawaiian and Other Pacific Islander only	*	*	. . .	*	*	. . .	*	*	. . .
Two or more races	6.3	6.0	. . .	*6.7	*	. . .	*6.0	*7.9	. . .
Hispanic Origin and Race [4]									
Hispanic or Latino	12.1	14.2	14.3	8.3	9.3	9.3	14.3	17.0	17.7
Not Hispanic or Latino	4.3	4.8	6.7	3.0	3.2	4.4	5.0	5.6	7.8
White only	3.4	3.9	5.7	2.7	2.8	3.7	3.7	4.4	6.7
Black or African American only	6.7	7.4	10.2	3.3	4.0	7.7	8.2	8.9	11.6
Poverty Status [5]									
Poor	10.6	12.5	13.9	7.1	7.6	9.4	12.6	15.2	16.8
Near poor	8.4	9.9	9.8	6.6	7.3	6.7	9.5	11.3	11.6
Nonpoor	3.3	3.5	3.7	1.9	2.2	1.8	3.9	4.1	4.6
Hispanic Origin, Race, and Poverty Status [4,5]									
Hispanic or Latino									
Poor	15.0	20.0	19.6	10.1	12.3	12.7	18.1	24.7	24.8
Near poor	15.0	16.4	15.3	10.6	11.6	9.9	17.6	19.2	18.9
Nonpoor	7.0	7.1	5.0	*4.4	4.2	*2..7	8.3	8.6	6.5
Not Hispanic or Latino									
White only									
Poor	7.2	9.2	10.2	*6.2	*	6.5	7.7	11.0	12.7
Near poor	5.2	6.5	8.7	*4.8	5.1	6.3	5.5	7.2	10.1
Nonpoor	2.4	2.6	3.4	1.4	1.7	1.6	2.8	3.0	4.2
Black or African American only									
Poor	9.6	9.1	13.7	*	*4.7	10.9	12.7	11.3	15.5
Near poor	6.7	9.3	9.1	*	*5.8	*6.0	7.6	11.0	10.8
Nonpoor	4.3	4.7	4.6	*2.7	*	*	5.1	5.7	5.8
Health Insurance Status [6]									
Insured	3.1	3.5	5.0	2.0	2.5	3.3	3.6	4.0	5.9
Private	2.4	2.9	3.8	1.3	1.9	1.9	2.8	3.4	4.6
Medicaid	5.0	5.1	8.9	3.3	3.9	6.4	6.1	5.9	11.3
Uninsured	29.2	29.3	23.5	25.5	20.9	18.0	30.6	32.9	26.0
Poverty Status and Health Insurance Status [5]									
Poor									
Insured	5.1	5.7	9.1	3.2	3.4	6.0	6.2	7.1	11.5
Uninsured	39.0	37.6	29.4	34.4	26.2	25.0	40.8	42.9	31.5
Near poor									
Insured	4.2	5.2	6.0	3.1	4.2	4.0	4.8	5.8	7.2
Uninsured	30.3	29.0	22.9	27.6	21.2	18.0	31.5	32.6	25.3
Nonpoor									
Insured	2.2	2.4	2.9	1.2	1.6	1.5	2.7	2.8	3.6
Uninsured	19.9	20.6	14.5	15.0	13.8	6.4	21.5	23.0	18.1
Geographic Region									
Northeast	2.6	2.4	4.1	*2.2	2.1	2.9	2.7	2.5	4.8
Midwest	3.6	4.8	5.2	3.5	3.6	4.1	3.7	5.4	5.9
South	7.2	7.7	10.9	4.4	4.9	7.3	8.6	9.1	12.7
West	8.1	9.6	8.6	5.5	6.3	5.3	9.4	11.3	10.6
Location of Residence									
Within MSA [7]	5.6	6.5	7.7	4.0	4.6	5.0	6.4	7.4	9.2
Outside MSA [7]	6.1	6.4	7.8	4.2	3.5	6.0	6.9	7.6	8.7

[1]Persons who reported the emergency department as the place of their usual source of care are defined as having no usual source of care.

[2]Data prior to 1997 are not strictly comparable with data for later years due to the 1997 questionnaire redesign.

[3]Includes all other races not shown separately, unknown poverty status, and unknown health insurance status.

[4]The race groups, White, Black, American Indian and Alaska Native (AI/AN), Asian, Native Hawaiian and Other Pacific Islander, and two or more races, include persons of Hispanic and non-Hispanic origin. Persons of Hispanic origin may be of any race.

[5]Poor persons are defined as having a total income below the poverty threshold. Near poor persons have incomes of 100 percent to less than 200 percent of the poverty threshold. Nonpoor persons have incomes of 200 percent or more than the poverty threshold.

[6]Health insurance categories are mutually exclusive. Persons who reported both Medicaid and private coverage are classified as having private coverage. Starting in 1997, Medicaid includes state-sponsored health plans and the State Children's Health Insurance Program (SCHIP).

[7]MSA = Metropolitan Statistical Area.

* = Figure does not meet standards of reliability or precision.

. . . = Not available.

Table III-34. Emergency Department Visits Within the Past 12 Months Among Children Under 18 Years of Age, According to Selected Characteristics, Selected Years, 1997–2003

(Percent.)

Characteristic	Under 18 years of age			Under 6 years of age			6–17 years of age		
	2003	2002	1997	2003	2002	1997	2003	2002	1997
PERCENT OF CHILDREN WITH 1 OR MORE EMERGENCY DEPARTMENT VISITS									
All children [1]	20.9	22.4	19.9	26.5	28.0	24.3	18.2	19.7	17.7
Race [2]									
White only	20.3	21.3	19.4	25.2	26.1	22.6	17.9	19.1	17.8
Black or African American only	23.9	27.9	24.0	32.0	36.6	33.1	20.2	23.8	19.4
American Indian and Alaska Native only	*22.7	*	*24.1	*	*	*24.3	*21.0	*	*24.0
Asian only	14.2	14.4	12.6	*20.7	*19.5	20.8	*11.0	*11.5	8.6
Native Hawaiian and Other Pacific Islander only	*	*	. . .	*	*	. . .	*	*	. . .
Two or more races	26.1	28.4	. . .	34.0	37.5	. . .	20.3	20.3	. . .
Hispanic Origin and Race [2]									
Hispanic or Latino	20.3	20.6	21.1	27.9	26.8	25.7	16.0	17.1	18.1
Not Hispanic or Latino	21.0	22.8	19.7	26.1	28.3	24.0	18.7	20.3	17.6
White only	20.4	21.7	19.2	24.6	26.3	22.2	18.5	19.7	17.7
Black or African American only	23.8	27.8	23.6	31.9	36.3	32.7	20.1	23.9	19.2
Poverty Status [3]									
Poor	27.0	26.7	25.1	34.7	34.3	29.5	22.7	22.3	22.2
Near poor	22.8	26.6	22.0	28.8	32.8	28.0	19.4	23.4	19.0
Nonpoor	18.3	19.6	17.3	22.5	23.9	20.5	16.5	17.7	15.8
Hispanic Origin and Race and Poverty Status [2,3]									
Hispanic or Latino									
Poor	23.7	22.3	21.9	31.5	30.3	25.0	18.9	17.2	19.6
Near poor	19.8	21.5	20.8	27.8	25.4	28.8	14.8	19.5	15.6
Nonpoor	17.6	18.4	20.4	24.2	24.8	23.4	14.3	15.0	18.7
Not Hispanic or Latino									
White only									
Poor	28.1	27.1	25.5	34.1	36.2	27.2	24.8	22.1	24.4
Near poor	23.4	27.9	22.3	27.0	33.8	25.8	21.3	25.0	20.7
Nonpoor	18.6	19.4	17.2	22.2	22.6	20.1	17.0	18.1	15.9
Black or African American only									
Poor	27.2	30.3	29.3	33.7	38.6	39.5	24.0	26.2	23.0
Near poor	27.5	32.2	22.5	44.4	40.8	31.7	21.1	27.8	18.5
Nonpoor	18.8	23.0	17.7	23.5	30.9	22.6	16.6	19.6	15.9
Health Insurance Status [4]									
Insured	21.4	22.9	19.8	26.7	28.7	24.4	18.7	20.1	17.5
Private	18.1	20.0	17.5	21.6	24.5	20.9	16.6	18.1	15.9
Medicaid'	28.9	30.7	28.2	35.1	37.6	33.0	24.5	26.2	24.1
Uninsured	17.1	18.2	20.2	23.9	22.0	23.0	14.7	16.6	18.9
Poverty Status and Health Insurance Status [3]									
Poor									
Insured	29.2	28.3	26.6	36.6	36.5	31.3	24.7	23.5	23.1
Uninsured	16.7	17.7	19.9	22.6	*21.5	19.8	14.7	15.9	20.0
Near poor									
Insured	23.8	28.0	22.2	29.5	34.7	28.5	20.4	24.5	18.9
Uninsured	17.5	19.3	21.3	23.9	23.2	26.2	15.2	17.4	19.2
Nonpoor									
Insured	18.5	19.8	17.1	22.4	24.0	20.2	16.7	17.9	15.7
Uninsured	16.9	17.6	18.9	25.0	*20.9	22.6	14.3	16.3	17.3
Geographic Region									
Northeast	21.8	23.3	18.5	26.3	27.4	20.7	19.7	21.4	17.4
Midwest	21.4	22.7	19.5	27.2	28.4	26.0	18.7	20.0	16.4
South	21.7	24.4	21.8	27.8	31.4	25.6	18.6	21.0	19.9
West	18.3	17.9	18.5	23.6	22.4	23.5	15.8	15.6	15.9
Location of Residence									
Within MSA[5]	20.2	21.7	19.7	25.2	27.1	23.9	17.8	19.0	17.4
Outside MSA[5]	23.6	25.4	20.8	31.8	32.3	26.2	19.7	22.4	18.6

[1]Includes all other races not shown separately, unknown poverty status, and unknown health insurance status.

[2]The race groups, White, Black, American Indian and Alaska Native (AI/AN), Asian, Native Hawaiian and Other Pacific Islander, and two or more races, include persons of Hispanic and non-Hispanic origin. Persons of Hispanic origin may be of any race.

[3]Poor persons are defined as having a total income below the poverty threshold. Near poor persons have incomes of 100 percent to less than 200 percent of the poverty threshold. Nonpoor persons have incomes of 200 percent or more than the poverty threshold.

[4]Health insurance categories are mutually exclusive. Persons who reported both Medicaid and private coverage are classified as having private coverage. Starting in 1997, Medicaid includes state-sponsored health plans and the State Children's Health Insurance Program (SCHIP).

[5]MSA = Metropolitan Statistical Area.

* = Figure does not meet standards of reliability or precision.

. . . = Not available.

Table III-34. Emergency Department Visits Within the Past 12 Months Among Children Under 18 Years of Age, According to Selected Characteristics, Selected Years, 1997–2003—*Continued*

(Percent.)

Characteristic	Under 18 years of age			Under 6 years of age			6–17 years of age		
	2003	2002	1997	2003	2002	1997	2003	2002	1997
PERCENT OF CHILDREN WITH 2 OR MORE EMERGENCY DEPARTMENT VISITS									
All children [1]	7.0	7.5	7.1	8.7	10.2	9.6	6.2	6.2	5.8
Race [2]									
White only	6.3	6.6	6.6	7.6	8.8	8.4	5.7	5.6	5.7
Black or African American only	10.4	11.1	9.6	13.9	17.4	14.9	8.8	8.1	6.9
American Indian and Alaska Native only	*	*	*	*	*	*	*	*	*
Asian only	*6.7	*	*5.7	*	*	*12.9	*	*	*
Native Hawaiian and Other Pacific Islander only	*	*	...	*	*	...	*	*	...
Two or more races	8.7	12.5	...	*10.1	17.2	...	*7.6	*8.2	...
Hispanic Origin and Race [2]									
Hispanic or Latino	7.4	8.0	8.9	10.8	11.7	11.8	5.5	5.9	7.0
Not Hispanic or Latino	6.9	7.4	6.8	8.2	9.8	9.2	6.4	6.2	5.7
White only	6.0	6.3	6.2	6.6	7.8	7.8	5.8	5.7	5.5
Black or African American only	10.6	11.2	9.3	14.4	17.5	14.6	8.9	8.2	6.8
Poverty Status [3]									
Poor	11.6	12.3	11.1	12.9	17.2	14.5	10.8	9.5	8.9
Near poor	8.6	8.8	8.3	10.7	11.2	12.2	7.4	7.6	6.3
Nonpoor	5.1	5.5	5.3	6.3	7.3	6.5	4.5	4.8	4.7
Hispanic Origin and Race and Poverty Status [2, 3]									
Hispanic or Latino									
Poor	9.9	8.8	10.4	13.5	14.2	13.9	7.7	*5.4	8.0
Near poor	7.2	9.2	8.2	11.7	12.9	12.0	4.5	*7.3	5.7
Nonpoor	5.3	6.2	7.6	7.0	8.5	8.4	4.5	*5.0	7.1
Not Hispanic or Latino									
White only									
Poor	10.1	12.0	10.7	*9.7	15.8	12.2	*10.3	*9.9	9.8
Near poor	8.8	8.1	8.0	8.0	8.8	11.2	9.2	7.7	6.4
Nonpoor	4.8	5.1	5.0	5.7	6.2	5.8	4.4	4.6	4.6
Black or African American only									
Poor	14.5	15.4	12.7	14.7	23.0	19.1	14.4	11.6	8.8
Near poor	11.8	10.4	9.2	21.9	*14.6	*13.5	*7.9	*8.3	*7.2
Nonpoor	6.8	8.1	5.5	*9.8	14.6	*8.2	*5.4	*5.3	*4.5
Health Insurance Status [4]									
Insured	7.1	7.5	7.0	8.7	10.2	9.6	6.3	6.2	5.7
Private	5.1	5.6	5.2	5.4	7.2	6.8	4.9	4.9	4.5
Medicaid	11.7	12.7	13.1	14.0	16.5	16.2	10.1	10.3	10.4
Uninsured	6.6	7.0	7.7	*8.8	9.1	9.8	5.9	6.2	6.8
Poverty Status and Health Insurance Status [3]									
Poor									
Insured	12.3	13.1	12.1	13.4	18.3	15.7	11.7	10.1	9.5
Uninsured	*8.1	*8.0	7.6	*	*	*8.3	*7.3	*	*7.3
Near poor									
Insured	9.1	9.1	8.4	10.8	11.4	12.3	8.0	7.9	6.3
Uninsured	*6.1	*7.0	7.9	*	*10.9	*11.1	*5.0	*	6.5
Nonpoor									
Insured	5.0	5.5	5.1	6.3	7.3	6.2	4.5	4.7	4.6
Uninsured	*5.8	*6.3	7.7	*	*	*10.1	*5.5	*6.5	*6.7
Geographic Region									
Northeast	7.8	7.2	6.2	8.0	9.3	7.6	7.6	6.3	5.4
Midwest	6.3	6.9	6.6	8.5	8.3	10.4	5.3	6.3	4.8
South	8.0	8.7	8.0	9.5	12.3	10.1	7.3	7.0	6.9
West	5.5	6.1	7.1	8.1	9.5	10.0	4.2	4.4	5.6
Location of Residence									
Within MSA [5]	6.7	7.1	7.2	8.3	9.9	9.6	6.0	5.8	5.9
Outside MSA [5]	8.2	8.8	6.8	10.3	11.4	9.7	7.2	7.6	5.6

[1] Includes all other races not shown separately, unknown poverty status, and unknown health insurance status.

[2] The race groups, White, Black, American Indian and Alaska Native (AI/AN), Asian, Native Hawaiian and Other Pacific Islander, and two or more races, include persons of Hispanic and non-Hispanic origin. Persons of Hispanic origin may be of any race.

[3] Poor persons are defined as having a total income below the poverty threshold. Near poor persons have incomes of 100 percent to less than 200 percent of the poverty threshold. Nonpoor persons have incomes of 200 percent or more than the poverty threshold.

[4] Health insurance categories are mutually exclusive. Persons who reported both Medicaid and private coverage are classified as having private coverage. Starting in 1997, Medicaid includes state-sponsored health plans and the State Children's Health Insurance Program (SCHIP).

[5] MSA = Metropolitan Statistical Area.

* = Figure does not meet standards of reliability or precision.

. . . = Not available.

TABLE III-35. NO USUAL SOURCE OF HEALTH CARE AMONG ADULTS 18–64 YEARS OF AGE, ACCORDING TO SELECTED CHARACTERISTICS, ANNUAL AVERAGES, 1993–2003

Approximately 16.6 percent of adults between ages of 18 and 64 years indicated that they had no usual source of medical care in 2002–2003. If the respondents indicated that they would seek medical care at a hospital's emergency department, the answer was counted as having no usual source of health care. Males were nearly twice as likely as females to have no usual source of health care in

2002–2003 (22 percent as compared to 12 percent after age adjustments). While non-Hispanic Blacks had a slightly higher frequency of lacking a usual source of health care than non-Hispanic Whites, Hispanics—especially poor Hispanics—had much higher percentages than either group.

Insurance status was an important factor in these data. About 46.7 percent of persons without health insurance lacked a usual place for health care, and this percentage rose to 49.9 percent for the uninsured poor. For those with health insurance, only 9.3 percent lacked a usual

Table III-35. No Usual Source of Health Care Among Adults 18–64 Years of Age, According to Selected Characteristics, Annual Averages, 1993–2003

(Percent.)

Characteristic	2002–2003	2000–2001	1997–1998	1995–1996 [1]	1993–1994 [1]
PERCENT OF ADULTS WITHOUT A USUAL SOURCE OF HEALTH CARE [2]					
All adults 18–64 years old [3, 4]	16.6	16.5	17.5	16.6	18.5
Age					
18–44 years	20.7	20.3	21.1	19.6	21.7
18–24 years	27.0	26.1	27.0	22.6	26.6
25–44 years	18.6	18.4	19.3	18.8	20.3
45–64 years	9.5	9.9	11.2	11.3	12.8
45–54 years	10.8	10.9	12.6	12.2	14.1
55–64 years	7.6	8.3	9.0	9.8	11.1
Sex [4]					
Male	21.8	21.8	23.2	21.0	23.3
Female	11.6	11.4	11.9	12.5	13.9
Race [4,5]					
White only	16.1	15.8	16.9	16.3	18.2
Black or African American only	17.6	16.8	18.7	17.6	19.2
American Indian and Alaska Native only	19.1	15.9	20.7	15.9	19.1
Asian only	20.9	18.5	21.1	20.7	24.0
Native Hawaiian and Other Pacific Islander only	*	*	...	...	...
Two or more races	17.3	21.1	...	...	...
American Indian and Alakan Native; White	17.1	24.0	...	...	...
Hispanic Origin and Race [4,5]					
Hispanic or Latino	29.4	30.8	28.6	26.2	28.8
Mexican	31.6	34.6	33.4	28.1	30.5
Not Hispanic or Latino	14.5	14.6	16.1	15.5	17.5
White only	13.6	13.9	15.4	15.0	17.0
Black or African American only	17.4	16.7	18.6	17.4	18.9
Poverty Status [4,6]					
Poor	22.7	27.8	28.2	24.9	28.2
Near poor	21.7	25.1	24.7	22.3	24.6
Nonpoor	14.0	12.7	13.9	13.5	14.8
Hispanic Origin and Race and Poverty Status [4,5,6]					
Hispanic or Latino					
Poor	35.2	43.9	40.8	32.6	38.0
Near poor	32.6	37.3	33.3	31.6	35.7
Nonpoor	24.5	20.8	19.0	18.2	18.3
Not Hispanic or Latino					
White only					
Poor	17.1	22.3	24.5	22.8	27.1
Near poor	17.9	21.8	21.8	20.3	22.7
Nonpoor	12.1	11.7	13.3	13.0	14.4
Black or African American only					
Poor	21.7	21.9	23.1	21.1	23.8
Near poor	21.1	20.9	24.7	21.2	21.6
Nonpoor	14.6	13.2	14.4	13.6	14.6

[1]Data prior to 1997 are not strictly comparable with data for later years due to the 1997 questionnaire redesign.
[2]Persons who report the emergency department as the place of their usual source of care are defined as having no usual source of care.
[3]Includes all other races not shown separately, unknown poverty status, and unknown health insurance status.
[4]Estimates are for persons 18-64 years of age and are age adjusted to the year 2000 standard population using three age groups: 18–44 years, 45–54 years, and 55–64 years of age.
[5]The race groups, White, Black, American Indian and Alaska Native (AI/AN), Asian, Native Hawaiian and Other Pacific Islander, and two or more races, include persons of Hispanic and non-Hispanic origin. Persons of Hispanic origin may be of any race.
[6]Poor persons are defined as having a total income below the poverty threshold. Near poor persons have incomes of 100 percent to less than 200 percent of the poverty threshold. Nonpoor persons have incomes of 200 percent or more than the poverty threshold.
* = Figure does not meet standards of reliability or precision.
. . . = Not available.

place for medical care. On a regional basis, the West had the greatest percentage of residents (19.5 percent) who lacked an usual place for medical care. The Northeast, with 12.2 percent, had the lowest proportion of residents without a usual place for medical care.

TABLE III-36. EMERGENCY DEPARTMENT VISITS WITHIN THE PAST 12 MONTHS AMONG ADULTS 18 YEARS OF AGE AND OVER, ACCORDING TO SELECTED CHARACTERISTICS, SELECTED YEARS, 1997–2003

In 2003, 20.0 percent of adults age 18 years and over made 1 or more visits to an emergency department of a hospital, and 7.0 percent made 2 or more visits. The fewest visits were made by Asians and Hispanics. Blacks made substantially more visits than Whites. By age, the most frequent visitors were between 18 and 24 years old

and 75 years old and over. Additional information on injury-related emergency department visits is given in Table III-42. Separate data for older teenagers, not shown here, indicated a peak for that age group—undoubtedly associated with adolescent behavior.

Insurance status did not cause a significant difference in the utilization of emergency departments, except for persons covered by Medicaid. As many as 39.7 percent of Medicaid-insured persons between 18 and 64 years old went to the emergency room 1 or more times in 2003, while 21.6 percent went 2 times or more. By comparison, 17.4 percent of privately insured persons in this age bracket made 1 or more visits to the emergency room, while only 5.0 percent made 2 or more visits. For persons 65 years old and over, the percentages were 34.9 percent for 1 or more visits and 17.8 percent for 2 or more visits.

Table III-35. No Usual Source of Health Care Among Adults 18–64 Years of Age, According to Selected Characteristics, Annual Averages, 1993–2003—Continued

(Percent.)

Characteristic	2002–2003	2000–2001	1997–1998	1995–1996 [1]	1993–1994 [1]
Health Insurance Status [4,7]					
Insured	9.3	9.7	11.4	11.4	13.3
Private	9.4	9.7	11.5	11.3	13.1
Medicaid	8.9	9.6	10.0	12.5	15.2
Uninsured	46.7	46.3	45.3	40.9	41.5
Poverty Status and Health Insurance Status [4,6]					
Poor					
Insured	9.8	12.0	13.8	13.6	16.8
Uninsured	49.9	51.7	50.4	42.1	45.7
Near poor					
Insured	10.4	12.3	13.9	13.1	15.3
Uninsured	46.3	48.4	46.2	41.5	42.9
Nonpoor					
Insured	8.8	9.1	10.7	10.8	12.3
Uninsured	44.0	41.7	41.2	39.4	37.0
Geographic Region					
Northeast	12.2	12.1	13.2	13.3	14.5
Midwest	14.3	15.2	14.9	14.5	15.8
South	18.9	17.8	20.5	18.4	21.6
West	19.5	20.0	19.8	19.5	20.5
Location of Residence					
Within MSA [8]	16.8	16.7	17.6	16.9	18.8
Outside MSA [8]	16.1	15.8	17.1	15.4	17.4

[1]Data prior to 1997 are not strictly comparable with data for later years due to the 1997 questionnaire redesign.

[4]Estimates are for persons 18-64 years of age and are age adjusted to the year 2000 standard population using three age groups: 18–44 years, 45–54 years, and 55–64 years of age.

[6]Poor persons are defined as having a total income below the poverty threshold. Near poor persons have incomes of 100 percent to less than 200 percent of the poverty threshold. Nonpoor persons have incomes of 200 percent or more than the poverty threshold.

[7]Health insurance categories are mutually exclusive. Persons who reported both Medicaid and private coverage are classified as having private coverage. Persons 65 years of age and over who reported Medicare HMO (health maintenance organization) and some other type of health insurance coverage are classified as having Medicare HMO.

[8]MSA = Metropolitan Statistical Area.

Table III-36. Emergency Department Visits Within the Past 12 Months Among Adults 18 Years of Age and Over, According to Selected Characteristics, Selected Years, 1997–2003

(Percent.)

Characteristic	2003	2002	2000	1997
PERCENT OF ADULTS WITH 1 OR MORE EMERGENCY DEPARTMENT VISITS				
All adults 18 years of age and over [1]	20.0	20.5	20.2	19.6
Age				
18–44 years	20.0	20.7	20.5	20.7
18–24 years	23.9	24.7	25.7	26.3
25–44 years	18.6	19.4	18.8	19.0
45–64 years	18.5	18.2	17.6	16.2
45–54 years	17.8	18.1	17.9	15.7
55–64 years	19.3	18.4	17.0	16.9
65 years and over	22.9	24.0	23.7	22.0
65–74 years	19.7	21.2	21.6	20.3
75 years and over	26.6	27.1	26.2	24.3
Sex				
Male	18.2	19.6	18.7	19.1
Female	21.8	21.5	21.6	20.2
Race [2]				
White only	19.2	19.6	19.4	19.0
Black or African American only	27.8	27.8	26.5	25.9
American Indian and Alaska Native only	22.5	25.3	30.3	24.8
Asian only	12.9	13.6	13.6	11.6
Native Hawaiian and Other Pacific Islander only	*	*	*	. . .
Two or more races	25.2	30.8	32.5	. . .
American Indian and Alaska Native; White	29.7	37.7	33.9	. . .
Hispanic Origin and Race [2]				
Hispanic or Latino	18.5	18.4	18.3	19.2
Mexican American	17.0	18.1	17.4	17.8
Not Hispanic or Latino	20.3	20.9	20.6	19.7
White only	19.5	20.0	19.8	19.1
Black or African American only	27.7	27.9	26.5	25.9
Poverty Status [3]				
Poor	26.3	28.6	29.0	28.1
Near poor	23.2	24.7	23.9	23.8
Nonpoor	18.2	18.2	18.0	17.0
Hispanic Origin, Race, and Poverty Status [2, 3]				
Hispanic or Latino				
Poor	21.2	22.3	22.4	22.1
Near poor	17.6	19.5	18.1	19.2
Nonpoor	17.9	16.7	16.8	17.6
Not Hispanic or Latino				
White only				
Poor	27.0	30.2	30.1	29.5
Near poor	24.0	25.9	25.5	24.3
Nonpoor	17.8	17.7	17.7	16.8
Black or African American only				
Poor	33.4	35.3	35.4	34.6
Near poor	31.2	29.7	28.5	29.2
Nonpoor	24.0	24.3	22.6	19.7
Health Insurance Status [4]				
18–64 years of age				
Insured	19.7	19.6	19.5	18.8
Private	17.4	17.4	17.6	16.9
Medicaid	39.7	40.4	42.2	37.6
Uninsured	18.1	20.4	19.3	20.0
65 years and over				
Medicare HMO	25.6	20.3	24.4	20.2
Private	21.2	24.0	23.3	21.3
Medicaid	34.9	33.1	36.0	35.2
Medicare fee-for-service only	22.2	22.4	20.1	22.0

[1] Includes all other races not shown separately, unknown poverty status, and unknown health insurance status.

[2] The race groups, White, Black, American Indian and Alaska Native (AI/AN), Asian, Native Hawaiian and Other Pacific Islander, and two or more races, include persons of Hispanic and non-Hispanic origin. Persons of Hispanic origin may be of any race.

[3] Poor persons are defined as having a total income below the poverty threshold. Near poor persons have incomes of 100 percent to less than 200 percent of the poverty threshold. Nonpoor persons have incomes of 200 percent or greater than the poverty threshold.

[4] Health insurance categories are mutually exclusive. Persons who reported both Medicaid and private coverage are classified as having private coverage. Persons 65 years of age and over who reported Medicare HMO (health maintenance organization) and some other type of health insurance coverage are classified as having Medicare HMO.

* = Figure does not meet standards of reliability or precision.

. . . = Not available.

Table III-36. Emergency Department Visits Within the Past 12 Months Among Adults 18 Years of Age and Over, According to Selected Characteristics, Selected Years, 1997–2003—*Continued*

(Percent.)

Characteristic	2003	2002	2000	1997
Poverty Status and Health Insurance Status [3]				
18–64 years of age				
Poor				
Insured	30.1	32.7	33.0	31.0
Unsured	19.9	23.4	24.2	22.8
Near poor				
Insured	25.5	26.1	25.9	25.3
Uninsured	18.8	21.1	18.7	20.2
Nonpoor				
Insured	17.5	17.0	17.2	16.2
Uninsured	16.7	18.5	17.4	18.0
Geographic Region				
Northeast	20.3	20.5	20.0	19.5
Midwest	20.0	20.9	20.1	19.3
South	20.9	21.4	21.2	20.9
West	18.2	18.4	18.6	17.7
Location of Residence				
Within MSA [5]	19.5	19.8	19.6	19.1
Outside MSA [5]	22.3	23.4	22.5	21.5
PERCENT OF ADULTS WITH 2 OR MORE EMERGENCY DEPARTMENT VISITS				
All adults 18 years of age and over [1]	7.0	7.1	6.9	6.7
Age				
18–44 years	6.8	7.1	7.0	6.8
18–24 years	8.2	8.5	8.8	9.1
25–44 years	6.4	6.6	6.4	6.2
45–64 years	6.4	6.3	5.6	5.6
45–54 years	5.9	6.7	5.8	5.5
55–64 years	7.0	5.7	5.3	5.7
65 years and over	8.7	8.3	8.6	8.1
65–74 years	7.1	7.7	7.4	7.1
75 years and over	10.4	9.0	10.0	9.3
Sex				
Male	5.6	6.2	5.7	5.9
Female	8.4	7.9	7.9	7.5
Race [2]				
White only	6.4	6.5	6.4	6.2
Black or African American only	12.4	11.7	10.8	11.1
American Indian and Alaska Native only	*9.1	*10.0	*12.6	13.1
Asian only	*3.5	*2.6	*3.8	*2.9
Native Hawaiian and Other Pacific Islander only	*	*	*	. . .
Two or more races	11.1	13.3	11.3	. . .
American Indian and Alaska Native; White	*15.1	15.9	*9.4	. . .
Hispanic Origin and Race [2]				
Hispanic or Latino	7.3	6.8	7.0	7.4
Mexican American	6.4	6.3	7.1	6.4
Not Hispanic or Latino	7.0	7.2	6.9	6.7
White only	6.3	6.6	6.4	6.2
Black or African American only	12.3	11.6	10.8	11.0
Poverty Status [3]				
Poor	12.6	12.6	13.3	12.8
Near poor	9.9	9.7	9.6	9.3
Nonpoor	5.4	5.6	5.2	4.9
Hispanic Origin, Race, and Poverty Status [2, 3]				
Hispanic or Latino				
Poor	9.6	9.0	9.7	9.8
Near poor	7.3	8.6	6.7	8.1
Nonpoor	6.4	5.0	6.1	5.4
Not Hispanic or Latino				
White only				
Poor	12.7	13.4	13.9	13.0
Near poor	10.0	9.6	10.4	9.1
Nonpoor	5.0	5.3	5.0	4.8
Black or African American only				
Poor	18.1	16.7	17.4	17.5
Near poor	15.7	13.8	12.2	12.8
Nonpoor	8.7	9.1	8.0	7.2

[1] Includes all other races not shown separately, unknown poverty status, and unknown health insurance status.
[2] The race groups, White, Black, American Indian and Alaska Native (AI/AN), Asian, Native Hawaiian and Other Pacific Islander, and two or more races, include persons of Hispanic and non-Hispanic origin. Persons of Hispanic origin may be of any race.
[3] Poor persons are defined as having a total income below the poverty threshold. Near poor persons have incomes of 100 percent to less than 200 percent of the poverty threshold. Nonpoor persons have incomes of 200 percent or greater than the poverty threshold.
[5] MSA = Metropolitan Statistical Area.
* = Figure does not meet standards of reliability or precision.
. . . = Not available.

Table III-36. Emergency Department Visits Within the Past 12 Months Among Adults 18 Years of Age and Over, According to Selected Characteristics, Selected Years, 1997–2003—Continued

(Percent.)

Characteristic	2003	2002	2000	1997
Health Insurance Status [4]				
18–64 years of age				
Insured	6.7	6.7	6.4	6.1
Private	5.0	5.0	5.1	4.7
Medicaid	21.6	21.9	21.0	19.7
Uninsured	6.7	7.4	6.9	7.5
65 years and over				
Medicare HMO	10.8	7.4	8.5	6.7
Private	7.1	7.9	7.8	6.9
Medicaid	17.8	12.8	18.3	20.2
Medicare fee-for-service only	9.4	8.6	7.2	9.4
Poverty Status and Health Insurance Status [3]				
18–64 years of age				
Poor				
Insured	15.2	15.0	16.2	15.2
Unsured	8.7	10.3	9.9	9.1
Near poor				
Insured	11.2	10.5	10.6	9.6
Uninsured	7.5	8.1	6.9	8.6
Nonpoor				
Insured	4.9	5.1	4.8	4.4
Uninsured	5.0	5.7	5.5	5.5
Geographic Region				
Northeast	6.9	6.2	6.2	6.9
Midwest	6.4	6.7	6.9	6.2
South	8.1	8.2	7.6	7.3
West	5.9	6.2	6.3	6.0
Location of Residence				
Within MSA [5]	6.6	6.6	6.6	6.4
Outside MSA [5]	8.6	8.9	7.8	7.8

[3] Poor persons are defined as having a total income below the poverty threshold. Near poor persons have incomes of 100 percent to less than 200 percent of the poverty threshold. Nonpoor persons have incomes of 200 percent or greater than the poverty threshold.

[4] Health insurance categories are mutually exclusive. Persons who reported both Medicaid and private coverage are classified as having private coverage. Persons 65 years of age and over who reported Medicare HMO (health maintenance organization) and some other type of health insurance coverage are classified as having Medicare HMO.

[5] MSA = Metropolitan Statistical Area.

TABLE III-37. DENTAL VISITS IN THE PAST YEAR, ACCORDING TO SELECTED CHARACTERISTICS, SELECTED YEARS, 1997–2003

In 2003, 64.8 percent of persons between the ages of 18 and 64 years old had gone to a dentist's office at some time during the previous year. For persons between 2 and 17 years of age, 75 percent visited a dental office. Persons age 65 years and over had a 58 percent rate of dental office visits. A survey showed that 25–30 percent of persons in the older age group had lost their natural teeth; this considerably reduced their dental visits. Seniors with natural teeth had a 70 percent rate of dental visits.

Approximately 69.3 percent of non-Hispanic Whites age 18–64 years, 58.3 percent of non-Hispanic Blacks age 18–64 years, and 48.3 percent of Hispanics age 18–64 years had a dental visit. For persons classified as poor, the rate of visits was 44.5 percent; for poor Hispanics, this rate dropped to 35.5 percent.

TABLE III-38. UNTREATED DENTAL CARIES (CAVITIES), ACCORDING TO AGE, SEX, RACE, HISPANIC ORIGIN, AND POVERTY STATUS, SELECTED ANNUAL AVERAGES, 1971–2002

Persons between 18 and 64 years of age during the 1999–2002 survey period had a 23.8 percent incidence rate of untreated dental caries. This rate was considerably less than the 48.4 percent rate reported for the 1971–1974 period. In the more recent survey, the percentages of untreated cavities were somewhat smaller for children and for persons age 65 years and over.

Untreated caries were much more frequent among minorities reported in the survey, including Blacks and Mexicans. The percentage of persons with untreated caries was especially large among poor respondents 18 to 64 years old. Of the poor respondents, 33.9 percent of non-Hispanic Whites, 53.5 percent of non-Hispanic Blacks, and 43.1 percent of persons of Mexican origin had untreated cavities. Poor children were more likely to have untreated caries than children in families with incomes above the poverty level. In 1999–2002, 33 percent of poor children age 6 to 17 years had untreated caries, compared with 13 percent of children in families with incomes equal to 200 percent or more than the poverty level.

Table III-37. Dental Visits in the Past Year, According to Selected Characteristics, Selected Years, 1997–2003

(Percent.)

Characteristic	2 years of age and over			2–17 years of age			18–64 years of age			65 years of age and over		
	2003	2002	1997	2003	2002	1997	2003	2002	1997	2003	2002	1997
PERCENT OF PERSONS WITH A DENTAL VISIT IN THE PAST YEAR												
Total [1]	66.3	64.4	64.9	75.0	74.2	72.7	64.8	62.6	64.1	58.0	55.5	54.8
Sex												
Male	63.6	61.5	62.6	74.1	73.7	72.3	60.9	58.4	60.4	58.4	55.4	55.4
Female	68.9	67.1	67.2	75.9	74.8	73.0	68.6	66.7	67.7	57.7	55.5	54.4
Race [2]												
White only	67.5	66.3	66.5	76.0	76.3	74.0	65.9	64.5	65.7	59.8	58.0	56.8
Black or African American only	58.4	54.5	56.5	70.5	68.8	68.8	58.1	53.5	57.0	38.7	33.9	35.4
American Indian and Alaska Native only	59.9	51.2	51.5	69.9	66.6	66.8	58.0	50.3	49.9	*49.2	*	*
Asian only	65.1	61.3	61.8	72.9	66.8	69.9	63.6	62.7	60.3	57.4	45.4	53.9
Native Hawaiian and Other Pacific Islander only	*	*	...	*	*	...	*	*	...	*	*	...
Two or more races	61.6	59.5	...	74.5	71.4	...	59.6	57.9	...	51.0	44.7	...
Black or African American; White	63.6	70.1	...	71.3	67.2	...	60.3	65.4	...	*80.7	*	...
American Indian and Alaska Native; White	50.0	51.9	...	52.8	64.3	...	53.7	50.2	...	*	*42.7	...
Hispanic Origin and Race [2]												
Hispanic or Latino	52.4	52.7	52.9	64.5	62.5	61.0	48.3	49.2	50.8	46.0	47.9	47.8
Not Hispanic or Latino	68.6	66.3	66.4	77.3	76.7	74.7	67.4	64.6	65.7	58.7	55.9	55.2
White only	70.5	68.6	68.2	79.4	79.4	76.4	69.3	66.7	67.5	60.9	58.4	57.2
Black or African American only	58.5	54.3	56.5	70.6	68.6	68.8	58.3	53.4	56.9	38.3	33.7	35.3
Poverty Status [3]												
Poor	48.2	47.5	47.7	65.8	64.4	62.0	44.5	44.3	46.9	37.1	35.0	31.5
Near poor	52.3	51.4	50.6	66.6	66.9	62.5	49.1	47.5	48.3	43.6	43.0	40.8
Nonpoor	73.4	70.7	72.5	80.8	79.6	80.1	72.0	68.9	71.2	67.8	64.7	65.9
Hispanic Origin, Race, and Poverty Status [2,3]												
Hispanic or Latino												
Poor	42.0	43.8	42.1	62.1	60.0	55.9	35.5	38.6	39.2	33.2	38.1	33.6
Near poor	45.5	45.1	46.4	59.1	57.8	53.8	40.8	40.1	43.5	39.4	40.6	47.9
Nonpoor	62.7	61.1	64.9	71.6	68.4	73.7	59.4	58.0	62.3	60.7	61.3	58.8
Not Hispanic or Latino												
White only												
Poor	52.8	51.9	50.6	69.1	69.5	64.4	50.4	48.6	50.6	39.9	38.2	32.0
Near poor	55.8	55.3	52.9	69.6	71.3	66.1	52.8	51.4	50.4	45.9	45.2	42.2
Nonpoor	75.6	73.1	73.9	83.2	82.7	81.3	74.2	71.1	72.7	69.1	66.5	67.0
Black or African American only												
Poor	45.1	42.9	47.7	66.7	63.5	66.1	40.8	39.8	46.2	27.6	23.8	27.7
Near poor	52.0	47.7	46.9	69.1	68.9	61.2	50.6	45.0	46.3	29.3	26.0	26.9
Nonpoor	66.7	61.8	66.0	74.5	72.5	77.1	67.2	61.4	66.1	51.9	45.6	49.8
Geographic Region												
Northeast	72.4	70.1	69.6	81.5	80.5	77.5	71.4	69.2	69.6	61.1	55.8	55.5
Midwest	68.8	68.0	68.3	77.6	77.9	76.4	67.6	66.6	67.4	58.8	56.9	57.6
South	61.4	58.8	60.0	70.7	69.1	68.0	59.6	56.7	59.4	53.3	50.7	49.0
West	66.7	65.0	64.9	74.1	73.5	71.5	64.7	62.3	62.9	62.8	63.2	61.9
Location of Residence												
Within MSA [4]	67.9	66.0	66.5	75.5	74.8	73.6	66.5	64.4	65.7	61.3	58.5	57.6
Outside MSA [4]	60.0	58.1	59.1	72.9	71.9	69.3	57.9	55.4	58.0	46.7	45.9	46.1

[1]Includes all other races not shown separately, unknown poverty status, and unknown health insurance status.

[2]The race groups, White, Black, American Indian and Alaska Native (AI/AN), Asian, Native Hawaiian and Other Pacific Islander, and two or more races, include persons of Hispanic and non-Hispanic origin. Persons of Hispanic origin may be of any race.

[3]Poor persons are defined as having a total income below the poverty threshold. Near poor persons have incomes of 100 percent to less than 200 percent of the poverty threshold. Nonpoor persons have incomes of 200 percent or greater than the poverty threshold.

[4]MSA = Metropolitan Statistical Area.

* = Figure does not meet standards of reliability or precision.

. . . = Not available.

Table III-38. Untreated Dental Caries (Cavities), According to Age, Sex, Race, Hispanic Origin, and Poverty Status, Selected Annual Averages, 1971–2002

(Percent.)

Sex, race, Hispanic origin, and poverty status	2–5 years of age			6–17 years of age		
	1999–2002	1988–1994	1971–1974	1999–2002	1988–1994	1971–1974
PERCENT OF PESONS WITH UNTREATED DENTAL CARIES						
Total [1]	19.4	19.6	25.1	21.9	23.9	55.3
Sex						
Male	20.4	20.0	26.6	23.0	23.0	55.2
Female	18.4	19.3	23.6	20.8	24.8	55.4
Race and Hispanic Origin [2]						
Not Hispanic or Latino						
White only	16.9	14.4	23.7	18.0	19.2	52.3
Black or African American only	24.3	25.1	29.0	28.3	33.1	70.5
Mexican	31.4	35.0	34.1	32.5	37.1	60.2
Poverty Status [3]						
Poor	31.9	30.6	32.0	32.6	38.4	68.9
Near poor	20.1	25.1	29.9	29.2	28.9	60.9
Nonpoor	11.0	9.7	17.9	13.2	15.1	46.2
Race, Hispanic Origin, and Poverty Status [2,3]						
Not Hispanic or Latino						
White only						
Poor	34.2	26.5	32.1	29.7	34.8	68.5
Near poor and nonpoor	12.8	12.2	22.1	15.8	17.0	50.4
Black or African American only						
Poor	29.3	27.7	29.1	35.8	35.7	72.7
Near poor and nonpoor	20.1	22.7	27.9	24.4	31.3	67.5
Mexican						
Poor	39.1	38.9	*	39.2	46.4	57.1
Near poor and nonpoor	25.7	30.5	27.4	25.1	26.9	61.2

Sex, race, Hispanic origin, and poverty status	18–64 years of age			65–74 years of age		
	1999–2002	1988–1994	1971–1974	1999–2002	1988–1994	1971–1974
PERCENT OF PESONS WITH UNTREATED DENTAL CARIES						
Total [1]	23.8	28.2	48.4	17.0	25.4	29.7
Sex						
Male	25.9	31.2	50.9	20.1	29.8	32.6
Female	21.7	25.3	46.0	14.4	21.5	27.4
Race and Hispanic Origin [2]						
Not Hispanic or Latino						
White only	18.7	23.6	45.6	14.3	22.7	28.3
Black or African American only	41.7	48.0	68.2	35.0	46.7	41.5
Mexican	35.5	40.0	62.0	33.9	43.8	*
Poverty Status [3]						
Poor	40.1	47.4	63.6	27.9	46.6	34.3
Near poor	36.1	42.6	56.3	28.1	40.1	35.6
Nonpoor	16.1	19.5	43.1	12.2	19.2	26.2
Race, Hispanic Origin, and Poverty Status [2,3]						
Not Hispanic or Latino						
White only						
Poor	33.9	42.4	59.5	*	*39.0	33.3
Near poor and nonpoor	16.8	21.6	44.5	14.0	22.7	28.3
Black or African American only						
Poor	53.5	59.3	73.1	*31.0	49.7	39.8
Near poor and nonpoor	37.2	43.4	65.8	39.0	43.8	41.1
Mexican						
Poor	43.1	52.4	65.4	*45.0	55.5	*
Near poor and nonpoor	32.2	31.6	59.1	31.1	35.6	*

Note: Excludes persons without teeth, most of whom are 65 years old and over. In this age group, they are estimated to account for 46 percent of persons in 1971–1974; 33 percent in 1988–1994; and 27 percent in 1999–2002.

[1] Includes all other races not shown separately, unknown poverty status, and unknown health insurance status.
[2] Persons of Mexican origin may be of any race. Starting with data year 1999, race-specific estimates are tabulated according to 1997 Standards for Federal Data on Race and Ethnicity and are not strictly comparable with estimates for earlier years. The two non-Hispanic race categories shown in the table conform to 1997 standards. The 1999–2002 race-specific estimates are for persons who reported only one racial group. Prior to data year 1999, data were tabulated according to 1977 standards.
[3] Poor persons are defined as having a total income below the poverty threshold. Near poor persons have incomes of 100 percent to less than 200 percent of the poverty threshold. Nonpoor persons have incomes of 200 percent or more than the poverty threshold.
* = Figure does not meet standards of reliability or precision.

Table III-38. Untreated Dental Caries (Cavities), According to Age, Sex, Race, Hispanic Origin, and Poverty Status, Selected Annual Averages, 1971–2002—*Continued*

(Percent.)

Sex, race, Hispanic origin, and poverty status	75 years and over		
	1999–2002	1988–1994	1971–1974
PERCENT OF PESONS WITH UNTREATED DENTAL CARIES			
Total [1]	20.3	30.3	. . .
Sex			
Male	24.4	34.4	. . .
Female	17.4	28.1	. . .
Race and Hispanic Origin [2]			
Not Hispanic or Latino			
White only	18.3	27.8	. . .
Black or African American only	46.8	62.6	. . .
Mexican	48.2	55.6	. . .
Poverty Status [3]			
Poor	33.0	47.1	. . .
Near poor	23.0	34.5	. . .
Nonpoor	15.8	23.2	. . .
Race, Hispanic Origin, and Poverty Status [2,3]			
Not Hispanic or Latino			
White only			
Poor	*32.2	38.0	. . .
Near poor and nonpoor	17.2	26.1	. . .
Black or African American only			
Poor	*	68.6	. . .
Near poor and nonpoor	43.8	60.2	. . .
Mexican			
Poor	*	79.4	. . .
Near poor and nonpoor	49.7	*	. . .

Note: Excludes persons without teeth, most of whom are 65 years old and over. In this age group, they are estimated to account for 46 percent of persons in 1971–1974; 33 percent in 1988–1994; and 27 percent in 1999–2002.

[1] Includes all other races not shown separately, unknown poverty status, and unknown health insurance status.

[2] Persons of Mexican origin may be of any race. Starting with data year 1999, race-specific estimates are tabulated according to 1997 Standards for Federal Data on Race and Ethnicity and are not strictly comparable with estimates for earlier years. The two non-Hispanic race categories shown in the table conform to 1997 standards. The 1999–2002 race-specific estimates are for persons who reported only one racial group. Prior to data year 1999, data were tabulated according to 1977 standards.

[3] Poor persons are defined as having a total income below the poverty threshold. Near poor persons have incomes of 100 percent to less than 200 percent of the poverty threshold. Nonpoor persons have incomes of 200 percent or more than the poverty threshold.

* = Figure does not meet standards of reliability or precision.

. . . = Not available.

TABLE III-39. USE OF MAMMOGRAPHY FOR WOMEN 40 YEARS OF AGE AND OVER, ACCORDING TO SELECTED CHARACTERISTICS, SELECTED YEARS, 1987–2003

Mammography is a screening tool for breast cancer. Although there is scientific debate over the benefits of its use, the Institute of Medicine recently concluded that the test, despite its flaws, remains the best choice for detecting breast cancer at early and treatable stages.

This table shows the percentage of women age 40 years and over who reported having a mammogram during the past two years. For 2003, 69.5 percent of women had mammograms. This rate peaked in 2000 after consecutive increases since 1987 (when the frequency was 28.7 percent). Women in the 50- to 64-year-old age bracket were the most frequent users of mammograms, with 76.2 percent having had the test.

Participation by non-Hispanic Blacks age 40 years and over was the same as that for non-Hispanic Whites, (70.5 percent). Hispanics increased their rate of use to 65 percent in 2003. American Indian or Alaska Natives had a 63 percent participation rate, and 58 percent of Asian women over 40 years of age obtained mammograms in 2003. Among poor women age 40 years and over, 55.4 percent received a mammogram during 2003, but non-poor respondents reported obtaining this test much more frequently.

Frequency of testing was influenced by educational attainment. The proportion of women age 50 to 64 years who had the procedure included 82.7 percent of women with some college or more, 71.8 percent of women with a high school diploma (or equivalent), and 63.4 percent of women with less than a high school diploma.

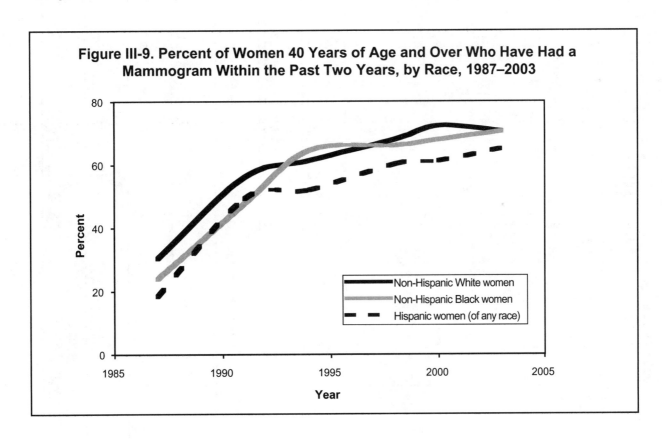

Figure III-9. Percent of Women 40 Years of Age and Over Who Have Had a Mammogram Within the Past Two Years, by Race, 1987–2003

Table III-39. Use of Mammography for Women 40 Years of Age and Over, According to Selected Characteristics, Selected Years, 1987–2003

(Percent.)

Characteristic	2003	2000	1999	1998	1994	1991	1990	1987
PERCENT OF WOMEN HAVING A MAMMOGRAM WITHIN THE PAST TWO YEARS								
40 years and over, age-adjusted [1]	69.5	70.4	70.3	67.0	61.0	54.7	51.7	29.0
40 years and over, crude [1]	69.7	70.4	70.3	66.9	60.9	54.6	51.4	28.7
Age								
40–49 years	64.4	64.3	67.2	63.4	61.3	55.6	55.1	31.9
50–64 years	76.2	78.7	76.5	73.7	66.5	60.3	56.0	31.7
65 years and over	67.7	67.9	66.8	63.8	55.0	48.1	43.4	22.8
65–74 years	74.6	74.0	73.9	69.4	63.0	55.7	48.7	26.6
75 years and over	60.6	61.3	58.9	57.2	44.6	37.8	35.8	17.3
Race [2]								
White only	70.1	71.4	70.6	67.4	60.6	55.6	52.2	29.6
Black or African American only	70.4	67.8	71.0	66.0	64.3	48.0	46.4	24.0
American Indian and Alaska Native only	63.1	47.4	63.0	45.2	65.8	54.5	43.2	*
Asian only	57.6	53.5	58.3	60.2	55.8	45.9	46.0	*
Native Hawaiian and Other Pacific Islander only	*	*	*	...	...	...	...	...
Two or more races	65.3	69.2	70.2	...	...	...	...	...
Hispanic Origin and Race [2]								
40 years and over, crude								
Hispanic or Latino	65.0	61.2	65.7	60.2	51.9	49.2	45.2	18.3
Not Hispanic or Latino	70.1	71.1	70.7	67.5	61.5	54.9	51.8	29.4
White only	70.5	72.2	71.1	68.0	61.3	56.0	52.7	30.3
Black or African American only	70.5	67.9	71.0	66.0	64.4	47.7	46.0	23.8
Age, Race, and Hispanic Origin [2]								
40–49 years								
Hispanic or Latino	59.4	54.1	61.6	55.2	47.5	44.0	45.1	*15.3
Not Hispanic or Latino								
White only	65.2	67.2	68.3	64.4	62.0	58.1	57.0	34.3
Black or African American only	68.2	60.9	69.2	65.0	67.2	48.0	48.4	27.8
50–64 years								
Hispanic or Latino	69.4	66.5	69.7	67.2	60.1	61.7	47.5	23.0
Not Hispanic or Latino								
White only	77.2	80.6	77.9	75.3	67.5	61.5	58.1	33.6
Black or African American only	76.2	77.7	75.0	71.2	63.6	52.4	48.4	26.4
65 years and older								
Hispanic or Latino	69.5	68.3	67.2	59.0	48.0	40.9	41.1	*
Not Hispanic or Latino								
White only	68.1	68.3	66.8	64.3	54.9	49.1	43.8	24.0
Black or African American only	65.4	65.5	68.1	60.6	61.0	41.6	39.7	14.1
Age and Poverty Status [3]								
40 years and over, crude								
Poor	55.4	54.8	57.4	50.1	44.2	35.2	30.8	14.6
Near poor	60.8	58.1	59.5	56.1	48.6	44.4	39.1	20.9
Nonpoor	74.3	75.9	75.0	72.6	68.5	62.2	59.2	35.2
40–49 years								
Poor	50.6	47.4	51.3	44.8	43.0	33.0	32.2	18.6
Near poor	54.0	43.6	52.8	46.9	47.6	43.8	39.0	18.4
Nonpoor	68.3	69.9	71.6	68.4	66.5	61.2	60.1	36.8
50–64 years								
Poor	58.3	61.7	63.3	52.7	46.2	37.3	29.9	14.6
Near poor	64.0	68.3	64.9	61.8	49.0	50.2	39.8	24.2
Nonpoor	80.9	82.6	80.2	78.7	73.7	66.0	63.3	37.0
65 years and over								
Poor	57.0	54.8	57.6	51.9	43.9	35.2	30.8	13.1
Near poor	62.8	60.3	60.2	57.8	48.8	41.8	38.6	19.9
Nonpoor	72.6	75.0	72.5	70.1	64.0	57.8	51.5	29.7
Health Insurance Staus [4]								
40–64 years of age								
Insured	75.1	76.0	75.5	72.3	68.3	...	...	...
Private	76.3	77.1	76.3	73.4	69.4	...	...	...
Medicaid	63.5	61.7	62.5	59.7	54.5	...	...	...
Uninsured	41.5	40.7	44.8	40.1	34.0	...	...	...
65 years and over								
Medicare HMO	70.2	73.2	76.3	70.4	...	...	...	...
Private	72.4	71.2	70.2	67.3	59.0	...	...	...
Medicaid	61.2	57.6	53.8	51.1	46.2	...	...	...
Medicare fee-for-service only	53.4	55.8	51.3	48.1	36.8	...	...	...

[1] Includes all other races not shown separately, unknown poverty status, and unknown education.

[2] The race groups White, Black, American Indian and Alaska Native (AI/AN), Asian, Native Hawaiian and Other Pacific Islander, and two or more races, include persons of Hispanic and Non-Hispanic origin. Persons of Hispanic origin may be of any race.

[3] Poor persons are defined as having a total income below the poverty threshold. Near poor persons have incomes of 100 percent to less than 200 percent of the poverty threshold. Nonpoor persons have incomes of 200 percent or more than the poverty threshold.

[4] Health insurance categories are mutually exclusive. Persons who reported both Medicaid and private coverage are classified as having private coverage. Starting in 1997, Medicaid includes state-sponsored health plans and State Children's Health Insurance Program (SCHIP). In addition to private and Medicaid, the category "insured" also includes military plans, other government-sponsored health plans, and Medicare, not shown separately. Persons 65 years of age and over who reported Medicare HMO (health maintenance organization) and some other type of health insurance coverage are classified as having Medicare HMO.

* = Figure does not meet standards of reliability or precision.

... = Not available.

Table III-39. Use of Mammography for Women 40 Years of Age and Over, According to Selected Characteristics, Selected Years, 1987–2003—*Continued*

(Percent.)

Characteristic	2003	2000	1999	1998	1994	1991	1990	1987
Age and Education [5]								
40 years and over, crude								
No high school diploma or GED	58.1	57.7	56.7	54.5	48.2	40.0	36.4	17.8
High school diploma or GED	67.8	69.7	69.2	66.7	61.0	55.8	52.7	31.3
Some college or more	75.1	76.2	77.3	72.8	69.7	65.2	62.8	37.7
40–49 years of age								
No high school diploma or GED	53.3	46.8	48.8	47.3	50.4	40.8	38.5	15.1
High school diploma or GED	60.8	59.0	60.8	59.1	55.8	52.0	53.1	32.6
Some college or more	68.1	70.6	74.4	68.3	68.7	63.7	62.3	39.2
50–64 years of age								
No high school diploma or GED	63.4	66.5	62.3	58.8	51.6	43.6	41.0	21.2
High school diploma or GED	71.8	76.6	77.2	73.3	67.8	60.8	56.5	33.8
Some college or more	82.7	84.2	81.2	79.8	74.7	72.7	68.0	40.5
65 years and over								
No high school diploma or GED	56.9	57.4	56.6	54.7	45.6	37.7	33.0	16.5
High school diploma or GED	69.7	71.8	68.4	66.8	59.1	54.0	47.5	25.9
Some college or more	75.1	74.1	77.1	71.3	64.3	57.9	56.7	32.3

[5]Education quantities shown are for 1998 and subsequent years. GED stands for General Educational Development high school equivalency diploma. In years prior to 1998, the following categories based on number of years of school completed were used: less than 12 years, 12 years, and 13 years or more.

TABLE III-40. USE OF PAP SMEARS FOR WOMEN 18 YEARS OF AGE AND OVER, ACCORDING TO SELECTED CHARACTERISTICS, SELECTED YEARS, 1987–2003

The Pap smear is a screening tool for cervical cancer, which causes about 4,000 deaths among women in the United States every year. The test has few false positives, but can result in a false negative. Nevertheless, it is an important public health measure for reducing the incidence rate of cervical cancer. A high percentage of women (79.2 percent) had a Pap smear test between 2000 and 2003. This percentage has held fairly steady since 1998. Women between 25 and 44 years of age were the most likely to obtain Pap smears.

Non-Hispanic Blacks had Pap smears more frequently than any other population group. This group was followed by non-Hispanic Whites and Hispanics. Persons classified as poor, especially those 65 years old and over, took the test less frequently. Low to moderate levels of educational attainment were also associated with a reduced frequency of Pap smears.

Table III-40. Use of Pap Smears for Women 18 Years of Age and Over, According to Selected Characteristics, Selected Years, 1987–2003

(Percent.)

Characteristic	2003	2000	1999	1998	1994	1993	1987
PERCENT OF WOMEN HAVING A PAP SMEAR WITHIN THE PAST THREE YEARS							
18 years and over, age-adjusted [1]	79.2	81.3	80.8	79.3	76.8	77.7	74.1
18 years and over, crude [1]	79.0	81.2	80.8	79.1	76.8	77.7	74.4
Age							
18–44 years	83.9	84.9	86.8	84.4	82.8	84.6	83.3
18–24 years	75.1	73.5	76.8	73.6	76.6	78.8	74.8
25–44 years	86.8	88.5	89.9	87.6	84.6	86.3	86.3
45–64 years	81.3	84.6	81.7	81.4	77.4	77.2	70.5
45–54 years	83.6	86.3	83.8	83.7	81.9	82.1	75.7
55–64 years	77.8	82.0	78.4	78.0	71.0	70.6	65.2
65 years and over	60.8	64.5	61.0	59.8	57.3	57.6	50.8
65–74 years	70.1	71.6	70.0	67.0	64.9	64.7	57.9
75 years and over	51.1	56.7	50.8	51.2	47.3	48.0	40.4
Race [2]							
White only	78.7	81.3	80.6	78.9	76.2	77.3	74.1
Black or African American only	84.0	85.1	85.7	84.2	83.5	82.7	80.7
American Indian and Alaska Native only	84.8	76.8	92.2	74.6	73.5	78.1	85.4
Asian only	68.3	66.4	64.4	68.5	66.4	68.8	51.9
Native Hawaiian and Other Pacific Islander only	*	*	*	...	...	...	...
Two or more races	81.6	80.0	86.9	...	...	...	...
Hispanic Origin and Race [2]							
18 years and over, crude							
Hispanic or Latino	75.4	77.0	76.3	75.2	74.4	77.2	67.6
Not Hispanic or Latino	79.5	81.7	81.3	79.6	77.0	77.8	74.9
White only	79.3	81.8	81.0	79.3	76.5	77.3	74.7
Black or African American only	83.8	85.1	86.0	84.2	83.8	82.7	80.9
Age, Hispanic Origin and Race [2]							
18–44 years							
Hispanic or Latino	75.9	78.1	77.0	76.4	80.6	80.9	73.9
Not Hispanic or Latino							
White only	85.8	86.6	88.7	85.7	82.9	85.3	84.5
Black or African American only	88.6	88.5	90.8	88.9	89.1	88.0	89.1
45–64 years							
Hispanic or Latino	77.9	77.8	79.5	78.3	70.1	75.8	57.7
Not Hispanic or Latino							
White only	81.4	85.9	81.9	81.7	77.5	77.2	71.2
Black or African American only	84.7	85.7	84.6	84.1	82.2	80.3	76.2
65 years and older							
Hispanic or Latino	64.6	66.8	63.7	59.8	43.8	57.1	41.7
Not Hispanic or Latino							
White only	60.7	64.2	60.5	59.7	58.2	57.1	51.8
Black or African American only	59.6	67.2	64.5	61.7	59.5	61.2	44.8
Age and Poverty Status [3]							
18 years and over, crude							
Below poverty	70.5	72.0	73.6	69.8	68.8	70.3	64.3
Near poor	71.4	73.4	72.5	70.6	68.8	71.2	68.2
Nonpoor	83.0	85.0	84.3	83.5	81.9	82.1	80.0
18–44 years							
Below poverty	77.1	77.1	79.7	77.1	78.9	77.0	77.1
Near poor	79.5	79.4	84.0	79.2	78.2	81.9	80.4
Nonpoor	86.9	88.0	89.0	87.6	85.7	87.9	86.4
45–64 years							
Below poverty	66.0	73.6	73.1	67.6	62.0	66.5	53.6
Near poor	71.4	76.1	70.4	69.9	66.2	64.8	60.4
Nonpoor	85.1	87.4	84.6	85.1	82.0	81.4	74.9
65 years and over							
Below poverty	52.6	53.7	51.9	48.2	44.0	47.4	33.2
Near poor	55.4	61.0	54.7	55.1	51.5	55.7	50.4
Nonpoor	65.4	68.8	66.4	65.3	66.8	62.0	60.0

[1]Includes all other races not shown separately, unknown poverty status, and unknown education.

[2]The race groups, White, Black, American Indian and Alaska Native (AI/AN), Asian, Native Hawaiian and Other Pacific Islander, and two or more races, include persons of Hispanic and non-Hispanic origin. Persons of Hispanic origin may be of any race.

[3]Poor persons are defined as having a total income below the poverty threshold. Near poor persons have incomes of 100 percent to less than 200 percent of poverty threshold. Nonpoor persons have incomes of 200 percent or more than the poverty threshold.

* = Figure does not meet standards of reliability or precision.

. . . = Not available.

Table III-40. Use of Pap Smears for Women 18 Years of Age and Over, According to Selected Characteristics, Selected Years, 1987–2003—*Continued*

(Percent.)

Characteristic	2003	2000	1999	1998	1994	1993	1987
Health Insurance Staus [4]							
18–64 years of age							
Insured	86.4	87.8	87.2	86.0	83.8	84.7	...
Private	87.0	88.0	87.5	86.5	83.6	84.8	...
Medicaid	82.8	85.8	84.2	83.0	86.2	82.7	...
Uninsured	66.6	70.4	73.3	69.6	68.6	69.4	...
65 years and over							
Medicare HMO	61.4	67.6	69.6	66.1	...	...	...
Private	63.0	67.2	62.9	61.3	61.2	60.6	...
Medicaid	53.9	57.8	54.8	49.9	44.9	47.8	...
Medicare fee-for-service only	53.8	55.1	48.4	49.8	42.4	43.6	...
Age and Education [5]							
25 years and over, crude							
No high school diploma or GED	64.9	69.9	66.1	65.0	60.9	61.9	57.1
High school diploma or GED	75.9	79.8	79.3	77.4	76.0	78.2	76.4
Some college or more	86.2	88.0	87.8	86.9	85.2	84.4	84.0
25–44 years							
No high school diploma or GED	71.7	79.6	79.0	76.8	73.6	73.6	75.1
High school diploma or GED	84.3	86.2	87.6	83.9	82.4	85.4	85.6
Some college or more	90.8	91.4	93.0	91.5	89.1	89.8	90.1
45–64 years							
No high school diploma or GED	71.4	75.7	71.6	69.2	66.1	65.6	58.0
High school diploma or GED	77.6	81.8	79.8	81.0	75.9	77.6	72.3
Some college or more	86.2	89.1	85.7	85.5	84.7	83.0	80.1
65 years and over							
No high school diploma or GED	52.5	56.6	51.8	52.4	47.7	50.7	44.0
High school diploma or GED	61.2	66.9	63.7	60.7	61.2	61.6	55.4
Some college or more	67.8	69.8	68.8	67.9	66.5	62.3	59.4

[4]Health insurance categories are mutually exclusive. Persons who reported both Medicaid and private coverage are classified as having private coverage. Starting in 1997, Medicaid includes state-sponsored health plans and State Children's Health Insurance Program (SCHIP). In addition to private and Medicaid, the category "insured" also includes military plans, other government-sponsored health plans, and Medicare, not shown separately. Persons 65 years of age and over who reported Medicare HMO (health maintenance organization) and some other type of health insurance coverage are classified as having Medicare HMO.

[5]Education categories shown are for 1998 and subsequent years. GED stands for General Educational Development high school equivalency diploma. In years prior to 1998 the following categories based on number of years of school completed were used: less than 12 years, 12 years, and 13 years or more.

. . . = Not available.

TABLE III-41. VISTS TO PHYSICIANS' OFFICES AND HOSPITAL OUTPATIENT AND EMERGENCY DEPARTMENTS, BY SELECETD CHARACTERISTICS, SELECETD YEARS, 1995–2003

Total visits to doctors, outpatient facilities, and emergency departments were estimated at about 1.1 billion in 2003. This astoundingly large figure is the result of 3.9 visits per year to all facilities combined by the average American resident. Visits to physicians' offices averaged 317 per 100 persons, visits to hospital outpatient departments averaged 33 per 100 persons, and those to emergency departments averaged 40 per 100 persons.

Females made about one-third more visits to physicians' offices, hospital outpatient facilities, and emergency departments than males. The rate of all visits for males age 18 to 44 years to all places is lowest (202 per 100 persons). Thereafter, it rises steadily with age, reaching an average of 830 visits per 100 males age 75 years and over. The pattern is somewhat different for females, as their frequency of visits increases during their main reproductive years (18 to 44 years of age). Thus, females average 297 visits per 100 persons when they are under 18 years of age, 396 visits per 100 persons between 18 and 44 years of age, and 474 visits per 100 persons between 45 and 54 years of age.

The number of visits by Blacks to all three venues was not markedly different than that of Whites, although Blacks under 18 years old had fewer medical visits than their White counterparts. Blacks had more visits than Whites to hospital outpatient and emergency departments. However, Blacks had fewer visits to physicians' offices.

Table III-41. Visits to Physicians' Offices and Hospital Outpatient and Emergency Departments, by Selected Characteristics, Selected Years, 1995–2003

(Number in thousands, rate per 100 population.)

Age, sex, and race	All places [1]				Physicians' offices			
	2003	2002	2001	1995	2003	2002	2001	1995
NUMBER OF VISITS (Thousands)								
Total	1 114 504	1 157 798	1 142 420	860 859	906 023	964 304	951 214	697 082
Under 18 years	223 964	238 571	220 921	194 644	169 392	188 933	173 383	150 351
18–44 years	330 687	337 681	341 383	285 184	251 853	263 672	267 844	219 065
45–64 years	301 477	308 627	300 567	188 320	257 258	267 249	259 718	159 531
45–54 years	164 383	169 871	165 321	104 891	138 634	145 767	141 598	88 266
55–64 years	137 094	138 756	135 247	83 429	118 624	121 482	118 120	71 264
65 years and over	258 375	272 919	279 548	192 712	227 520	244 451	250 269	168 135
65–74 years	120 817	132 116	136 819	102 605	106 424	118 971	122 970	90 544
75 years and over	137 558	140 802	142 729	90 106	121 096	125 479	127 299	77 591
NUMBER OF VISITS PER 100 PERSONS								
Total, age-adjusted [2]	391	410	410	334	317	342	342	271
Total, crude	390	409	408	329	317	341	340	266
Under 18 years	307	328	305	275	232	260	239	213
18–44 years	300	306	311	264	229	239	244	203
45–64 years	442	466	469	364	377	404	406	309
45–54 years	406	427	425	339	343	367	364	286
55–64 years	494	525	538	401	428	459	470	343
65 years and over	754	804	829	612	664	720	742	534
65–74 years	668	733	757	560	588	660	680	494
75 years and over	850	884	913	683	748	788	814	588
Sex and Age								
Male, age-adjusted [2]	338	353	356	290	273	293	294	232
Male, crude	329	343	343	277	264	283	281	220
Under 18 years	317	329	306	273	241	262	238	209
18–44 years	202	214	217	190	147	161	163	139
45–54 years	335	351	349	275	280	298	294	229
55–64 years	422	448	457	351	365	393	399	300
65–74 years	633	703	726	508	558	631	654	445
75 years and over	881	850	934	711	777	762	840	616
Female, age-adjusted [2]	442	465	463	377	360	388	388	309
Female, crude	449	472	470	378	368	396	395	310
Under 18 years	297	327	304	277	223	258	240	217
18–44 years	396	397	402	336	309	316	323	265
45–54 years	474	500	498	400	403	433	431	339
55–64 years	561	596	612	446	486	521	535	382
65–74 years	697	757	782	603	613	684	702	534
75 years and over	830	905	900	666	730	804	798	571
Race and Age [3]								
White, age-adjusted [2]	399	421	428	339	332	359	364	282
White, crude	405	426	433	338	337	364	369	281
Under 18 years	330	346	330	295	260	282	268	237
18–44 years	308	317	327	267	242	256	264	211
45–54 years	409	439	434	334	352	385	378	286
55–64 years	500	534	552	397	439	476	490	345
65–74 years	654	734	778	557	582	669	708	496
75 years and over	844	880	938	689	747	790	845	598
Black or African American, age-adjusted [2]	391	427	357	309	261	301	242	204
Black or African American, crude	363	392	329	281	236	269	217	178
Under 18 years	247	307	210	193	131	198	110	100
18–44 years	326	316	291	260	199	191	178	158
45–54 years	442	422	454	387	315	306	342	281
55–64 years	486	563	519	414	349	421	383	294
65–74 years	761	842	633	553	602	*687	492	429
75 years and over	774	*1 019	676	534	608	*842	517	395

[1] All places includes visits to physicians' offices and hospital outpatient and emergency departments.
[2] Estimates are age adjusted to the 2000 standard population using six age groups: under 18 years, 18–44 years, 45–54 years, 55–64 years, 65–74 years, and 75 years and over.
[3] Beginning in 1999, the instruction for the race item on the Patient Record Form was changed so that more than one race could be recorded. In previous years, only one racial category could be checked.
* = Figure does not meet standards of reliability or precision.

Table III-41. Visits to Physicians' Offices and Hospital Outpatient and Emergency Departments, by Selected Characteristics, Selected Years, 1995–2003—*Continued*

(Number in thousands, rate per 100 population.)

Age, sex, and race	Hospital outpatient departments				Hospital emergency rooms			
	2003	2002	2001	1995	2003	2002	2001	1995
NUMBER OF VISITS (Thousands)								
Total	94 578	83 339	83 715	67 232	113 903	110 155	107 490	96 545
Under 18 years	25 652	21 707	21 299	17 636	28 920	27 932	26 239	26 657
18–44 years	32 386	28 216	27 430	24 299	46 449	45 792	46 109	41 820
45–64 years	23 227	21 436	21 590	14 811	20 992	19 943	19 260	13 978
45–54 years	12 889	12 054	12 016	8 029	12 861	12 050	11 707	8 595
55–64 years	10 338	9 382	9 574	6 782	8 132	7 892	7 552	5 383
65 years and over	13 313	11 980	13 396	10 486	17 542	16 488	15 883	14 090
65–74 years	7 240	6 386	7 299	6 004	7 153	6 759	6 551	6 057
75 years and over	6 073	5 595	6 097	4 482	10 389	9 728	9 332	8 033
NUMBER OF VISITS PER 100 PERSONS								
Total, age-adjusted [2]	33	29	30	26	40	39	39	37
Total, crude	33	29	30	26	40	39	38	37
Under 18 years	35	30	29	25	40	38	36	38
18–44 years	29	26	25	22	42	42	42	39
45–64 years	34	32	34	29	31	30	30	27
45–54 years	32	30	31	26	32	30	30	28
55–64 years	37	36	38	33	29	30	30	26
65 years and over	39	35	40	33	51	49	47	45
65–74 years	40	35	40	33	40	38	36	33
75 years and over	38	35	39	34	64	61	60	61
Sex and Age								
Male, age-adjusted [2]	27	24	25	21	39	37	37	37
Male, crude	26	23	24	21	38	37	37	36
Under 18 years	35	28	29	25	41	39	38	40
18–44 years	18	16	16	14	37	37	39	37
45–54 years	25	25	26	20	30	29	29	26
55–64 years	29	28	30	26	29	28	28	25
65–74 years	35	34	35	29	41	38	38	34
75 years and over	38	31	37	34	67	58	57	61
Female, age-adjusted [2]	40	35	35	31	42	41	40	37
Female, crude	40	35	35	31	42	41	40	37
Under 18 years	36	31	29	25	38	38	34	35
18–44 years	41	35	34	31	47	46	45	40
45–54 years	38	36	36	32	33	32	31	29
55–64 years	45	43	45	38	30	32	32	26
65–74 years	45	36	45	36	39	37	35	32
75 years and over	37	38	40	34	63	63	61	61
Race and Age [3]								
White, age-adjusted [2]	30	27	28	23	38	36	36	34
White, crude	30	27	28	23	37	36	36	34
Under 18 years	33	28	28	23	38	36	34	35
18–44 years	27	23	23	20	39	38	40	36
45–54 years	28	27	28	23	29	27	28	25
55–64 years	33	31	34	28	28	27	28	24
65–74 years	36	30	37	29	36	35	33	32
75 years and over	35	31	36	31	62	59	58	60
Black or African American, age-adjusted [2]	59	55	51	48	71	71	65	58
Black or African American, crude	58	53	49	45	69	70	64	58
Under 18 years	55	46	44	39	61	63	55	53
18–44 years	51	46	41	38	77	79	71	64
45–54 years	62	57	56	55	65	59	56	51
55–64 years	84	78	79	73	53	65	56	47
65–74 years	82	87	70	*77	77	68	71	47
75 years and over	64	85	67	66	103	92	91	73

[2]Estimates are age adjusted to the 2000 standard population using six age groups: under 18 years, 18–44 years, 45–54 years, 55–64 years, 65–74 years, and 75 years and over.

[3]Beginning in 1999, the instruction for the race item on the Patient Record Form was changed so that more than one race could be recorded. In previous years, only one racial category could be checked.

* = Figure does not meet standards of reliability or precision.

TABLE III-42. INJURY-RELATED VISITS TO HOSPITAL EMERGENCY DEPARTMENTS, BY SEX, AGE, AND INTENT AND MECHANISM OF INJURY, SELECTED ANNUAL AVERAGES, 1995–2003

Almost 40 million injury-related visits to hospital emergency departments took place, taking the average from 2002 and 2003. There were about 14 visits for every 100 persons, with rates of 15.5 by males and 12.5 by females (the table expresses these rates per 10,000 persons).

The most injury-prone age group was young men between 18 and 24 years of age; they made 21.3 visits to emergency departments for each representative 100 persons. This rate consisted of 14.6 visits for unintentional injuries and 2.1 visits for intentional injuries (consisting

of suicide attempts and assaults). In addition, the total includes unclassified unintentional injuries and some injuries resulting from adverse effects of medical treatment. The two largest accident categories for this age group were motor vehicle traffic accidents (2.7 per 100 males) and "struck by or against objects or persons" (3.1 per 100 males).

Females 18 to 24 years old incurred 16.7 visits per 100 persons to emergency departments, substantially fewer than their male contemporaries. However, for injuries from motor vehicle traffic, females had 3.3 visits per 100 persons, more than the 2.7 per 100 figure for males. It should be noted that those categorized as injured in motor vehicle accidents consisted of passengers as well as drivers.

Table III-42. Injury-Related Visits to Hospital Emergency Departments, by Sex, Age, and Intent and Mechanism of Injury, Selected Annual Averages, 1995–2003

(Number, rate per 10,000 population.)

Sex, age, and intent and mechanism of injury [1]	Injury-related visits in thousands			Injury-related visits per 10,000 persons		
	2002–2003	1998–1999	1995–1996	2002–2003	1998–1999	1995–1996
BOTH SEXES						
All Ages [2]	39 676	37 361	36 081	1 401.4	1 378.3	1 360.9
MALE						
All Ages [2]	21 467	20 445	20 030	1 548.1	1 535.2	1 530.7
Under 18 Years [2]	5 974	6 054	6 238	1 604.5	1 644.3	1 720.2
Unintentional injuries [3]	4 781	5 190	5 478	1 284.2	1 409.7	1 510.5
Falls	1 228	1 247	1 402	329.9	338.7	386.5
Struck by or against objects or persons	1 315	1 398	1 011	353.2	379.7	278.9
Motor vehicle traffic	369	388	453	99.2	105.5	125.0
Cut or pierce	348	505	493	93.5	137.1	136.0
Intentional injuries	202	222	290	54.4	60.3	80.0
18–24 Years [2]	2 956	2 948	2 980	2 134.3	2 295.1	2 396.9
Unintentional injuries [3]	2 019	2 319	2 423	1 457.7	1 805.3	1 948.7
Falls	289	333	299	208.3	259.5	240.8
Struck by or against objects or persons	433	389	387	312.8	303.1	311.0
Motor vehicle traffic	376	412	347	271.9	320.9	279.4
Cut or pierce	286	344	304	206.4	268.2	244.8
Intentional injuries	287	291	335	207.0	226.5	269.2
25–44 Years [2]	7 157	7 112	7 245	1 758.7	1 751.7	1 767.4
Unintentional injuries [3]	4 701	5 391	5 757	1 155.2	1 327.8	1 404.3
Falls	840	847	817	206.5	208.6	199.4
Struck by or against objects or persons	698	819	619	171.5	201.6	151.0
Motor vehicle traffic	766	839	912	188.3	206.6	222.6
Cut or pierce	615	786	860	151.1	193.7	209.8
Intentional injuries	479	473	701	117.7	116.5	171.0
45–64 Years [2]	3 528	2 822	2 240	1 082.8	1 011.9	883.4
Unintentional injuries [3]	2 207	2 213	1 845	677.5	793.4	727.6
Falls	518	569	445	159.0	204.0	175.6
Struck by or against objects or persons	247	197	186	75.8	70.6	73.3
Motor vehicle traffic	343	322	244	105.3	115.5	96.3
Cut or pierce	276	290	203	84.6	104.1	79.9
Intentional injuries	123	73	86	37.9	26.2	33.8
65 Years and Over [2]	1 854	1 509	1 327	1 285.9	1 100.3	1 000.7
Unintentional injuries [3]	1 232	1 151	1 009	854.4	839.3	760.6
Falls	649	584	505	450.4	426.0	380.9
Struck by or against objects or persons	77	101	*39	53.4	73.3	*29.4
Motor vehicle traffic	128	113	99	88.5	82.7	74.7
Cut or pierce	91	85	*81	62.8	*61.7	*61.1
Intentional injuries	22	16	*	*	*	*

[1] Intent and mechanism of injury are based on the first-listed external cause of injury code. Intentional injuries include suicide attempts and assaults.
[2] Includes all injury-related visits not shown separately in table, including those with undetermined intent (less than 0.5 percent in 2000–2001), insufficient or no information to code cause of injury (about 16.9 percent in 2000–2001), and resulting from adverse effects of medical treatment (about 3.3 percent in 2000–2001).
[3] Includes unintentional injury-related visits with mechanism of injury not shown in table.
* = Figure does not meet standards of reliability or precision.

Table III-42. Injury-Related Visits to Hospital Emergency Departments, by Sex, Age, and Intent and Mechanism of Injury, Selected Annual Averages, 1995–2003—*Continued*

(Number, rate per 10,000 population.)

Sex, age, and intent and mechanism of injury [1]	Injury-related visits in thousands			Injury-related visits per 10,000 persons		
	2002–2003	1998–1999	1995–1996	2002–2003	1998–1999	1995–1996
FEMALE						
All Ages [2]	18 208	16 917	16 051	1 253.1	1 217.6	1 186.4
Under 18 Years [2]	4 321	4 290	4 372	1 214.5	1 220.4	1 263.9
Unintentional injuries [3]	3 204	3 598	3 760	900.4	1 023.4	1 087.0
Falls	908	964	1 040	255.3	274.2	300.7
Struck by or against objects or persons	627	689	477	176.1	196.1	137.9
Motor vehicle traffic	368	394	447	103.5	112.1	129.3
Cut or pierce	198	258	253	55.7	73.4	73.0
Intentional injuries	216	147	220	60.7	41.7	63.6
18–24 Years [2]	2 307	2 049	1 900	1 672.9	1 589.6	1 523.4
Unintentional injuries [3]	1 492	1 464	1 430	1 081.5	1 135.8	1 146.7
Falls	260	208	268	188.2	161.7	214.5
Struck by or against objects or persons	201	169	134	145.9	130.8	107.4
Motor vehicle traffic	456	442	373	330.9	342.7	298.8
Cut or pierce	129	122	131	93.2	94.8	105.3
Intentional injuries	202	230	239	146.2	178.6	191.7
25–44 Years [2]	5 527	5 257	5 098	1 320.9	1 246.7	1 205.8
Unintentional injuries [3]	3 470	3 820	3 877	829.4	906.1	916.8
Falls	802	908	817	191.8	215.5	193.3
Struck by or against objects or persons	381	405	380	91.0	95.9	89.8
Motor vehicle traffic	819	794	872	195.8	188.4	206.2
Cut or pierce	337	472	338	80.4	111.9	79.8
Intentional injuries	401	422	422	95.8	100.2	99.8
45–64 Years [2]	3 335	2 802	2 369	963.4	940.4	873.7
Unintentional injuries [3]	2 272	2 109	1 857	656.4	707.9	685.2
Falls	791	706	600	228.4	237.0	221.5
Struck by or against objects or persons	213	193	160	61.5	64.8	58.8
Motor vehicle traffic	388	317	343	111.9	106.4	126.5
Cut or pierce	205	214	127	59.1	71.8	46.9
Intentional injuries	119	111	*64	34.3	37.4	*23.5
65 Years and Over [2]	2 718	2 518	2 313	1 379.3	1 346.8	1 256.1
Unintentional injuries [3]	1 957	2 016	1 931	993.2	1 078.1	1 049.0
Falls	1 225	1 258	1 230	621.9	672.7	667.9
Struck by or against objects or persons	170	119	82	86.1	63.6	44.8
Motor vehicle traffic	175	148	169	88.6	79.3	91.6
Cut or pierce	48	73	*42	24.4	*39.0	*22.7
Intentional injuries	12	34	*	*	*	*

[1] Intent and mechanism of injury are based on the first-listed external cause of injury code. Intentional injuries include suicide attempts and assaults.

[2] Includes all injury-related visits not shown separately in table, including those with undetermined intent (less than 0.5 percent in 2000–2001), insufficient or no information to code cause of injury (about 16.9 percent in 2000–2001), and resulting from adverse effects of medical treatment (about 3.3 percent in 2000–2001).

[3] Includes unintentional injury-related visits with mechanism of injury not shown in table.

* = Figure does not meet standards of reliability or precision.

TABLE III-43. VISITS TO PRIMARY CARE AND SPECIALIST PHYSICIANS, ACCORDING TO SELECTED CHARACTERISTICS AND TYPE OF PHYSICIAN, SELECTED YEARS, 1980–2003

In 2003, 58.5 percent of all physicians' office visits were to primary care physicians, including physicians in general and family practice, internal medicine, obstetrics and gynecology, and pediatrics. There has been a decline in the share of office visits to general and family practice physicians since 1980.

The other 41.5 percent of visits were to specialists. A significant number of adult visits were to specialists, while children predominantly saw pediatricians. About 22 percent of children under 18 years old visited a specialist.

Table III-43. Visits to Primary Care and Specialist Physicians, According to Selected Characteristics and Type of Physician, Selected Years, 1980–2003

(Percent.)

| Age, sex, and race | Type of primary care generalist physician | | | | | | | | | | | |
| | All primary care | | | | General and family practice | | | | Internal medicine | | | |
	2003	2000	1990	1980	2003	2000	1990	1980	2003	2000	1990	1980
PERCENT OF ALL PHYSICIANS' OFFICE VISITS												
All Persons	58.5	58.9	63.6	66.2	24.5	24.1	29.9	33.5	15.6	15.3	13.8	12.1
Under 18 years	78.3	79.7	79.5	77.8	19.3	19.9	26.5	26.1	*	*	2.9	2.0
18–44 years	63.7	62.1	65.2	65.3	28.5	28.2	31.9	34.3	13.0	12.7	11.8	8.6
45–64 years	52.2	51.2	55.5	60.2	27.3	26.4	32.1	36.3	19.0	20.1	18.6	19.5
45–54 years	55.1	52.3	55.6	60.2	29.7	27.8	32.0	37.4	18.3	18.7	17.1	17.1
55–64 years	48.9	49.9	55.5	60.2	24.5	24.7	32.1	35.4	19.9	21.7	20.0	21.8
65 years and over	45.2	46.5	52.6	61.6	20.6	20.2	28.1	37.5	22.4	24.5	23.3	22.7
65–74 years	46.6	46.6	52.7	61.2	20.8	19.7	28.1	37.4	22.9	24.5	23.0	22.1
75 years and over	44.0	46.4	52.4	62.3	20.5	20.8	28.0	37.6	22.0	24.5	23.7	23.5
SEX AND AGE												
Male												
Under 18 years	76.5	77.7	78.1	77.3	17.3	18.3	24.1	25.6	*	*	3.0	2.0
18–44 years	54.2	51.5	51.8	50.8	35.6	34.2	35.9	38.0	17.3	14.4	15.0	11.5
45–64 years	50.1	49.4	50.6	55.6	30.3	28.7	31.0	34.4	19.2	19.8	19.2	20.5
65 years and over	40.4	43.1	51.2	58.2	20.0	19.3	27.7	35.6	20.1	23.8	23.3	22.3
Female												
Under 18 years	80.4	82.0	81.1	78.5	21.5	21.7	29.1	26.6	*	*	2.8	2.0
18–44 years	68.2	67.2	71.3	72.1	25.2	25.3	30.0	32.5	10.9	11.9	10.3	7.3
45–64 years	53.7	52.5	58.8	63.4	25.3	24.9	32.8	37.7	18.9	20.2	18.2	18.9
65 years and over	48.6	48.9	53.5	63.9	21.0	20.9	28.3	38.7	24.1	25.0	23.3	22.9
RACE AND AGE [1]												
White												
Under 18 years	78.1	78.5	79.2	77.6	19.8	21.2	27.1	26.4	*	*	2.3	2.0
18–44 years	63.3	61.4	64.4	64.8	29.1	29.2	31.9	34.5	12.1	11.0	10.6	8.6
45–64 years	51.9	49.3	54.2	59.6	27.5	27.3	31.5	36.0	18.4	17.1	17.6	19.2
65 years and over	43.1	45.1	51.9	61.4	20.3	20.3	27.5	36.6	20.8	23.0	23.1	23.3
Black or African American												
Under 18 years	77.3	87.3	85.5	79.9	*18.8	*	20.2	23.7	*	*	9.8	*2.2
18–44 years	66.5	65.0	68.3	68.5	25.0	22.0	31.9	31.7	*	20.9	18.1	9.0
45–64 years	56.7	61.7	61.6	66.1	26.2	23.3	31.2	38.6	23.8	35.9	26.9	22.6
65 years and over	56.0	52.8	58.6	64.6	*20.9	*18.5	28.9	49.0	31.4	33.4	28.7	14.2

[1] Beginning in 1999, the instruction for the race item on the Patient Record Form was changed so that more than one race could be recorded. In previous years, only one racial category could be checked.

* = Figure does not meet standards of reliability or precision.

Table III-43. Visits to Primary Care and Specialist Physicians, According to Selected Characteristics and Type of Physician, Selected Years, 1980–2003—*Continued*

(Percent.)

Age, sex, and race	Type of primary care generalist physician — Obstetrics and gynecology 2003	2000	1990	1980	Pediatrics 2003	2000	1990	1980	Specialty care physicians 2003	2000	1990	1980
PERCENT OF ALL PHYSICIANS' OFFICE VISITS												
All Persons	8.4	7.8	8.7	9.6	10.1	11.7	11.2	10.9	41.5	41.1	36.4	33.8
Under 18 years	*1.5	*1.1	1.2	1.3	52.4	57.3	48.9	48.5	21.7	20.3	20.5	22.2
18–44 years	21.5	20.4	20.8	21.7	*0.7	*0.9	0.7	0.7	36.3	37.9	34.8	34.7
45–64 years	5.6	4.5	4.6	4.2	*	*	*	*	47.8	48.8	44.5	39.8
45–54 years	6.7	5.6	6.3	5.6	*	*	*	*	44.9	47.7	44.4	39.8
55–64 years	*4.4	3.3	3.1	2.9	*	*	*	*	51.1	50.1	44.5	39.8
65 years and over	*2.0	1.5	1.1	1.4	*	*	*	*	54.8	53.5	47.4	38.4
65–74 years	*2.7	2.0	1.6	1.7	*	*	*	*	53.4	53.4	47.3	38.8
75 years and over	*1.4	*1.0	*0.6	1.0	*	*	*	*	56.0	53.6	47.6	37.7
SEX AND AGE												
Male												
Under 18 years	X	X	X	X	53.2	58.0	50.7	49.4	23.5	22.3	21.9	22.7
18–44 years	X	X	X	X	*1.2	*1.7	0.7	1.0	45.8	48.5	48.2	49.2
45–64 years	X	X	X	X	*	*	*	*	49.9	50.6	49.4	44.4
65 years and over	X	X	X	X	*	*	*	*	59.6	56.9	48.8	41.8
Female												
Under 18 years	*3.2	2.1	2.3	2.5	51.4	56.5	46.9	47.4	19.6	18.0	18.9	21.5
18–44 years	31.6	29.6	30.4	31.7	*	*	0.7	0.6	31.8	32.8	28.7	27.9
45–64 years	9.2	7.3	7.7	6.7	*	*	*	*	46.3	47.5	41.2	36.6
65 years and over	*3.4	2.6	1.8	2.1	*	*	*	*	51.4	51.1	46.5	36.1
RACE AND AGE [1]												
White												
Under 18 years	*1.5	*1.2	1.0	1.1	52.4	54.7	48.8	48.2	21.9	21.5	20.8	22.4
18–44 years	21.3	20.4	21.1	21.0	*0.8	*0.8	0.7	0.7	36.7	38.6	35.6	35.2
45–64 years	5.7	4.7	4.8	4.1	*	*	*	*	48.1	50.7	45.8	40.4
65 years and over	*1.9	1.5	1.2	1.4	*	*	*	*	56.9	54.9	48.1	38.6
Black or African American												
Under 18 years	*	*	*3.4	2.8	51.3	75.0	52.1	51.2	22.7	*12.7	14.5	20.1
18–44 years	*25.8	20.7	17.9	27.1	*	*	*	*	33.5	35.0	31.7	31.5
45–64 years	*	*2.4	3.5	4.8	*	*	*	*	43.3	38.3	38.4	33.9
65 years and over	*	*	*	*	*	*	*	*	44.0	47.2	41.4	35.4

[1]Beginning in 1999, the instruction for the race item on the Patient Record Form was changed so that more than one race could be recorded. In previous years, only one racial category could be checked.

* = Figure does not meet standards of reliability or precision.

X = Category not applicable.

TABLE III-44. PRESCRIPTION DRUG USE IN THE PAST MONTH, BY SEX, AGE, RACE, AND HISPANIC ORIGIN, 1988–1994 AND 1999–2002

During the 1999–2002 period, 45 percent of the population reported using at least one prescription drug in the past month, an increase of 16 percent from the 1988–1994 survey period. Women used prescription drugs more frequently than men, and Whites used prescription drugs more often than Blacks and Mexicans.

Percentages are also given in this table for persons using three or more prescription drugs per month. Of the total population, 18 percent used three or more prescription drugs per month; this percentage rose to almost 52 percent for persons age 65 years and over. In this age group, over 50 percent of both Whites and Blacks were using three or more prescription drugs per month, compared to just under 40 percent of Mexicans.

Table III-44. Prescription Drug Use in the Past Month, by Sex, Age, Race, and Hispanic Origin, 1988–1994 and 1999–2002

(Percent.)

Sex and age	All persons [1]		Not Hispanic or Latino				Mexican [2]	
			White		Black or African American			
	1999–2002	1988–1994	1999–2002	1988–1994	1999–2002	1988–1994	1999–2002	1988–1994
PERCENT OF POPULATION WITH AT LEAST ONE PRESCRIPTION DRUG IN PAST MONTH								
Both sexes, age-adjusted [3]	45.3	39.1	48.9	41.1	40.1	36.9	31.7	31.7
Male	39.9	32.7	43.1	34.2	35.4	31.1	25.8	27.5
Female	50.4	45.0	54.5	47.6	43.8	41.4	37.8	36.0
Both sexes, crude	45.1	37.8	50.9	41.4	36.0	31.2	23.7	24.0
Male	38.7	30.6	43.9	33.5	30.8	25.5	18.8	20.1
Female	51.2	44.6	57.6	48.9	40.6	36.2	28.9	28.1
Under 18 years	24.2	20.5	27.6	22.9	18.6	14.8	15.9	16.1
18–44 years	35.9	31.3	41.3	34.3	28.5	27.8	19.2	21.1
45–64 years	64.1	54.8	66.1	55.5	62.3	57.5	49.3	48.1
65 years and over	84.7	73.6	85.4	74.0	81.1	74.5	72.0	67.7
Male								
Under 18 years	26.2	20.4	30.6	22.3	19.8	15.5	16.2	16.3
18–44 years	27.1	21.5	31.2	23.5	21.5	21.1	13.0	14.9
45–64 years	55.6	47.2	57.4	48.1	54.0	48.2	36.4	43.8
65 years and over	80.1	67.2	81.0	67.4	78.1	64.4	66.8	61.3
Female								
Under 18 years	22.0	20.6	24.4	23.6	17.3	14.2	15.6	16.0
18–44 years	44.6	40.7	51.7	44.7	34.2	33.4	26.2	28.1
45–64 years	72.0	62.0	74.7	62.6	69.0	64.4	62.4	52.2
65 years and over	88.1	78.3	88.8	78.8	83.1	81.3	76.3	73.0
PERCENT OF POPULATION WITH THREE OR MORE PRESCRIPTION DRUGS IN PAST MONTH								
Both sexes, age-adjusted [3]	17.7	11.8	18.9	12.4	16.5	12.6	11.2	9.0
Male	14.8	9.4	15.9	9.9	14.4	10.2	9.5	7.0
Female	20.4	13.9	21.7	14.6	18.0	14.3	12.9	11.0
Both sexes, crude	17.6	11.0	20.5	12.5	13.4	9.2	6.1	4.8
Male	13.9	8.3	16.4	9.5	10.9	7.0	4.8	3.4
Female	21.1	13.6	24.5	15.4	15.6	11.1	7.5	6.4
Under 18 years	4.1	2.4	4.9	3.2	2.5	1.5	2.1	*1.2
18–44 years	8.4	5.7	10.1	6.3	6.5	5.4	2.7	3.0
45–64 years	30.8	20.0	31.6	20.9	31.1	21.9	20.7	16.0
65 years and over	51.6	35.3	52.5	35.0	50.1	41.2	39.5	31.3
Male								
Under 18 years	4.3	2.6	5.2	3.3	3.0	1.7	1.9	*
18–44 years	6.7	3.6	8.4	4.1	4.4	4.2	*1.7	*1.8
45–64 years	23.5	15.1	24.0	15.8	26.3	18.7	18.2	11.6
65 years and over	46.0	31.3	47.0	30.9	48.2	31.7	34.2	27.6
Female								
Under 18 years	3.9	2.3	4.7	3.0	*2.0	*1.2	2.2	*1.5
18–44 years	10.2	7.6	11.9	8.5	8.3	6.4	4.0	4.3
45–64 years	37.4	24.7	39.1	25.8	35.0	24.3	23.3	20.3
65 years and over	55.7	38.2	56.6	38.0	51.3	47.7	44.0	34.5

Note: Starting with data year 1999, race-specific estimates are tabulated according to 1997 standards for Federal Data on Race and Ethnicity and are not strictly comparable with earlier years. The two non-Hispanic race categories shown in the table conform to 1997 standards. The 1999–2000 race-specific data are for persons who reported only one racial group.

[1] Includes persons of all races and Hispanic origins, not just those shown separately.
[2] Persons of Mexican origin may be of any race.
[3] Age adjusted to the 2000 standard population using four age groups: under 18 years, 18–44 years, 45–64 years, and 65 years and over.
* = Figure does not meet standards of reliability or precision.

TABLE III-45. SELECTED PRESCRIPTION AND NONPRE-SCRIPTION DRUGS RECORDED DURING PHYSICIANS' OFFICE VISITS AND HOSPITAL OUTPATIENT DEPARTMENT VISITS, BY AGE AND SEX, 1995–1996 AND 2002–2003

During the two-year period ending in 2003, doctors prescribed, ordered (for nonprescription), or provided a total of 586 drugs, when measured at an annual rate per 100 of the United States population. The underlying records were prepared during 235 patient visits that involved at least one drug, also per 100 of the U.S. population.

Table III-45. Selected Prescription and Nonprescription Drugs Recorded During Physicians' Office Visits and Hospital Outpatient Department Visits, by Age and Sex, 1995–1996 and 2002–2003

(Number per 100 population.)

Age group and National Drug Code (NDC) therapeutic class (common reasons for use) [1]	Total		Men		Women	
	2002–2003	1995–1996	2002–2003	1995–1996	2002–2003	1995–1996
All Ages						
Drug visits with at least one drug per 100 population [2,3]	234.9	189.8	193.7	156.5	274.1	221.5
Number of Drugs per 100 Population [4]						
Total number of drugs [5]	585.7	400.3	477.6	321.1	688.8	475.6
NSAID(pain relief) [6]	30.0	19.9	24.1	16.0	35.6	23.7
Antidepressants (depression and related disorders)	27.8	13.8	19.2	9.1	36.0	18.2
Antihistamines (allergies)	23.8	13.7	18.7	10.8	28.6	16.4
Antiasthmatics/bronchodilators (asthma, breathing)	22.9	13.0	19.9	11.7	25.7	14.3
Nonnarcotic analgesics (pain relief)	21.8	14.4	20.4	13.0	23.2	15.7
Hyperlipidemia (high cholesterol)	20.8	5.4	21.5	5.4	20.2	5.4
Hypertension control drugs, not otherwise specified	20.7	6.0	17.6	4.1	23.6	7.8
Acid/peptic disorders (gastrointestinal reflux, ulcers)	19.2	12.0	15.6	9.8	22.6	14.1
Blood glucose/sugar regulators (diabetes)	18.5	9.5	17.5	8.6	19.4	10.4
ACE inhibitors (high blood pressure, heart disease)	16.6	9.6	16.3	9.0	16.9	10.2
Diuretics (high blood pressure, heart disease)	15.9	10.2	12.8	7.8	18.8	12.6
Penicillins (bacterial infections)	15.2	16.6	14.3	15.5	15.9	17.7
Narcotic analgesics (pain relief)	15.3	11.2	12.3	10.3	18.2	12.2
Vitamins/minerals (dietary supplements)	14.5	9.2	8.3	3.4	20.5	14.8
Estrogens/progestins (menopause, hot flashes)	X	X	X	X	19.2	19.8
Under 18 Years						
Drug visits with at least one drug per 100 population [2,3]	177.9	153.9	181.6	152.3	174.1	155.6
Number of Drugs per 100 Population [4]						
Total number of drugs [5]	334.8	261.3	340.1	255.6	329.3	267.3
Penicillins (bacterial infections)	34.3	37.2	34.0	36.4	34.6	38.0
Antiasthmatics/bronchodilators (asthma, breathing)	26.0	13.4	27.7	14.8	24.3	11.9
Antihistamines (allergies)	25.9	17.5	26.0	16.7	25.8	18.4
Erythromycins/lincosamides (infections)	13.6	10.2	13.3	11.0	13.9	9.4
NSAID (pain relief) [6]	13.1	7.4	12.4	6.9	13.8	7.9
Cephalosporins (bacterial infections)	12.7	18.1	13.7	18.8	11.6	17.3
Nonnarcotic analgesics (pain relief)	12.0	12.1	12.5	10.4	11.4	13.9
Antitussives/expectorants (cough and cold, congestion)	10.3	11.8	10.3	11.0	10.3	12.7
Nasal corticosteroid inhalants (asthma, breathing)	9.3	3.5	9.3	3.5	9.3	3.5
Anorexiants/CNS stimulants (attention deficit disorder, hyperactivity)	8.8	3.9	12.5	5.6	4.9	2.1
Nasal decongestants (congestion)	8.3	14.0	8.0	12.4	8.5	15.7
Antidepressants (depression and related disorders)	6.8	1.9	7.7	1.9	5.9	1.9
18–44 Years						
Drug visits with at least one drug per 100 population [2,3]	161.4	136.2	108.4	90.9	213.3	180.4
Number of Drugs per 100 Population [4]						
Total number of drugs [5]	330.5	251.0	227.5	168.8	431.5	331.2
Antidepressants (depression and related disorders)	26.6	14.0	17.9	9.3	35.0	18.5
NSAID (pain relief) [6]	22.2	16.7	16.7	14.5	27.6	18.8
Antihistamines (allergies)	19.0	10.8	12.8	7.5	25.0	14.1
Narcotic analgesics (pain)	14.0	11.7	10.6	10.8	17.4	12.7
Antiasthmatics/bronchodilator (asthma, breathing)	11.5	6.8	7.4	3.3	15.6	10.2
Vitamins/minerals (dietary supplements)	11.3	11.8	2.1	1.1	20.2	22.2
Acid/peptic disorders (gastrointestinal reflux, ulcers)	9.4	6.6	8.5	5.3	10.2	7.9
Penicillins (bacterial infections)	8.8	9.5	6.2	7.0	11.3	11.9
Nasal corticosteroid inhalants (asthma, breathing, allergies)	8.7	4.7	6.7	3.3	10.6	6.1
Erythromycins/lincosamides (infections)	8.4	7.5	5.9	5.4	10.9	9.5
Antitussives/expectorants (cough and cold, congestion)	8.1	7.7	5.4	5.8	10.7	9.5
Nonnarcotic analgesics (pain relief)	7.7	6.0	5.4	4.5	9.9	7.4
Contraceptive agents (prevent pregnancy)	X	X	X	X	22.8	13.4
Age 45–64 Years						
Drug visits with at least one drug per 100 population [2,3]	284.1	222.4	231.7	185.0	333.3	257.4
Number of Drugs per 100 Population [4]						
Total number of drugs [5]	757.7	505.1	612.5	403.2	894.3	600.4
Antidepressants (depression and related disorders)	44.5	23.5	29.6	14.9	58.4	31.5
NSAID (pain relief) [6]	42.6	30.3	37.0	23.9	47.8	36.4
Hyperlipidemia (high cholesterol)	36.9	10.4	40.2	12.0	33.7	8.8
Hypertension control drugs, not otherwise specified (high blood pressure)	33.7	9.4	31.6	6.9	35.7	11.7
Blood glucose/sugar regulators (diabetes)	33.0	17.7	32.3	16.7	33.6	18.7
Acid/peptic disorders (gastrointestinal reflux, ulcers)	29.8	19.8	24.8	18.3	34.5	21.3
ACE inhibitors (high blood pressure, heart disease)	26.2	16.8	28.1	17.7	24.3	16.0
Antiasthmatics/bronchodilator (asthma, breathing)	26.2	14.4	20.1	11.4	32.0	17.1
Antihistamines (allergies)	25.5	13.5	17.3	9.1	33.2	17.7
Narcotic analgesics (pain relief)	25.5	17.5	22.8	17.0	28.1	18.0
Nonnarcotic analgesics (pain relief)	25.2	16.3	26.4	15.6	24.1	17.0
Diuretics (high blood pressure, heart disease)	22.6	13.5	18.7	11.2	26.3	15.7
Beta blockers (high blood pressure, heart disease)	20.8	10.6	18.6	10.0	22.8	11.2
Calcium channel blockers (high blood pressure, heart disease)	19.4	19.3	19.5	19.9	19.3	18.8
Estrogens/progestins (menopause, hot flashes)	X	X	X	X	43.8	55.7

Note: Drugs recorded on the patient record form are those prescribed, continued, administered, or provided during a physician office visit or hospital outpatient department visit.

[1] The National Drug Code (NDC) therapeutic class is a general therapeutic or pharmacological classification scheme for drug products reported to the Food and Drug Administration (FDA) under the provisions of the Drug Listing Act.
[2] Estimated number of drug visits during the 2-year period divided by the sum of population estimates for both years times 100.
[3] Drug visits are physicians' office and hospital outpatient department visits in which at least one prescription or nonprescription drug was recorded on the patient record form.
[4] Estimated number of drugs recorded during visits during the 2-year period divided by the sum of population estimates for both years times 100.
[5] Up to six prescription and nonprescription drugs may be recorded per visit.
[6] NSAID is nonsteroidal anti-inflammatory drug. Aspirin was not included as an NSAID in this analysis.
X = Not applicable.

Major types of drugs included NSAIDs (non-steroidal anti-inflammatory drugs, excluding aspirin), antidepressants, blood glucose regulators, high cholesterol drugs, and penicillin. Since the 1995–1996 survey, the usage of these particular drugs, except for penicillin, have increased significantly. Overall, the rate of recorded drug prescriptions has increased from 400 per 100 persons to 586. Women obtained more drugs than men, beginning with childbearing age. For both sexes, the largest number of drugs was obtained at age 75 years and over. In this age group, men obtained 1,732 drugs and women 1,915 drugs per year per 100 persons.

Table III-45. Selected Prescription and Nonprescription Drugs Recorded During Physicians' Office Visits and Hospital Outpatient Department Visits, by Age and Sex, 1995–1996 and 2002–2003 —Continued

(Number per 100 population.)

Age group and National Drug Code (NDC) therapeutic class (common reasons for use) [1]	Total		Men		Women	
	2002–2003	1995–1996	2002–2003	1995–1996	2002–2003	1995–1996
Age 65 Years and Over						
Drug visits with at least one drug per 100 population [2,3]	496.7	399.4	462.0	378.1	522.2	414.7
Number of Drugs per 100 Population [4]						
Total number of drugs [5]	1 606.2	1 047.4	1 473.8	956.9	1 703.1	1 112.5
Hypertension control drugs, not otherwise specified (high blood pressure)	91.8	29.1	81.3	22.7	99.5	33.8
Hyperlipidemia (high cholesterol)	90.4	24.7	101.5	25.1	82.3	24.5
Nonnarcotic analgesics (pain relief)	81.8	44.9	83.6	49.0	80.4	42.0
Diuretics (high blood pressure, heart disease)	77.7	55.2	74.5	48.5	70.0	60.0
ACE inhibitors (high blood pressure, heart disease)	74.1	42.6	79.8	41.2	63.1	43.6
Blood glucose/sugar regulators (diabetes)	69.0	37.5	76.9	38.0	67.7	37.1
Beta blockers (high blood pressure, heart disease)	66.9	25.5	65.7	23.6	76.0	26.8
NSAID (pain relief) [6]	66.2	41.8	52.7	31.9	71.7	49.0
Acid/peptic disorders (gastrointestinal reflux, ulcers)	64.5	42.2	54.8	36.0	66.9	46.6
Calcium channel blockers (high blood pressure, heart disease)	60.4	57.3	51.6	52.2	45.8	60.9
Antiasthmatics/bronchodilators (asthma, breathing)	46.2	31.3	46.7	37.1	50.2	27.0
Vitamins/minerals (dietary supplements)	44.1	17.1	35.8	13.1	53.5	20.0
Antidepressants (depression and related disorders)	43.7	23.5	30.4	16.7	37.6	28.5
Anticoagulants/thrombolytics (blood thinning, reduce or prevent clots)	42.0	20.7	48.0	24.0	38.5	18.3
Estrogens/progestins (menopause, hot flashes)	X	X	X	X		37.1
Age 65–74 Years						
Drug visits with at least one drug per 100 population [2,3]	444.3	362.8	408.4	323.0	474.3	394.9
Number of Drugs per 100 Population [4]						
Total number of drugs [5]	1 394.7	930.5	1 278.8	804.7	1 491.4	1 032.1
Hyperlipidemia (high cholesterol)	93.3	27.3	102.2	27.1	85.9	27.4
Hypertension control drugs, not otherwise specified (high blood pressure)	83.1	24.8	68.4	19.2	95.4	29.3
Blood glucose/sugar regulators (diabetes)	72.6	35.7	82.4	32.4	64.5	38.4
Nonnarcotic analgesics (pain relief)	70.0	38.0	73.6	40.5	67.0	35.9
ACE inhibitors (high blood pressure, heart disease)	67.5	37.1	73.0	35.6	62.8	38.3
NSAID (pain relief) [6]	61.2	42.0	54.0	31.2	67.1	50.8
Beta blockers (high blood pressure, heart disease)	59.1	23.7	58.2	20.7	59.8	26.1
Acid/peptic disorders (gastrointestinal reflux, ulcers)	57.1	38.7	50.8	30.6	62.3	45.2
Diuretics (high blood pressure, heart disease)	55.8	40.0	52.2	32.3	58.8	46.3
Calcium channel blockers (high blood pressure, heart disease)	52.6	48.9	44.5	46.2	59.3	51.2
Antiasthmatics/bronchodilators (asthma, breathing)	44.2	31.1	38.5	33.0	48.9	29.5
Antidepressants (depression and related disorders)	39.0	22.7	29.4	14.2	47.1	29.6
Vitamins/minerals (dietary supplements)	35.9	14.1	31.1	10.1	39.8	17.4
Antihistamines (allergies)	34.1	14.7	27.8	12.3	39.3	16.6
Estrogens/progestins (menopause, hot flashes)	X	X	X	X	45.2	47.5
Age 75 Years and Over						
Drug visits with at least one drug per 100 population [2,3]	555.6	449.2	532.8	466.3	570.0	438.7
Number of Drugs per 100 Population [4]						
Total number of drugs [5]	1 844.1	1 206.8	1 732.0	1 200.9	1 914.7	1 210.4
Diuretics (high blood pressure, heart disease)	102.4	75.8	104.1	74.5	101.3	76.6
Hypertension control drugs, not otherwise specified (high blood pressure)	101.6	35.1	98.5	28.4	103.5	39.2
Nonnarcotic analgesics (pain relief)	95.0	54.4	96.8	62.6	93.9	49.4
Hyperlipidemia (high cholesterol)	87.2	21.3	100.7	21.8	78.7	21.0
ACE inhibitors (high blood pressure, heart disease)	81.6	50.2	88.7	50.2	77.1	50.1
Beta blockers (high blood pressure, heart disease)	75.7	27.9	75.7	28.3	81.0	27.6
Acid/peptic disorders (gastrointestinal reflux, ulcers)	72.9	47.0	60.1	44.7	84.9	46.7
NSAID (pain relief) [6]	71.8	41.5	51.0	33.1	74.5	72.7
Calcium channel blockers (high blood pressure, heart disease)	69.3	68.6	61.0	61.8	61.8	35.5
Blood glucose/sugar regulators (diabetes)	64.8	39.8	69.7	46.9	61.8	24.7
Anticoagulants/thrombolytics (blood thinning, reduce or prevent clots)	57.5	28.6	68.8	34.9	50.3	23.2
Vitamins/minerals (dietary supplements)	53.4	21.2	42.0	18.0	60.6	27.0
Antidepressants (depression and related disorders)	49.0	24.6	31.7	20.7	59.9	24.0
Antiasthmatics/bronchodilators (asthma, breathing)	48.4	31.5	57.5	43.7	42.7	34.4
Thyroid/antrithyroid (hyper- and hypothyroidism)	45.1	27.1	25.0	15.1	57.8	

Note: Drugs recorded on the patient record form are those prescribed, continued, administered, or provided during a physician office visit or hospital outpatient department visit.

[1] The National Drug Code (NDC) therapeutic class is a general therapeutic or pharmacological classification scheme for drug products reported to the Food and Drug Administration (FDA) under the provisions of the Drug Listing Act.
[2] Estimated number of drug visits during the 2-year period divided by the sum of population estimates for both years times 100.
[3] Drug visits are physicians' office and hospital outpatient department visits in which at least one prescription or nonprescription drug was recorded on the patient record form.
[4] Estimated number of drugs recorded during visits during the 2-year period divided by the sum of population estimates for both years times 100.
[5] Up to six prescription and nonprescription drugs may be recorded per visit.
[6] NSAID is nonsteroidal anti-inflammatory drug. Aspirin was not included as an NSAID in this analysis.
X = Not applicable.

TABLE III-46. HOME HEALTH CARE PATIENTS, ACCORDING TO AGE, SEX, AND DIAGNOSIS, SELECTED YEARS, 1992–2000

Home health care is provided by home health care agencies to individuals and families in their place of residence, in order to promote health or to minimize the effects of disability and illness (including terminal illness). Almost 1.4 million home health care patients were reported at the time of the survey in 2000, a slightly higher number than in 1992 but below the levels of intervening years. Almost 30 percent of home health care patients were under 65 years of age. In terms of rates per 10,000 persons, the largest client group was 85 years old and over. Female clients were much more frequent than males. Care for diseases of the circulatory system ranked as the most frequent reason for home health care, and accounted for 23.6 percent of diagnosed illnesses.

Table III-46 Home Health Care Patients, According to Age, Sex, and Diagnosis, Selected Years, 1992–2000

(Number, rate per 10,000 population, percent.)

Age, sex, and diagnosis	2000	1998	1996	1994	1992
NUMBER OF CURRENT PATIENTS					
Total home health care patients	1 355 290	1 881 768	2 427 483	1 889 327	1 232 200
CURRENT PATIENTS PER 10,000 POPULATION					
Total	48.7	69.6	90.6	71.8	47.8
Age at Time of Survey					
Under 65 years, crude	16.4	25.0	27.8	21.0	12.6
65 years and over, crude	277.0	375.7	526.3	424.9	295.4
65 years and over, age-adjusted [1]	276.5	381.0	546.6	449.6	315.8
65–74 years	130.2	202.0	240.1	209.1	151.7
75–84 years	347.6	470.3	753.6	542.2	398.3
85 years and over	694.1	885.4	1 253.4	1 206.1	775.9
Sex					
Male, total	35.1	47.9	60.9	47.8	32.6
Under 65 years, crude	15.6	22.9	22.1	17.8	10.9
65 years and over, crude	199.6	255.2	386.4	303.1	219.2
65 years and over, age-adjusted [1]	216.4	277.6	438.3	350.0	255.8
65–74 years	100.7	159.7	187.0	169.9	121.8
75–84 years	270.0	321.4	598.7	427.5	322.0
85 years and over	553.9	653.0	1 044.3	893.1	635.2
Female, total	61.8	90.4	118.9	94.7	62.4
Under 65 years, crude	17.2	27.0	33.6	24.2	14.3
65 years and over, crude	332.6	460.4	623.9	508.9	347.4
65 years and over, age-adjusted [1]	315.5	445.8	615.0	506.6	351.5
65–74 years	154.6	236.3	283.2	240.6	175.3
75–84 years	400.4	568.8	854.0	614.5	445.3
85 years and over	754.9	981.7	1 337.0	1 327.6	830.7
PERCENT DISTRIBUTION					
Age at Time of Survey [2]					
Under 65 years	29.5	31.3	27.0	25.7	23.1
65 years and over	70.5	68.7	73.0	74.3	76.9
65–74 years	17.3	19.7	18.4	20.6	22.6
75–84 years	31.3	29.9	35.3	31.2	33.9
85 years and over	21.9	19.1	19.4	22.4	20.4
Sex					
Male	35.2	33.6	32.9	32.5	33.2
Female	64.8	66.4	67.1	67.5	66.8
Primary Admission Diagnosis [3]					
Malignant neoplasms	4.9	3.8	4.8	5.7	5.7
Diabetes	7.8	6.1	8.5	8.1	7.7
Diseases of the nervous system and sense organs	6.1	7.6	5.8	8.0	6.3
Diseases of the circulatory system	23.6	23.6	25.6	27.2	25.9
Diseases of heart	10.9	12.3	10.9	14.3	12.6
Cerebrovascular diseases	7.3	5.1	7.8	6.1	5.8
Diseases of the respiratory system	6.8	7.9	7.7	6.1	6.6
Decubitus ulcers	1.9	1.2	1.0	1.1	1.9
Diseases of the musculoskeletal system and connective tissue	9.8	8.3	8.8	8.3	9.4
Osteoarthritis	3.5	2.7	3.2	2.8	2.5
Fractures, all sites	4.1	4.0	3.3	3.7	3.8
Fracture of neck of femur (hip)	1.5	1.1	1.3	1.7	1.4
Other	34.9	37.5	34.6	31.8	32.7

[1] Age adjusted by the direct method to the year 2000 standard population using the following three age groups: 65–74 years, 75–84 years, and 85 years and over.
[2] Denominator excludes persons with unknown age.
[3] Denominator excludes persons with unknown diagnosis.

INPATIENT CARE

TABLE III-47. ADDITIONS TO MENTAL HEALTH ORGANIZATIONS, ACCORDING TO TYPE OF SERVICE AND ORGANIZATION, SELECTED YEARS, 1986–2002

An "addition" is a new admission, readmission, return from long-term leave, or transfer from another service. This table indicates the volume of care by state and local mental hospitals, Department of Veterans Affairs medical centers, and various private organizations.

In 2002, there were 2.2 million additions to residential or 24-hour hospital treatment and 3.6 million additions to less than 24-hour care. This represented a rate of 760 per 100,000 persons (or a rate of somewhat less than 1 percent) for the former type of care, and a rate of 1,240 per 100,000 persons for the latter treatment. The largest providers of 24-hour treatment were general hospitals (other than federal), but the top providers for less than overnight care were "all other organizations," consisting of freestanding psychiatric outpatient clinics, partial care organizations, and multi-service mental health organizations.

Table III-47. Additions to Mental Health Organizations, According to Type of Service and Organization, Selected Years, 1986–2002

(Number.)

Service and organization	Additions in thousands					Additions per 100,000 civilian population [1]				
	2002 [2]	2000	1994 [3]	1990	1986	2002 [2]	2000	1994 [3]	1990	1986
24-Hour Hospital and Residential Treatment [4]										
All organizations	2 193	2 029	2 267	2 035	1 819	760.4	719.3	874.6	833.7	759.9
State and county mental hospitals	239	236	238	276	333	82.7	83.6	92.0	113.2	139.1
Private psychiatric hospitals	477	451	485	407	235	165.6	159.8	187.1	166.5	98.0
Non-federal general hospital psychiatric services	1 095	994	1 067	960	849	379.6	352.3	411.5	393.2	354.8
Department of Veterans Affairs medical centers [5]	182	171	173	198	180	63.1	60.5	66.9	81.2	75.1
Residential treatment centers for emotionally disturbed children	60	46	47	42	25	20.7	16.2	18.0	17.0	10.2
All other organizations [6]	141	132	257	153	198	48.7	46.8	99.0	62.6	82.7
Less than 24-Hour Care [7]										
All organizations	3 575	4 057	3 516	3 298	2 955	1 239.7	1 438.1	1 356.8	1 352.4	1 233.4
State and county mental hospitals	53	49	42	48	68	18.3	17.2	16.1	19.8	28.4
Private psychiatric hospitals	426	265	214	163	132	147.6	94.1	82.4	66.9	55.2
Non-federal general hospital psychiatric services	546	1 103	498	659	533	189.4	391.0	192.0	270.0	222.4
Department of Veterans Affairs medical centers [5]	80	139	132	184	133	27.7	49.1	51.1	75.3	55.3
Residential treatment centers for emotionally disturbed children	208	199	167	100	67	72.0	70.6	64.6	40.8	28.1
All other organizations [6]	2 263	2 302	2 464	2 145	2 022	784.7	816.0	950.7	879.6	844.0

[1]Civilian population estimates for 2000 and beyond are based on 2000 census as of July 1; population estimates for 1992–1998 are 1990 postcensal estimates.

[2]Preliminary data.

[3]Beginning in 1994, data for supportive residential clients (moderately staffed housing arrangements such as supervised apartments, group homes, and halfway houses) are included in the totals and "all other organizations." This change affects the comparability of trend data prior to 1994 with data for 1994 and later years.

[4]These data exclude mental health care provided in nonpsychiatric units of hospitals, such as general medical units.

[5]Includes Department of Veterans Affairs (VA) neuropsychiatric hospitals, VA general hospital psychiatric services, and VA psychiatric outpatient clinics.

[6]Includes freestanding psychiatric outpatient clinics, partial care organizations, and multiservice mental health organizations.

[7]Formerly reported as partial care and outpatient treatment, the survey format was changed in 1994 and the reporting of these services was combined due to similarities in the care provided. These data exclude office-based mental health care (psychiatrists, psychologists, licensed clinical social workers, and psychiatric nurses).

TABLE III-48. HOSPICE PATIENTS, ACCORDING TO AGE, SEX, AND DIAGNOSIS, SELECTED YEARS, 1992–2000

Hospice services consist of palliative (noncurative) care for terminally ill patients, which usually includes psychological and spiritual support for patients and their families. Hospice care is provided in the patient's home or on an inpatient basis. At the time of the survey in 2000, there were a little over 100,000 hospice patients. The number of patients had doubled since 1992, representing a rate of 3.8 per 10,000 persons. Rates of attendance increased with age and tended to be somewhat higher for women than for men. About 52 percent of hospice patients had cancer; 13 percent had heart disease.

TABLE III-49. DISCHARGES, DAYS OF CARE, AND AVERAGE LENGTH OF STAY IN SHORT-STAY HOSPITALS, ACCORDING TO SELECTED CHARACTERISTICS, SELECTED YEARS, 1997–2003

Discharges occur when inpatient hospitalizations are complete, and thus give a measure of the number of hospital stays per year. Discharges and their characteristics were collected for this table from household interviews. In 2003, there were 120 discharges per 1,000 persons. On average, patients stayed in the hospital for 4.7 days, giving a rate of 559 days in the hospital per 1,000 persons.

In 2003, among persons under 65 years of age, the hospital discharge rate for the poor was nearly twice the rate for nonpoor (150 versus 82 per 1,000 persons, respectively). Poor persons had longer hospital stays on average than the nonpoor (4.6 versus 3.9 days, respectively, among persons under 65 years of age). By race, non-Hispanic Blacks had longer stays than non-Hispanic Whites. Medicaid patients had both a higher rate of discharge and a longer length of stay, spending more than four times as many days in the hospital (per 1,000 persons) as privately insured persons. This table also gives separate statistics for persons age 65 years and over.

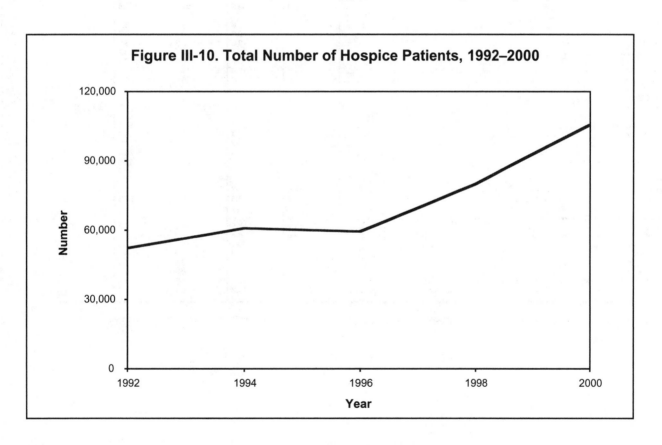

Figure III-10. Total Number of Hospice Patients, 1992–2000

Table III-48. Hospice Patients, According to Age, Sex, and Diagnosis, Selected Years, 1992–2000

(Number, number per 10,000 population, percent.)

Age, sex, and diagnosis	2000	1998	1996	1994	1992
NUMBER OF CURRENT PATIENTS					
Total hospice patients	105 496	79 837	59 363	60 783	52 100
CURRENT PATIENTS PER 10,000 POPULATION					
Total	3.8	3.0	2.2	2.3	2.0
Age at Time of Survey					
Under 65 years, crude	0.8	0.7	0.5	0.8	0.5
65 years and over, crude	24.9	18.2	13.9	12.9	13.1
65 years and over, age-adjusted [1]	24.9	18.4	14.4	13.6	13.7
65–74 years	10.1	9.9	7.8	7.3	7.8
75–84 years	31.9	22.0	16.9	16.9	19.2
85 years and over	67.3	44.7	34.7	30.6	23.4
Sex					
Male, total	3.3	2.6	2.0	2.1	1.9
Under 65 years, crude	0.8	0.7	0.5	0.9	0.5
65 years and over, crude	24.8	18.5	14.8	12.5	13.9
65 years and over, age-adjusted [1]	26.9	20.3	16.1	14.4	16.0
65–74 years	13.0	10.2	10.4	7.0	6.3
75–84 years	32.6	25.2	18.5	18.2	25.8
85 years and over	69.9	49.2	33.9	34.8	28.8
Female, total	4.3	3.3	2.4	2.5	2.1
Under 65 years, crude	0.9	0.8	0.6	0.7	0.4
65 years and over, crude	25.0	18.0	13.2	13.2	12.6
65 years and over, age-adjusted [1]	23.3	17.3	12.9	13.2	12.6
65–74 years	7.6	9.6	5.8	7.5	8.9
75–84 years	31.5	19.9	15.9	16.1	15.1
85 years and over	66.2	42.9	35.0	29.0	21.4
PERCENT DISTRIBUTION					
Age at Time of Survey [2]					
Under 65 years	18.6	21.6	21.3	30.1	19.5
65 years and over	81.4	78.4	78.7	69.9	80.5
65–74 years	17.2	22.7	24.5	22.2	27.3
75–84 years	37.0	32.9	32.4	30.1	38.6
85 years and over	27.3	22.7	21.9	17.6	14.6
Sex					
Male	42.6	42.7	44.9	44.7	46.1
Female	57.4	57.3	55.1	55.3	53.9
Primary Admission Diagnosis [3]					
Malignant neoplasms	51.9	55.5	58.3	57.2	65.7
Large intestine and rectum	4.9	6.4	4.0	8.0	9.0
Trachea, bronchus, and lung	12.3	13.0	15.8	12.5	21.1
Breast	4.8	4.9	6.2	4.8	3.9
Prostate	7.7	6.1	6.6	5.9	6.0
Diseases of the heart	12.8	9.7	8.3	9.3	10.2
Diseases of the respiratory system	6.5	10.6	7.3	6.6	4.3
Other	28.8	24.3	26.1	27.0	19.8

[1]Age adjusted by the direct method to the year 2000 standard population using the following three age groups: 65–74 years, 75–84 years, and 85 years and over.
[2]Denominator excludes persons with unknown age.
[3]Denominator excludes persons with unknown diagnosis.

Table III-49. Discharges, Days of Care, and Average Length of Stay in Short-Stay Hospitals, According to Selected Characteristics, Selected Years, 1997–2003

(Number per 1,000 population, number.)

Characteristic	Number per 1,000 population						Number of days		
	Discharges			Days of care			Average length of stay		
	2003	2002	1997	2003	2002	1997	2003	2002	1997
TOTAL [1]	119.9	122.9	124.3	558.9	541.3	601.2	4.7	4.4	4.8
Age									
Under 18 years	72.0	81.0	90.8	258.7	269.3	319.0	3.6	3.3	3.5
Under 6 years	169.8	188.9	203.5	610.9	601.0	632.6	3.6	3.2	3.1
6–17 years	24.3	29.2	34.0	86.9	110.3	163.1	3.6	3.8	4.8
18–44 years	93.2	94.7	96.8	352.7	311.2	358.8	3.8	3.3	3.7
45–64 years	129.5	124.3	124.9	676.5	574.5	631.1	5.2	4.6	5.1
45–54 years	107.5	106.8	99.2	543.4	495.8	527.5	5.1	4.6	5.3
55–64 years	161.6	150.7	164.8	871.1	693.0	792.4	5.4	4.6	4.8
65 years and over	283.9	293.2	274.4	1 607.8	1 745.3	1 852.5	5.7	6.0	6.8
65–74 years	242.9	250.5	249.1	1 261.7	1 269.6	1 595.2	5.2	5.1	6.4
75 years and over	330.3	342.0	307.3	2 000.4	2 290.1	2 188.4	6.1	6.7	7.1
UNDER 65 YEARS OF AGE									
Total [1]	96.0	98.1	102.2	406.2	365.5	416.4	4.2	3.7	4.1
Sex									
Male	74.1	72.8	79.1	363.1	312.9	374.9	4.9	4.3	4.7
Female	117.5	122.9	124.7	448.7	416.7	456.6	3.8	3.4	3.7
Race [2]									
White only	93.2	96.4	100.8	378.3	342.5	385.8	4.1	3.6	3.8
Black or African American only	124.8	121.3	126.3	623.7	536.4	688.6	5.0	4.4	5.5
American Indian and Alaska Native only	*	*	*	*	*	*	*	*	*
Asian only	53.2	45.0	61.7	*	*	*	*	*	*
Native Hawaiian and Other Pacific Islander only	*	*	...	*	*	...	*	*	...
Two or more races	*135.9	*	...	*	*	...	*	*	...
Hispanic Origin and Race [2]									
Hispanic or Latino	95.6	94.9	109.9	393.5	377.4	416.7	4.1	4.0	3.8
Not Hispanic or Latino	96.3	98.8	101.2	407.1	365.2	415.4	4.2	3.7	4.1
White only	93.7	97.2	99.6	376.7	345.0	382.7	4.0	3.5	3.8
Black or African American only	124.2	121.2	125.7	629.3	517.9	692.6	5.1	4.3	5.5
Poverty Status [3]									
Poor	150.3	157.9	186.0	694.9	747.1	922.0	4.6	4.7	5.0
Near poor	117.2	124.0	119.3	571.1	491.7	530.5	4.9	4.0	4.4
Nonpoor	82.4	83.1	82.7	323.5	283.3	308.9	3.9	3.4	3.7
Hispanic Origin, Race and Poverty Status [2, 3]									
Hispanic or Latino									
Poor	132.3	132.8	152.3	*557.3	*	592.3	*4.2	*	3.9
Near poor	99.3	103.6	92.7	*378.9	*377.7	*415.0	*3.8	*3.6	*4.5
Nonpoor	78.6	72.8	92.1	*335.0	*289.1	294.5	*4.3	*4.0	3.2
Not Hispanic or Latino									
White only									
Poor	144.2	159.6	205.2	*721.7	695.9	955.5	*5.0	4.4	4.7
Near poor	125.9	129.1	124.3	*557.4	488.1	503.4	*4.4	3.8	4.0
Nonpoor	82.9	85.3	83.1	311.9	287.1	303.0	3.8	3.4	3.6
Black or African American only									
Poor	*207.2	199.4	199.0	*	*	*	*	*	*
Near poor	*121.4	*129.8	139.1	*	*	*819.0	*	*	*5.9
Nonpoor	93.1	93.3	85.2	*418.8	292.6	*402.1	*4.5	3.1	*4.7
Health Insurance Status [4]									
Insured	101.5	104.2	108.1	441.5	390.4	442.5	4.3	3.7	4.1
Private	80.1	84.3	85.6	323.0	275.1	310.2	4.0	3.3	3.6
Medicaid	268.8	277.4	311.6	1 397.1	1 301.2	1 575.3	5.2	4.7	5.1
Uninsured	69.3	68.7	75.3	251.2	247.2	296.3	3.6	3.6	3.9
Poverty Status and Health Insurance Status [3]									
Poor									
Insured	184.5	193.0	234.6	912.3	958.1	1 243.1	4.9	5.0	5.3
Uninsured	*86.7	90.2	102.8	*306.8	*355.3	*407.7	*3.5	*3.9	*4.0
Near poor									
Insured	139.5	146.1	141.2	*714.3	603.7	640.0	*5.1	4.1	4.5
Uninsured	69.4	75.2	72.0	*	*252.9	*285.3	*	*3.4	*4.0
Nonpoor									
Insured	85.6	86.8	85.5	340.4	294.4	315.6	4.0	3.4	3.7
Uninsured	59.3	54.5	*58.5	*201.5	*193.4	*	*3.4	*3.6	*

Note: Data are based on household interviews.

[1] Includes all other races not shown separately, unknown poverty status, and unknown health insurance status.

[2] The race groups, White, Black, American Indian and Alaska Native (AI/AN), Asian, Native Hawaiian and Other Pacific Islander, and two or more races, include persons of Hispanic and non-Hispanic origin. Persons of Hispanic origin may be of any race.

[3] Poor persons are defined as having a total income below the poverty threshold. Near poor persons have incomes of 100 percent to less than 200 percent of poverty threshold. Nonpoor persons have incomes of 200 percent or more than the poverty threshold.

[4] Health insurance categories are mutually exclusive. Persons who reported both Medicaid and private coverage are classified as having private coverage. Persons 65 years of age and over who reported Medicare HMO (health maintenance organization) and some other type of health insurance coverage are classified as having Medicare HMO.

* = Figure does not meet standards of reliability or precision.

... = Not available.

Table III-49. Discharges, Days of Care, and Average Length of Stay in Short-Stay Hospitals, According to Selected Characteristics, Selected Years, 1997–2003—*Continued*

(Number per 1,000 population, number.)

Characteristic	Number per 1,000 population						Number of days		
	Discharges			Days of care			Average length of stay		
	2003	2002	1997	2003	2002	1997	2003	2002	1997
Geographic region									
Northeast	82.3	92.8	96.0	384.4	348.0	455.4	4.7	3.8	4.7
Midwest	95.7	104.9	108.7	368.1	382.6	384.4	3.8	3.6	3.5
South	112.5	106.6	111.8	467.4	400.6	466.1	4.2	3.8	4.2
West	79.0	80.9	82.9	359.8	300.8	327.2	4.6	3.7	3.9
Location of Residence									
Within MSA [5]	91.7	94.6	99.3	406.6	355.4	411.8	4.4	3.8	4.1
Outside MSA [5]	113.8	112.4	113.2	405.8	407.5	435.9	3.6	3.6	3.8
65 YEARS OF AGE AND OVER									
Total [1]	284.6	294.2	276.9	1 614.4	1 756.9	1 878.4	5.7	6.0	6.8
Sex									
Male	273.0	312.5	291.6	1 614.1	1 804.6	2 077.4	5.9	5.8	7.1
Female	293.7	280.6	265.2	1 609.3	1 708.5	1 727.4	5.5	6.1	6.5
Hispanic Origin and Race [2]									
Hispanic or Latino	311.2	290.8	312.7	*1 725.2	1 489.4	*2 512.1	*5.5	5.1	*8.0
Not Hispanic or Latino	283.0	294.6	274.6	1 603.4	1 771.4	1 846.3	5.7	6.0	6.7
White only	280.6	293.0	274.8	1 547.2	1 683.5	1 808.2	5.5	5.7	6.6
Black or African American only	349.4	*373.3	290.8	*2 327.8	*	2 423.5	*6.7	*	8.3
Poverty status [3]									
Poor	359.5	361.2	342.3	2 110.0	*	2 566.3	5.9	*	7.5
Near poor	329.1	314.8	311.5	1 724.6	1 836.0	2 269.4	5.2	5.8	7.3
Nonpoor	256.5	273.8	251.5	1 501.8	1 575.4	1 606.7	5.9	5.8	6.4
Health Insurance Status [4]									
Medicare HMO	290.5	239.7	217.8	1 508.4	1 072.2	1 355.3	5.2	4.5	6.2
Private	265.6	295.7	271.9	1 537.6	1 782.6	1 756.1	5.8	6.0	6.5
Medicaid	463.2	487.1	539.7	3 008.3	2 505.1	3 810.6	6.5	5.1	7.1
Medicare fee-for-service only	*294.1	258.2	252.9	1 442.7	*	1 906.6	*4.9	*	7.5
Geographic Region									
Northeast	*300.4	281.8	265.0	1 604.1	1 659.3	1 828.5	*5.3	5.9	6.9
Midwest	275.2	306.3	285.2	1 588.6	1 765.3	1 971.1	5.8	5.8	6.9
South	298.5	319.7	298.1	1 834.8	2 075.3	2 140.2	6.1	6.5	7.2
West	249.4	243.6	237.2	1 200.3	1 234.8	1 299.2	4.8	5.1	5.5
Location of Residence									
Within MSA [5]	286.9	283.5	271.3	1 593.8	1 661.8	1 875.9	5.6	5.9	6.9
Outside MSA [5]	276.7	329.5	295.1	1 683.6	*2 070.2	1 893.6	6.1	*6.3	6.4

Note: Data are based on household interviews.

[1] Includes all other races not shown separately, unknown poverty status, and unknown health insurance status.

[2] The race groups, White, Black, American Indian and Alaska Native (AI/AN), Asian, Native Hawaiian and Other Pacific Islander, and two or more races, include persons of Hispanic and non-Hispanic origin. Persons of Hispanic origin may be of any race.

[3] Poor persons are defined as having a total income below the poverty threshold. Near poor persons have incomes of 100 percent to less than 200 percent of poverty threshold. Nonpoor persons have incomes of 200 percent or more than the poverty threshold.

[4] Health insurance categories are mutually exclusive. Persons who reported both Medicaid and private coverage are classified as having private coverage. Persons 65 years of age and over who reported Medicare HMO (health maintenance organization) and some other type of health insurance coverage are classified as having Medicare HMO.

[5] MSA = Metropolitan Statistical Area.

* = Figure does not meet standards of reliability or precision.

TABLE III-50. DISCHARGES, DAYS OF CARE, AND AVERAGE LENGTH OF STAY IN NON-FEDERAL SHORT-STAY HOSPITALS, ACCORDING TO SELECTED CHARACTERISTICS, SELECTED YEARS, 1980–2003

The data in this table are based on a sample of hospital records, and thus are slightly different from those shown in Table III-49, the previous table on discharges, which were based on household interviews. Hospital discharges in 2003 are shown at the rate of 120 per 1,000 persons, 21 percent lower than the average in 1985 (with age-adjusted data). The decline in the discharge rate had occurred by 1995. In 2003, the average length of stay was 4.8 days, which was 1.8 days shorter than in 1985. The discharge rate increased considerably with age. For persons under 18 years old, the discharge rate per 1,000 persons was 44, but

for persons 75 years and over, the rate increased to 475 per 1,000 persons. The rate of female discharges was about one-third higher than the rate for males, but the average length of stay for females was substantially shorter.

TABLE III-51. RATES OF DISCHARGES AND DAYS OF CARE IN NON-FEDERAL SHORT-STAY HOSPITALS, ACCORDING TO SEX, AGE, AND SELECTED FIRST-LISTED DIAGNOSIS, SELECTED YEARS, 1990–2003

This table—based on hospital records—focuses on the first-listed diagnosis of hospital patients, subdivided by age group. The table also shows that days of care for patients declined substantially during the 1990s, before rising moderately between 2000 and 2003.

In 2003, for hospitalized children under 18 years old, the leading cause of hospital stays was pneumonia. For male patients between 18 and 44 years old, injuries and poisoning and mental illnesses were the most frequent diagnoses. For females in this age group, deliveries were by far the most frequent cause of hospitalization, followed by mental illnesses and injuries and poisoning

Those between 45 and 64 years of age were predominantly hospitalized for heart disease, followed by injuries and poisoning and cancer. Hospitalizations increased markedly for the 65- to 74-year-old age group, but the ranking of diagnoses was similar to that of the previous age group for both males and females.

Table III-50. Discharges, Days of Care, and Average Length of Stay in Non-Federal Short-Stay Hospitals, According to Selected Characteristics, Selected Years, 1980–2003

(Rate per 1,000 population, number.)

Characteristic	2003	2002	2001	2000	1998	1995	1990	1985 [1]	1980 [1]
DISCHARGES PER 1,000 POPULATION									
Total [2]	119.5	117.3	115.1	113.3	117.9	118.0	125.2	151.4	173.4
Age									
Under 18 years	43.6	43.4	43.4	40.3	40.4	42.4	46.4	61.4	75.6
18–44 years	91.3	90.3	87.3	84.9	88.8	91.4	102.7	128.0	155.3
45–54 years	99.5	95.6	94.4	92.1	92.7	98.5	112.4	146.8	174.8
55–64 years	145.7	146.5	139.3	141.5	155.1	148.3	163.3	194.8	215.4
65 years and over	367.9	357.5	354.3	353.4	365.3	347.7	334.1	369.8	383.7
65–74 years	265.1	254.0	256.1	254.6	267.6	260.0	261.6	297.2	315.8
75 years and over	475.2	466.6	460.0	462.0	477.4	459.1	434.0	475.6	489.3
Sex [2]									
Male	104.4	102.4	100.0	99.1	102.8	104.8	113.0	137.3	153.2
Female	135.1	132.9	130.6	127.7	133.3	131.7	139.0	167.3	195.0
Geographic region [2]									
Northeast	127.6	123.5	125.2	127.5	127.3	133.5	133.2	142.6	162.0
Midwest	117.1	113.6	113.5	110.9	116.4	113.3	128.8	158.1	192.1
South	125.8	126.7	126.3	120.9	126.4	125.2	132.5	155.5	179.7
West	103.9	99.7	88.8	89.4	97.1	96.7	100.7	145.7	150.5
DAYS OF CARE PER 1,000 POPULATION									
Total [2]	574.6	570.9	562.2	557.7	598.6	638.6	818.9	997.5	1 297.0
Age									
Under 18 years	195.5	195.2	192.5	179.0	182.4	184.7	226.3	281.2	341.4
18–44 years	339.7	333.9	322.7	309.4	328.3	351.7	467.7	619.2	818.6
45–54 years	477.2	456.7	455.4	437.4	452.9	516.2	699.7	967.8	1 314.9
55–64 years	735.9	752.2	732.2	729.1	836.1	867.2	1 172.3	1 436.9	1 889.4
65 years and over	2 088.3	2 085.1	2 064.2	2 111.9	2 264.2	2 373.7	2 895.6	3 228.0	4 098.3
65–74 years	1 428.9	1 411.9	1 449.5	1 439.0	1 596.1	1 684.7	2 087.8	2 437.3	3 147.0
75 years and over	2 776.1	2 795.0	2 725.5	2 851.9	3 030.8	3 247.8	4 009.1	4 381.3	5 578.8
Sex [2]									
Male	546.7	549.5	534.5	535.9	576.7	623.9	805.8	973.3	1 239.7
Female	605.2	596.0	591.9	581.0	622.9	654.9	840.5	1 033.1	1 365.2
Geographic Region [2]									
Northeast	694.4	690.0	697.7	718.6	731.0	839.0	1 026.7	1 113.0	1 400.6
Midwest	507.9	502.1	491.6	500.5	552.5	590.9	830.6	1 078.6	1 484.8
South	609.8	618.6	623.6	592.5	643.9	666.0	820.4	957.7	1 262.3
West	476.4	454.7	408.3	408.2	450.4	451.1	575.5	824.7	956.9
AVERAGE LENGTH OF STAY IN DAYS									
Total [2]	4.8	4.9	4.9	4.9	5.1	5.4	6.5	6.6	7.5
Age									
Under 18 years	4.5	4.5	4.4	4.4	4.5	4.4	4.9	4.6	4.5
18–44 years	3.7	3.7	3.7	3.6	3.7	3.8	4.6	4.8	5.3
45–54 years	4.8	4.8	4.8	4.8	4.9	5.2	6.2	6.6	7.5
55–64 years	5.1	5.1	5.3	5.2	5.4	5.8	7.2	7.4	8.8
65 years and over	5.7	5.8	5.8	6.0	6.2	6.8	8.7	8.7	10.7
65–74 years	5.4	5.6	5.7	5.7	6.0	6.5	8.0	8.2	10.0
75 years and over	5.8	6.0	5.9	6.2	6.3	7.1	9.2	9.2	11.4
Sex [2]									
Male	5.2	5.4	5.3	5.4	5.6	6.0	7.1	7.1	8.1
Female	4.5	4.5	4.5	4.6	4.7	5.0	6.0	6.2	7.0
Geographic Region [2]									
Northeast	5.4	5.6	5.6	5.6	5.7	6.3	7.7	7.8	8.6
Midwest	4.3	4.4	4.3	4.5	4.7	5.2	6.5	6.8	7.7
South	4.8	4.9	4.9	4.9	5.1	5.3	6.2	6.2	7.0
West	4.6	4.6	4.6	4.6	4.6	4.7	5.7	5.7	6.4

Note: Data are based on a sample of hospital records.

[1]Comparisons of data from 1980–1985 with data from later years should be made with caution, as estimates of change may reflect improvements in the design rather than true changes in hospital use.

[2]Estimates are age adjusted to the year 2000 standard population using six age groups: under 18 years, 18–44 years, 45–54 years, 55–64 years, 65–74 years, and 75 years and over.

Hospital patients age 75 years and over were in the hospital most frequently for heart disease. Other frequent diagnoses included pneumonia, stroke, and injuries and poisoning. Hospital discharges for cancer declined considerably between 1990 and 2003, partly reflecting sizable declines in prostate and breast cancer hospitalizations.

Table III-51. Rates of Discharges and Days of Care in Non-Federal Short-Stay Hospitals, According to Sex, Age, and Selected First-Listed Diagnosis, Selected Years, 1990–2003

(Number per 1,000 population.)

Sex, age, and first-listed diagnosis	Discharges			Days of care		
	2003	2000	1990	2003	2000	1990
BOTH SEXES [1, 2]	119.5	113.3	125.2	574.6	557.7	818.9
MALE						
All Ages [1, 2]	104.4	99.1	113.0	546.7	535.9	805.8
Under 18 Years [2]	44.9	40.9	46.3	200.0	195.6	233.6
Pneumonia	5.9	5.4	5.3	19.1	17.3	22.6
Asthma	2.0	3.5	3.3	4.7	7.4	9.3
Injuries and poisoning	5.5	5.0	6.8	21.6	21.4	30.1
Fracture, all sites	2.0	1.8	2.2	6.1	7.2	9.3
18–44 Years [2]	47.7	45.0	57.9	236.0	217.5	351.7
HIV infection	0.5	0.6	*0.3	4.3	*5.4	*3.0
Alcohol and drug [3]	3.6	4.0	3.7	14.9	19.1	33.1
Serious mental illness [4]	5.8	*5.3	3.4	46.2	*43.6	47.1
Diseases of heart	3.0	2.7	3.0	*13.5	9.4	16.3
Intervertebral disc disorders	1.2	1.5	2.6	2.9	3.2	10.7
Injuries and poisoning	8.4	7.3	13.1	40.8	33.2	65.7
Fracture, all sites	3.0	2.5	4.0	15.5	12.8	22.7
45–64 Years [2]	120.1	112.7	140.3	605.0	570.4	943.4
HIV infection	*0.7	*0.5	*0.1	*	*	*
Malignant neoplasms	6.6	6.2	10.6	44.7	42.1	99.1
Trachea, bronchus, and lung	0.9	0.9	2.7	6.1	5.2	19.1
Diabetes	3.1	3.7	2.9	14.8	22.5	21.2
Alcohol and drug [3]	4.2	3.5	3.5	18.7	15.8	29.7
Serious mental illness [4]	4.4	*4.0	2.5	39.9	*34.6	34.8
Diseases of heart	24.7	26.4	31.7	99.0	101.5	185.0
Ischemic heart disease	14.8	17.7	22.6	56.1	63.8	128.2
Acute myocardial infarction	4.8	5.9	7.4	25.0	27.8	55.8
Congestive heart failure	3.9	3.3	3.0	18.5	17.2	19.7
Cerebrovascular diseases	3.8	3.8	4.1	16.6	19.8	40.7
Pneumonia	4.1	3.4	3.5	24.9	20.5	27.4
Injuries and poisoning	11.0	8.8	11.6	60.9	49.8	82.6
Fracture, all sites	3.1	2.5	3.3	18.0	16.2	24.2
65–74 Years [2]	276.5	264.9	287.8	1 465.3	1 489.7	2 251.5
Malignant neoplasms	19.3	17.6	27.9	124.7	121.2	277.6
Large intestine and rectum	2.1	3.0	3.0	17.0	27.3	34.2
Trachea, bronchus, and lung	3.6	2.8	6.4	21.0	19.2	55.7
Prostate	3.9	3.7	5.1	12.7	14.0	33.1
Diabetes	5.1	4.7	4.4	27.9	29.0	39.8
Serious mental illness [4]	2.8	*3.4	2.5	28.6	39.9	43.8
Diseases of heart	66.3	70.6	69.4	290.0	331.9	487.2
Ischemic heart disease	35.2	39.7	42.0	147.4	171.2	285.2
Acute myocardial infarction	12.5	12.5	14.0	66.9	66.5	122.4
Congestive heart failure	13.5	13.4	11.4	65.6	76.8	90.2
Cerebrovascular diseases	13.4	13.2	13.8	57.8	59.0	114.8
Pneumonia	12.9	12.8	11.4	77.2	82.0	107.8
Hyperplasia of prostate	3.8	5.4	14.4	10.5	15.0	65.0
Osteoarthritis	8.7	9.6	5.0	34.7	46.7	44.9
Injuries and poisoning	19.2	17.9	17.6	105.6	105.7	139.0
Fracture, all sites	4.6	4.7	4.5	27.5	29.9	45.9
Fracture of neck of femur (hip)	*1.5	*2.0	1.5	*10.4	*15.9	*18.1
75 Years and Over [2]	483.1	467.4	478.5	2 844.9	2 888.0	4 231.6
Malignant neoplasms	24.1	21.9	41.0	166.8	165.2	408.3
Large intestine and rectum	4.0	4.2	5.4	36.9	44.1	80.7
Trachea, bronchus, and lung	4.1	3.0	5.4	29.3	18.3	53.4
Prostate	2.3	3.2	9.7	*10.4	*19.4	65.6
Diabetes	6.6	6.5	4.6	*36.5	43.2	51.2
Serious mental illness [4]	2.5	2.9	*2.6	*25.2	*32.6	*40.5
Diseases of heart	110.3	113.3	106.2	560.2	600.9	855.7
Ischemic heart disease	47.2	53.0	49.1	238.8	276.1	398.1
Acute myocardial infarction	21.6	23.0	23.1	142.6	136.5	227.5
Congestive heart failure	31.1	30.5	31.0	170.6	175.4	242.3
Cerebrovascular diseases	29.1	30.2	30.2	142.2	171.2	298.3
Pneumonia	39.7	37.2	38.6	245.2	233.3	393.6
Hyperplasia of prostate	5.4	6.8	17.9	17.0	21.6	109.2
Osteoarthritis	9.7	6.2	5.8	42.3	28.7	60.7
Injuries and poisoning	34.6	33.6	31.2	226.1	257.7	341.3
Fracture, all sites	15.3	14.4	13.7	108.0	*119.2	145.1
Fracture of neck of femur (hip)	9.7	8.4	8.5	67.2	63.3	97.8

Note: Excludes newborn infants.

[1] Estimates are age adjusted to the year 2000 standard population using six age groups: under 18 years, 18–44 years, 45–54 years, 55–64 years, 65–74 years, and 75 years and over.
[2] Includes discharges with first-listed diagnoses not shown in table.
[3] Includes abuse, dependence, and withdrawal. These estimates are for non-federal short-stay hospitals and do not include alcohol and drug discharges from other types of facilities or programs, such as the Department of Veterans Affairs or day treatment programs.
[4] These estimates are for non-federal short-stay hospitals and do not include serious mental illness discharges from other types of facilities or programs, such as the Department of Veterans Affairs or long-term hospitals.
* = Figure does not meet standards of reliability or precision.

Table III-51. Rates of Discharges and Days of Care in Non-Federal Short-Stay Hospitals, According to Sex, Age, and Selected First-Listed Diagnosis, Selected Years, 1990–2003—Continued

(Number per 1,000 population.)

Sex, age, and first-listed diagnosis	Discharges			Days of care		
	2003	2000	1990	2003	2000	1990
FEMALE						
All Ages, [1,2]	135.1	127.7	139.0	605.2	581.0	840.5
Under 18 years [2]	42.2	39.6	46.4	190.9	161.5	218.7
Pneumonia	4.5	4.8	4.0	13.9	17.2	17.4
Asthma	1.3	2.4	2.2	*3.1	5.5	6.8
Injuries and poisoning	3.6	3.1	4.3	*15.4	*12.0	16.7
Fracture, all sites	1.1	0.9	1.3	3.6	2.3	6.4
18–44 Years [2]	135.2	124.8	146.8	444.2	401.1	582.0
HIV infection	0.3	0.3	*	2.5	*2.1	*
Delivery	69.5	64.5	69.9	179.6	160.2	195.0
Alcohol and drug [3]	1.9	*2.1	1.6	*9.5	*10.8	14.1
Serious mental illness [4]	6.0	*5.4	3.7	48.2	*41.1	54.3
Diseases of heart	1.8	1.7	1.3	7.5	6.3	7.2
Intervertebral disc disorders	1.1	1.0	1.5	2.6	2.4	7.3
Injuries and poisoning	4.8	4.3	6.7	18.9	18.1	36.6
Fracture, all sites	1.0	1.0	1.6	4.8	4.5	10.7
45–64 Years [2]	116.5	110.2	131.0	560.9	533.6	886.5
HIV infection	*	*	*	*	*	*
Malignant neoplasms	6.4	6.1	12.7	37.9	34.7	107.4
Trachea, bronchus, and lung	0.8	0.5	1.7	5.3	3.4	14.8
Breast	1.0	1.3	2.8	2.5	2.6	12.1
Diabetes	2.8	2.9	2.9	15.3	15.0	25.8
Alcohol and drug [3]	1.6	1.5	1.0	*8.2	*7.1	8.0
Serious mental illness [4]	5.4	4.6	4.0	48.1	42.7	60.5
Diseases of heart	14.1	14.6	16.6	59.7	59.5	101.1
Ischemic heart disease	6.9	7.8	9.9	25.0	29.5	57.4
Acute myocardial infarction	1.9	2.0	2.8	8.2	10.0	21.6
Congestive heart failure	3.1	2.9	2.1	14.5	13.6	15.8
Cerebrovascular diseases	3.0	3.5	3.0	15.3	19.5	32.1
Pneumonia	3.9	3.6	3.4	21.3	20.8	26.5
Injuries and poisoning	8.8	7.7	9.4	48.8	41.2	63.3
Fracture, all sites	2.0	2.7	3.1	9.5	13.3	25.0
65–74 Years [2]	255.5	246.1	241.1	1 398.4	1 397.1	1 959.3
Malignant neoplasms	14.5	14.1	20.9	98.5	101.0	189.8
Large intestine and rectum	2.0	1.7	2.4	17.1	15.2	34.9
Trachea, bronchus, and lung	2.5	2.4	2.6	16.8	*17.5	26.9
Breast	2.2	2.8	3.9	*4.3	*	17.6
Diabetes	5.1	4.6	5.8	26.8	26.1	46.8
Serious mental illness [4]	4.4	4.0	3.9	44.1	46.3	62.8
Diseases of heart	48.0	52.1	45.1	229.6	256.0	316.9
Ischemic heart disease	20.5	23.3	24.4	86.8	113.9	153.8
Acute myocardial infarction	7.6	8.0	7.5	40.6	52.8	58.1
Congestive heart failure	11.6	12.7	9.2	61.8	68.4	81.8
Cerebrovascular diseases	11.1	12.3	11.3	58.4	59.4	96.0
Pneumonia	11.8	11.7	8.7	65.6	73.5	81.8
Osteoarthritis	13.2	9.3	6.9	54.7	43.6	68.9
Injuries and poisoning	18.5	18.3	17.8	103.2	109.9	166.2
Fracture, all sites	7.3	7.7	8.4	39.8	43.8	97.3
Fracture of neck of femur (hip)	2.8	3.2	3.6	16.8	21.1	*59.6
75 Years and Over [2]	470.5	458.8	409.6	2 734.8	2 830.8	3 887.1
Malignant neoplasms	15.9	17.6	22.1	124.5	125.7	257.3
Large intestine and rectum	2.8	3.4	4.6	26.8	28.4	69.8
Trachea, bronchus, and lung	2.0	1.9	2.1	*16.2	14.0	20.6
Breast	1.4	2.5	3.9	*4.4	*8.9	22.0
Diabetes	6.2	6.3	4.6	28.6	34.0	55.3
Serious mental illness [4]	3.3	4.7	4.2	37.2	49.2	78.4
Diseases of heart	97.2	99.1	84.6	480.1	523.4	672.8
Ischemic heart disease	32.1	35.5	33.7	150.8	185.5	253.2
Acute myocardial infarction	15.8	16.5	13.1	95.1	110.7	125.9
Congestive heart failure	29.6	32.2	28.0	159.4	181.7	236.6
Cerebrovascular diseases	24.5	27.6	29.6	138.3	156.8	302.0
Pneumonia	29.7	30.5	23.9	189.9	209.7	260.1
Osteoarthritis	10.6	8.7	5.3	45.8	40.4	54.1
Injuries and poisoning	46.2	44.7	46.3	271.0	275.4	489.2
Fracture, all sites	29.4	30.0	31.5	173.5	190.0	352.7
Fracture of neck of femur (hip)	15.5	17.9	18.8	98.6	125.3	236.3

Note: Excludes newborn infants.

[1] Estimates are age adjusted to the year 2000 standard population using six age groups: under 18 years, 18–44 years, 45–54 years, 55–64 years, 65–74 years, and 75 years and over.

[2] Includes discharges with first-listed diagnoses not shown in table.

[3] Includes abuse, dependence, and withdrawal. These estimates are for non-federal short-stay hospitals and do not include alcohol and drug discharges from other types of facilities or programs, such as the Department of Veterans Affairs or day treatment programs.

[4] These estimates are for non-federal short-stay hospitals and do not include serious mental illness discharges from other types of facilities or programs, such as the Department of Veterans Affairs or long-term hospitals.

* = Figure does not meet standards of reliability or precision.

TABLE III-52. NUMBER OF DISCHARGES AND DAYS OF CARE IN NON-FEDERAL SHORT-STAY HOSPITALS, ACCORDING TO SEX, AGE, AND SELECTED FIRST-LISTED DIAGNOSIS, SELECTED YEARS, 1990–2003

In this table, the number of discharges and days of hospital care are broken down by sex and by age group. The previous table, Table III-51, provided information in terms of rates per 1,000 persons, while this table shows the number of discharges (in thousands) and the days of

Table III-52. Number of Discharges and Days of Care in Non-Federal Short-Stay Hospitals, According to Sex, Age, and Selected First-Listed Diagnosis, Selected Years, 1990–2003

(Number.)

Sex, age, and first-listed diagnosis	Discharges (in thousands)			Average number of days		
	2003	2000	1990	2003	2000	1990
BOTH SEXES [1,2]	34 738	31 706	30 788	4.8	4.9	6.5
MALE						
All Ages [1,2]	13 874	12 514	12 280	5.2	5.4	7.1
Under 18 Years [2]	1 679	1 515	1 572	4.5	4.8	5.0
Pneumonia	221	199	178	3.2	3.2	4.3
Asthma	74	129	111	2.4	2.1	2.8
Injuries and poisoning	207	185	232	3.9	4.3	4.4
Fracture, all sites	77	68	76	3.0	3.9	4.2
18–44 Years [2]	2 683	2 498	3 120	4.9	4.8	6.1
HIV infection	28	32	*15	8.6	*9.4	*10.6
Alcohol and drug [3]	203	224	201	4.1	4.7	8.9
Serious mental illness [4]	323	*296	184	8.0	*8.2	13.8
Diseases of heart	169	148	163	*4.5	3.5	5.4
Intervertebral disc disorders	69	81	138	2.3	2.2	4.2
Injuries and poisoning	470	408	704	4.9	4.5	5.0
Fracture, all sites	171	141	217	5.1	5.0	5.6
45–64 Years [2]	4 016	3 424	3 115	5.0	5.1	6.7
HIV infection	*22	*15	*3	*	*	*7.1
Malignant neoplasms	221	188	235	6.7	6.8	9.4
Trachea, bronchus, and lung	30	26	60	6.9	6.0	7.1
Diabetes	105	114	65	4.7	6.0	7.3
Alcohol and drug [3]	140	106	77	4.5	4.5	8.5
Serious mental illness [4]	147	*120	56	9.1	*8.8	13.7
Diseases of heart	827	802	704	4.0	3.8	5.8
Ischemic heart disease	494	539	502	3.8	3.6	5.7
Acute myocardial infarction	161	178	165	5.2	4.7	7.5
Congestive heart failure	129	101	66	4.8	5.2	6.7
Cerebrovascular diseases	126	116	91	4.4	5.2	10.0
Pneumonia	137	104	77	6.1	6.0	7.9
Injuries and poisoning	369	266	257	5.5	5.7	7.2
Fracture, all sites	102	77	74	5.9	6.4	7.2
65–74 Years [2]	2 309	2 199	2 268	5.3	5.6	7.8
Malignant neoplasms	161	146	220	6.5	6.9	9.9
Large intestine and rectum	18	24	24	8.0	9.2	11.4
Trachea, bronchus, and lung	30	23	50	5.8	6.8	8.7
Prostate	33	31	40	3.2	3.8	6.5
Diabetes	42	39	34	5.5	6.2	9.1
Serious mental illness [4]	24	*28	20	10.1	*11.7	17.4
Diseases of heart	553	586	547	4.4	4.7	7.0
Ischemic heart disease	294	329	331	4.2	4.3	6.8
Acute myocardial infarction	105	104	110	5.3	5.3	8.8
Congestive heart failure	113	112	90	4.9	5.7	7.9
Cerebrovascular diseases	112	109	108	4.3	4.5	8.3
Pneumonia	108	106	90	6.0	6.4	9.5
Hyperplasia of prostate	32	45	113	2.8	2.8	4.5
Osteoarthritis	72	80	39	4.0	4.9	9.0
Injuries and poisoning	160	149	139	5.5	5.9	7.9
Fracture, all sites	38	39	36	6.0	6.4	10.2
Fracture of neck of femur (hip)	*12	*17	12	*7.1	*7.9	*11.8
75 Years and Over [2]	3 188	2 878	2 203	5.9	6.2	8.8
Malignant neoplasms	159	135	189	6.9	7.6	10.0
Large intestine and rectum	26	26	25	9.2	10.6	15.0
Trachea, bronchus, and lung	27	18	25	7.2	6.1	10.0
Prostate	16	20	45	*4.4	*6.1	6.8
Diabetes	44	40	21	*5.5	6.6	11.0
Serious mental illness [4]	17	18	*12	*10.0	*11.2	*15.5
Diseases of heart	728	697	489	5.1	5.3	8.1
Ischemic heart disease	311	326	226	5.1	5.2	8.1
Acute myocardial infarction	142	141	106	6.6	5.9	9.9
Congestive heart failure	205	188	143	5.5	5.7	7.8
Cerebrovascular diseases	192	186	139	4.9	5.7	9.9
Pneumonia	262	229	178	6.2	6.3	10.2
Hyperplasia of prostate	36	42	82	3.1	3.2	6.1
Osteoarthritis	64	38	27	4.4	4.6	10.5
Injuries and poisoning	228	207	144	6.5	7.7	10.9
Fracture, all sites	101	89	63	7.1	*8.3	10.6
Fracture of neck of femur (hip)	64	52	39	6.9	7.5	11.5

Note: Excludes newborn infants.

[1] Average length of stay estimates are age adjusted to the year 2000 standard population using six age groups: under 18 years, 18–44 years, 45–54 years, 55–64 years, 65–74 years, and 75 years and over.
[2] Includes discharges with first-listed diagnoses not shown in table.
[3] Includes abuse, dependence, and withdrawal. These estimates are for non-federal short-stay hospitals and do not include alcohol and drug discharges from other types of facilities or programs, such as the Department of Veterans Affairs or day treatment programs.
[4] These estimates are for non-federal short-stay hospitals and do not include serious mental illness discharges from other types of facilities or programs, such as the Department of Veterans Affairs or long-term hospitals.
* = Figure does not meet standards of reliability or precision.

care (in number of days). For males, the average length of hospitalization was 5.2 days in 2003, down considerably from 7.1 days in 1990. The average length of stay for females was 4.5 days.

For serious mental illnesses and for cancer, the length of stay tended to be longer than average. Fractures also resulted in relatively long hospital stays for men.

Table III-52. Number of Discharges and Days of Care in Non-Federal Short-Stay Hospitals, According to Sex, Age, and Selected First-Listed Diagnosis, Selected Years, 1990–2003—Continued

(Number.)

Sex, age, and first–listed diagnosis	Discharges (in thousands)			Average number of days		
	2003	2000	1990	2003	2000	1990
FEMALE						
All Ages, [1,2]	20 864	19 192	18 508	4.5	4.5	6.0
Under 18 years [2]	1 504	1 397	1 500	4.5	4.1	4.7
Pneumonia	159	168	129	3.1	3.6	4.4
Asthma	46	85	71	*2.4	2.3	3.1
Injuries and poisoning	128	111	138	*4.3	*3.8	3.9
Fracture, all sites	38	32	42	3.4	2.5	5.0
18–44 Years [2]	7 537	6 941	8 018	3.3	3.2	4.0
HIV infection	19	15	*	7.4	*7.5	*
Delivery	3 874	3 588	3 815	2.6	2.5	2.8
Alcohol and drug [3]	106	*116	85	*5.0	*5.2	9.1
Serious mental illness [4]	333	*300	200	8.1	*7.6	14.8
Diseases of heart	102	95	73	4.1	3.7	5.4
Intervertebral disc disorders	60	58	84	2.4	2.3	4.7
Injuries and poisoning	268	237	366	3.9	4.2	5.5
Fracture, all sites	57	57	85	4.7	4.4	6.9
45–64 Years [2]	4 104	3 534	3 129	4.8	4.8	6.8
HIV infection	*	*	*	*	*	*
Malignant neoplasms	226	195	303	5.9	5.7	8.5
Trachea, bronchus, and lung	27	17	41	6.8	6.4	8.6
Breast	37	40	67	2.4	2.1	4.3
Diabetes	99	93	70	5.4	5.2	8.9
Alcohol and drug [3]	55	47	23	*5.2	*4.8	8.2
Serious mental illness [4]	191	146	95	8.8	9.4	15.2
Diseases of heart	498	470	397	4.2	4.1	6.1
Ischemic heart disease	242	251	237	3.6	3.8	5.8
Acute myocardial infarction	66	64	68	4.4	5.0	7.6
Congestive heart failure	110	94	51	4.6	4.6	7.4
Cerebrovascular diseases	104	113	72	5.2	5.5	10.7
Pneumonia	136	117	80	5.5	5.7	7.9
Injuries and poisoning	310	248	225	5.5	5.3	6.7
Fracture, all sites	71	87	75	4.7	4.9	7.9
65–74 Years [2]	2 552	2 479	2 421	5.5	5.7	8.1
Malignant neoplasms	144	142	210	6.8	7.2	9.1
Large intestine and rectum	20	17	24	8.4	9.0	14.5
Trachea, bronchus, and lung	25	25	26	6.8	*7.1	10.2
Breast	22	29	40	*2.0	*	4.5
Diabetes	51	47	59	5.2	5.6	8.0
Serious mental illness [4]	43	40	39	10.1	11.7	16.3
Diseases of heart	480	525	453	4.8	4.9	7.0
Ischemic heart disease	205	235	245	4.2	4.9	6.3
Acute myocardial infarction	76	81	75	5.4	6.6	7.8
Congestive heart failure	116	128	92	5.3	5.4	8.9
Cerebrovascular diseases	111	124	114	5.3	4.8	8.5
Pneumonia	117	117	87	5.6	6.3	9.4
Osteoarthritis	132	94	69	4.1	4.7	10.0
Injuries and poisoning	184	185	179	5.6	6.0	9.3
Fracture, all sites	73	77	85	5.4	5.7	11.5
Fracture of neck of femur (hip)	28	32	36	5.9	6.7	*16.7
75 Years and Over [2]	5 168	4 840	3 440	5.8	6.2	9.5
Malignant neoplasms	175	186	185	7.8	7.1	11.7
Large intestine and rectum	31	36	39	9.6	8.4	15.1
Trachea, bronchus, and lung	22	20	18	*8.1	7.3	9.9
Breast	15	27	33	*3.2	*3.5	5.7
Diabetes	68	67	39	4.6	5.4	11.9
Serious mental illness [4]	37	49	35	11.2	10.5	18.7
Diseases of heart	1 067	1 045	711	4.9	5.3	8.0
Ischemic heart disease	352	375	283	4.7	5.2	7.5
Acute myocardial infarction	174	174	110	6.0	6.7	9.6
Congestive heart failure	325	339	235	5.4	5.6	8.5
Cerebrovascular diseases	269	292	249	5.6	5.7	10.2
Pneumonia	327	322	201	6.4	6.9	10.9
Osteoarthritis	117	91	45	4.3	4.7	10.2
Injuries and poisoning	507	472	389	5.9	6.2	10.6
Fracture, all sites	323	316	265	5.9	6.3	11.2
Fracture of neck of femur (hip)	171	189	158	6.3	7.0	12.5

Note: Excludes newborn infants.

[1] Average length of stay estimates are age adjusted to the year 2000 standard population using six age groups: under 18 years, 18–44 years, 45–54 years, 55–64 years, 65–74 years, and 75 years and over.

[2] Includes discharges with first-listed diagnoses not shown in table.

[3] Includes abuse, dependence, and withdrawal. These estimates are for non-federal short-stay hospitals and do not include alcohol and drug discharges from other types of facilities or programs, such as the Department of Veterans Affairs or day treatment programs.

[4] These estimates are for non-federal short-stay hospitals and do not include serious mental illness discharges from other types of facilities or programs, such as the Department of Veterans Affairs or long-term hospitals.

* = Figure does not meet standards of reliability or precision.

TABLE III-53. SELECTED INPATIENT PROCEDURES, ACCORDING TO SEX, AGE, AND TYPE OF PROCEDURE, ANNUAL AVERAGES, 1992–1993 AND 2002–2003

This table shows the frequency of different medical procedures performed in the hospital, classified by age group.

Inpatient procedures in 2002–2003 totaled 19.3 million annually for patients 18 years old and over. The frequency of inpatient procedures increased substantially with age. For persons 75 years old and over, there were 2,425 procedures completed per 10,000 persons, while 647 procedures per 10,000 persons were completed on those 18–44 years old. Frequently, procedures were done in car-

Table III-53. Selected Inpatient Procedures, According to Sex, Age, and Type of Procedure, Annual Averages, 1992–1993 and 2002–2003

(Number in thousands, number per 10,000 population.)

Sex, age, and procedure category	Both sexes		Male		Female	
	2002–2003	1992–1993	2002–2003	1992–1993	2002–2003	1992–1993
18 YEARS OF AGE AND OVER						
Number of hospital stays with at least one procedure (in thousands) [1,2]	19 283	18 700	7 084	6 953	12 199	11 748
18 YEARS OF AGE AND OVER, AGE-ADJUSTED [3]						
Number Per 10,000 Population [4]						
Hospital stays with at least one procedure [2]	897.3	992.3	729.0	845.8	1 076.2	1 152.6
Cardiac catheterization	58.8	54.6	78.8	74.4	42.2	37.9
Insertion, replacement, removal, and revision of pacemaker leads or device	10.4	8.8	12.2	10.9	9.1	7.4
Incision, excision, and occlusion of vessels	64.1	40.3	68.2	46.9	61.1	35.5
Angiocardiography using contrast material	47.5	45.6	61.5	61.3	35.8	32.3
Operations on vessels of heart	43.1	37.0	64.4	56.4	25.4	20.8
Removal of coronary artery obstruction and insertion of stent	30.2	21.0	43.5	30.7	18.9	12.7
Insertion of coronary artery stent(s) [5]	25.0	X	36.8	X	15.1	X
Coronary artery bypass graft	13.2	16.9	21.3	27.1	6.6	8.6
Diagnostic procedures on small intestine	47.1	44.8	46.7	47.1	47.8	43.1
Diagnostic procedures on large intestine	26.7	28.7	24.8	27.7	28.3	29.6
Diagnostic radiology	35.1	78.0	34.9	80.4	35.6	76.6
Computerized axial tomography	28.4	54.9	28.5	59.2	28.1	51.2
Diagnostic ultrasound	32.7	66.1	33.8	61.5	32.2	71.1
Joint replacement of lower extremity	35.6	22.6	30.9	18.2	39.3	25.7
Total hip replacement	9.5	6.8	9.2	6.2	9.6	7.1
Partial hip replacement	5.0	4.9	3.5	2.9	6.0	6.1
Total knee replacement	17.7	8.9	15.1	6.9	20.0	10.5
Reduction of fracture and dislocation	24.2	27.5	23.3	24.7	23.6	28.3
Excision or destruction of intervertebral disc	14.4	17.3	16.2	19.6	12.9	15.2
Cholecystectomy	19.7	27.2	14.9	18.9	24.4	35.4
Laparoscopic cholecystectomy	14.5	18.1	9.6	10.9	19.3	25.0
Lysis of peritoneal adhesions	15.2	18.0	5.9	7.3	24.1	28.1
18–44 YEARS OF AGE						
Number of hospital stays with at least one procedure (in thousands) [1,2]	7 238	7 855	1 481	1 874	5 757	5 981
Number Per 10,000 Population [4]						
Hospital stays with at least one procedure [2]	646.5	719.2	263.8	344.9	1 031.3	1 089.5
Repair of hernia	4.2	4.7	2.6	5.0	5.9	4.3
Cesarean section and removal of fetus	X	X	X	X	191.0	163.1
Forceps, vacuum, and breech delivery	X	X	X	X	55.6	77.1
Other procedures inducing or assisting delivery	X	X	X	X	399.5	399.6
Dilation and curettage of uterus	X	X	X	X	7.1	20.9
Total abdominal hysterectomy	X	X	X	X	36.5	38.5
Vaginal hysterectomy	X	X	X	X	18.8	20.3
Cardiac catheterization	9.1	8.3	12.3	12.3	5.9	4.4
Incision, excision, and occlusion of vessels	20.2	11.9	20.2	12.3	20.3	11.4
Angiocardiography using contrast material	8.2	7.4	10.6	11.0	5.7	3.8
Operations on vessels of heart	4.5	3.6	7.0	6.2	2.0	1.0
Removal of coronary artery obstruction and insertion of stent	3.6	2.6	5.5	4.5	1.7	*0.7
Insertion of coronary artery stent(s) [5]	3.0	X	4.7	X	1.2	X
Coronary artery bypass graft	0.9	1.0	1.5	1.8	*	*
Diagnostic procedures on small intestine	13.4	12.9	11.4	13.8	15.5	12.1
Diagnostic procedures on large intestine	6.3	6.7	5.7	6.6	6.9	6.9
Diagnostic radiology	14.7	33.2	12.7	32.4	16.6	33.9
Computerized axial tomography	11.4	21.2	11.4	24.7	11.3	17.6
Diagnostic ultrasound	10.6	29.0	7.7	15.8	13.6	42.0
Reduction of fracture and dislocation	13.4	15.9	18.9	21.3	7.9	10.5
Excision or destruction of intervertebral disc	10.6	15.0	11.6	18.7	9.7	11.5
Cholecystectomy	12.0	16.1	5.0	6.3	19.0	25.8
Laparoscopic cholecystectomy	10.2	11.9	3.7	4.1	16.8	19.5
Lysis of peritoneal adhesions	12.4	15.2	1.6	2.1	23.2	28.2

[1]Average number of stays per year.
[2]Includes stays for procedures not shown separately.
[3]Estimates are age adjusted to the year 2000 standard population using five age groups: 18–44 years, 45–54 years, 55–64 years, 65–74 years, and 75 years and over.
[4]Average annual rate.
[5]The procedure code for insertion of coronary artery stents was not available in 1991–1992.
* = Figure does not meet standards of reliability or precision.
X = Not applicable.

diology (especially angiocardiography), gastroenterology, and hip and knee replacement. The use of angioplasty and stents to repair vessels of the heart increased markedly between 1992–1993 and 2002–2003, while the frequency of coronary artery bypass graft (CABG) declined between those periods. However, in persons 75 years old and over, hospital stays with at least one operation on vessels of the heart performed increased from 79 to 129 hospital stays per 10,000 persons, mainly reflecting increases in stent insertion. Hospital stays including diag-

Table III-53. Selected Inpatient Procedures, According to Sex, Age, and Type of Procedure, Annual Averages, 1992–1993 and 2002–2003—*Continued*

(Number in thousands, number per 10,000 population.)

Sex, age, and procedure category	Both sexes		Male		Female	
	2002–2003	1992–1993	2002–2003	1992–1993	2002–2003	1992–1993
45–64 YEARS OF AGE						
Number of hospital stays with at least one procedure (in thousands) [1,2]	4 924	4 227	2 457	2 105	2 467	2 122
Number Per 10,000 Population [4]						
Hospital stays with at least one procedure [2]	727.8	866.5	746.2	892.3	710.4	842.2
Transurethral prostatectomy	X	X	6.5	21.2	X	X
Repair of hernia	13.5	15.7	12.2	18.6	14.6	12.9
Total abdominal hysterectomy	X	X	X	X	47.2	49.6
Vaginal hysterectomy	X	X	X	X	21.1	19.4
Cardiac catheterization	79.8	86.5	106.7	120.3	54.3	54.9
Insertion, replacement, removal, and revision of pacemaker leads or device	4.3	6.1	5.5	7.6	3.1	4.8
Incision, excision, and occlusion of vessels	65.0	43.2	68.5	48.1	61.6	38.6
Angiocardiography using contrast material	64.4	72.9	83.2	99.1	46.5	48.3
Operations on vessels of heart	58.6	59.5	88.4	91.8	30.3	29.3
Removal of coronary artery obstruction and insertion of stent	41.4	35.3	61.2	52.2	22.6	19.5
Insertion of coronary artery stent(s) [5]	34.4	X	52.0	X	17.6	X
Coronary artery bypass graft	17.6	25.8	27.7	42.1	8.0	10.7
Diagnostic procedures on small intestine	41.5	42.2	41.7	44.2	41.3	40.3
Diagnostic procedures on large intestine	20.9	27.2	18.0	26.3	23.7	28.1
Diagnostic radiology	31.5	76.8	31.4	77.7	31.5	75.9
Computerized axial tomography	24.0	48.8	25.5	51.1	22.7	46.6
Diagnostic ultrasound	30.4	60.6	34.2	63.3	26.9	58.2
Joint replacement of lower extremity	34.8	18.0	31.0	15.2	38.4	20.7
Total hip replacement	10.4	6.5	11.6	7.1	9.4	5.9
Partial hip replacement	1.2	1.6	*1.0	*	1.3	2.2
Total knee replacement	20.2	7.8	16.1	5.2	24.1	10.2
Reduction of fracture and dislocation	16.4	21.1	17.8	18.4	15.0	23.6
Excision or destruction of intervertebral disc	21.0	23.7	23.2	25.1	18.9	22.4
Cholecystectomy	20.5	31.9	17.3	21.1	23.4	41.9
Laparoscopic cholecystectomy	14.6	23.0	11.1	14.2	17.8	31.4
Lysis of peritoneal adhesions	14.9	16.6	5.7	7.6	23.6	25.0
65–74 YEARS OF AGE						
Number of hospital stays with at least one procedure (in thousands) [1,2]	2 889	3 216	1 421	1 605	1 468	1 611
Number Per 10,000 Population [4]						
Hospital stays with at least one procedure [2]	1 578.4	1 749.6	1 707.4	1 974.0	1 470.7	1 571.7
Transurethral prostatectomy	X	X	50.5	128.6	X	X
Repair of hernia	27.1	36.2	29.5	51.1	25.0	24.4
Total abdominal hysterectomy	X	X	X	X	18.0	23.8
Vaginal hysterectomy	X	X	X	X	13.9	14.2
Cardiac catheterization	178.1	175.7	230.0	227.5	134.8	134.7
Insertion, replacement, removal, and revision of pacemaker leads or device	27.8	24.3	28.6	28.9	27.0	20.6
Incision, excision, and occlusion of vessels	154.9	109.5	167.1	131.5	144.7	92.0
Angiocardiography using contrast material	139.4	144.0	174.3	185.2	110.2	111.3
Operations on vessels of heart	144.8	127.5	208.5	184.6	91.7	82.1
Removal of coronary artery obstruction and insertion of stent	97.3	67.0	134.5	91.8	66.3	47.4
Insertion of coronary artery stent(s) [5]	81.8	X	113.9	X	55.0	X
Coronary artery bypass graft	48.6	64.0	75.9	97.8	25.9	37.1
Diagnostic procedures on small intestine	110.7	104.6	114.9	104.2	107.2	105.0
Diagnostic procedures on large intestine	67.9	64.4	64.4	57.9	70.8	69.6
Diagnostic radiology	75.8	159.7	77.9	169.5	74.1	151.9
Computerized axial tomography	59.1	120.6	56.5	129.4	61.3	113.7
Diagnostic ultrasound	75.5	142.7	78.5	152.2	73.0	135.2
Joint replacement of lower extremity	120.3	79.0	95.2	61.2	141.2	93.1
Total hip replacement	30.5	24.4	26.5	20.5	33.8	27.6
Partial hip replacement	8.3	8.0	5.9	X	10.3	11.5
Total knee replacement	70.1	40.4	52.9	30.7	84.4	48.1
Reduction of fracture and dislocation	36.8	38.4	26.7	28.4	45.2	46.4
Excision or destruction of intervertebral disc	16.8	17.6	19.1	15.6	15.0	19.3
Cholecystectomy	40.1	54.5	38.8	48.7	41.1	59.1
Laparoscopic cholecystectomy	27.5	31.6	24.9	24.2	29.6	37.5
Lysis of peritoneal adhesions	20.9	24.5	16.8	21.3	24.3	27.0

[1] Average number of stays per year.
[2] Includes stays for procedures not shown separately.
[4] Average annual rate.
[5] The procedure code for insertion of coronary artery stents was not available in 1991–1992.
* = Figure does not meet standards of reliability or precision.
X = Not applicable.

nostic ultrasound performed on persons 18 years old and over decreased substantially, dropping from 66 to 33 hospital stays per 10,000 persons (age-adjusted), which reflected the shifting of ultrasound procedures (and many other diagnostic tools) to outpatient settings.

Table III-53. Selected Inpatient Procedures, According to Sex, Age, and Type of Procedure, Annual Averages, 1992–1993 and 2002–2003—*Continued*

(Number in thousands, number per 10,000 population.)

Sex, age, and procedure category	Both sexes		Male		Female	
	2002–2003	1992–1993	2002–2003	1992–1993	2002–2003	1992–1993
75 YEARS OF AGE AND OVER						
Number of hospital stays with at least one procedure (in thousands) [1, 2]	4 232	3 402	1 725	1 369	2 507	2 033
Number Per 10,000 Population [4]						
Hospital stays with at least one procedure [2]	2 424.5	2 455.5	2 638.9	2 756.6	2 296.1	2 287.3
Transurethral prostatectomy	X	X	81.2	225.9	X	X
Repair of hernia	27.2	41.5	32.1	58.4	24.3	32.0
Total abdominal hysterectomy	X	X	X	X	13.0	13.8
Vaginal hysterectomy	X	X	X	X	6.8	9.1
Cardiac catheterization	176.7	114.2	246.0	150.0	135.2	94.2
Insertion, replacement, removal, and revision of pacemaker leads or device	78.7	57.6	94.5	72.6	69.2	49.3
Incision, excision, and occlusion of vessels	249.1	143.6	272.4	180.2	235.1	123.1
Angiocardiography using contrast material	142.8	93.2	191.7	120.2	113.4	78.1
Operations on vessels of heart	128.3	78.9	194.3	120.6	88.8	55.6
Removal of coronary artery obstruction and insertion of stent	90.0	41.0	127.5	59.2	67.5	30.8
Insertion of coronary artery stent(s) [5]	73.3	X	106.7	X	53.3	X
Coronary artery bypass graft	39.1	39.0	67.7	63.5	22.0	25.4
Diagnostic procedures on small intestine	219.1	200.0	220.8	214.9	218.2	191.6
Diagnostic procedures on large intestine	136.2	141.0	131.2	138.8	139.2	142.1
Diagnostic radiology	137.9	289.9	146.2	309.1	132.8	279.2
Computerized axial tomography	121.8	228.9	121.2	240.8	122.2	222.2
Diagnostic ultrasound	139.2	248.8	155.0	258.0	129.8	243.6
Joint replacement of lower extremity	162.9	118.1	145.6	91.7	173.3	132.8
Total hip replacement	37.1	27.7	33.2	22.4	39.4	30.7
Partial hip replacement	48.0	44.7	32.0	27.7	57.6	54.2
Total knee replacement	63.3	36.1	64.7	30.8	62.5	39.1
Reduction of fracture and dislocation	109.9	115.7	68.9	65.9	134.4	143.6
Excision or destruction of intervertebral disc	12.1	8.1	16.7	9.4	9.3	7.4
Cholecystectomy	44.9	54.4	44.0	61.8	45.4	50.2
Laparoscopic cholecystectomy	28.1	26.6	25.9	28.7	29.4	25.4
Lysis of peritoneal adhesions	28.1	34.0	23.3	25.8	31.0	38.7

[1]Average number of stays per year.

[2]Includes stays for procedures not shown separately.

[4]Average annual rate.

[5]The procedure code for insertion of coronary artery stents was not available in 1991–1992.

X = Not applicable.

TABLE III-54. NURSING HOME RESIDENTS 65 YEARS OF AGE AND OVER, ACCORDING TO AGE, SEX, AND RACE, SELECTED YEARS, 1973–1999

In 1999, there were about 1.5 million residents in nursing homes, including some 500,000 persons between 75 and 84 years of age and 750,000 persons age 85 years and over. Women were much more frequent residents than men: per 1,000 persons age 65 years and over, 55 women were in nursing homes, but only 27 men. Because these figures are rates, they adjust for the fact that the female population is substantially larger than the male population in the top age brackets. When a head count is used to measure nursing home residents, the dominance of female clients becomes apparent. Female clients made up 1.092 million of nursing home residents in 1999, while male residents made up 378,000 of nursing home residents.

The rate of Black clients in nursing homes is greater than the rate of Whites. In 1999, there were 55.6 Blacks (per 1,000 persons age 65 years and over) in nursing homes, compared to 41.9 Whites (per 1,000 persons, age-adjusted). This represents a remarkable reversal, in which the rate for Blacks has increased steadily from a low of 28.2 per 1,000 persons over 65 years old in 1972–1974, while the rate for Whites has decreased steadily from a high of 61.2 per 1,000 persons (age-adjusted) during that same period.

Table III-54. Nursing Home Residents 65 Years of Age and Over, According to Age, Sex, and Race, Selected Years, 1973–1999

(Number, rate per 1,000 population.)

Age, sex, and race	Residents				Residents per 1,000 population			
	1999	1995	1985	1973–1974	1999	1995	1985	1973–1974
All Persons								
65 years and over, age-adjusted [1]	X	X	X	X	43.3	45.9	54.0	58.5
65 years and over, crude	1 469 500	1 422 600	1 318 300	961 500	42.9	42.4	46.2	44.7
65–74 years	194 800	190 200	212 100	163 100	10.8	10.1	12.5	12.3
75–84 years	517 600	511 900	509 000	384 900	43.0	45.9	57.7	57.7
85 years and over	757 100	720 400	597 300	413 600	182.5	198.6	220.3	257.3
Male								
65 years and over, age-adjusted [1]	X	X	X	X	30.6	32.8	38.8	42.5
65 years and over, crude	377 800	356 800	334 400	265 700	26.5	26.1	29.0	30.0
65–74 years	84 100	79 300	80 600	65 100	10.3	9.5	10.8	11.3
75–84 years	149 500	144 300	141 300	102 300	30.8	33.3	43.0	39.9
85 years and over	144 200	133 100	112 600	98 300	116.5	130.8	145.7	182.7
Female								
65 years and over, age-adjusted [1]	X	X	X	X	49.8	52.3	61.5	67.5
65 years and over, crude	1 091 700	1 065 800	983 900	695 800	54.6	53.7	57.9	54.9
65–74 years	110 700	110 900	131 500	98 000	11.2	10.6	13.8	13.1
75–84 years	368 100	367 600	367 700	282 600	51.2	53.9	66.4	68.9
85 years and over	612 900	587 300	484 700	315 300	210.5	224.9	250.1	294.9
White [2]								
65 years and over, age-adjusted [1]	X	X	X	X	41.9	45.4	55.5	61.2
65 years and over, crude	1 279 600	1 271 200	1 227 400	920 600	42.1	42.3	47.7	46.9
65–74 years	157 200	154 400	187 800	150 100	10.0	9.3	12.3	12.5
75–84 years	440 600	453 800	473 600	369 700	40.5	44.9	59.1	60.3
85 years and over	681 700	663 000	566 000	400 800	181.8	200.7	228.7	270.8
Black or African American [2]								
65 years and over, age-adjusted [1]	X	X	X	X	55.6	50.4	41.5	28.2
65 years and over, crude	145 900	122 900	82 000	37 700	51.1	45.2	35.0	22.0
65–74 years	30 300	29 700	22 500	12 200	18.2	18.4	15.4	11.1
75–84 years	58 700	47 300	30 600	13 400	66.5	57.2	45.3	26.7
85 years and over	56 900	45 800	29 000	12 100	183.1	167.1	141.5	105.7

Note: Excludes residents in personal care or domiciliary care homes.

[1] Age adjusted by the direct method to the year 2000 population standard using the following three age groups: 65–74 years, 75–84 years, and 85 years and over.

[2] Beginning in 1999, the instruction for the race item on the Current Resident Questionnaire was changed so that more than one race could be recorded. In previous years, only one racial category could be checked. Estimates in this table are for single race residents.

X = Not applicable.

TABLE III-55. NURSING HOME RESIDENTS 65 YEARS OF AGE AND OVER, ACCORDING TO SELECTED FUNCTIONAL STATUS AND AGE, SEX, AND RACE, 1985, 1995, AND 1999

This table shows the percentage of nursing home residents who are functionally dependent in regard to mobility or eating or who are incontinent. Residents are considered dependent if they require assistance or special equipment for mobility or eating. In 1999, 80.4 percent of nursing home residents age 65 years and over were dependent in regard to mobility; 65.7 percent were incontinent; 47.4 percent were dependent in regard to eating; and 37.0 percent were dependent in all three functions. The percentages of impairment for Blacks were higher than those for Whites in each of the functional categories and in each separate age group.

TABLE III-56. NURSING HOMES, BEDS, OCCUPANCY, AND RESIDENTS, ACCORDING TO GEOGRAPHIC DIVISION AND STATE, SELECTED YEARS, 1995–2003

Of the nearly 1.5 million nursing home residents in 2003, 113,000 were located in New York, 108,000 in California, and 87,000 in Texas. There were 16,300 nursing homes in the United States. By state, the largest number of nursing homes—over 1,300—was in California, followed by Texas with more than 1,100.

The resident rate, or the number of nursing home residents (all ages) per 1,000 persons age 85 years and over, was highest in Louisiana at 470. The lowest resident rates were in Oregon (131) and Arizona (164). Resident rates declined in most states between 1995 and 2003, with the exception of Vermont. The occupancy rate (percent of beds occupied) was relatively stable, averaging 82.6 percent in 2003.

Table III-55. Nursing Home Residents 65 Years of Age and Over, According to Selected Functional Status and Age, Sex, and Race, 1985, 1995, and 1999

(Percent.)

Age, sex, and race	Functional status [1]											
	Dependent mobility			Incontinent			Dependent eating			Dependent mobility, eating, and incontinent		
	1999	1995	1985	1999	1995	1985	1999	1995	1985	1999	1995	1985
All Persons												
65 years and over, age-adjusted [2]	80.3	79.0	75.7	65.7	63.8	55.0	47.3	44.9	40.9	36.9	36.5	32.5
65 years and over, crude	80.4	79.0	74.8	65.7	63.8	54.5	47.4	44.9	40.5	37.0	36.5	32.1
65–74 years	73.9	73.0	61.2	58.5	61.9	42.9	43.1	43.8	33.5	31.7	35.8	25.7
75–84 years	77.8	76.5	70.5	64.2	62.5	55.1	46.6	45.2	39.4	35.4	35.3	30.6
85 years and over	83.8	82.4	83.3	68.6	65.3	58.1	49.0	45.0	43.9	39.4	37.5	35.6
Male												
65 years and over, age-adjusted [2]	76.6	76.6	71.2	66.6	63.8	54.2	45.2	42.1	36.0	35.0	34.3	28.0
65 years and over, crude	75.9	75.8	67.8	66.0	63.9	51.9	45.1	42.7	34.9	35.0	34.8	26.9
65–74 years	70.5	70.6	55.8	59.6	63.4	38.8	45.0	44.2	32.8	34.8	36.9	24.1
75–84 years	76.9	76.6	65.7	68.9	64.6	54.4	44.7	44.1	32.6	35.2	35.5	25.5
85 years and over	78.1	78.2	79.2	66.8	63.4	58.1	45.7	40.2	39.2	34.9	32.7	30.9
Female												
65 years and over, age-adjusted [2]	81.5	79.7	77.3	65.0	63.6	55.4	47.8	45.6	42.4	37.2	36.9	33.9
65 years and over, crude	81.9	80.1	77.1	65.6	63.8	55.4	48.1	45.6	42.4	37.7	37.0	33.8
65–74 years	76.4	74.8	64.5	57.7	60.9	45.4	41.6	43.6	34.0	29.3	35.0	26.7
75–84 years	78.2	76.5	72.3	62.2	61.7	55.3	47.4	45.7	42.0	35.6	35.2	32.6
85 years and over	85.2	83.3	84.3	69.0	65.7	58.1	49.7	46.0	45.0	40.4	38.6	36.7
White [3]												
65 years and over, age-adjusted [2]	79.9	78.5	75.2	64.9	63.2	54.6	46.1	44.2	40.4	35.7	35.7	32.1
65 years and over, crude	80.2	78.7	74.3	65.1	63.3	54.2	46.2	44.2	40.1	35.8	35.7	31.7
65–74 years	72.6	71.4	60.2	57.1	60.2	42.2	40.7	41.9	32.6	28.8	33.8	24.9
75–84 years	77.5	76.4	69.6	63.8	61.8	54.2	45.8	44.9	38.9	34.8	34.7	30.1
85 years and over	83.6	81.9	83.1	67.8	65.0	58.2	47.7	44.3	43.5	38.1	36.9	35.5
Black or African American [3]												
65 years and over, age-adjusted [2]	82.1	83.2	83.4	71.9	69.3	61.0	55.9	52.2	49.2	46.8	44.0	38.2
65 years and over, crude	81.5	82.1	81.1	70.6	69.1	59.9	54.9	51.7	47.9	45.7	43.7	37.7
65–74 years	78.7	79.6	70.9	64.6	68.3	48.6	53.3	51.2	43.1	42.6	43.1	33.8
75–84 years	80.1	77.8	82.5	67.5	68.9	70.1	49.7	49.5	47.9	41.0	42.3	40.6
85 years and over	84.5	88.0	87.4	77.0	69.8	57.9	61.0	54.3	51.7	52.1	45.5	37.6

Note: Excludes residents in personal care or domiciliary care homes.

[1] Nursing home residents who are dependent in mobility and eating require the assistance of a person or special equipment. Nursing home residents who are incontinent have difficulty in controlling bowels and/or bladder or have an ostomy or indwelling catheter.

[2] Age adjusted by the direct method to the 1995 National Nursing Home Survey population using the following three age groups: 65–74 years, 75–84 years, and 85 years and over.

[3] Beginning in 1999, the instruction for the race item on the Current Resident Questionnaire was changed so that more than one race could be recorded. In previous years, only one racial category could be checked. Estimates in this table are for single race residents.

Table III-56. Nursing Homes, Beds, Occupancy, and Residents, According to Geographic Division and State, Selected Years, 1995–2003

(Number, percent, rate per 1,000 population 85 years of age and over.)

Geographic division and state	Nursing homes			Beds			Residents			Occupancy rate (percent) [1]			Resident rate per 1,000 [2]		
	2003	2000	1995	2003	2000	1995	2003	2000	1995	2003	2000	1995	2003	2000	1995
UNITED STATES	16 323	16 886	16 389	1 756 699	1 795 388	1 751 302	1 451 672	1 480 076	1 479 550	82.6	82.4	84.5	308.0	349.1	404.5
New England	1 067	1 137	1 140	111 892	118 562	115 488	101 561	106 308	105 792	90.8	89.7	91.6	359.2	419.5	474.2
Connecticut	252	259	267	31 248	32 433	32 827	28 622	29 657	29 948	91.6	91.4	91.2	386.8	461.4	541.7
Maine	119	126	132	7 552	8 248	9 243	6 954	7 298	8 587	92.1	88.5	92.9	274.9	313.0	417.9
Massachusetts	478	526	550	52 323	56 030	54 532	46 993	49 805	49 765	89.8	88.9	91.3	366.8	426.8	477.3
New Hampshire	81	83	74	7 811	7 837	7 412	7 145	7 158	6 877	91.5	91.3	92.8	346.7	392.6	434.1
Rhode Island	94	99	94	9 376	10 271	9 612	8 528	9 041	8 823	91.0	88.0	91.8	363.1	432.6	476.9
Vermont	43	44	23	3 582	3 743	1 862	3 319	3 349	1 792	92.7	89.5	96.2	296.7	335.0	207.0
Middle Atlantic	1 767	1 796	1 650	264 041	267 772	244 342	239 286	242 674	228 649	90.6	90.6	93.6	313.8	354.2	384.0
New Jersey	356	361	300	50 551	52 195	43 967	44 356	45 837	40 397	87.7	87.8	91.9	290.3	337.0	351.6
New York	671	665	624	122 633	120 514	107 750	113 456	112 957	103 409	92.5	93.7	96.0	330.5	362.6	371.8
Pennsylvania	740	770	726	90 857	95 063	92 625	81 474	83 880	84 843	89.7	88.2	91.6	305.9	353.1	419.2
East North Central	3 182	3 301	3 171	360 504	369 657	367 879	278 339	289 404	294 319	77.2	78.3	80.0	358.1	414.3	476.1
Illinois	827	869	827	106 734	110 766	103 230	79 833	83 604	83 696	74.8	75.5	81.1	377.4	435.4	495.3
Indiana	527	564	556	55 475	56 762	59 538	40 623	42 328	44 328	73.2	74.6	74.5	401.9	462.3	548.9
Michigan	431	439	432	49 225	50 696	49 473	41 547	42 615	43 271	84.4	84.1	87.5	256.5	299.1	345.0
Ohio	989	1 009	943	106 426	105 038	106 884	79 839	81 946	79 026	75.0	78.0	73.9	406.5	463.5	499.5
Wisconsin	408	420	413	42 644	46 395	48 754	36 497	38 911	43 998	85.6	83.9	90.2	343.2	406.9	518.9
West North Central	2 212	2 281	2 258	186 548	193 754	200 109	149 004	157 224	164 660	79.9	81.1	82.3	378.5	429.8	489.6
Iowa	454	467	419	35 428	37 034	39 959	27 805	29 204	27 506	78.5	78.9	68.8	394.8	448.5	458.0
Kansas	374	392	429	27 045	27 067	30 016	21 085	22 230	25 140	78.0	82.1	83.8	384.5	429.4	528.9
Minnesota	425	433	432	39 336	42 149	43 865	36 231	38 813	41 163	92.1	92.1	93.8	380.0	453.4	537.4
Missouri	534	551	546	54 415	54 829	52 679	37 345	38 586	39 891	68.6	70.4	75.7	361.1	391.5	432.8
Nebraska	228	236	231	16 378	17 877	18 169	13 598	14 989	16 166	83.0	83.8	89.0	376.0	441.5	501.4
North Dakota	84	88	87	6 582	6 954	7 125	6 137	6 343	6 868	93.2	91.2	96.4	380.8	430.7	522.0
South Dakota	113	114	114	7 364	7 844	8 296	6 803	7 059	7 926	92.4	90.0	95.5	391.4	438.8	543.3
South Atlantic	2 374	2 418	2 215	263 651	264 147	243 069	232 185	227 818	217 303	88.1	86.2	89.4	264.6	291.9	335.4
Delaware	42	43	42	4 679	4 906	4 739	3 962	3 900	3 819	84.7	79.5	80.6	318.6	369.7	448.7
District of Columbia	21	20	19	3 114	3 078	3 206	2 861	2 858	2 576	91.9	92.9	80.3	306.0	318.4	297.6
Florida	693	732	627	82 546	83 365	72 656	71 987	69 050	61 845	87.2	82.8	85.1	193.7	208.4	228.2
Georgia	360	363	352	39 998	39 817	38 097	36 372	36 559	35 933	90.9	91.8	94.3	375.4	416.1	496.0
Maryland	243	255	218	29 362	31 495	28 394	25 270	25 629	24 716	86.1	81.4	87.0	326.1	383.1	432.7
North Carolina	423	410	391	43 022	41 376	38 322	37 936	36 658	35 511	88.2	88.6	92.7	320.1	347.6	401.1
South Carolina	178	178	166	18 306	18 102	16 682	16 220	15 739	14 568	88.6	86.9	87.3	278.1	313.1	366.0
Virginia	278	278	271	31 472	30 595	30 070	27 614	27 091	28 119	87.7	88.5	93.5	277.9	310.4	385.2
West Virginia	136	139	129	11 152	11 413	10 903	9 963	10 334	10 216	89.3	90.5	93.7	298.4	325.2	355.2
East South Central	1 065	1 071	1 014	108 105	106 250	99 707	95 938	96 348	91 563	88.7	90.7	91.8	363.2	385.5	416.6
Alabama	228	225	221	26 369	25 248	23 353	23 564	23 089	21 691	89.4	91.4	92.9	329.6	343.1	370.1
Kentucky	296	307	288	25 629	25 341	23 221	22 814	22 730	20 696	89.0	89.7	89.1	370.5	390.1	391.9
Mississippi	204	190	183	18 149	17 068	16 059	16 057	15 815	15 247	88.5	92.7	94.9	366.8	368.7	405.3
Tennessee	337	349	322	37 958	38 593	37 074	33 503	34 714	33 929	88.3	89.9	91.5	383.6	426.1	479.6
West South Central	2 069	2 199	2 264	217 469	224 100	224 695	156 297	159 160	169 047	71.9	71.0	75.2	368.7	397.6	486.1
Arkansas	242	255	256	24 791	25 715	29 952	17 997	19 317	20 823	72.6	75.1	69.5	365.9	415.5	508.3
Louisiana	314	337	337	38 397	39 430	37 769	29 151	30 735	32 493	75.9	77.9	86.0	470.0	523.8	639.3
Oklahoma	370	392	405	32 733	33 903	33 918	21 679	23 833	26 377	66.2	70.3	77.8	372.6	416.8	499.1
Texas	1 143	1 215	1 266	121 548	125 052	123 056	87 470	85 275	89 354	72.0	68.2	72.6	343.7	358.4	439.9
Mountain	785	827	800	73 464	75 152	70 134	58 451	59 379	58 738	79.6	79.0	83.8	229.4	271.2	335.9
Arizona	135	150	152	16 451	17 458	16 162	13 245	13 253	12 382	80.5	75.9	76.6	163.7	193.4	233.3
Colorado	215	225	219	20 127	20 240	19 912	16 344	17 045	17 055	81.2	84.2	85.7	300.7	353.5	420.6
Idaho	80	84	76	6 258	6 181	5 747	4 754	4 640	4 697	76.0	75.1	81.7	224.2	257.0	321.7
Montana	101	104	100	7 489	7 667	7 210	5 739	5 973	6 415	76.6	77.9	89.0	328.1	389.5	491.4
Nevada	44	51	42	5 197	5 547	3 998	4 308	3 657	3 645	82.9	65.9	91.2	195.3	215.3	312.0
New Mexico	81	80	83	7 443	7 289	6 969	6 280	6 503	6 051	84.4	89.2	86.8	236.9	279.0	332.0
Utah	90	93	91	7 438	7 651	7 101	5 306	5 703	5 832	71.3	74.5	82.1	213.3	262.2	323.5
Wyoming	39	40	37	3 061	3 119	3 035	2 475	2 605	2 661	80.9	83.5	87.7	334.2	386.8	468.2
Pacific	1 802	1 856	1 877	171 025	175 994	185 879	140 611	141 761	149 479	82.2	80.5	80.4	207.7	241.3	302.4
Alaska	14	15	15	806	821	814	619	595	634	76.8	72.5	77.9	185.2	225.9	348.0
California	1 342	1 369	1 382	129 658	131 762	140 203	107 578	106 460	109 805	83.0	80.8	78.3	220.2	250.1	302.9
Hawaii	45	45	34	4 059	4 006	2 513	3 806	3 558	2 413	93.8	88.8	96.0	172.4	202.6	178.5
Oregon	141	150	161	12 789	13 500	13 885	8 640	9 990	11 673	67.6	74.0	84.1	131.0	173.9	244.9
Washington	260	277	285	23 713	25 905	28 464	19 968	21 158	24 954	84.2	81.7	87.7	205.9	251.6	362.5

Note: Annual numbers of nursing homes, beds, and residents are based on a 15-month Online Survey Certification and Reporting Database (OSCAR) reporting cycle.

[1] Percent of beds occupied (number of nursing home residents per 100 nursing home beds).

[2] Number of nursing home residents (all ages) per 1,000 resident population 85 years of age and over. Resident rates for 1995–1999 are based on population estimates projected from the 1990 census. Starting with 2000, resident rates are based on the 2000 census.

HEALTH PERSONNEL

TABLE III-57. PERSONS EMPLOYED IN HEALTH SERVICE SITES, ACCORDING TO SEX, 2000–2004

Health service sites provided work for 13.8 million persons in 2004, an increase of about 1.6 million from 2000. These health service jobs represented almost 10 percent of all civilian employment. Hospitals accounted for the largest portion of health service jobs (41.3 percent), followed by nursing care facilities (13.4 percent) and offices and clinics of physicians (12.5 percent).

Women were predominant in health care work; they filled 10.8 million jobs in 2003, compared to the 3.1 million jobs filled by men.

Table III-57. Persons Employed in Health Service Sites, According to Sex, 2000–2004

(Number in thousands, percent.)

Site and sex	2004	2003	2002	2001	2000
BOTH SEXES (IN THOUSANDS)					
All Employed Civilians [1]	139 252	137 736	136 485	136 933	136 891
All Health Service Sites [2]	13 817	13 615	13 069	12 558	12 211
Offices and clinics of physicians	1 727	1 673	1 533	1 499	1 387
Offices and clinics of dentists	780	771	734	701	672
Offices and clinics of chiropractors	156	142	132	111	120
Offices and clinics of optometrists	93	92	113	102	95
Offices and clinics of other health practitioners [3]	274	250	149	140	143
Outpatient care centers	885	873	850	830	772
Home health care services	750	741	636	582	548
Other health care services [4]	976	943	1 188	1 101	1 027
Hospitals	5 700	5 652	5 330	5 256	5 202
Nursing care facilities	1 858	1 877	1 715	1 568	1 593
Residential care facilities, without nursing	618	601	689	668	652
MEN					
All Health Service Sites [2]	3 067	2 986	2 838	2 778	2 756
Offices and clinics of physicians	424	414	370	379	354
Offices and clinics of dentists	158	163	151	150	158
Offices and clinics of chiropractors	63	53	47	39	32
Offices and clinics of optometrists	24	29	29	27	26
Offices and clinics of other health practitioners [3]	69	63	42	41	38
Outpatient care centers	203	200	172	185	186
Home health care services	65	56	54	51	45
Other health care services [4]	314	297	362	345	304
Hospitals	1 333	1 263	1 195	1 187	1 241
Nursing care facilities	251	267	223	189	195
Residential care facilities, without nursing	164	181	193	185	177
WOMEN					
All Health Service Sites	10 750	10 631	10 232	9 782	9 457
Offices and clinics of physicians	1 302	1 259	1 164	1 120	1 034
Offices and clinics of dentists	623	607	584	551	514
Offices and clinics of chiropractors	93	90	85	72	88
Offices and clinics of optometrists	69	64	84	75	69
Offices and clinics of other health practitioners [3]	204	186	106	99	106
Outpatient care centers	683	673	678	646	586
Home health care services	685	685	582	531	503
Other health care services [4]	662	646	826	756	723
Hospitals	4 366	4 390	4 135	4 069	3 961
Nursing care facilities	1 607	1 611	1 492	1 380	1 398
Residential care facilities, without nursing	454	420	496	483	475
BOTH SEXES					
All Health Service Sites (Percent of Employed Civilians)	9.9	9.9	9.6	9.2	8.9
All Health Service Sites (Percent Distribution)	100.0	100.0	100.0	100.0	100.0
Offices and clinics of physicians	12.5	12.3	11.7	11.9	11.4
Offices and clinics of dentists	5.6	5.7	5.6	5.6	5.5
Offices and clinics of chiropractors	1.1	1.0	1.0	0.9	1.0
Offices and clinics of optometrists	0.7	0.7	0.9	0.8	0.8
Offices and clinics of other health practitioners [3]	2.0	1.8	1.1	1.1	1.2
Outpatient care centers	6.4	6.4	6.5	6.6	6.3
Home health care services	5.4	5.4	4.9	4.6	4.5
Other health care services [4]	7.1	6.9	9.1	8.8	8.4
Hospitals	41.3	41.5	40.8	41.9	42.6
Nursing care facilities	13.4	13.8	13.1	12.5	13.0
Residential care facilities, without nursing	4.5	4.4	5.3	5.3	5.3

[1] Excludes workers under the age of 16 years.
[2] Data for all health service sites for men and women may not sum to the total of all health service sites due to rounding.
[3] Includes health service sites such as acupuncture, nutritionists' offices, speech defect clinics, and other offices and clinics.
[4] Includes health service sites such as ambulance services, blood banks, CT SCAN (computer tomography) centers, and other offices and clinics.

TABLE III-58. ACTIVE PHYSICIANS AND DOCTORS OF MEDICINE IN PATIENT CARE, ACCORDING TO SELECTED GEOGRAPHIC DIVISION AND STATE, SELECTED YEARS, 1975–2003

The number of physicians per every 10,000 civilians has increased significantly since 1975. For the United States as a whole, there were 15.3 physicians (per 10,000 persons) in 1975; this rate increased to 26.6 in 2003. The number of physicians per 10,000 persons varied considerably by state. Massachusetts (40.8) had the highest number in 2003, followed by Maryland (39.1) and New York (37.1). In addition, the District of Columbia reported a rate of 70.7 physicians per 10,000 persons. States with low numbers of physicians were Idaho (17.7 per 10,000 persons) and Mississippi (18.3). This table presents separate data for all physicians and for doctors of medicine in patient care. It excludes doctors in teaching, research, and administration.

Table III-58. Active Physicians and Doctors of Medicine in Patient Care, According to Selected Geographic Division and State, Selected Years, 1975–2003

(Number per 10,000 civilian population.)

Geographic division and state	Total physicians [1]				Doctors of medicine in patient care [2]			
	2003 [3,4]	1995 [5]	1985	1975	2003 [4]	1995	1985	1975
UNITED STATES	26.6	24.2	20.7	15.3	23.5	21.3	18.0	13.5
New England	36.3	32.5	26.7	19.1	32.3	28.8	22.9	16.9
Connecticut	34.9	32.8	27.6	19.8	31.2	29.5	24.3	17.7
Maine	29.9	22.3	18.7	12.8	24.1	18.2	15.6	10.7
Massachusetts	40.8	37.5	30.2	20.8	36.5	33.2	25.4	18.3
New Hampshire	26.3	21.5	18.1	14.3	24.0	19.8	16.7	13.1
Rhode Island	34.3	30.4	23.3	17.8	30.7	26.7	20.2	16.1
Vermont	35.0	26.9	23.8	18.2	32.1	24.2	20.3	15.5
Middle Atlantic	34.3	32.4	26.1	19.5	29.6	28.0	22.2	17.0
New Jersey	32.1	29.3	23.4	16.2	27.3	24.9	19.8	14.0
New York	37.1	35.3	29.0	22.7	33.1	31.6	25.2	20.2
Pennsylvania	31.5	30.1	23.6	16.6	25.7	24.6	19.2	13.9
East North Central	25.9	23.3	19.3	13.9	22.2	19.8	16.4	12.0
Illinois	27.1	24.8	20.5	14.5	23.9	22.1	18.2	13.1
Indiana	21.8	18.4	14.7	10.6	19.7	16.6	13.2	9.6
Michigan	26.7	24.8	20.8	15.4	20.9	19.0	16.0	12.0
Ohio	26.5	23.8	19.9	14.1	22.6	20.0	16.8	12.2
Wisconsin	24.8	21.5	17.7	12.5	22.8	19.6	15.9	11.4
West North Central	24.6	21.8	18.3	13.3	21.3	18.9	15.6	11.4
Iowa	21.6	19.2	15.6	11.4	16.6	15.1	12.4	9.4
Kansas	23.0	20.8	17.3	12.8	19.8	18.0	15.1	11.2
Minnesota	27.0	23.4	20.5	14.9	24.8	21.5	18.5	13.7
Missouri	25.7	23.9	20.5	15.0	21.3	19.7	16.3	11.6
Nebraska	23.6	19.8	15.7	12.1	21.9	18.3	14.4	10.9
North Dakota	23.5	20.5	15.8	9.7	21.8	18.9	14.9	9.2
South Dakota	21.3	16.7	13.4	8.2	19.9	15.7	12.3	7.7
South Atlantic	26.4	23.4	19.7	14.0	23.6	21.0	17.6	12.6
Delaware	26.6	23.4	19.7	14.3	22.6	19.7	17.1	12.7
District of Columbia	70.7	63.6	55.3	39.6	60.2	53.6	45.6	34.6
Florida	25.4	22.9	20.2	15.2	22.4	20.3	17.8	13.4
Georgia	21.8	19.7	16.2	11.5	19.8	18.0	14.7	10.6
Maryland	39.1	34.1	30.4	18.6	33.6	29.9	24.9	16.5
North Carolina	24.5	21.1	16.9	11.7	22.6	19.4	15.0	10.6
South Carolina	22.5	18.9	14.7	10.0	20.9	17.6	13.6	9.3
Virginia	26.4	22.5	19.5	12.9	24.4	20.8	17.8	11.9
West Virginia	24.2	21.0	16.3	11.0	20.5	17.9	14.6	10.0
East South Central	22.3	19.2	15.0	10.5	20.5	17.8	14.0	9.7
Alabama	21.1	18.4	14.2	9.2	19.3	17.0	13.1	8.6
Kentucky	22.4	19.2	15.1	10.9	20.6	18.0	13.9	10.1
Mississippi	18.3	13.9	11.8	8.4	16.7	13.0	11.1	8.0
Tennessee	25.1	22.5	17.7	12.4	23.3	20.8	16.2	11.3

Source: American Medical Association (AMA). Physician distribution and medical licensure in the U.S., 1975; Physician characteristics and distribution in the U.S., 1986, 1996–1997, and 2005 editions; Department of Physician Practice and Communication Information, Division of Survey and Data Resources, AMA. (Copyrights 1976, 1986, 1997, 2005: Used with the permission of the AMA); American Osteopathic Association: 1975–1976 Yearbook and Directory of Osteopathic Physicians, 1985–1986 Yearbook and Directory of Osteopathic Physicians; American Association of Colleges of Osteopathic Medicine: 2003 Annual Report on Osteopathic Medical Education, 2004.

Note: Data for doctors of medicine are as December 31.

[1] Includes active non-federal doctors of medicine and active doctors of osteopathy.

[2] Excludes doctors of osteopathy (D.O.'s). States with more than 2,500 active D.O.'s are Pennsylvania, Michigan, Ohio, Florida, New York, Texas, California, and New Jersey. States with fewer than 100 active D.O.'s are the District of Columbia, Wyoming, Vermont, North Dakota, South Dakota, Louisiana, Montana, and Alaska. Excludes doctors of medicine in medical teaching, administration, research, and other nonpatient care activities.

[3] Data for doctors of osteopathy are as of June 2003.

[4] Data for the year 2003 include federal and non-federal physicians. Prior to the year 2003, the data include non-federal physicians only.

[5] Data for doctors of osteopathy are as of July 1996.

TABLE III-59. DOCTORS OF MEDICINE, ACCORDING TO ACTIVITY AND PLACE OF MEDICAL EDUCATION, UNITED STATES AND OUTLYING U.S. AREAS, SELECTED YEARS, 1975–2003

Of the 736,000 active doctors of medicine in 2003, 178,000 were medical graduates from schools outside the United States and Canada. Most doctors in patient care had office-based practices, while others, particularly interns and residents, were based in hospitals. There was a large number of medical specializations; the most practiced included internal medicine, general and family practice, pediatrics, and obstetrics and gynecology. The number of professionals in certain specialties, such as diagnostic radiology and emergency medicine, continued to grow. However, specialties such as neurology, pathology, and psychiatry showed little growth.

Table III-59. Doctors of Medicine, According to Activity and Place of Medical Education, United States and Outlying U.S. Areas, Selected Years, 1975–2003

(Number.)

Activity and place of medical eduation	2003 [1]	2002	2001	2000	1999	1995	1985	1975
DOCTORS OF MEDICINE	871 535	853 187	836 156	813 770	797 634	720 325	552 716	393 742
Professionally Active [2]	736 211	719 431	713 375	692 368	669 949	625 443	497 140	340 280
Place of Medical Education								
U.S. medical graduates	558 167	544 779	537 529	525 691	510 738	481 137	392 007	. . .
International medical graduates [3]	178 044	172 770	171 639	164 437	158 211	144 306	105 133	. . .
Activity								
Non-federal	. . .	699 249	693 358	672 987	650 899	604 364	475 573	312 089
Patient care [4]	691 873	658 123	652 328	631 431	610 656	564 074	431 527	287 837
Office-based practice	529 836	516 246	514 016	490 398	473 241	427 275	329 041	213 334
General and family practice	73 508	71 696	70 030	67 534	66 246	59 932	53 862	46 347
Cardiovascular diseases	17 301	16 989	16 991	16 300	15 586	13 739	9 054	5 046
Dermatology	8 477	8 282	8 199	7 969	7 788	6 959	5 325	3 442
Gastroenterology	9 326	9 044	8 905	8 515	8 185	7 300	4 135	1 696
Internal medicine	99 670	96 496	94 674	88 699	84 633	72 612	52 712	28 188
Pediatrics	47 996	46 097	44 824	42 215	40 502	33 890	22 392	12 687
Pulmonary diseases	6 919	6 672	6 596	6 095	5 745	4 964	3 035	1 166
General surgery	25 284	24 902	25 632	24 475	26 822	24 086	24 708	19 710
Obstetrics and gynecology	33 636	32 738	32 582	31 726	31 103	29 111	23 525	15 613
Ophthalmology	16 240	16 052	15 994	15 598	15 238	14 596	12 212	8 795
Orthopedic surgery	18 423	18 118	17 829	17 367	16 974	17 136	13 033	8 148
Otolaryngology	8 103	8 001	7 866	7 581	7 282	7 139	5 751	4 297
Plastic surgery	5 725	5 593	5 545	5 308	5 127	4 612	3 299	1 706
Urological surgery	8 804	8 615	8 636	8 460	8 229	7 991	7 081	5 025
Anesthesiology	29 254	28 661	28 868	27 624	26 635	23 770	15 285	8 970
Diagnostic radiology	16 403	15 896	15 596	14 622	14 259	12 751	7 735	1 978
Emergency medicine	17 727	16 907	15 823	14 541	13 932	11 700	. . .	. . .
Neurology	9 304	9 034	9 156	8 559	8 065	7 623	4 691	1 862
Pathology, anatomical/clinical	10 209	10 103	10 554	10 267	10 074	9 031	6 877	4 195
Psychiatry	25 656	25 350	25 653	24 955	24 393	23 334	18 521	12 173
Radiology	7 010	6 916	6 830	6 674	6 523	5 994	7 355	6 970
Other specialty	34 861	34 084	37 233	35 314	29 900	29 005	28 453	15 320
Hospital-based practice	162 037	141 877	138 312	141 033	137 225	136 799	102 486	74 503
Residents and interns [5]	100 033	96 547	92 935	95 125	92 461	93 650	72 159	53 527
Full-time hospital staff	62 004	45 330	45 377	45 908	44 764	43 149	30 327	20 976
Other professional activity [6]	44 338	41 126	41 118	41 556	41 243	40 290	44 046	24 252
Federal [7]	. . .	20 182	20 017	19 381	18 050	21 079	21 567	28 191
Patient care	. . .	16 701	16 611	15 999	14 678	18 057	17 293	24 100
Office-based practice	. . .	X	X	X	X	X	1 156	2 095
Hospital-based practice	. . .	16 701	16 611	15 999	14 678	18 057	16 137	22 005
Residents and interns	. . .	390	739	600	375	2 702	3 252	4 275
Full-time hospital staff	. . .	16 311	15 872	15 399	14 303	15 355	12 885	17 730
Other professional activity [6]	. . .	3 481	3 406	3 382	3 372	3 022	4 274	4 091
Inactive	84 360	84 166	81 520	75 168	75 893	72 326	38 646	21 449
Not classified	50 447	49 067	38 314	45 136	50 906	20 579	13 950	26 145
Unknown address	517	523	2 947	1 098	886	1 977	2 980	5 868

Source: American Medical Association (AMA). Distribution of physicians in the United States, 1970; Physician distribution and medical licensure in the U.S., 1975; Physician characteristics and distribution in the U.S., 1981, 1986, 1989, 1990, 1992, 1993, 1994, 1995–1996, 1996–1997, 1997–1998, 1999, 2000–2001, 2001–2002, 2002–2003, 2003–2004, 2004, 2005 editions, Department of Physician Practice and Communications Information, Division of Survey and Data Resources, AMA. (Copyrights 1971, 1976, 1982, 1986, 1989, 1990, 1992, 1993, 1994, 1996, 1997, 1997, 1999, 2000, 2001, 2002, 2003, 2004, 2005: Used with the permission of the AMA.)

Note: Data for doctors of medicine are as of December 31.

[1] Activity data for the year 2003 include federal and non-federal physicians.
[2] Excludes inactive, not classified, and address unknown.
[3] International medical graduates received their medical education in schools outside the United States and Canada.
[4] Specialty information based on the physician's self-designated primary area of practice. Categories include generalists and specialists.
[5] Beginning in 1990, clinical fellows are included in this category. In prior years, clinical fellows were included in "Other professional activity."
[6] Includes medical teaching, administration, research, and other. Prior to 1990, this category also included clinical fellows.
[7] Beginning in 1993, data collection for federal physicians was revised.
X = Not applicable.
. . . = Not available.

TABLE III-60. DOCTORS OF MEDICINE IN PRIMARY CARE, ACCORDING TO SPECIALTY, UNITED STATES AND OUTLYING U.S. AREAS, SELECTED YEARS, 1949–2003

This table provides detail on the number of primary care doctors in the United States, with data going back to 1949. By 1980, the number of doctors of internal medi-cine (both those who are classified as generalists and those who are classified as specialists) surpassed the number of doctors in general and family practice. The number of pediatricians was much smaller at 29,500. By 2003, 19.1 percent of all active doctors of medicine were practitioners of internal medicine, while 11.7 percent had a general and family practice.

Table III-60. Doctors of Medicine in Primary Care, According to Specialty, United States and Outlying U.S. Areas, Selected Years, 1949–2003

(Number, percent.)

Age, sex, and race	2003	2002	2001	2000	1995	1990	1980	1970	1960 [1]	1949 [1]
Number										
Total doctors of medicine [2]	871 535	853 187	836 156	813 770	720 325	615 421	467 679	334 028	260 484	201 277
Active doctors of medicine [3]	786 658	768 498	751 689	737 504	646 022	559 988	435 545	310 929	247 257	191 577
General primary care specialists	293 701	286 294	283 583	274 653	241 329	213 514	170 705	134 354	125 359	113 222
General practice/family medicine	91 545	89 357	88 597	86 312	75 976	70 480	60 049	57 948	88 023	95 980
Internal medicine	109 317	106 499	105 229	101 353	88 240	76 295	58 462	39 924	26 209	12 453
Obstetrics/gynecology	37 725	36 810	36 869	35 922	33 519	30 220	24 612	18 532	. . .	. . .
Pediatrics	55 114	53 628	52 888	51 066	43 594	36 519	27 582	17 950	11 127	4 789
Primary care specialists	60 589	57 929	55 871	52 294	39 659	30 911	16 642	3 161	. . .	. . .
Family medicine	691	627	564	483	236	. . .	. . .	. . .	. . .	. . .
Internal medicine	40 598	38 821	37 558	34 831	26 928	22 054	13 069	1 948	. . .	. . .
Obstetrics/gynecology	4 191	4 228	4 173	4 319	4 133	3 477	1 693	344	. . .	. . .
Pediatrics	15 109	14 253	13 576	12 661	8 362	5 380	1 880	869	. . .	. . .
Percent										
General primary care specialists	37.3	37.3	37.7	37.2	37.4	38.1	39.2	43.2	50.7	59.1
General practice/family medicine	11.6	11.6	11.8	11.7	11.8	12.6	13.8	18.6	35.6	50.1
Internal medicine	13.9	13.9	14.0	13.7	13.7	13.6	13.4	12.8	10.6	6.5
Obstetrics/gynecology	4.8	4.8	4.9	4.9	5.2	5.4	5.7	6.0	. . .	. . .
Pediatrics	7.0	7.0	7.0	6.9	6.7	6.5	6.3	5.8	4.5	2.5
Primary care specialists	7.7	7.5	7.4	7.1	6.1	5.5	3.8	1.0	. . .	. . .
Family medicine	0.1	0.1	0.1	0.1	0.0	. . .	. . .	. . .	. . .	. . .
Internal medicine	5.2	5.1	5.0	4.7	4.2	3.9	3.0	0.6	. . .	. . .
Obstetrics/gynecology	0.5	0.6	0.6	0.6	0.6	0.6	0.4	0.1	. . .	. . .
Pediatrics	1.9	1.9	1.8	1.7	1.3	1.0	0.4	0.3	. . .	. . .

Source: Health Manpower Source Book: Medical Specialists, USDHEW, 1962; American Medical Association (AMA). Distribution of physicians in the United States, 1970; Physician characteristics and distribution in the U.S., 1981, 1992, 1996–1997, 1997–1998, 1999, 2000–2001, 2001–2002, 2002–2003, 2003–2004, 2004, 2005 editions, Department of Data Survey and Planning, Division of Survey and Data Resources, AMA. (Copyrights 1971, 1982, 1992, 1996, 1997, 1997, 1999, 2000, 2001, 2002, 2003, 2004, 2005: Used with the permission of the AMA.)

Note: Data are as of December 31 except for 1990–1994 data, which are as of January 1, and 1949 data, which are as of midyear.

[1] Estimated by the Bureau of Health Professions, Health Resources Administration. Active doctors of medicine (M.D.'s) include those with address unknown and primary specialty not classified.

[2] Includes M.D.'s engaged in federal and non-federal patient care (office-based or hospital-based) and other professional activities.

[3] Beginning in 1970, M.D.'s who are inactive, have unknown address, or primary specialty not classified are excluded.

. . . = Not available.

TABLE III-61. ACTIVE HEALTH PROFESSIONALS, ACCORDING TO OCCUPATION, SELECTED YEARS, 1980–2001

This table shows the number of health practitioners in various occupations. Data are given for professionals such as chiropractors, podiatrists, dieticians, and speech therapists, which are not readily available in other tables.

Data in this table are incomplete for 2000 and 2001.

The 2.2 million nurses in 1999 made up the largest health profession. In comparison, there were 753,000 physicians, 193,000 pharmacists, and 165,000 dentists practicing that year. In regard to alternative medicine, 62,000 chiropractors are listed.

Table III-61. Active Health Professionals, According to Occupation, Selected Years, 1980–2001

(Number, number per 100,000 population.)

Occupation	2001	2000 [1]	1999	1995	1990	1985 [2]	1980
Number							
Chiropractors	66 800	64 100	61 500	52 100	42 400	35 000	25 600
Dentists [3]	...	168 000	164 700	158 600	147 500	133 500	121 900
Nurses, registered [4]	...	...	2 201 800	2 115 800	1 789 600	1 538 100	1 272 900
Associate and diploma	...	...	1 237 400	1 235 100	1 107 300	1 024 500	908 300
Baccalaureate	...	...	731 200	673 200	549 000	419 900	297 300
Master's and doctorate	...	...	229 200	207 500	133 300	93 700	67 300
Nutritionists/dietitians	...	90 000	...	...	57 000	...	32 000
Occupational therapists	...	72 000	...	...	42 000	...	25 000
Optometrists	...	32 200	31 500	28 900	26 000	24 000	21 900
Pharmacists	...	196 000	193 400	181 000	168 000	153 500	142 400
Physical therapists	...	130 000	...	...	92 000	...	50 000
Physicians	793 263	772 296	753 176	672 859	567 610	542 653	427 122
Federal	20 017	19 228	17 338	21 153	20 784	23 305	17 642
Doctors of medicine [5]	20 017	19 110	17 224	19 830	19 166	21 938	16 585
Doctors of osteopathy [6]	...	118	114	1 323	1 618	1 367	1 057
Non-federal	773 246	753 068	735 838	651 706	546 826	519 348	409 480
Doctors of medicine [5]	731 672	708 463	693 345	617 362	520 450	497 473	393 407
Doctors of osteopathy [6]	41 574	44 605	42 493	34 344	26 376	21 875	16 073
Podiatrists [7]	...	12 242	11 853	10 304	10 353	9 620	7 780
Speech therapists	...	121 000	...	...	65 000	...	50 000
Number per 100,000 Population							
Chiropractors	23.5	22.8	22.0	19.6	17.0	14.6	11.3
Dentists	...	59.5	59.0	59.6	59.1	56.5	54.0
Nurses, registered	...	...	789.1	794.6	716.9	641.4	560.0
Associate and diploma	...	...	443.4	463.8	443.6	425.8	399.9
Baccalaureate	...	...	262.0	252.8	219.9	175.6	130.9
Master's and doctorate	...	...	82.1	77.9	53.4	39.9	29.6
Nutritionists/dietitians	...	31.9	...	...	22.8	...	14.0
Occupational therapists	...	25.5	...	...	16.8	...	10.9
Optometrists	...	11.4	11.3	10.9	10.4	10.1	9.6
Pharmacists	...	69.5	69.3	68.0	67.3	66.3	62.5
Physical therapists	...	46.1	...	...	36.9	...	21.8
Physicians	274.3	269.7	265.9	248.9	223.9	221.3	189.8
Federal	6.9	6.7	6.1	7.8	8.2	9.5	7.8
Doctors of medicine [5]	6.9	6.7	6.1	7.3	7.6	8.9	7.4
Doctors of osteopathy [6]	...	0.0	0.0	0.5	0.6	0.6	0.5
Non-federal	267.3	263.0	259.8	241.1	215.7	211.8	182.0
Doctors of medicine [5]	253.0	247.4	244.8	228.4	205.3	202.9	174.9
Doctors of osteopathy [6]	14.4	15.6	15.0	12.7	10.4	8.9	7.1
Podiatrists [7]	...	4.4	4.3	3.9	4.1	4.0	3.4
Speech therapists	...	42.9	...	...	26.0	...	21.8

Source: National Center for Health Workforce Analysis, Bureau of Health Professions: United States Health Personnel FACTBOOK. Health Resources and Services Administration. Rockville, MD, June 2003, and unpublished data; American Medical Association. Physician characteristics and distribution in the U.S., 1981, 1986, 1992, 1996–1997, 2001–2002, 2002–2003, and 2003–2004 editions. Chicago, IL, 1982, 1986, 1992, 1997, 2001, 2002, and 2003; American Osteopathic Association. 1980–1981 Yearbook and Directory of Osteopathic Physicians. Chicago, IL, 1980. American Association of Colleges of Osteopathic Medicine. Annual statistical report, 1990, 1997 1999, 2000, and 2001 editions. Rockville, MD, 1990, 1997, 2000, 2001, and 2002; Bureau of Labor Statistics: unpublished data.

[1] Data for speech therapists are for 1996.

[2] Osteopath, podiatric, and chiropractic data are for 1986.

[3] Excludes dentists in military service, U.S. Public Health Service, and Department of Veterans Affairs.

[4] In 1999, the total number of registered nurses includes an estimated 4,000 nurses whose highest nursing-related educational preparation was not known.

[5] Excludes physicians with unknown addresses and those who do not practice or practice fewer than 20 hours per week. 1990 data for doctors of medicine are as of January 1; in other years, these data are as of December 31.

[6] Beginning in 2001, doctors of osteopathy include federal and non-federal doctors of osteopathy.

[7] Podiatrists in patient care.

... = Not available.

TABLE III-62. FIRST-YEAR ENROLLMENT AND GRADUATES OF HEALTH PROFESSIONAL SCHOOLS AND NUMBER OF SCHOOLS, ACCORDING TO PROFESSION, SELECTED YEARS, 1980–2003

There were almost 15,500 medical school (allopathic) graduates in 2003, a number that has mostly held steady since 1990. First-year enrollment was usually higher than the number of graduates by more than 1,000 students, a discrepancy that most likely reflects attrition.

Graduates of registered nursing programs numbered almost 73,000 in 2002, reflecting a slight decline since 1980. Graduates in public health numbered 5,900 in 2003.

The table also shows the number of schools for health professionals. For 2003, it lists 125 medical schools (allopathic) and 1,459 schools with registered nursing programs. Since 1980, there has been a notable growth in the number of occupational therapy schools and in the number of schools of public health.

Table III-62. First-Year Enrollment and Graduates of Health Professional Schools and Number of Schools, According to Profession, Selected Years, 1980–2003

(Number.)

Profession	2003	2002	2000	1995	1990	1985	1980
First-Year Enrollment							
Dentistry	4 448	4 407	4 314	4 121	3 979	5 047	6 132
Medicine (allopathic)	16 953	16 875	16 856	17 085	16 756	16 997	16 930
Medicine (osteopathic)	3 079	3 043	2 848	2 217	1 844	1 750	1 426
Nursing							
Licensed practical	...	...	...	57 906	52 969	47 034	56 316
Registered, total	...	...	...	127 184	108 580	118 224	105 952
Baccalaureate	...	...	...	43 451	29 858	39 573	35 414
Associate degree	...	...	...	76 016	68 634	63 776	53 633
Diploma	...	...	...	7 717	10 088	14 875	16 905
Optometry	1 416	...	1 410	1 390	1 258	1 187	1 202
Pharmacy	9 909	9 128	8 382	8 740	8 267	6 986	8 035
Podiatry	441	419	475	630	561	811	695
Public Health [1]	6 786	6 329	5 840	5 332	4 392	...	...
Graduates							
Dentistry	4 443	4 349	4 171	3 908	4 233	5 353	5 256
Medicine (allopathic)	15 499	15 648	15 718	15 883	15 398	16 318	15 113
Medicine (osteopathic)	2 607	2 536	2 279	1 843	1 529	1 474	1 059
Nursing [2]							
Licensed practical	...	...	...	44 234	35 417	36 955	41 892
Registered, total	...	72 882	...	97 052	66 088	82 075	75 523
Baccalaureate	...	30 522	...	31 254	18 571	24 975	24 994
Associate degree	...	40 073	...	58 749	42 318	45 208	36 034
Diploma	...	2 287	...	7 049	5 199	11 892	14 495
Occupational therapy	...	...	...	3 473	2 424	...	...
Optometry	1 305	1 309	1 315	1 219	1 115	1 114	1 073
Pharmacy	7 488	7 573	7 260	7 837	6 956	5 735	7 432
Podiatry	436	478	583	558	679	582	597
Public Health	5 906	5 664	5 879	4 636	3 549	3 047	3 326
Schools							
Dentistry	56	56	55	54	58	60	60
Medicine (allopathic)	126	125	125	125	127	127	126
Medicine (osteopathic)	19	19	19	16	15	15	14
Nursing [3]							
Licensed practical	...	...	...	1 210	1 154	1 165	1 299
Registered, total	...	1 459	...	1 516	1 470	1 473	1 385
Baccalaureate	...	526	...	521	489	441	377
Associate degree	...	857	...	876	829	776	697
Diploma	...	76	...	119	152	256	311
Occupational therapy	...	...	142	98	69	61	50
Optometry	17	17	17	17	17	17	16
Pharmacy	89	83	81	75	74	72	72
Podiatry	7	7	7	7	7	7	5
Public Health	33	32	28	27	25	23	21

Source: Association of American Medical Colleges: AAMC Data Book, Statistical Information Related to Medical Schools and Teaching Hospitals, 2004. Washington, DC, 2004, and unpublished data (Copyright 2005: Used with the permission of the AMA); Bureau of Health Professions: United States Health Personnel FACTBOOK. Health Resources and Services Administration. Rockville, MD, 2003; National League for Nursing: unpublished data; American Dental Association: 2002–2003 Survey of Predoctoral Dental Education, vol. 1, Academic Programs, Enrollments, and Graduates. Chicago, IL, 2004; American Dental Education Association: <http://www.adea.org/ADEA.html>; American Association of Colleges of Osteopathic Medicine. 2003 Annual Report on Osteopathic Medical Education. Chevy Chase, MD, 2004; Association of Schools of Public Health: 2003 Annual Data Report. Washington, DC, 2004; Association of Schools and Colleges of Optometry: Annual Student Data Report Academic Year 2003–2004, and unpublished data; American Association of Colleges of Pharmacy: Academic Pharmacy's Vital Statistics, 2004, and unpublished data; American Association of Colleges of Podiatric Medicine: unpublished data; American Medical Association: Health Professions Career and Education Directory, 29th edition. Chicago, IL, 2001.

Note: Data on the number of schools are reported as of the beginning of the academic year while data on first-year enrollment and number of graduates are reported as of the end of the academic year.

[1] Number of students entering schools of public health for the first time.

[2] Data for 2000–2002 exclude American Samoa, Guam, Puerto Rico, and the Virgin Islands.

[3] Some nursing schools offer more than one type of program. Numbers shown for nursing are number of nursing programs.

. . . = Not available.

HEALTH EXPENDITURES

TABLE III-63. TOTAL HEALTH EXPENDITURES AS A PERCENT OF GROSS DOMESTIC PRODUCT, AND PER CAPITA HEALTH EXPENDITURES IN CURRENT DOLLARS, SELECTED COUNTRIES AND YEARS, 1960–2002

In 2002, the United States spent 14.9 percent of its gross domestic product (GDP) on health expenditures, a larger share than any other major industrialized country. (As shown in Table III-64, this ratio increased to 15.3 percent in 2003.) The share of health expenditures in GDP has increased from 5.1 percent in 1960 and 12.0 percent in 1990, a development that reflects both the introduction of many new treatments and inefficiencies in the delivery system. Among other major countries, Switzerland and Germany had the highest percentages of health expendi-

tures, amounting to 11.2 and 10.9 percent, respectively. More moderate shares of health outlays in 2002 occurred in Canada (9.6 percent), France (9.7 percent), Japan (7.8 percent in 2001), and the United Kingdom (7.7 percent).

On a per capita basis in 2002, U.S. residents averaged just over $5,300 in health care costs, whether privately or government financed (latter expenditures included research and construction costs). Outlays for health have risen considerably since the $143 per capita total in 1960. This increase was due to inflation and the growth in real GDP, combined with the increased share of health expenditures as a percentage of GDP. The per capita health expenditures of other countries have been converted to U.S. dollars on the basis of a GDP purchasing power comparison.

Table III-63. Total Health Expenditures as a Percent of Gross Domestic Product, and Per Capita Health Expenditures in Current Dollars, Selected Countries and Years, 1960–2002

(Percent, dollar.)

Country	2002	2001	2000	1999	1998	1995	1990	1980	1970	1960
Health Expenditures as a Percent of Gross Domestic Product										
Australia	. . .	9.1	9.0	8.8	8.6	8.2	7.8	7.0	. . .	4.1
Austria	7.7	7.6	7.7	7.8	7.7	8.2	7.1	7.6	5.3	4.3
Belgium	9.1	9.0	8.8	8.7	8.6	8.7	7.4	6.4	4.0	. . .
Canada	9.6	9.4	8.9	9.0	9.2	9.2	9.0	7.1	7.0	5.4
Czech Republic	7.4	7.3	7.1	7.1	7.1	7.3	5.0	. . .	. . .	. . .
Denmark	8.8	8.6	8.4	8.5	8.4	8.2	8.5	9.1	. . .	. . .
Finland	7.3	7.0	6.7	6.9	6.9	7.5	7.8	6.4	5.6	3.8
France	9.7	9.4	9.3	9.3	9.3	9.5	8.6	7.1	5.4	3.8
Germany	10.9	10.8	10.6	10.6	10.6	10.6	8.5	8.7	6.2	. . .
Greece	9.5	9.4	9.7	9.6	9.4	9.6	7.4	6.6	6.1	. . .
Hungary	7.8	7.4	7.1	7.4	7.3	7.5	. . .	. . .	. . .	. . .
Iceland	9.9	9.2	9.2	9.4	8.6	8.4	8.0	6.2	4.7	3.0
Ireland	7.3	6.9	6.4	6.3	6.2	6.8	6.1	8.4	5.1	3.7
Italy	8.5	8.3	8.1	7.8	7.7	7.4	8.0	. . .	. . .	. . .
Japan	. . .	7.8	7.6	7.4	7.2	6.8	5.9	6.5	4.5	3.0
Korea	5.1	5.3	4.6	4.7	4.4	4.1	4.2	. . .	. . .	. . .
Luxembourg	6.2	5.9	5.5	6.2	5.8	6.4	6.1	5.9	3.6	. . .
Mexico	6.1	6.0	5.6	5.6	5.4	5.6	4.8	. . .	. . .	. . .
Netherlands	9.1	8.5	8.2	8.2	8.1	8.4	8.0	7.5	. . .	. . .
New Zealand	8.5	8.0	7.9	7.8	7.9	7.2	6.9	5.9	5.1	. . .
Norway	9.6	8.9	7.7	8.5	8.5	7.9	7.7	7.0	4.4	2.9
Poland	6.1	6.0	5.7	5.9	6.0	5.6	4.9	. . .	. . .	. . .
Portugal	9.3	9.3	9.2	8.7	8.4	8.2	6.2	5.6	2.6	. . .
Slovak Republic	5.7	5.6	5.5	5.8	5.7	. . .	. . .	. . .	. . .	. . .
Spain	7.6	7.5	7.5	7.5	7.5	7.6	6.7	5.4	3.6	1.5
Sweden	9.2	8.8	8.4	8.4	8.3	8.1	8.4	9.1	6.9	. . .
Switzerland	11.2	10.9	10.4	10.5	10.3	9.7	8.3	7.3	5.4	4.9
Turkey	. . .	. . .	6.6	6.4	4.8	3.4	3.6	3.3	2.4	. . .
United Kingdom	7.7	7.5	7.3	7.2	6.9	7.0	6.0	5.6	4.5	3.9
United States	14.9	14.1	13.3	13.2	13.2	13.4	12.0	8.8	7.0	5.1

. . . = Not available.

Table III-63. Total Health Expenditures as a Percent of Gross Domestic Product, and Per Capita Health Expenditures in Current Dollars, Selected Countries and Years, 1960–2002—*Continued*

(Percent, dollar.)

Country	2002	2001	2000	1999	1998	1995	1990	1980	1970	1960
Per Capita Health Expenditures [1]										
Australia	...	2 504	2 379	2 231	2 077	1 737	1 300	684	...	93
Austria	2 220	2 174	2 147	2 069	1 953	1 865	1 344	762	190	77
Belgium	2 515	2 441	2 288	2 139	2 041	1 882	1 340	627	147	...
Canada	2 931	2 743	2 541	2 400	2 291	2 044	1 714	770	289	121
Czech Republic	1 118	1 083	977	932	918	876	553	...	...	...
Denmark	2 583	2 520	2 353	2 297	2 141	1 843	1 554	943		
Finland	1 943	1 841	1 698	1 641	1 607	1 428	1 414	584	190	62
France	2 736	2 588	2 416	2 306	2 231	2 025	1 555	699	206	69
Germany	2 817	2 735	2 640	2 563	2 470	2 263	1 729	955	266	...
Greece	1 814	1 670	1 617	1 517	1 428	1 269	838	464	171	...
Hungary	1 079	961	847	820	775	674	...	...		
Iceland	2 807	2 680	2 559	2 540	2 252	1 853	1 598	698	163	57
Ireland	2 367	2 059	1 774	1 623	1 487	1 208	791	511	117	42
Italy	2 166	2 107	2 001	1 853	1 800	1 524	1 397	...		
Japan	...	2 077	1 958	1 829	1 742	1 530	1 105	559	144	29
Korea	996	943	777	714	589	491	329	...	...	...
Luxembourg	3 065	2 900	2 682	2 734	2 291	2 053	1 533	637	161	...
Mexico	553	536	494	463	427	380	290	...	...	...
Netherlands	2 643	2 455	2 196	2 098	2 016	1 827	1 419	750	...	...
New Zealand	1 857	1 710	1 611	1 527	1 441	1 238	987	488	205	...
Norway	3 409	3 258	2 747	2 561	2 314	1 892	1 385	659	140	49
Poland	654	629	578	571	563	423	298	...	...	...
Portugal	1 702	1 662	1 570	1 424	1 290	1 080	661	283	54	...
Slovak Republic	698	633	591	578	559	...	...	...	...	...
Spain	1 646	1 567	1 493	1 467	1 371	1 195	865	363	97	16
Sweden	2 517	2 370	2 243	2 119	1 961	1 733	1 566	924	305	...
Switzerland	3 446	3 288	3 111	2 985	2 967	2 555	2 040	1 031	350	166
Turkey	...	...	446	392	312	184	165	76	24	...
United Kingdom	2 160	2 012	1 839	1 725	1 607	1 393	977	472	160	84
United States	5 317	4 914	4 560	4 302	4 098	3 698	2 738	1 067	348	143

[1]Per capita health expenditures for each country have been adjusted to U.S. dollars using gross domestic product purchasing power parities for each year.

. . . = Not available.

TABLE III-64. GROSS DOMESTIC PRODUCT, FEDERAL AND STATE AND LOCAL GOVERNMENT EXPENDITURES, NATIONAL HEALTH EXPENDITURES, AND AVERAGE ANNUAL PERCENT CHANGE, SELECTED YEARS, 1960–2003

In 2003, national health expenditures increased 7.7 percent (compared with a 4.9 percent growth in gross domestic product, not adjusted for inflation) reaching a total of $1.7 trillion; this represented 15.3 percent of gross domestic product (GDP). The health care share of GDP has increased steadily since 1960, except for a period of plateau in the late 1990s. About 54 percent of these outlays came from private sources, with the rest financed by government. Federal health expenditures, including Medicare, amounted to $540 billion in 2003. State and local spending was about $225 billion in that same year.

TABLE III-65. CONSUMER PRICE INDEX AND AVERAGE ANNUAL PERCENT CHANGE FOR ALL ITEMS, SELECTED ITEMS AND MEDICAL CARE COMPONENTS, SELECTED YEARS, 1960–2004

Many of the medical care components in the Consumer Price Index have increased substantially faster than the price index as a whole. All of the items in the index are calibrated to equal 100 over the 3-year period from 1982–1984. On this basis, the average of all items in the Consumer Price Index was 189 in 2003. However, medical care services measured 310, with hospital and related services showing an index level of 418. Among medical care commodities, prescription drugs and medical supplies reached a level of 337.

Estimation of the Consumer Price Index is inherently complicated, because quality changes in the components are quite difficult to measure. This is especially true for medical care services.

Table III-64. Gross Domestic Product, Federal and State and Local Government Expenditures, National Health Expenditures, and Average Annual Percent Change, Selected Years, 1960–2003

(Dollar, percent.)

Gross domestic product, government expenditures, and national health expenditures	2003	2002	2001	2000	1995	1990	1980	1970	1960
Amount in Billions									
Gross domestic product (GDP)	11 004	10 487	10 128	9 817	7 401	5 803	2 796	1 040	527
Federal government expenditures	2 242.0	2 102.0	1 970.0	1 864.0	1 576.0	1 229.0	576.6	198.6	85.8
State and local government expenditures	1 498.0	1 437.0	1 368.0	1 270.0	903.0	661.0	307.8	107.5	38.1
National health expenditures	1 679.0	1 559.0	1 426.0	1 310.0	990.0	696.0	245.8	73.1	26.7
Private	913.2	841.0	771.8	717.5	533.6	413.5	140.9	45.4	20.1
Public	765.7	718.0	654.6	592.4	456.6	282.5	104.8	27.6	6.6
Federal government	541.7	508.6	463.8	416.0	322.4	192.7	71.3	17.6	2.8
State and local government	224.0	209.4	190.8	176.4	134.2	89.8	33.5	10.0	3.8
Amount per Capita									
National health expenditures	5 671	5 317	4 914	4 560	3 698	2 738	1 067	348	143
Private	3 084	2 869	2 659	2 498	1 993	1 627	612	216	108
Public	2 586	2 449	2 255	2 062	1 705	1 111	455	131	35
National Health Expenditures as Percent of GDP	15.3	14.9	14.1	13.3	13.4	12.0	8.8	7.0	5.1
Health Expenditures as Percent of Total Government Expenditures									
Federal	24.2	24.2	23.5	22.3	20.5	15.7	12.4	8.9	3.3
State and local	15.0	14.6	13.9	13.9	14.9	13.6	10.9	9.3	9.9
National Health Expenditures, Percent Distribution	100.0	100.0	100.0	100.0	100.0	100.0	100.0	100.0	100.0
Private	54.4	53.9	54.1	54.8	53.9	59.4	57.3	62.2	75.2
Public	45.6	46.1	45.9	45.2	46.1	40.6	42.7	37.8	24.8
Average Annual Percent Change from Previous Year Shown									
Gross domestic product	4.9	3.5	3.2	5.8	5.0	7.6	10.4	7.0	X
Federal government expenditures	6.7	6.7	5.6	3.1	5.1	7.9	11.2	8.8	X
State and local government expenditures	4.3	5.0	7.8	5.4	6.4	7.9	11.1	10.9	X
National health expenditures	7.7	9.3	8.9	5.8	7.3	11.0	12.9	10.6	X
Private	8.6	9.0	7.6	6.1	5.2	11.4	12.0	8.5	X
Public	6.6	9.7	10.5	5.3	10.1	10.4	14.3	15.4	X
Federal government	6.5	9.7	11.5	5.2	10.8	10.5	15.0	20.1	X
State and local government	7.0	9.7	8.2	5.6	8.4	10.4	12.8	10.2	X
National health expenditures, per capita	6.6	8.2	7.8	4.5	6.2	9.9	11.9	9.3	X
Private	7.5	7.9	6.5	4.9	4.1	10.3	11.0	7.2	X
Public	5.6	8.6	9.4	4.1	8.9	9.3	13.2	14.0	X

X = Not applicable.

Table III-65. Consumer Price Index and Average Annual Percent Change for All Items, Selected Items and Medical Care Components, Selected Years, 1960–2004

(Number, percent.)

Items and medical care components	2004	2003	2002	2001	2000	1995	1990	1980	1970	1960
Consumer Price Index										
All items	188.9	184.0	179.9	177.1	172.2	152.4	130.7	82.4	38.8	29.6
All items, excluding medical care	182.7	178.1	174.3	171.9	167.3	148.6	128.8	82.8	39.2	30.2
All services	222.8	216.5	209.8	203.4	195.3	168.7	139.2	77.9	35.0	24.1
Food	186.2	180.0	176.2	173.1	167.8	148.4	132.4	86.8	39.2	30.0
Apparel	120.4	120.9	124.0	127.3	129.6	132.0	124.1	90.9	59.2	45.7
Housing	189.5	184.8	180.3	176.4	169.6	148.5	128.5	81.1	36.4	. . .
Energy	151.4	136.5	121.7	129.3	124.6	105.2	102.1	86.0	25.5	22.4
Medical care	310.1	297.1	285.6	272.8	260.8	220.5	162.8	74.9	34.0	22.3
Components of Medical Care										
Medical care services	321.3	306.0	292.9	278.8	266.0	224.2	162.7	74.8	32.3	19.5
Professional services	271.5	261.2	253.9	246.5	237.7	201.0	156.1	77.9	37.0	. . .
Physicians' services	278.3	267.7	260.6	253.6	244.7	208.8	160.8	76.5	34.5	21.9
Dental services	306.9	292.5	281.0	269.0	258.5	206.8	155.8	78.9	39.2	27.0
Eye glasses and eye care [1]	159.3	155.9	155.5	154.5	149.7	137.0	117.3	. . .	. . .	. . .
Services by other medical professionals [1]	181.9	177.1	171.8	167.3	161.9	143.9	120.2	. . .	. . .	. . .
Hospital and related services	417.9	394.8	367.8	338.3	317.3	257.8	178.0	69.2	. . .	. . .
Hospital services [2]	153.4	144.7	134.7	123.6	115.9	. . .	. . .	. . .	. . .	. . .
Inpatient hospital services [2,3]	148.1	140.1	131.2	121.0	113.8	. . .	. . .	. . .	. . .	. . .
Outpatient hospital services [1,3]	356.3	337.9	309.8	281.1	263.8	204.6	138.7	. . .	. . .	. . .
Hospital rooms	. . .	. . .	. . .	. . .	. . .	251.2	175.4	68.0	23.6	9.3
Other inpatient services [1]	. . .	. . .	. . .	. . .	. . .	206.8	142.7	. . .	. . .	. . .
Nursing homes and adult day care [2]	140.4	135.2	127.9	121.8	117.0	. . .	. . .	. . .	. . .	. . .
Medical care commodities	269.3	262.8	256.4	247.6	238.1	204.5	163.4	75.4	46.5	46.9
Prescription drugs and medical supplies	337.1	326.3	316.5	300.9	285.4	235.0	181.7	72.5	47.4	54.0
Nonprescription drugs and medical supplies [1]	152.3	152.0	150.4	150.6	149.5	140.5	120.6	. . .	. . .	. . .
Internal and respiratory over-the-counter drugs	180.9	181.2	178.8	178.9	176.9	167.0	145.9	74.9	42.3	. . .
Nonprescription medical equipment and supplies [1]	179.7	178.1	177.5	178.2	178.1	166.3	138.0	79.2	. . .	. . .
Average Annual Percent Change from Previous Year Shown										
All items	2.7	2.3	1.6	2.8	2.5	3.1	4.7	7.8	2.7	X
All items excluding medical care	2.6	2.2	1.4	2.7	2.4	2.9	4.5	7.8	2.6	X
All services	2.9	3.2	3.1	4.1	3.0	3.9	6.0	8.3	3.8	X
Food	3.4	2.2	1.8	3.2	2.5	2.3	4.3	8.3	2.7	X
Apparel	-0.4	-2.5	-2.6	-1.8	-0.4	1.2	3.2	4.4	2.6	X
Housing	2.5	2.5	2.2	4.0	2.7	2.9	4.7	8.3	. . .	X
Energy	10.9	12.2	-5.9	3.8	3.4	0.6	1.7	12.9	1.3	X
Medical care	4.4	4.0	4.7	4.6	3.4	6.3	8.1	8.2	4.3	X
Components of Medical Care										
Medical care services	5.0	4.5	5.1	4.8	3.5	6.6	8.1	8.8	5.2	X
Professional services	3.9	2.9	3.0	3.7	3.4	5.2	7.2	7.7	. . .	X
Physicians' services	4.0	2.7	2.8	3.6	3.2	5.4	7.7	8.3	4.6	X
Dental services	4.9	4.1	4.5	4.1	4.6	5.8	7.0	7.2	3.8	X
Eye glasses and eye care [1]	2.2	0.3	0.6	3.2	1.8	3.2	. . .	. . .	. . .	X
Services by other medical professionals [1]	2.7	3.1	2.7	3.3	2.4	3.7	. . .	. . .	. . .	X
Hospital and related services	5.9	7.3	8.7	6.6	4.2	7.7	9.9	. . .	. . .	X
Hospital services [2]	6.0	7.4	9.0	6.6	. . .	. . .	. . .	. . .	. . .	X
Inpatient hospital services [2,3]	5.7	6.8	8.4	6.3	. . .	. . .	. . .	. . .	. . .	X
Outpatient hospital services [1,3]	5.4	9.1	10.2	6.6	5.2	8.1	. . .	. . .	. . .	X
Hospital rooms	. . .	. . .	. . .	. . .	. . .	7.4	9.9	11.2	9.8	X
Other inpatient services [1]	. . .	. . .	. . .	. . .	. . .	7.7	. . .	. . .	. . .	X
Nursing homes and adult day care [2]	3.8	5.7	5.0	4.1	. . .	. . .	. . .	. . .	. . .	X
Medical care commodities	2.5	2.5	3.6	4.0	3.1	4.6	8.0	5.0	-0.1	X
Prescription drugs and medical supplies	3.3	3.1	5.2	5.4	4.0	5.3	9.6	4.3	-1.3	X
Nonprescription drugs and medical supplies [1]	0.2	1.1	-0.1	0.7	1.2	3.1	. . .	. . .	. . .	X
Internal and respiratory over-the-counter drugs	-0.2	1.3	-0.1	1.1	1.2	2.7	6.9	5.9	. . .	X
Nonprescription medical equipment and supplies	0.9	0.3	-0.4	0.1	1.4	3.8	5.7	. . .	. . .	X

Note: Consumer Price Index for all urban consumers (CPI-U), U.S. city average, detailed expenditure categories 1982–1984 = 100, except where noted. Data are not seasonally adjusted.

[1] December 1986 = 100.
[2] December 1996 = 100.
[3] Special index based on a substantially smaller sample.
X = Not applicable.
. . . = Not available.

TABLE III-66. NATIONAL HEALTH EXPENDITURES, AVERAGE ANNUAL PERCENT CHANGE, AND PERCENT DISTRIBUTION, ACCORDING TO TYPE OF EXPENDITURE, SELECTED YEARS, 1960–2003

National health expenditures increased 7.7 percent in 2003. The biggest components of these expenditures were hospital care (30.7 percent) and professional services (32.3 percent), of which physician and clinical services accounted for 22 percent of the total. Prescription drugs amounted to 10.7 percent of total spending, and nursing home care was 6.6 percent of the total. Between 1990 and 2003, prescription drug expenditures increased more than fourfold, compared to a better than twofold increase in total health expenditures.

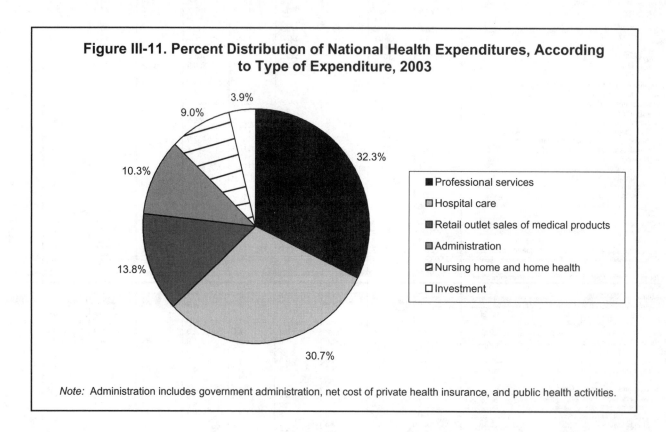

Figure III-11. Percent Distribution of National Health Expenditures, According to Type of Expenditure, 2003

3.9%
9.0%
10.3%
32.3%
13.8%
30.7%

- Professional services
- Hospital care
- Retail outlet sales of medical products
- Administration
- Nursing home and home health
- Investment

Note: Administration includes government administration, net cost of private health insurance, and public health activities.

Table III-66. National Health Expenditures, Average Annual Percent Change, and Percent Distribution, According to Type of Expenditure, Selected Years, 1960–2003

(Dollars, percent.)

Type of national health expenditure	2003	2002	2001	2000	1995	1990	1980	1970	1960
Amount in Billions of Dollars									
National health expenditures	1 678.9	1 559.0	1 426.4	1 309.9	990.2	696.0	245.8	73.1	26.7
Health services and supplies	1 614.2	1 499.8	1 373.8	1 260.9	957.6	669.6	233.5	67.3	25.0
Personal health care	1 440.8	1 342.9	1 235.5	1 136.1	865.7	609.4	214.6	63.2	23.4
Hospital care	515.9	484.2	446.4	413.1	343.6	253.9	101.5	27.6	9.2
Professional services	542.0	503.0	464.4	426.4	316.5	216.9	67.3	20.7	8.3
Physician and clinical services	369.7	340.8	315.1	290.2	220.5	157.5	47.1	14.0	5.4
Other professional services	48.5	46.1	42.6	38.8	28.6	18.2	3.6	0.7	0.4
Dental services	74.3	70.9	65.6	60.7	44.5	31.5	13.3	4.7	2.0
Other personal health care	49.5	45.3	41.1	36.7	22.9	9.6	3.3	1.3	0.6
Nursing home and home health	150.8	143.1	134.9	126.9	105.1	65.3	20.1	4.4	0.9
Home health care [1]	40.0	36.5	33.7	31.6	30.5	12.6	2.4	0.2	0.1
Nursing home care [1]	110.8	106.6	101.2	95.3	74.6	52.7	17.7	4.2	0.8
Retail outlet sales of medical products	232.1	212.6	189.7	169.7	100.5	73.3	25.7	10.5	5.0
Prescription drugs	179.2	161.8	140.8	121.5	60.8	40.3	12.0	5.5	2.7
Other medical products	52.9	50.7	48.9	48.1	39.7	33.1	13.7	5.0	2.3
Government administration and net cost of private health insurance	119.7	105.7	90.9	81.0	60.5	40.0	12.1	2.8	1.2
Government public health activities [2]	53.8	51.2	47.4	43.9	31.4	20.2	6.7	1.4	0.4
Investment	64.6	59.2	52.6	49.0	32.6	26.4	12.3	5.7	1.7
Research [3]	40.2	36.5	32.9	29.1	17.1	12.7	5.5	2.0	0.7
Construction	24.5	22.7	19.7	19.8	15.5	13.7	6.8	3.8	1.0
Average Annual Percent Change from Previous Year									
National health expenditures	7.7	9.3	8.9	5.8	7.3	11.0	12.9	10.6	X
Health services and supplies	7.6	9.2	9.0	5.7	7.4	11.1	13.2	10.4	X
Personal health care	7.3	8.7	8.7	5.6	7.3	11.0	13.0	10.5	X
Hospital care	6.5	8.5	8.1	3.8	6.2	9.6	13.9	11.7	X
Professional services	7.8	8.3	8.9	6.1	7.9	12.4	12.5	9.5	X
Physician and clinical services	8.5	8.2	8.6	5.6	7.0	12.8	12.9	10.1	X
Other professional services	5.3	8.0	9.9	6.3	9.5	17.5	17.1	6.6	X
Dental services	4.8	8.0	8.0	6.4	7.1	9.0	11.1	9.1	X
Other personal health care	9.2	10.1	12.1	9.9	18.9	11.4	10.0	7.2	X
Nursing home and home health	5.4	6.1	6.3	3.8	10.0	12.5	16.3	17.2	X
Home health care [1]	9.5	8.5	6.5	0.7	19.4	18.1	26.9	14.5	X
Nursing home care [1]	4.0	5.3	6.2	5.0	7.2	11.5	15.4	17.4	X
Retail outlet sales of medical products	9.2	12.0	11.8	11.0	6.5	11.1	9.4	7.8	X
Prescription drugs	10.7	14.9	15.9	14.9	8.6	12.8	8.2	7.5	X
Other medical products	4.2	3.6	1.7	3.9	3.8	9.2	10.6	8.1	X
Government administration and net cost of private health insurance	13.2	16.3	12.3	6.0	8.6	12.7	15.9	8.6	X
Government public health activities	5.1	7.9	8.1	6.9	9.2	11.6	17.4	13.2	X
Investment	9.1	12.7	7.4	8.5	4.3	8.0	7.9	12.9	X
Research [3]	10.0	11.0	12.9	11.3	6.2	8.8	10.8	10.9	X
Construction	7.7	15.5	-0.7	5.1	2.4	7.3	6.1	14.1	X
Percent Distribution									
National health expenditures	100.0	100.0	100.0	100.0	100.0	100.0	100.0	100.0	100.0
Health services and supplies	96.1	96.2	96.3	96.3	96.7	96.2	95.0	92.2	93.6
Personal health care	85.8	86.1	86.6	86.7	87.4	87.6	87.3	86.5	87.6
Hospital care	30.7	31.1	31.3	31.5	34.7	36.5	41.3	37.8	34.4
Professional services	32.3	32.3	32.6	32.6	32.0	31.2	27.4	28.3	31.3
Physician and clinical services	22.0	21.9	22.1	22.2	22.3	22.6	19.2	19.1	20.1
Other professional services	2.9	3.0	3.0	3.0	2.9	2.6	1.5	1.0	1.5
Dental services	4.4	4.5	4.6	4.6	4.5	4.5	5.4	6.4	7.4
Other personal health care	2.9	2.9	2.9	2.8	2.3	1.4	1.3	1.7	2.4
Nursing home and home health	9.0	9.2	9.5	9.7	10.6	9.4	8.2	6.1	3.4
Home health care [1]	2.4	2.3	2.4	2.4	3.1	1.8	1.0	0.3	0.2
Nursing home care [1]	6.6	6.8	7.1	7.3	7.5	7.6	7.2	5.8	3.2
Retail outlet sales of medical products	13.8	13.6	13.3	13.0	10.2	10.5	10.5	14.3	18.6
Prescription drugs	10.7	10.4	9.9	9.3	6.1	5.8	4.9	7.5	10.0
Other medical products	3.1	3.3	3.4	3.7	4.0	4.7	5.6	6.8	8.5
Government administration and net cost of private health insurance	7.1	6.8	6.4	6.2	6.1	5.7	4.9	3.8	4.5
Government public health activities	3.2	3.3	3.3	3.3	3.2	2.9	2.7	1.9	1.5
Investment	3.9	3.8	3.7	3.7	3.3	3.8	5.0	7.8	6.4
Research [3]	2.4	2.3	2.3	2.2	1.7	1.8	2.2	2.7	2.6
Construction	1.5	1.5	1.4	1.5	1.6	2.0	2.8	5.2	3.8

[1] Freestanding facilities only. Additional services of this type are provided in hospital-based facilities and counted as hospital care.

[2] Includes personal care services delivered by government public health agencies.

[3] Research and development expenditures of drug companies and other manufacturers and providers of medical equipment and supplies are excluded from "research expenditures," but are included in the expenditure class into which the product falls, in that they are covered by the payment received for that product.

X = Not applicable.

HEALTH INSURANCE

TABLE III-67. PEOPLE WITH OR WITHOUT HEALTH INSURANCE COVERAGE, BY SELECTED CHARACTERISTICS, 2003 AND 2004

In 2004, 45.8 million people were without health insurance coverage, up from 45.0 million people in 2003. However, the Census Bureau warns that health insurance coverage is likely to be more underreported on the Current Population Survey (CPS) than in other national surveys that ask about insurance. There was virtually no change in the proportion of people without health insurance coverage (15.7 percent) between 2003 and 2004. The percent and number of children (under 18 years old) without health insurance in 2004 were 11.2 percent and 8.3 million, respectively. Neither changed significantly from 2003.

By race, the rate and number of uninsured in 2004 was 11.3 percent and 22.0 million, respectively, for non-Hispanic Whites, and 19.7 percent and 7.2 million, respectively, for

Blacks. The figures for both groups were virtually unchanged from 2003. The uninsured rate for Asians decreased from 18.8 percent to 16.8 percent. The number of uninsured Hispanics increased in 2004 (from 13.2 million in 2003 to 13.7 million); their rate was unchanged at 32.7 percent. The uninsured rate for the native-born population increased to 13.3 percent in 2004 from 13.0 percent in 2003. The uninsured rate for the foreign-born population in 2004 (33.7 percent) declined slightly from the 2003 rate.

The likelihood of being covered by health insurance rises with income. Among people in households with annual incomes of less than $25,000 in 2004, 75.7 percent had health insurance; the level increased to 91.6 percent for those in households with incomes of $75,000 or more. Among 18- to 64-year-olds in 2004, full-time workers were more likely to be covered by health insurance (82.2 percent) than part-time workers (75.0 percent) or non-workers (74.2 percent). During 2004, the number of uninsured increased for both full-time workers (from 20.6 million to 21.1 million) and part-time workers (5.9 million to 6.3 million).

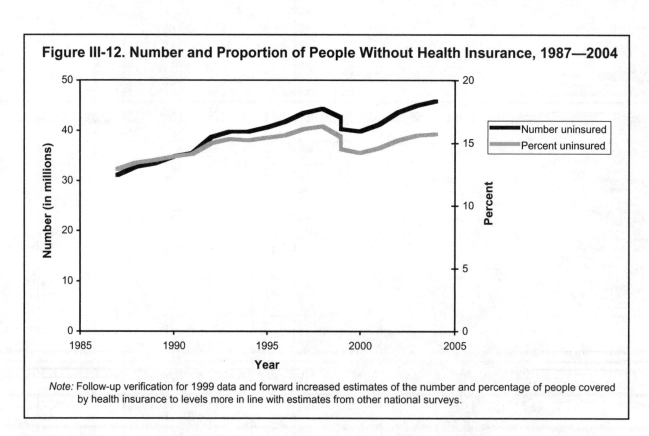

Figure III-12. Number and Proportion of People Without Health Insurance, 1987—2004

Note: Follow-up verification for 1999 data and forward increased estimates of the number and percentage of people covered by health insurance to levels more in line with estimates from other national surveys.

The historical record is marked by a 12-year period, from 1987 to 1998, in which the rate of uninsured persons (beginning at 12.9 percent in 1987) increased in most years. After peaking at 16.3 percent in 1998, this rate declined for two years in a row—dropping to 14.2 percent in 2000—before increasing for three years. It finally stabilized at 15.7 percent in 2004. The two estimates for 1999 reflect the results of follow-up verification questions related to the 2000 census.

Table III-67. People With or Without Health Insurance Coverage, by Selected Characteristics, 2003 and 2004

(Number in thousands, percent.)

| Characteristic | Uninsured | | | | | | | | Change (2004 less than 2003) [1] | | | | | |
| | 2004 | | | | 2003 | | | | Uninsured | | | | Insured | |
	Number	90-percent C.I. (±) [2]	Percentage	90-percent C.I. (±) [2]	Number	90-percent C.I. (±) [2]	Percentage	90-percent C.I.(±) [2]	Number	90-percent C.I. (±) [2]	Percentage	90-percent C.I. (±) [2]	Number	90-percent C.I. (±) [2]
TOTAL	45 820	527	15.7	0.2	44 961	523	15.6	0.2	^860	621	0.1	0.2	^2 015	648
Family Status														
In families	35 698	523	14.8	0.2	35 198	520	14.7	0.2	500	617	0.1	0.3	^1 750	868
Householder	10 634	271	13.8	0.3	10 511	270	13.8	0.3	123	308	-	0.4	663	691
Related children under 18 years	7 803	233	10.8	0.3	7 915	235	11.0	0.3	-112	277	-0.2	0.4	369	710
Related children under 6 years	2 325	129	9.8	0.5	2 369	130	10.1	0.5	-44	153	-0.3	0.6	339	445
In unrelated subfamilies	348	50	27.8	3.4	338	49	28.1	3.5	10	59	-0.4	4.1	43	94
Unrelated individual	9 774	260	20.1	0.5	9 424	256	19.6	0.5	^350	294	0.5	0.6	223	561
Race and Hispanic Origin [3]														
White	34 788	469	14.9	0.2	33 983	464	14.6	0.2	^804	552	0.2	0.2	^1 019	806
White, not Hispanic	21 983	382	11.3	0.2	21 582	379	11.1	0.2	401	450	0.2	0.2	24	847
Black	7 186	254	19.7	0.7	7 080	252	19.6	0.7	107	300	0.1	0.8	319	451
Asian	2 070	138	16.8	1.1	2 228	143	18.8	1.2	-158	166	^-2.0	1.3	^600	269
Hispanic origin (any race)	13 678	308	32.7	0.7	13 237	303	32.7	0.7	^442	321	-0.1	0.8	^972	321
Age														
Under 18 years	8 269	240	11.2	0.3	8 373	242	11.4	0.3	-105	285	-0.2	0.4	346	715
18–24 years	8 772	247	31.4	0.7	8 414	242	30.2	0.7	^358	290	^1.1	0.9	-209	426
25–34 years	10 177	266	25.9	0.6	10 345	268	26.0	1.0	-168	315	-0.5	1.0	274	512
35–44 years	8 110	238	18.7	0.5	7 885	235	18.1	0.5	226	280	^0.6	0.6	-449	560
45–64 years	10 196	266	14.3	0.4	9 657	259	13.9	0.4	^539	310	0.4	0.4	^1 510	695
65 years and older	297	46	0.8	0.1	286	45	0.8	0.1	11	54	-	0.2	543	554
Nativity														
Native	33 962	464	13.3	0.2	33 146	459	13.0	0.0	^816	547	^0.2	0.0	^1 146	743
Foreign-born	11 858	326	34.0	1.0	11 815	325	35.0	1.0	44	385	-0.8	1.0	^869	524
Naturalized citizen	2 317	146	17.2	1.0	2 243	144	17.0	1.0	73	172	0.1	1.0	297	372
Not a citizen	9 542	293	44.0	1.0	9 571	294	45.0	1.0	-29	347	^-1.3	1.0	^573	385
Region														
Northeast	7 106	216	13.2	0.4	6 919	196	12.9	0.4	187	244	0.3	0.5	128	240
Midwest	7 737	224	11.9	0.3	7 748	211	12.0	0.3	-11	258	-	0.4	94	262
South	19 262	350	18.3	0.3	18 621	354	18.0	0.3	^641	416	0.4	0.0	^874	423
West	11 715	276	17.4	0.4	11 674	292	17.6	0.4	41	336	-0.2	0.5	^919	333
Household Income														
Less than $25,000	15 102	321	24.3	0.5	15 331	323	24.2	0.5	-229	381	0.1	0.5	^-896	633
$25,000 to $49,999	14 784	317	20.0	0.4	14 823	318	19.9	0.4	-39	376	0.1	0.5	-673	691
$50,000 to $74,999	7 842	234	13.3	0.4	7 226	225	13.0	0.0	^616	272	^0.7	0.0	^782	650
$75,000 or more	8 092	238	8.0	0.0	7 580	230	8.0	0.0	^512	277	0.3	0.0	^2 802	783
Work Experience														
Total, 18–64 years	37 255	499	20.5	0.0	36 301	478	20.0	0.0	^954	578	0.3	0.0	^1 1 26	765
Worked during year	27 353	441	19.0	0.0	26 581	417	19.0	0.0	^772	508	^0.4	0.0	352	789
Worked full-time	21 092	395	17.8	0.3	20 636	371	17.5	0.3	^456	454	0.2	0.4	673	779
Worked part-time	6 261	224	25.0	0.8	5 945	204	23.8	0.7	^316	254	^1.3	0.9	-320	434
Did not work	9 902	279	25.8	0.6	9 720	260	26.0	0.6	182	319	-0.2	1.0	^774	516

[1] Details may not sum to totals because of rounding.

[2] A 90-percent confidence interval is a measure of an estimate's variability. The larger the confidence interval in relation to the size of the estimate, the less reliable the estimate.

[3] Federal surveys now give respondents the option of reporting more than one race. Therefore, two basic ways of defining a race group are possible. A group such as Asian may be defined as those who reported Asian and no other race (the race-alone or single-race concept) or as those who reported Asian regardless of whether they also reported another race (the race-alone-or-in-combination concept). This table shows data using the first approach (race alone).

0.0 = Quantity more than zero but less than 0.05.

- = Quantity zero.

^ = Statistically different from zero at the 90-percent confidence level.

TABLE III-68. PERCENT OF PEOPLE WITHOUT HEALTH INSURANCE COVERAGE, BY STATE, USING 2- AND 3-YEAR AVERAGES, 2002–2004

A comparison of states using 3-year average uninsured rates for 2002–2004 shows that Texas (25.1 percent) had the highest proportion of uninsured persons. The next highest rate was in New Mexico (21.4 percent, consider-

Table III-68. Percent of People Without Health Insurance Coverage, by State, Using 2- and 3-Year Averages, 2002–2004

(Percent.)

Characteristic	3-year average 2002–2004		2-year average				Change in percentage points (2003–2004 less than 2002–2003 average) [1]	
			2003–2004		2002–2003			
	Percentage	90-percent confidence interval (±) [2]	Percentage	90-percent confidence interval (±) [2]	Percentage	90-percent confidence interval (±) [2]	Percentage	90-percent confidence interval (±) [2]
UNITED STATES	15.5	0.1	15.7	0.1	15.4	0.1	^0.2	0.1
Alabama	13.5	0.9	13.8	1.1	13.4	1.0	0.4	0.9
Alaska	18.2	1.0	18.0	1.3	18.8	1.2	-0.8	1.1
Arizona	17.0	1.0	17.1	1.2	16.9	1.2	0.2	1.1
Arkansas	16.7	1.1	16.9	1.3	16.9	1.2	-	1.1
California	18.4	0.5	18.5	0.5	18.3	0.6	0.3	0.5
Colorado	16.8	0.9	17.1	1.2	16.7	1.0	0.4	1.0
Connecticut	10.9	0.8	11.0	1.0	10.5	0.8	0.6	0.9
Delaware	11.8	0.9	12.8	1.1	10.5	1.0	^2.3	1.0
District of Columbia	13.5	1.0	13.8	1.3	13.7	1.2	0.2	1.1
Florida	18.5	0.6	19.0	0.7	17.7	0.7	^1.3	0.6
Georgia	16.6	0.9	16.9	1.0	16.3	1.1	0.7	0.9
Hawaii	9.9	0.8	9.9	0.9	10.1	0.9	-0.2	0.8
Idaho	17.3	1.1	17.0	1.3	18.3	1.3	^-1.3	1.1
Illinois	14.2	0.6	14.2	0.7	14.3	0.7	-0.1	0.6
Indiana	13.7	0.8	14.0	1.0	13.5	0.9	0.6	0.8
Iowa	10.1	0.8	10.4	1.0	10.4	0.9	-	0.8
Kansas	10.8	0.8	11.0	1.0	10.7	0.9	0.3	0.9
Kentucky	13.9	0.9	14.1	1.1	13.8	1.0	0.4	1.0
Louisiana	18.8	1.1	18.9	1.3	19.5	1.3	-0.6	1.1
Maine	10.6	0.8	10.2	1.0	10.9	0.8	-0.7	0.9
Maryland	14.0	0.8	14.2	1.0	13.6	0.9	0.6	0.9
Massachusetts	10.8	0.7	11.2	0.8	10.3	0.8	^0.9	0.7
Michigan	11.4	0.6	11.2	0.7	11.3	0.7	-	0.6
Minnesota	8.5	0.7	8.8	0.8	8.3	0.8	0.5	0.7
Mississippi	17.2	1.1	17.5	1.3	17.3	1.3	0.2	1.1
Missouri	11.7	0.8	11.8	0.9	11.3	0.9	0.5	0.8
Montana	17.9	1.1	19.2	1.4	17.3	1.3	^1.9	1.1
Nebraska	11.0	0.8	11.4	1.0	10.7	0.9	0.6	0.9
Nevada	19.1	1.0	18.7	1.3	19.3	1.1	-0.6	1.1
New Hampshire	10.6	0.8	11.0	1.0	10.1	0.8	^0.9	0.9
New Jersey	14.4	0.7	14.6	0.8	14.0	0.8	0.7	0.7
New Mexico	21.4	1.3	21.5	1.5	21.6	1.5	-0.1	1.3
New York	15.0	0.5	14.7	0.6	15.4	0.6	^-0.8	0.5
North Carolina	16.6	0.8	16.5	0.9	17.0	0.9	-0.5	0.8
North Dakota	11.0	0.8	11.0	1.0	10.9	0.9	0.1	0.9
Ohio	11.8	0.6	11.7	0.7	12.0	0.7	-0.3	0.6
Oklahoma	19.2	1.1	20.1	1.3	18.8	1.2	^1.3	1.1
Oregon	16.1	1.0	16.8	1.2	15.9	1.1	1.0	1.1
Pennsylvania	11.5	0.5	11.7	0.6	11.4	0.6	0.3	0.6
Rhode Island	10.5	0.8	10.8	1.0	10.0	0.8	0.8	0.9
South Carolina	13.8	0.9	14.5	1.1	13.4	1.0	^1.1	1.0
South Dakota	11.9	0.8	12.1	1.0	11.8	0.9	0.2	0.9
Tennessee	12.7	0.9	13.7	1.0	12.0	1.0	^1.7	0.9
Texas	25.1	0.6	24.8	0.7	25.2	0.8	-0.4	0.7
Utah	13.4	0.9	13.4	1.1	13.0	1.0	0.3	1.0
Vermont	10.5	0.8	10.3	1.0	10.1	0.9	0.2	0.9
Virginia	13.6	0.8	13.7	0.9	13.3	1.0	0.4	0.8
Washington	14.2	0.9	14.2	1.0	14.8	1.1	-0.6	0.9
West Virginia	15.9	0.9	16.5	1.1	15.6	1.1	0.9	1.0
Wisconsin	10.4	0.7	10.6	0.9	10.4	0.8	0.3	0.8
Wyoming	15.9	1.0	15.0	1.2	16.8	1.2	^-1.8	1.1

[1]Details may not sum to totals because of rounding.

[2]A 90-percent confidence interval is a measure of an estimate's variability. The larger the confidence interval in relation to the size of the estimate, the less reliable the estimate.

- = Quantity zero.

^ = Statistically different from zero at the 90-percent confidence level.

ably lower than the rate in Texas), followed by Oklahoma (19.2 percent), Nevada (19.1 percent), Louisiana (18.8 percent), Florida (18.5 percent), and California (18.4 percent). Thus, three of the four most populous states were among the top seven in proportion of residents lacking insurance. The lowest proportions of uninsured persons occurred in Minnesota (8.5 percent), Hawaii (9.9 percent), Iowa (10.1 percent), Wisconsin (10.4 percent), and Vermont (10.5 percent). Comparisons of 2-year moving averages (2002–2003 and 2003–2004) show that the proportion of persons without coverage experienced a statistically significant increase in eight states and a decrease in three states. Four of the states that experienced significant increases were in the South (Florida, Oklahoma, South Carolina, and Tennessee); the others were Delaware, Montana, Massachusetts and New Hampshire. The rate of uninsured persons decreased significantly for Idaho, New York, and Wyoming.

TABLE III-69. HEALTH INSURANCE COVERAGE STATUS AND TYPE OF COVERAGE, BY RACE AND HISPANIC ORIGIN, 1987–2004

This table presents insured populations and percentages from 1987 to 2004 by private and government health insurance categories, race, and Hispanic origin. Private health insurance is divided into employment-based versus direct purchase, while government health insurance is divided into Medicaid, Medicare, and military health care (including programs for active duty, retired, families of servicemen, and Department of Veterans Affairs). The survey was based on data that underreported Medicare and Medicaid coverage as compared with enrollment and participation data from the Centers for Medicare and Medicaid Services. Changes in Medicaid coverage estimates from one year to the next should be viewed with caution.

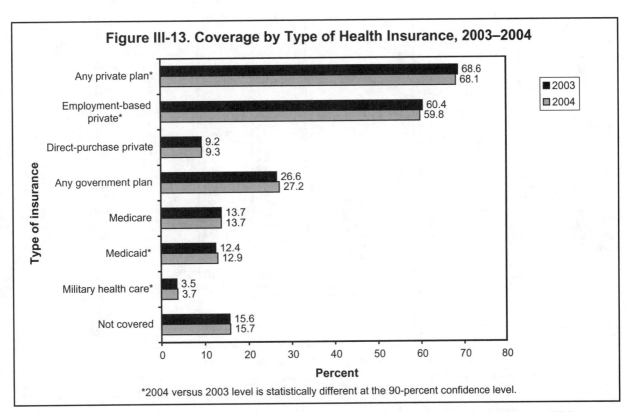

Figure III-13. Coverage by Type of Health Insurance, 2003–2004

The percentage of the population covered by employment-based health insurance decreased to 59.8 percent in 2004, down from 60.4 percent in 2003. The rate and number of people covered by government health insurance programs increased between 2003 and 2004, rising from 26.6 percent and 76.8 million, respectively, to 27.2 percent and 79.1 million. This increase was driven by the greater proportion and number of people covered by Medicaid (up from 12.4 percent and 35.6 million, respectively, to 12.9 percent and 37.5 million.)

Table III-69. Health Insurance Coverage Status and Type of Coverage, by Race and Hispanic Origin, 1987–2004

(Number in thousands, percent.)

Year, race, and Hispanic origin	Total population	Covered by private or government health insurance									Not covered
		Total	Private health insurance			Government health insurance				
			Total	Employment-based	Direct purchase	Total	Medicaid	Medicare	Military health care [1]	

ALL RACES

Number

2004	291 155	245 335	198 262	174 174	26 961	79 086	37 514	39 745	10 680	45 820
2003	288 280	243 320	197 869	174 020	26 486	76 755	35 647	39 456	9 979	44 961
2002	285 933	242 360	198 973	175 296	26 639	73 624	33 246	38 448	10 063	43 574
2001	282 082	240 875	199 860	176 551	26 057	71 295	31 601	38 043	9 552	41 207
2000 [2]	279 517	239 714	201 060	177 848	26 524	69 037	29 533	37 740	9 099	39 804
1999 [3]	276 804	236 576	198 841	175 101	27 415	67 683	28 506	36 923	8 648	40 228
1999	274 087	231 533	194 599	172 023	26 179	66 176	27 890	36 066	8 530	42 554
1998	271 743	227 462	190 861	168 576	25 948	66 087	27 854	35 887	8 747	44 281
1997 [4]	269 094	225 646	188 532	165 091	27 158	66 685	28 956	35 590	8 527	43 448
1996	266 792	225 077	187 395	163 221	28 335	69 000	31 451	35 227	8 712	41 716
1995	264 314	223 733	185 881	161 453	30 188	69 776	31 877	34 655	9 375	40 582
1994 [5]	262 105	222 387	184 318	159 634	31 349	70 163	31 645	33 901	11 165	39 718
1993 [6]	259 753	220 040	182 351	148 318	...	68 554	31 749	33 097	9 560	39 713
1992 [7]	256 830	218 189	181 466	148 796	...	66 244	29 416	33 230	9 510	38 641
1991	251 447	216 003	181 375	150 077	...	63 882	26 880	32 907	9 820	35 445
1990	248 886	214 167	182 135	150 215	...	60 965	24 261	32 260	9 922	34 719
1989	246 191	212 807	183 610	151 644	...	57 382	21 185	31 495	9 870	33 385
1988	243 685	211 005	182 019	150 940	...	56 850	20 728	30 925	10 105	32 680
1987 [8]	241 187	210 161	182 160	149 739	...	56 282	20 211	30 458	10 542	31 026

Percent

2004	100.0	84.3	68.1	59.8	9.3	27.2	12.9	13.7	3.7	15.7
2003	100.0	84.4	68.6	60.4	9.2	26.6	12.4	13.7	3.5	15.6
2002	100.0	84.8	69.6	61.3	9.3	25.7	11.6	13.4	3.5	15.2
2001	100.0	85.4	70.9	62.6	9.2	25.3	11.2	13.5	3.4	14.6
2000 [2]	100.0	85.8	71.9	63.6	9.5	24.7	10.6	13.5	3.3	14.2
1999 [3]	100.0	85.5	71.8	63.3	9.9	24.5	10.3	13.3	3.1	14.5
1999	100.0	84.5	71.0	62.8	9.6	24.1	10.2	13.2	3.1	15.5
1998	100.0	83.7	70.2	62.0	9.5	24.3	10.3	13.2	3.2	16.3
1997 [4]	100.0	83.9	70.1	61.4	10.1	24.8	10.8	13.2	3.2	16.1
1996	100.0	84.4	70.2	61.2	10.6	25.9	11.8	13.2	3.3	15.6
1995	100.0	84.6	70.3	61.1	11.4	26.4	12.1	13.1	3.5	15.4
1994 [5]	100.0	84.8	70.3	60.9	12.0	26.8	12.1	12.9	4.3	15.2
1993 [6]	100.0	84.7	70.2	57.1	...	26.4	12.2	12.7	3.7	15.3
1992 [7]	100.0	85.0	70.7	57.9	...	25.8	11.5	12.9	3.7	15.0
1991	100.0	85.9	72.1	59.7	...	25.4	10.7	13.1	3.9	14.1
1990	100.0	86.1	73.2	60.4	...	24.5	9.7	13.0	4.0	13.9
1989	100.0	86.4	74.6	61.6	...	23.3	8.6	12.8	4.0	13.6
1988	100.0	86.6	74.7	61.9	...	23.3	8.5	12.7	4.1	13.4
1987 [8]	100.0	87.1	75.5	62.1	...	23.3	8.4	12.6	4.4	12.9

WHITE ALONE [9]

Number

2004	234 077	199 289	165 327	144 246	23 511	61 311	25 586	34 084	8 567	34 788
2003	232 254	198 270	165 852	144 780	23 253	59 495	23 959	33 765	8 105	33 983
2002	230 809	198 103	167 151	146 210	23 511	57 072	22 171	33 135	8 065	32 706

Percent

2004	100.0	85.1	70.6	61.6	10.0	26.2	10.9	14.6	3.7	14.9
2003	100.0	85.4	71.4	62.3	10.0	25.6	10.3	14.5	3.5	14.6
2002	100.0	85.8	72.4	63.3	10.2	24.7	9.6	14.4	3.5	14.2

[1] Includes CHAMPUS (Comprehensive Health and Medical Plan for Uniformed Services)/Tricare, veterans', and military health care.
[2] Implementation of a 28,000 household sample expansion.
[3] Estimates reflect the results of follow-up verification questions and implementation of Census 2000-based population controls.
[4] Beginning with the 1998 CPS ASEC, people with no coverage other than access to Indian Health Service are no longer considered covered by health insurance; instead, they are considered to be uninsured. The effect of this change on the overall estimates of health insurance coverage is negligible; however, the decrease in the number of people covered by Medicaid may be partially due to this change.
[5] Health insurance questions were redesigned. Increases in estimates of employment-based and military health care coverage may be partially due to questionnaire changes. Overall coverage estimates were not affected.
[6] Data collection method changed from paper and pencil to computer-assisted interviewing.
[7] Implementation of 1990 census population controls.
[8] Implementation of a new CPS ASEC processing system.
[9] The 2003 CPS asked respondents to choose one or more races. White alone refers to people who reported White and did not report any other race category. The use of this single-race population does not imply that it is the preferred method of presenting or analyzing data. The Census Bureau uses a variety of approaches. Information on people who reported more than one race, such as White and American Indian and Alaska Native or Asian and Black or African American, is available from Census 2000 through American FactFinder. About 2.6 percent of people reported more than one race in Census 2000.
. . . = Not available.

Table III-69. Health Insurance Coverage Status and Type of Coverage, by Race and Hispanic Origin, 1987–2004—*Continued*

(Number in thousands, percent.)

Year, race, and Hispanic origin	Total population	Covered by private or government health insurance								Not covered
		Total	Private health insurance			Government health insurance				
			Total	Employment-based	Direct purchase	Total	Medicaid	Medicare	Military health care [1]	

WHITE [10]

Number

2001	230 071	198 878	169 180	148 371	23 110	56 200	21 535	33 006	7 788	31 193
2000 [2]	228 208	198 133	170 071	149 364	23 474	54 287	19 889	32 695	7 158	30 075
1999 [3]	225 794	195 929	168 730	147 583	24 213	53 175	18 977	32 144	6 902	29 865
1999	224 806	192 943	166 191	145 878	23 315	52 139	18 676	31 416	6 848	31 863
1998	223 294	189 706	163 690	143 705	23 201	51 690	18 247	31 174	7 140	33 588
1997 [4]	221 650	188 409	161 682	140 601	24 347	52 975	19 652	31 108	6 994	33 241
1996	220 070	188 341	161 806	139 913	25 519	54 004	20 856	30 919	6 981	31 729
1995	218 442	187 337	161 303	139 151	27 337	54 141	20 528	30 580	7 656	31 105
1994 [5]	216 751	186 447	160 414	137 966	28 287	54 288	20 464	29 978	8 845	30 305
1993 [6]	215 221	184 732	158 586	128 855	. . .	53 222	20 642	29 297	7 689	30 489
1992 [7]	213 198	183 479	158 612	129 685	. . .	51 195	18 659	29 341	7 556	29 719
1991	210 257	183 130	159 628	131 646	. . .	49 699	17 058	28 940	7 867	27 127
1990	208 754	181 795	160 146	131 836	. . .	47 589	15 078	28 530	8 022	26 959
1989	206 983	181 126	161 363	132 882	. . .	44 868	12 779	27 859	8 116	25 857
1988	205 333	180 122	160 753	133 050	. . .	44 477	12 504	27 293	8 305	25 211
1987 [8]	203 745	179 845	161 338	132 264	. . .	44 028	12 163	27 044	8 482	23 900

Percent

2001	100.0	86.4	73.5	64.5	10.0	24.4	9.4	14.3	3.4	13.6
2000 [2]	100.0	86.8	74.5	65.5	10.3	23.8	8.7	14.3	3.1	13.2
1999 [3]	100.0	86.8	74.7	65.4	10.7	23.6	8.4	14.2	3.1	13.2
1999	100.0	85.8	73.9	64.9	10.4	23.2	8.3	14.0	3.0	14.2
1998	100.0	85.0	73.3	64.4	10.4	23.1	8.2	14.0	3.2	15.0
1997 [4]	100.0	85.0	72.9	63.4	11.0	23.9	8.9	14.0	3.2	15.0
1996	100.0	85.6	73.5	63.6	11.6	24.5	9.5	14.0	3.2	14.4
1995	100.0	85.8	73.8	63.7	12.5	24.8	9.4	14.0	3.5	14.2
1994 [5]	100.0	86.0	74.0	63.7	13.1	25.0	9.4	13.8	4.1	14.0
1993 [6]	100.0	85.8	73.7	59.9	. . .	24.7	9.6	13.6	3.6	14.2
1992 [7]	100.0	86.1	74.4	60.8	. . .	24.0	8.8	13.8	3.5	13.9
1991	100.0	87.1	75.9	62.6	. . .	23.6	8.1	13.8	3.7	12.9
1990	100.0	87.1	76.7	63.2	. . .	22.8	7.2	13.7	3.8	12.9
1989	100.0	87.5	78.0	64.2	. . .	21.7	6.2	13.5	3.9	12.5
1988	100.0	87.7	78.3	64.8	. . .	21.7	6.1	13.3	4.0	12.3
1987 [8]	100.0	88.3	79.2	64.9	. . .	21.6	6.0	13.3	4.2	11.7

WHITE ALONE, NOT HISPANIC [9]

Number

2004	195 301	173 319	148 069	128 368	21 944	50 806	17 241	31 640	7 952	21 983
2003	194 877	173 295	149 084	129 261	21 865	49 743	16 247	31 458	7 563	21 582
2002	194 421	173 639	150 422	130 801	22 128	47 736	14 984	30 718	7 465	20 782

Percent

2004	100.0	88.7	75.8	65.7	11.2	26.0	8.8	16.2	4.1	11.3
2003	100.0	88.9	76.5	66.3	11.2	25.5	8.3	16.1	3.9	11.1
2002	100.0	89.3	77.4	67.3	11.4	24.6	7.7	15.8	3.8	10.7

[1]Includes CHAMPUS (Comprehensive Health and Medical Plan for Uniformed Services)/Tricare, veterans', and military health care.
[2]Implementation of a 28,000 household sample expansion.
[3]Estimates reflect the results of follow-up verification questions and implementation of Census 2000-based population controls.
[4]Beginning with the 1998 CPS ASEC, people with no coverage other than access to Indian Health Service are no longer considered covered by health insurance; instead, they are considered to be uninsured. The effect of this change on the overall estimates of health insurance coverage is negligible; however, the decrease in the number of people covered by Medicaid may be partially due to this change.
[5]Health insurance questions were redesigned. Increases in estimates of employment-based and military health care coverage may be partially due to questionnaire changes. Overall coverage estimates were not affected.
[6]Data collection method changed from paper and pencil to computer-assisted interviewing.
[7]Implementation of 1990 census population controls.
[8]Implementation of a new CPS ASEC processing system.
[9]The 2003 CPS asked respondents to choose one or more races. White alone refers to people who reported White and did not report any other race category. The use of this single-race population does not imply that it is the preferred method of presenting or analyzing data. The Census Bureau uses a variety of approaches. Information on people who reported more than one race, such as White and American Indian and Alaska Native or Asian and Black or African American, is available from Census 2000 through American FactFinder. About 2.6 percent of people reported more than one race in Census 2000.
[10]The 2001 CPS and earlier years asked respondents to report only one race. The reference groups for these years are: White, White not Hispanic, Black, and Asian and Pacific Islander.
. . . = Not available.

Table III-69. Health Insurance Coverage Status and Type of Coverage, by Race and Hispanic Origin, 1987–2004—Continued

(Number in thousands, percent.)

Year, race, and Hispanic origin	Total population	Covered by private or government health insurance								Not covered
		Total	Private health insurance			Government health insurance				
			Total	Employment-based	Direct purchase	Total	Medicaid	Medicare	Military health care [1]	
WHITE, NOT HISPANIC [10]										
Number										
2001	194 822	175 412	152 821	133 295	21 796	47 661	15 035	30 811	7 144	19 409
2000 [2]	193 931	175 247	153 816	134 253	22 242	46 297	13 788	30 642	6 564	18 683
1999 [3]	192 858	173 958	152 984	133 123	22 882	45 540	13 157	30 256	6 326	18 901
1999	193 633	172 271	151 539	132 381	22 104	44 749	13 120	29 457	6 306	21 363
1998	193 074	170 184	149 910	130 956	22 110	44 699	12 985	29 222	6 675	22 890
1997 [4]	192 178	169 043	148 426	128 280	23 349	45 691	14 046	29 213	6 504	23 135
1996	191 791	169 699	149 262	128 355	24 456	46 772	15 082	29 211	6 537	22 092
1995	191 271	169 272	149 686	128 378	26 363	46 501	14 381	28 918	7 163	21 999
1994 [5]	192 771	170 541	150 181	128 633	27 205	47 475	15 052	28 467	8 318	22 230
1993 [6]	191 087	168 306	147 729	119 861	. . .	46 158	14 980	27 795	7 243	22 781
1992 [7]	189 113	167 394	147 967	120 482	. . .	44 649	13 390	27 853	7 104	21 719
1991	189 216	168 810	149 798	123 109	. . .	44 228	12 750	27 695	7 402	20 406
1990	188 240	168 015	150 306	123 261	. . .	42 732	11 423	27 313	7 528	20 224
1989	187 078	167 889	151 424	124 311	. . .	40 624	9 759	26 738	7 567	19 188
1988	186 047	167 048	151 009	124 622	. . .	40 259	9 522	26 224	7 743	19 000
1987 [8]	185 044	166 922	151 817	124 068	. . .	39 792	9 143	26 054	7 883	18 122
Percent										
2001	100.0	90.0	78.4	68.4	11.2	24.5	7.7	15.8	3.7	10.0
2000 [2]	100.0	90.4	79.3	69.2	11.5	23.9	7.1	15.8	3.4	9.6
1999 [3]	100.0	90.2	79.3	69.0	11.9	23.6	6.8	15.7	3.3	9.8
1999	100.0	89.0	78.3	68.4	11.4	23.1	6.8	15.2	3.3	11.0
1998	100.0	88.1	77.6	67.8	11.5	23.2	6.7	15.1	3.5	11.9
1997 [4]	100.0	88.0	77.2	66.8	12.1	23.8	7.3	15.2	3.4	12.0
1996	100.0	88.5	77.8	66.9	12.8	24.4	7.9	15.2	3.4	11.5
1995	100.0	88.5	78.3	67.1	13.8	24.3	7.5	15.1	3.7	11.5
1994 [5]	100.0	88.5	77.9	66.7	14.1	24.6	7.8	14.8	4.3	11.5
1993 [6]	100.0	88.1	77.3	62.7	. . .	24.2	7.8	14.5	3.8	11.9
1992 [7]	100.0	88.5	78.2	63.7	. . .	23.6	7.1	14.7	3.8	11.5
1991	100.0	89.2	79.2	65.1	. . .	23.4	6.7	14.6	3.9	10.8
1990	100.0	89.3	79.8	65.5	. . .	22.7	6.1	14.5	4.0	10.7
1989	100.0	89.7	80.9	66.4	. . .	21.7	5.2	14.3	4.0	10.3
1988	100.0	89.8	81.2	67.0	. . .	21.6	5.1	14.1	4.2	10.2
1987 [8]	100.0	90.2	82.0	67.0	. . .	21.5	4.9	14.1	4.3	9.8
BLACK ALONE OR IN COMBINATION [11]										
Number										
2004	38 161	30 714	20 457	18 885	1 825	13 501	9 451	4 000	1 446	7 447
2003	37 651	30 344	20 136	10 282	1 732	13 195	9 292	4 080	1 283	7 307
2002	37 350	29 921	20 231	18 837	1 621	12 624	8 744	3 851	1 342	7 429
Percent										
2004	100.0	80.5	53.6	49.5	4.8	35.4	24.8	10.5	3.8	19.5
2003	100.0	80.6	53.5	49.6	4.6	35.1	24.7	10.8	3.4	19.4
2002	100.0	80.1	54.2	50.4	4.3	33.8	23.4	10.3	3.6	19.9
BLACK ALONE [11]										
Number										
2004	36 546	29 360	19 596	18 122	1 732	12 878	8 943	3 925	1 369	7 186
2003	36 121	29 041	19 320	17 924	1 663	12 585	8 797	3 989	1 225	7 080
2002	35 806	28 578	19 347	18 002	1 571	12 058	8 289	3 776	1 268	7 228
Percent										
2004	100.0	80.3	53.6	49.6	4.7	35.2	24.5	10.7	3.7	19.7
2003	100.0	80.4	53.5	49.6	4.6	34.8	24.4	11.0	3.4	19.6
2002	100.0	79.8	54.0	50.3	4.4	33.7	23.1	10.5	3.5	20.2

[1]Includes CHAMPUS (Comprehensive Health and Medical Plan for Uniformed Services)/Tricare, veterans', and military health care.
[2]Implementation of a 28,000 household sample expansion.
[3]Estimates reflect the results of follow-up verification questions and implementation of Census 2000-based population controls.
[4]Beginning with the 1998 CPS ASEC, people with no coverage other than access to Indian Health Service are no longer considered covered by health insurance; instead, they are considered to be uninsured. The effect of this change on the overall estimates of health insurance coverage is negligible; however, the decrease in the number of people covered by Medicaid may be partially due to this change.
[5]Health insurance questions were redesigned. Increases in estimates of employment-based and military health care coverage may be partially due to questionnaire changes. Overall coverage estimates were not affected.
[6]Data collection method changed from paper and pencil to computer-assisted interviewing.
[7]Implementation of 1990 census population controls.
[8]Implementation of a new CPS ASEC processing system.
[10]The 2001 CPS and earlier years asked respondents to report only one race. The reference groups for these years are: White, White not Hispanic, Black, and Asian and Pacific Islander.
[11]Black alone refers to people who reported Black or African American and did not report any other race category.
. . . = Not available.

Table III-69. Health Insurance Coverage Status and Type of Coverage, by Race and Hispanic Origin, 1987–2004—Continued

(Number in thousands, percent.)

Year, race, and Hispanic origin	Total population	Covered by private or government health insurance									Not covered
		Total	Private health insurance			Government health insurance					
			Total	Employment-based	Direct purchase	Total	Medicaid	Medicare	Military health care [1]		
BLACK [10]											
Number											
2001	36 023	29 190	20 363	18 975	1 696	11 616	7 994	3 783	1 192		6 833
2000 [2]	35 597	28 915	20 485	18 922	1 893	11 579	7 735	3 871	1 372		6 683
1999 [3]	35 893	28 775	20 442	18 854	2 065	11 361	7 652	3 615	1 216		7 119
1999	35 509	27 973	19 805	18 363	1 912	11 165	7 495	3 588	1 198		7 536
1998	35 070	27 274	18 663	17 132	1 782	11 524	7 903	3 703	1 111		7 797
1997 [4]	34 598	27 166	18 544	17 077	1 841	11 157	7 750	3 573	1 100		7 432
1996	34 218	26 799	17 718	16 358	1 745	12 074	8 572	3 393	1 357		7 419
1995	33 889	26 781	17 106	15 683	1 815	12 465	9 184	3 316	1 171		7 108
1994 [5]	33 531	26 928	17 147	15 607	2 147	12 693	9 007	3 167	1 683		6 603
1993 [6]	33 040	26 279	16 590	13 693	. . .	12 588	9 283	3 072	1 331		6 761
1992 [7]	32 535	25 967	15 994	13 545	. . .	12 464	9 122	3 154	1 459		6 567
1991	31 439	24 932	15 466	13 297	. . .	11 776	8 352	3 248	1 482		6 507
1990	30 895	24 802	15 957	13 560	. . .	11 150	7 809	3 106	1 402		6 093
1989	30 392	24 550	16 520	14 187	. . .	10 443	7 123	3 043	1 340		5 843
1988	29 904	24 029	15 818	13 418	. . .	10 415	7 049	3 064	1 385		5 875
1987 [8]	29 417	23 555	15 358	13 055	. . .	10 380	7 046	2 918	1 497		5 862
Percent											
2001	100.0	81.0	56.5	52.7	4.7	32.2	22.2	10.5	3.3		19.0
2000 [2]	100.0	81.2	57.5	53.2	5.3	32.5	21.7	10.1	3.9		18.8
1999 [3]	100.0	80.2	57.0	52.5	5.8	31.7	21.3	10.1	3.4		19.8
1999	100.0	78.8	55.8	51.7	5.4	31.4	21.1	10.1	3.4		21.2
1998	100.0	77.8	53.2	48.9	5.1	32.9	22.5	10.6	3.2		22.2
1997 [4]	100.0	78.5	53.6	49.4	5.3	32.2	22.4	10.3	3.2		21.5
1996	100.0	78.3	51.8	47.8	5.1	35.3	25.1	9.9	4.0		21.7
1995	100.0	79.0	50.5	46.3	5.4	36.8	27.1	9.8	3.5		21.0
1994 [5]	100.0	80.3	51.1	46.5	6.4	37.9	26.9	9.4	5.0		19.7
1993 [6]	100.0	79.5	50.2	41.4	. . .	38.1	28.1	9.3	4.0		20.5
1992 [7]	100.0	79.8	49.2	41.6	. . .	38.3	28.0	9.7	4.5		20.2
1991	100.0	79.3	49.2	42.3	. . .	37.5	26.6	10.3	4.7		20.7
1990	100.0	80.3	51.6	43.9	. . .	36.1	25.3	10.1	4.5		19.7
1989	100.0	80.8	54.4	46.7	. . .	34.4	23.4	10.0	4.4		19.2
1988	100.0	80.4	52.9	44.9	. . .	34.8	23.6	10.2	4.6		19.6
1987 [8]	100.0	80.1	52.2	44.4	. . .	35.3	24.0	9.9	5.1		19.9
ASIAN ALONE OR IN COMBINATION [12]											
Number											
2004	13 373	11 157	9 486	8 305	1 324	2 597	1 377	1 127	433		2 217
2003	12 905	10 504	8 826	7 829	1 159	2 478	1 385	1 096	355		2 401
2002	12 504	10 256	8 639	7 576	1 194	2 341	1 322	1 008	347		2 248
Percent											
2004	100.0	83.4	70.9	62.1	9.9	19.4	10.3	8.4	3.2		16.6
2003	100.0	81.4	68.4	60.7	9.0	19.2	10.7	8.5	2.8		18.6
2002	100.0	82.0	69.1	60.6	9.5	18.7	10.6	8.1	2.8		18.0
ASIAN ALONE [12]											
Number											
2004	12 311	10 241	8 704	7 612	1 231	2 396	1 267	1 098	360		2 070
2003	11 869	9 641	8 143	7 210	1 095	2 244	1 229	1 067	295		2 228
2002	11 558	9 426	7 939	6 932	1 137	2 132	1 202	988	270		2 132
Percent											
2004	100.0	83.2	70.7	61.8	10.0	19.5	10.3	8.9	2.9		16.8
2003	100.0	81.2	68.6	60.7	9.2	18.9	10.4	9.0	2.5		18.8
2002	100.0	81.6	68.7	60.0	9.8	18.4	10.4	8.5	2.3		18.4

[1]Includes CHAMPUS (Comprehensive Health and Medical Plan for Uniformed Services)/Tricare, veterans', and military health care.
[2]Implementation of a 28,000 household sample expansion.
[3]Estimates reflect the results of follow-up verification questions and implementation of Census 2000-based population controls.
[4]Beginning with the 1998 CPS ASEC, people with no coverage other than access to Indian Health Service are no longer considered covered by health insurance; instead, they are considered to be uninsured. The effect of this change on the overall estimates of health insurance coverage is negligible; however, the decrease in the number of people covered by Medicaid may be partially due to this change.
[5]Health insurance questions were redesigned. Increases in estimates of employment-based and military health care coverage may be partially due to questionnaire changes. Overall coverage estimates were not affected.
[6]Data collection method changed from paper and pencil to computer-assisted interviewing.
[7]Implementation of 1990 census population controls.
[8]Implementation of a new CPS ASEC processing system.
[10]The 2001 CPS and earlier years asked respondents to report only one race. The reference groups for these years are: White, White not Hispanic, Black, and Asian and Pacific Islander.
[12]Asian alone refers to people who reported Asian and did not report any other race category.
. . . = Not available.

Table III-69. Health Insurance Coverage Status and Type of Coverage, by Race and Hispanic Origin, 1987–2004—*Continued*

(Number in thousands, percent.)

Year, race, and Hispanic origin	Total population	Covered by private or government health insurance								Not covered
		Total	Private health insurance			Government health insurance				
			Total	Employment-based	Direct purchase	Total	Medicaid	Medicare	Military health care [1]	
ASIAN AND PACIFIC ISLANDER [10]										
Number										
2001	12 500	10 222	8 643	7 684	1 088	2 312	1 257	949	414	2 278
2000 [2]	12 693	10 405	8 916	8 104	994	2 249	1 288	886	443	2 287
1999 [3]	11 964	9 673	8 189	7 331	964	2 204	1 179	897	450	2 292
1999	10 925	8 653	7 285	6 588	805	2 023	1 087	825	412	2 272
1998	10 897	8 596	7 202	6 511	857	2 113	1 201	819	351	2 301
1997 [4]	10 492	8 320	7 100	6 290	848	1 877	1 093	700	334	2 173
1996	10 071	7 946	6 718	5 888	962	1 768	1 071	667	275	2 125
1995	9 653	7 671	6 347	5 576	963	2 075	1 272	586	424	1 982
1994 [5]	6 656	5 312	4 267	3 774	698	1 551	883	501	426	1 344
1993 [6]	7 444	5 927	5 026	3 970	...	1 408	802	474	345	1 517
1992 [7]	7 782	6 230	5 202	4 207	...	1 460	823	507	314	1 552
1991	7 193	5 886	4 917	3 995	...	1 451	727	560	347	1 307
1990	7 023	5 832	4 887	3 883	...	1 410	771	463	364	1 191
1989	6 679	5 532	4 615	3 661	...	1 414	792	444	322	1 147
1988	6 447	5 329	4 392	3 599	...	1 353	763	401	322	1 118
1987 [8]	6 326	5 440	4 468	3 691	...	1 394	702	357	475	886
Percent										
2001	100.0	81.8	69.1	61.5	8.7	18.5	10.1	7.6	3.3	18.2
2000 [2]	100.0	82.0	70.2	63.8	7.8	17.7	10.1	7.0	3.5	18.0
1999 [3]	100.0	80.8	68.4	61.3	8.1	18.4	9.9	7.5	3.8	19.2
1999	100.0	79.2	66.7	60.3	7.4	18.5	9.9	7.5	3.8	20.8
1998	100.0	78.9	66.1	59.8	7.9	19.4	11.0	7.5	3.2	21.1
1997 [4]	100.0	79.3	67.7	60.0	8.1	17.9	10.4	6.7	3.2	20.7
1996	100.0	78.9	66.7	58.5	9.5	17.6	10.6	6.6	2.7	21.1
1995	100.0	79.5	65.8	57.8	10.0	21.5	13.2	6.1	4.4	20.5
1994 [5]	100.0	79.8	64.1	56.7	10.5	23.3	13.3	7.5	6.4	20.2
1993 [6]	100.0	79.6	67.5	53.3	...	18.9	10.8	6.4	4.6	20.2
1992 [7]	100.0	80.1	66.8	54.1	...	18.8	10.6	6.5	4.0	20.4
1991	100.0	81.8	68.4	55.5	...	20.2	10.1	7.8	4.8	18.2
1990	100.0	83.0	69.6	55.3	...	20.1	11.0	6.6	5.2	17.0
1989	100.0	82.8	69.1	54.8	...	21.2	11.9	6.6	4.8	17.2
1988	100.0	82.7	68.1	55.8	...	21.0	11.8	6.2	5.0	17.3
1987 [8]	100.0	86.0	70.6	58.3	...	22.0	11.1	5.6	7.5	14.0
HISPANIC [13]										
Number										
2004	41 839	28 160	18 714	17 208	1 698	11 462	9 123	2 618	694	13 678
2003	40 425	27 188	18 183	16 788	1 551	10 716	8 505	2 462	639	13 237
2002	39 384	26 627	18 108	16 714	1 469	10 280	7 946	2 535	724	12 756
2001	37 438	25 021	17 322	15 965	1 390	9 227	7 074	2 295	704	12 417
2000 [2]	36 093	24 210	17 114	15 893	1 337	8 566	6 552	2 141	682	11 883
1999 [3]	34 773	23 311	16 634	15 275	1 398	8 168	6 253	1 979	626	11 462
1999	32 804	21 853	15 424	14 214	1 264	7 875	5 946	2 047	589	10 951
1998	31 689	20 493	14 377	13 310	1 133	7 401	5 585	2 026	503	11 196
1997 [4]	30 773	20 239	13 751	12 790	1 028	7 718	5 970	1 974	526	10 534
1996	29 703	19 730	13 151	12 140	1 105	7 784	6 255	1 806	474	9 974
1995	28 438	18 964	12 187	11 309	1 011	8 027	6 478	1 732	516	9 474
1994 [5]	27 521	18 244	11 743	10 729	1 208	7 829	6 226	1 677	630	9 277
1993 [6]	26 646	18 235	12 021	9 981	...	7 873	6 328	1 613	530	8 411
1992 [7]	25 682	17 242	11 330	9 786	...	7 099	5 703	1 578	523	8 441
1991	22 096	15 128	10 336	8 972	...	5 845	4 597	1 309	522	6 968
1990	21 437	14 479	10 281	8 948	...	5 169	3 912	1 269	519	6 958
1989	20 779	13 846	10 348	8 914	...	4 526	3 221	1 180	595	6 932
1988	20 076	13 684	10 188	8 831	...	4 414	3 125	1 114	594	6 391
1987 [8]	19 428	13 456	9 845	8 490	...	4 482	3 214	1 029	631	5 972

[1] Includes CHAMPUS (Comprehensive Health and Medical Plan for Uniformed Services)/Tricare, veterans', and military health care.
[2] Implementation of a 28,000 household sample expansion.
[3] Estimates reflect the results of follow-up verification questions and implementation of Census 2000-based population controls.
[4] Beginning with the 1998 CPS ASEC, people with no coverage other than access to Indian Health Service are no longer considered covered by health insurance; instead, they are considered to be uninsured. The effect of this change on the overall estimates of health insurance coverage is negligible; however, the decrease in the number of people covered by Medicaid may be partially due to this change.
[5] Health insurance questions were redesigned. Increases in estimates of employment-based and military health care coverage may be partially due to questionnaire changes. Overall coverage estimates were not affected.
[6] Data collection method changed from paper and pencil to computer-assisted interviewing.
[7] Implementation of 1990 census population controls.
[8] Implementation of a new CPS ASEC processing system.
[10] The 2001 CPS and earlier years asked respondents to report only one race. The reference groups for these years are: White, White not Hispanic, Black, and Asian and Pacific Islander.
[13] May be of any race.
. . . = Not available.

Table III-69. Health Insurance Coverage Status and Type of Coverage, by Race and Hispanic Origin, 1987–2004—*Continued*

(Number in thousands, percent.)

Year, race, and Hispanic origin	Total population	Covered by private or government health insurance								Not covered
		Total	Private health insurance			Government health insurance				
			Total	Employment-based	Direct purchase	Total	Medicaid	Medicare	Military health care [1]	
Percent										
2004	100.0	67.3	44.7	41.1	4.1	27.4	21.8	6.3	1.7	32.7
2003	100.0	67.3	45.0	41.5	3.8	26.5	21.0	6.1	1.6	32.7
2002	100.0	67.6	46.0	42.4	3.7	26.1	20.2	6.4	1.8	32.4
2001	100.0	66.8	46.3	42.6	3.7	24.6	18.9	6.1	1.9	33.2
2000 [2]	100.0	67.1	47.4	44.0	3.7	23.7	18.2	5.9	1.9	32.9
1999 [3]	100.0	67.0	47.8	43.9	4.0	23.5	18.0	5.7	1.8	33.0
1999	100.0	66.6	47.0	43.3	3.9	24.0	18.1	6.2	1.8	33.4
1998	100.0	64.7	45.4	42.0	3.6	23.4	17.6	6.4	1.6	35.3
1997 [4]	100.0	65.8	44.7	41.6	3.3	25.1	19.4	6.4	1.7	34.2
1996	100.0	66.4	44.3	40.9	3.7	26.2	21.1	6.1	1.6	33.6
1995	100.0	66.7	42.9	39.8	3.6	28.2	22.8	6.1	1.8	33.3
1994 [5]	100.0	66.3	42.7	39.0	4.4	28.4	22.6	6.1	2.3	33.7
1993 [6]	100.0	68.4	45.1	37.5	...	29.5	23.7	6.1	2.0	31.6
1992 [7]	100.0	67.1	44.1	38.1	...	27.6	22.2	6.1	2.0	32.9
1991	100.0	68.5	46.8	40.6	...	26.5	20.8	5.9	2.4	31.5
1990	100.0	67.5	48.0	41.7	...	24.1	18.2	5.9	2.4	32.5
1989	100.0	66.6	49.8	42.9	...	21.8	15.5	5.7	2.9	33.4
1988	100.0	68.2	50.7	44.0	...	22.0	15.6	5.5	3.0	31.8
1987 [8]	100.0	69.3	50.7	43.7	...	23.1	16.5	5.3	3.2	30.7

[1] Includes CHAMPUS (Comprehensive Health and Medical Plan for Uniformed Services)/Tricare, veterans', and military health care.
[2] Implementation of a 28,000 household sample expansion.
[3] Estimates reflect the results of follow-up verification questions and implementation of Census 2000-based population controls.
[4] Beginning with the 1998 CPS ASEC, people with no coverage other than access to Indian Health Service are no longer considered covered by health insurance; instead, they are considered to be uninsured. The effect of this change on the overall estimates of health insurance coverage is negligible; however, the decrease in the number of people covered by Medicaid may be partially due to this change.
[5] Health insurance questions were redesigned. Increases in estimates of employment-based and military health care coverage may be partially due to questionnaire changes. Overall coverage estimates were not affected.
[6] Data collection method changed from paper and pencil to computer-assisted interviewing.
[7] Implementation of 1990 census population controls.
[8] Implementation of a new CPS ASEC processing system.
. . . = Not available.

TABLE III-70. HEALTH INSURANCE COVERAGE STATUS AND TYPE OF COVERAGE, BY AGE, 1987–2004

This table presents the number and percentage of insured persons from 1987 to 2004 by private and government health insurance categories and age categories. As in the previous table, private health insurance is divided into employment-based versus direct purchase insurance, while government health insurance is divided into Medicaid, Medicare, and military health care (including programs for active duty, retired, families of servicemen, and Department of Veterans Affairs). The survey was based on data that underreported Medicare and Medicaid coverage as compared with enrollment and participation data from the Centers for Medicare and Medicaid Services. Changes in Medicaid coverage estimates from one year to the next should be viewed with caution.

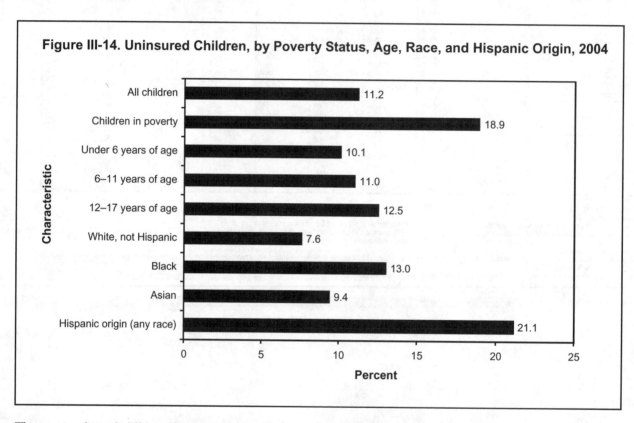

Figure III-14. Uninsured Children, by Poverty Status, Age, Race, and Hispanic Origin, 2004

The proportion of children (under 18 years of age) without health insurance in 2004 was 11.2 percent. The likelihood of health insurance coverage varied by poverty status, age, race, and Hispanic origin. Children in poverty had the highest rate (18.9 percent) of no health insurance coverage in 2004. Children 12 to 17 years old were more likely to be uninsured than those under 12 years of age (12.5 percent, compared with 10.5 percent). About 21.1 percent of Hispanic children lacked health insurance in 2004, compared with 7.6 percent of non-Hispanic White children, 13.0 percent of Black children, and 9.4 percent of Asian children.

Table III-70. Health Insurance Coverage Status and Type of Coverage, by Age, 1987–2004

(Number in thousands, percent.)

Year and age	Total population	Covered by private or government health insurance									Not covered
		Total	Private health insurance			Government health insurance					
			Total	Employment-based	Direct purchase	Total	Medicaid	Medicare	Military health care [1]	
ALL AGES											
Number											
2004	291 155	245 335	198 262	174 174	26 961	79 086	37 514	39 745	10 680	45 820
2003	288 280	243 320	197 869	174 020	26 486	76 755	35 647	39 456	9 979	44 961
2002	285 933	242 360	198 973	175 296	26 639	73 624	33 246	38 448	10 063	43 574
2001	282 082	240 875	199 860	176 551	26 057	71 295	31 601	38 043	9 552	41 207
2000 [2]	279 517	239 714	201 060	177 848	26 524	69 037	29 533	37 740	9 099	39 804
1999 [3]	276 804	236 576	198 841	175 101	27 415	67 683	28 506	36 923	8 648	40 228
1999	274 087	231 533	194 599	172 023	26 179	66 176	27 890	36 066	8 530	42 554
1998	271 743	227 462	190 861	168 576	25 948	66 087	27 854	35 887	8 747	44 281
1997 [4]	269 094	225 646	188 532	165 091	27 158	66 685	28 956	35 590	8 527	43 448
1996	266 792	225 077	187 395	163 221	28 335	69 000	31 451	35 227	8 712	41 716
1995	264 314	223 733	185 881	161 453	30 188	69 776	31 877	34 655	9 375	40 582
1994 [5]	262 105	222 387	184 318	159 634	31 349	70 163	31 645	33 901	11 165	39 718
1993 [6]	259 753	220 040	182 351	148 318	. . .	68 554	31 749	33 097	9 560	39 713
1992 [7]	256 830	218 189	181 466	148 796	. . .	66 244	29 416	33 230	9 510	38 641
1991	251 447	216 003	181 375	150 077	. . .	63 882	26 880	32 907	9 820	35 445
1990	248 886	214 167	182 135	150 215	. . .	60 965	24 261	32 260	9 922	34 719
1989	246 191	212 807	183 610	151 644	. . .	57 382	21 185	31 495	9 870	33 385
1988	243 685	211 005	182 019	150 940	. . .	56 850	20 728	30 925	10 105	32 680
1987 [8]	241 187	210 161	182 160	149 739	. . .	56 282	20 211	30 458	10 542	31 026
Percent											
2004	100.0	84.3	68.1	59.8	9.3	27.2	12.9	13.7	3.7	15.7
2003	100.0	84.4	68.6	60.4	9.2	26.6	12.4	13.7	3.5	15.6
2002	100.0	84.8	69.6	61.3	9.3	25.7	11.6	13.4	3.5	15.2
2001	100.0	85.4	70.9	62.6	9.2	25.3	11.2	13.5	3.4	14.6
2000 [2]	100.0	85.8	71.9	63.6	9.5	24.7	10.6	13.5	3.3	14.2
1999 [3]	100.0	85.5	71.8	63.3	9.9	24.5	10.3	13.3	3.1	14.5
1999	100.0	84.5	71.0	62.8	9.6	24.1	10.2	13.2	3.1	15.5
1998	100.0	83.7	70.2	62.0	9.5	24.3	10.3	13.2	3.2	16.3
1997 [4]	100.0	83.9	70.1	61.4	10.1	24.8	10.0	8.0	2.0	2.0
1996	100.0	84.4	70.2	61.2	10.6	25.9	11.0	8.0	2.0	3.0
1995	100.0	84.6	70.3	61.1	11.4	26.4	12.0	1.0	1.0	5.0
1994 [5]	100.0	84.8	70.3	60.9	12.0	26.8	12.0	1.0	9.0	3.0
1993 [6]	100.0	84.7	70.2	57.1	. . .	26.4	12.0	2.0	7.0	7.0
1992 [7]	100.0	85.0	70.7	57.9	. . .	25.8	11.0	5.0	9.0	7.0
1991	100.0	85.9	72.1	59.7	. . .	25.4	10.0	7.0	1.0	9.0
1990	100.0	86.1	73.2	60.4	. . .	24.5	9.7	13.0	4.0	13.9
1989	100.0	86.4	74.6	61.6	. . .	23.3	8.6	12.8	4.0	13.6
1988	100.0	86.6	74.7	61.9	. . .	23.3	8.5	13.0	4.0	13.4
1987 [8]	100.0	87.1	75.5	62.1	. . .	23.3	8.4	12.6	4.0	12.9
UNDER 18 YEARS											
Number											
2004	73 821	65 553	48 462	44 892	4 166	21 922	19 847	500	2 045	8 269
2003	73 580	65 207	48 475	45 004	3 893	21 389	19 392	483	2 021	8 373
2002	73 312	64 781	49 473	46 182	3 864	19 662	17 526	524	2 148	8 531
2001	72 628	64 118	49 647	46 439	3 624	18 822	16 502	423	2 381	8 509
2000 [2]	72 314	63 697	50 499	47 431	3 586	17 658	15 090	518	2 563	8 617
1999 [3]	72 281	62 996	50 300	46 834	4 052	16 793	14 697	364	2 076	9 285
1999	72 325	62 302	49 822	46 594	3 868	16 579	14 479	355	2 080	10 023
1998	72 022	60 949	48 627	45 593	3 666	16 400	14 274	325	2 240	11 073
1997 [4]	71 682	60 939	47 968	44 869	3 672	16 800	14 683	395	2 163	10 743
1996	71 224	60 670	47 219	44 054	3 865	17 749	15 502	484	2 291	10 554
1995	71 148	61 353	47 021	43 822	4 217	18 755	16 524	348	2 336	9 795
1994 [5]	70 509	60 505	46 266	42 966	4 634	18 559	16 132	228	2 708	10 003
1993 [6]	69 766	60 192	47 017	39 745	. . .	18 696	16 693	48	2 307	9 574
1992 [7]	68 720	60 005	47 183	40 382	. . .	17 294	15 109	97	2 378	8 716
1991	66 173	57 794	46 114	39 683	. . .	15 792	13 514	52	2 425	8 379
1990	65 290	56 786	46 436	39 981	. . .	14 300	12 094	88	2 408	8 504
1989	64 343	55 795	47 376	40 610	. . .	12 345	10 100	43	2 425	8 548
1988	63 902	55 552	46 944	40 750	. . .	12 270	9 961	62	2 469	8 350
1987 [8]	63 499	55 306	46 763	40 577	. . .	12 071	9 681	53	2 567	8 193

[1] Includes CHAMPUS (Comprehensive Health and Medical Plan for Uniformed Services)/Tricare, veterans', and military health care.
[2] Implementation of a 28,000 household sample expansion.
[3] Estimates reflect the results of follow-up verification questions and implementation of Census 2000-based population controls.
[4] Beginning with the 1998 CPS ASEC, people with no coverage other than access to Indian Health Service are no longer considered covered by health insurance; instead, they are considered to be uninsured. The effect of this change on the overall estimates of health insurance coverage is negligible; however, the decrease in the number of people covered by Medicaid may be partially due to this change.
[5] Health insurance questions were redesigned. Increases in estimates of employment-based and military health care coverage may be partially due to questionnaire changes. Overall coverage estimates were not affected.
[6] Data collection method changed from paper and pencil to computer-assisted interviewing.
[7] Implementation of 1990 census population controls.
[8] Implementation of a new CPS ASEC processing system.
. . . = Not available.

Table III-70. Health Insurance Coverage Status and Type of Coverage, by Age, 1987–2004—*Continued*

(Number in thousands, percent.)

Year and age	Total population	Covered by private or government health insurance								Not covered
		Total	Private health insurance			Government health insurance				
			Total	Employment-based	Direct purchase	Total	Medicaid	Medicare	Military health care[1]	
Percent										
2004	100.0	88.8	65.6	60.8	5.6	29.7	26.9	0.7	2.8	11.2
2003	100.0	88.6	65.9	61.2	5.3	29.1	26.4	0.7	2.7	11.4
2002	100.0	88.4	67.5	63.0	5.3	26.8	23.9	0.7	2.9	11.6
2001	100.0	88.3	68.4	63.9	5.0	25.9	22.7	0.6	3.3	11.7
2000[2]	100.0	88.1	69.8	65.6	5.0	24.4	20.9	0.7	3.5	11.9
1999[3]	100.0	87.2	69.6	64.8	5.6	23.2	20.3	0.5	2.9	12.8
1999	100.0	86.1	68.9	64.4	5.3	22.9	20.0	0.5	2.9	13.9
1998	100.0	84.6	67.5	63.3	5.1	22.8	19.8	0.5	3.1	15.4
1997[4]	100.0	85.0	66.9	62.6	5.1	23.4	20.5	0.6	3.0	15.0
1996	100.0	85.2	66.3	61.9	5.4	24.9	21.8	0.7	3.2	14.8
1995	100.0	86.2	66.1	61.6	5.9	26.4	23.2	0.5	3.3	13.8
1994[5]	100.0	85.8	65.6	60.9	6.6	26.3	22.9	0.3	3.8	14.2
1993[6]	100.0	86.3	67.4	57.0	...	26.8	23.9	0.1	3.3	13.7
1992[7]	100.0	87.3	68.7	58.8	...	25.2	22.0	0.1	3.5	12.7
1991	100.0	87.3	69.7	60.0	...	23.9	20.4	0.1	3.7	12.7
1990	100.0	87.0	71.1	61.2	...	21.9	18.5	0.1	3.7	13.0
1989	100.0	86.7	73.6	63.1	...	19.2	15.7	0.1	3.8	13.3
1988	100.0	86.9	73.5	63.8	...	19.2	15.6	0.1	3.9	13.1
1987[8]	100.0	87.1	73.6	63.9	...	19.0	15.2	0.1	4.0	12.9
18–24 YEARS										
Number										
2004	27 972	19 200	16 229	12 966	1 495	4 022	3 196	212	804	8 772
2003	27 824	19 410	16 526	13 434	1 596	3 929	3 016	176	902	8 414
2002	27 438	19 310	16 562	13 429	1 566	3 738	2 909	183	779	8 128
2001	27 312	19 640	17 012	13 766	1 634	3 642	2 831	180	742	7 673
2000[2]	26 815	19 409	17 086	14 151	1 533	3 361	2 508	207	805	7 406
1999[3]	26 326	18 990	16 542	13 558	1 564	3 485	2 684	152	787	7 336
1999	26 532	18 844	16 438	13 535	1 469	3 450	2 643	152	798	7 688
1998	25 967	18 191	15 872	13 108	1 514	3 347	2 538	149	795	7 776
1997[4]	25 201	17 619	15 256	12 638	1 558	3 283	2 555	155	692	7 582
1996	24 987	17 770	15 066	12 423	1 528	3 750	2 909	156	829	7 217
1995	24 843	17 847	14 961	12 492	1 688	4 018	3 003	129	1 034	6 997
1994[5]	25 158	18 446	15 528	12 895	1 854	4 246	3 179	89	1 179	6 712
1993[6]	25 475	18 645	15 668	11 133	...	4 087	2 976	148	1 115	6 830
1992[7]	25 717	18 146	15 155	10 981	...	3 826	2 875	178	964	7 570
1991	24 436	17 851	15 168	11 474	...	3 405	2 477	163	940	6 585
1990	24 901	18 408	15 913	11 999	...	3 270	2 204	161	1 094	6 493
1989	25 311	18 954	16 638	12 929	...	3 114	2 057	167	1 031	6 357
1988	25 628	19 354	16 965	13 098	...	3 082	2 033	170	1 007	6 274
1987[8]	26 053	19 945	17 434	13 429	...	3 280	1 968	196	1 273	6 108
Percent										
2004	100.0	68.6	58.0	46.4	5.3	14.4	11.4	0.8	2.9	31.4
2003	100.0	69.8	59.4	48.3	5.7	14.1	10.8	0.6	3.2	30.2
2002	100.0	70.4	60.4	48.9	5.7	13.6	10.6	0.7	2.8	29.6
2001	100.0	71.9	62.3	50.4	6.0	13.3	10.4	0.7	2.7	28.1
2000[2]	100.0	72.4	63.7	52.8	5.7	12.5	9.4	0.8	3.0	27.6
1999[3]	100.0	72.1	62.8	51.5	5.9	13.2	10.2	0.6	3.0	27.9
1999	100.0	71.0	62.0	51.0	5.5	13.0	10.0	0.6	3.0	29.0
1998	100.0	70.1	61.1	50.5	5.8	12.9	9.8	0.6	3.1	29.9
1997[4]	100.0	69.9	60.5	50.1	6.2	13.0	10.1	0.6	2.7	30.1
1996	100.0	71.1	60.3	49.7	6.1	15.0	11.6	0.6	3.3	28.9
1995	100.0	71.8	60.2	50.3	6.8	16.2	12.1	0.5	4.2	28.2
1994[5]	100.0	73.3	61.7	51.3	7.4	16.9	12.6	0.4	4.7	26.7
1993[6]	100.0	73.2	61.5	43.7	...	16.0	11.7	0.6	4.4	26.8
1992[7]	100.0	70.6	58.9	42.7	...	14.9	11.2	0.7	3.7	29.4
1991	100.0	73.1	62.1	47.0	...	13.9	10.1	0.7	3.8	26.9
1990	100.0	73.9	63.9	48.2	...	13.1	8.9	0.6	4.4	26.1
1989	100.0	74.9	65.7	51.1	...	12.3	8.1	0.7	4.1	25.1
1988	100.0	75.5	66.2	51.1	...	12.0	7.9	0.7	3.9	24.5
1987[8]	100.0	76.6	66.9	51.5	...	12.6	7.6	0.8	4.9	23.4

[1]Includes CHAMPUS (Comprehensive Health and Medical Plan for Uniformed Services)/Tricare, veterans', and military health care.
[2]Implementation of a 28,000 household sample expansion.
[3]Estimates reflect the results of follow-up verification questions and implementation of Census 2000-based population controls.
[4]Beginning with the 1998 CPS ASEC, people with no coverage other than access to Indian Health Service are no longer considered covered by health insurance; instead, they are considered to be uninsured. The effect of this change on the overall estimates of health insurance coverage is negligible; however, the decrease in the number of people covered by Medicaid may be partially due to this change.
[5]Health insurance questions were redesigned. Increases in estimates of employment-based and military health care coverage may be partially due to questionnaire changes. Overall coverage estimates were not affected.
[6]Data collection method changed from paper and pencil to computer-assisted interviewing.
[7]Implementation of 1990 census population controls.
[8]Implementation of a new CPS ASEC processing system.
. . . = Not available.

Table III-70. Health Insurance Coverage Status and Type of Coverage, by Age, 1987–2004—*Continued*

(Number in thousands, percent.)

Year and age	Total population	Covered by private or government health insurance								Not covered
		Total	Private health insurance			Government health insurance				
			Total	Employment-based	Direct purchase	Total	Medicaid	Medicare	Military health care [1]	
25–34 YEARS										
Number										
2004	39 307	29 130	25 765	24 027	2 266	4 578	3 408	482	982	10 177
2003	39 201	28 856	25 606	23 946	2 058	4 210	3 073	538	898	10 345
2002	39 243	29 474	26 492	24 800	2 098	3 944	2 801	455	922	9 769
2001	38 670	29 619	26 905	25 306	2 072	3 653	2 587	489	817	9 051
2000 [2]	38 865	30 358	27 755	26 211	2 033	3 551	2 480	403	922	8 507
1999 [3]	39 031	30 309	27 730	26 153	2 114	3 578	2 458	332	974	8 723
1999	37 786	29 031	26 567	25 150	1 939	3 429	2 344	323	940	8 755
1998	38 474	29 347	26 726	25 096	2 049	3 616	2 476	423	991	9 127
1997 [4]	39 354	30 192	27 138	25 496	2 157	3 956	2 842	365	1 011	9 163
1996	40 256	31 283	27 915	26 205	2 325	4 508	3 264	433	1 086	8 974
1995	40 919	31 561	27 938	26 020	2 601	4 722	3 496	364	1 146	9 357
1994 [5]	41 388	32 274	28 386	26 417	2 874	5 261	3 748	359	1 435	9 115
1993 [6]	41 946	32 869	28 629	25 432	. . .	5 345	4 002	515	1 176	9 076
1992 [7]	42 356	33 389	28 994	26 164	. . .	5 277	3 774	576	1 283	8 967
1991	42 496	33 940	29 808	27 103	. . .	5 031	3 542	495	1 327	8 555
1990	42 905	34 581	30 875	27 920	. . .	4 634	3 185	471	1 296	8 324
1989	43 240	35 326	31 912	28 867	. . .	4 217	2 692	363	1 396	7 914
1988	43 239	35 319	31 996	29 140	. . .	4 195	2 699	342	1 374	7 920
1987 [8]	42 953	35 645	32 296	29 198	. . .	4 247	2 702	405	1 423	7 308
Percent										
2004	100.0	74.1	65.5	61.1	5.8	11.6	8.7	1.2	2.5	25.9
2003	100.0	73.6	65.3	61.1	5.2	10.7	7.8	1.4	2.3	26.4
2002	100.0	75.1	67.5	63.2	5.3	10.1	7.1	1.2	2.3	24.9
2001	100.0	76.6	69.6	65.4	5.4	9.4	6.7	1.3	2.1	23.4
2000 [2]	100.0	78.1	71.4	67.4	5.2	9.1	6.4	1.0	2.4	21.9
1999 [3]	100.0	77.7	71.0	67.0	5.4	9.2	6.3	0.8	2.5	22.3
1999	100.0	76.8	70.3	66.6	5.1	9.1	6.2	0.9	2.5	23.2
1998	100.0	76.3	69.5	65.2	5.3	9.4	6.4	1.1	2.6	23.7
1997 [4]	100.0	76.7	69.0	64.8	5.5	10.1	7.2	0.9	2.6	23.3
1996	100.0	77.7	69.3	65.1	5.8	11.2	8.1	1.1	2.7	22.3
1995	100.0	77.1	68.3	63.6	6.4	11.5	8.5	0.9	2.8	22.9
1994 [5]	100.0	78.0	68.6	63.8	6.9	12.7	9.1	0.9	3.5	22.0
1993 [6]	100.0	78.4	68.3	60.6	. . .	12.7	9.5	1.2	2.8	21.6
1992 [7]	100.0	78.8	68.5	61.8	. . .	12.5	8.9	1.4	3.0	21.2
1991	100.0	79.9	70.1	63.8	. . .	11.8	8.3	1.2	3.1	20.1
1990	100.0	80.6	72.0	65.1	. . .	10.8	7.4	1.1	3.0	19.4
1989	100.0	81.7	73.8	66.8	. . .	9.8	6.2	0.8	3.2	18.3
1988	100.0	81.7	74.0	67.4	. . .	9.7	6.2	0.8	3.2	18.3
1987 [8]	100.0	83.0	75.2	68.0	. . .	9.9	6.3	0.9	3.3	17.0
35–44 YEARS										
Number										
2004	43 350	35 240	31 883	29 824	2 773	4 680	3 135	900	1 129	8 110
2003	43 573	35 688	32 533	30 386	2 793	4 420	2 860	940	1 111	7 885
2002	44 074	36 292	33 240	31 180	2 817	4 240	2 728	881	1 121	7 781
2001	44 284	37 153	34 315	32 386	2 649	4 003	2 532	860	1 066	7 131
2000 [2]	44 566	37 669	35 033	33 004	2 723	3 920	2 390	780	1 206	6 898
1999 [3]	44 474	37 748	34 908	32 620	3 151	4 028	2 390	825	1 257	6 726
1999	44 805	37 428	34 624	32 423	3 057	3 988	2 340	856	1 256	7 377
1998	44 744	37 036	34 134	32 019	2 937	4 190	2 579	749	1 232	7 708
1997 [4]	44 462	36 763	33 673	31 560	2 897	4 257	2 700	878	1 161	7 699
1996	43 960	36 809	33 448	31 231	3 074	4 657	3 109	767	1 173	7 152
1995	43 078	35 946	32 813	30 552	3 250	4 399	2 863	775	1 210	7 132
1994 [5]	42 334	35 555	32 271	29 894	3 714	4 628	2 918	711	1 415	6 780
1993 [6]	41 528	34 537	31 441	28 115	. . .	4 189	2 619	647	1 276	6 991
1992 [7]	40 747	34 332	31 261	28 252	. . .	3 990	2 310	718	1 324	6 415
1991	39 578	33 902	31 118	28 339	. . .	3 710	2 036	559	1 414	5 676
1990	38 665	33 534	31 046	28 136	. . .	3 542	1 894	578	1 368	5 131
1989	37 195	32 541	30 329	27 641	. . .	3 156	1 598	514	1 300	4 654
1988	35 873	31 294	29 168	26 651	. . .	3 126	1 506	463	1 397	4 579
1987 [8]	34 692	30 557	28 353	25 868	. . .	3 186	1 590	447	1 373	4 135

[1] Includes CHAMPUS (Comprehensive Health and Medical Plan for Uniformed Services)/Tricare, veterans', and military health care.
[2] Implementation of a 28,000 household sample expansion.
[3] Estimates reflect the results of follow-up verification questions and implementation of Census 2000-based population controls.
[4] Beginning with the 1998 CPS ASEC, people with no coverage other than access to Indian Health Service are no longer considered covered by health insurance; instead, they are considered to be uninsured. The effect of this change on the overall estimates of health insurance coverage is negligible; however, the decrease in the number of people covered by Medicaid may be partially due to this change.
[5] Health insurance questions were redesigned. Increases in estimates of employment-based and military health care coverage may be partially due to questionnaire changes. Overall coverage estimates were not affected.
[6] Data collection method changed from paper and pencil to computer-assisted interviewing.
[7] Implementation of 1990 census population controls.
[8] Implementation of a new CPS ASEC processing system.
. . . = Not available.

Table III-70. Health Insurance Coverage Status and Type of Coverage, by Age, 1987–2004—*Continued*

(Number in thousands, percent.)

Year and age	Total population	Covered by private or government health insurance									Not covered
		Total	Private health insurance			Government health insurance					
			Total	Employment-based	Direct purchase	Total	Medicaid	Medicare	Military health care [1]		

Percent

Year and age	Total population	Total	Total	Employment-based	Direct purchase	Total	Medicaid	Medicare	Military health care [1]	Not covered
2004	100.0	81.3	73.5	68.8	6.4	10.8	7.2	2.1	2.6	18.7
2003	100.0	81.9	74.7	69.7	6.4	10.1	6.6	2.2	2.6	18.1
2002	100.0	82.3	75.4	70.7	6.4	9.6	6.2	2.0	2.5	17.7
2001	100.0	83.9	77.5	73.1	6.0	9.0	5.7	1.9	2.4	16.1
2000[2]	100.0	84.5	78.6	74.1	6.1	8.8	5.4	1.8	2.7	15.5
1999[3]	100.0	84.9	78.5	73.3	7.1	9.1	5.4	1.9	2.8	15.1
1999	100.0	83.5	77.3	72.4	6.8	8.9	5.2	1.9	2.8	16.5
1998	100.0	82.8	76.3	71.6	6.6	9.4	5.8	1.7	2.8	17.2
1997[4]	100.0	82.7	75.7	71.0	6.5	9.6	6.1	2.0	2.6	17.3
1996	100.0	83.7	76.1	71.0	7.0	10.6	7.1	1.7	2.7	16.3
1995	100.0	83.4	76.2	70.9	7.5	10.2	6.6	1.8	2.8	16.6
1994[5]	100.0	84.0	76.2	70.6	8.8	10.9	6.9	1.7	3.3	16.0
1993[6]	100.0	83.2	75.7	67.7	...	10.1	6.3	1.6	3.1	16.8
1992[7]	100.0	84.3	76.7	69.3	...	9.8	5.7	1.8	3.2	15.7
1991	100.0	85.7	78.6	71.6	...	9.4	5.1	1.4	3.6	14.3
1990	100.0	86.7	80.3	72.8	...	9.2	4.9	1.5	3.5	13.3
1989	100.0	87.5	81.5	74.3	...	8.5	4.3	1.4	3.5	12.5
1988	100.0	87.2	81.3	74.3	...	8.7	4.2	1.3	3.9	12.8
1987[8]	100.0	88.1	81.7	74.6	...	9.2	4.6	1.3	4.0	11.9

45–54 YEARS

Number

Year and age	Total population	Total	Total	Employment-based	Direct purchase	Total	Medicaid	Medicare	Military health care [1]	Not covered
2004	41 960	35 700	32 414	30 088	3 215	4 847	2 595	1 548	1 425	6 260
2003	41 068	35 108	32 000	29 722	3 198	4 569	2 359	1 569	1 369	5 961
2002	40 234	34 648	31 724	29 617	3 087	4 345	2 227	1 382	1 351	5 586
2001	39 545	34 365	31 649	29 487	3 087	3 990	2 071	1 331	1 170	5 179
2000[2]	38 720	33 955	31 373	29 329	3 042	3 964	1 996	1 384	1 169	4 764
1999[3]	37 334	32 640	30 230	28 156	3 180	3 682	1 769	1 162	1 244	4 694
1999	36 631	31 737	29 440	27 489	3 034	3 544	1 693	1 124	1 209	4 893
1998	35 232	30 427	28 153	26 400	2 782	3 522	1 610	1 139	1 225	4 805
1997[4]	34 057	29 319	27 063	25 099	2 967	3 677	1 766	1 133	1 281	4 738
1996	33 013	28 504	26 266	24 329	2 889	3 705	1 875	948	1 282	4 509
1995	31 584	27 398	25 269	23 332	3 227	3 495	1 756	856	1 267	4 186
1994[5]	30 693	26 752	24 874	22 897	3 330	3 342	1 499	794	1 406	3 942
1993[6]	29 522	25 424	23 332	20 654	...	3 248	1 546	812	1 244	4 098
1992[7]	28 332	24 311	22 354	19 862	...	2 929	1 326	746	1 155	4 021
1991	27 025	23 695	21 973	19 751	...	2 797	1 186	671	1 174	3 331
1990	25 686	22 381	20 712	18 485	...	2 645	1 124	644	1 161	3 306
1989	25 304	22 167	20 658	18 437	...	2 497	1 017	582	1 123	3 137
1988	24 622	21 686	20 171	18 131	...	2 574	984	567	1 247	2 935
1987[8]	23 861	21 167	19 765	17 574	...	2 344	890	495	1 151	2 695

Percent

Year and age	Total population	Total	Total	Employment-based	Direct purchase	Total	Medicaid	Medicare	Military health care [1]	Not covered
2004	100.0	85.1	77.2	71.7	7.7	11.6	6.2	3.7	3.4	14.9
2003	100.0	85.5	77.9	72.4	7.8	11.1	5.7	3.8	3.3	14.5
2002	100.0	86.1	78.8	73.6	7.7	10.8	5.5	3.4	3.4	13.9
2001	100.0	86.9	80.0	74.6	7.8	10.1	5.2	3.4	3.0	13.1
2000[2]	100.0	87.7	81.0	75.7	7.9	10.2	5.2	3.6	3.0	12.3
1999[3]	100.0	87.4	81.0	75.4	8.5	9.9	4.7	3.1	3.3	12.6
1999	100.0	86.6	80.4	75.0	8.3	9.7	4.6	3.1	3.3	13.4
1998	100.0	86.4	79.9	74.9	7.9	10.0	4.6	3.2	3.5	13.6
1997[4]	100.0	86.1	79.5	73.7	8.7	10.8	5.2	3.3	3.8	13.9
1996	100.0	86.3	79.6	73.7	8.8	11.2	5.7	2.9	3.9	13.7
1995	100.0	86.7	80.0	73.9	10.2	11.1	5.6	2.7	4.0	13.3
1994[5]	100.0	87.2	81.0	74.6	10.8	10.9	4.9	2.6	4.6	12.8
1993[6]	100.0	86.1	79.0	70.0	...	11.0	5.2	2.8	4.2	13.9
1992[7]	100.0	85.8	78.9	70.1	...	10.3	4.7	2.6	4.1	14.2
1991	100.0	87.7	81.3	73.1	...	10.3	4.4	2.5	4.3	12.3
1990	100.0	87.1	80.6	72.0	...	10.3	4.4	2.5	4.5	12.9
1989	100.0	87.6	81.6	72.9	...	9.9	4.0	2.3	4.4	12.4
1988	100.0	88.1	81.9	73.6	...	10.5	4.0	2.3	5.1	11.9
1987[8]	100.0	88.7	82.8	73.7	...	9.8	3.7	2.1	4.8	11.3

[1]Includes CHAMPUS (Comprehensive Health and Medical Plan for Uniformed Services)/Tricare, veterans', and military health care.
[2]Implementation of a 28,000 household sample expansion.
[3]Estimates reflect the results of follow-up verification questions and implementation of Census 2000-based population controls.
[4]Beginning with the 1998 CPS ASEC, people with no coverage other than access to Indian Health Service are no longer considered covered by health insurance; instead, they are considered to be uninsured. The effect of this change on the overall estimates of health insurance coverage is negligible; however, the decrease in the number of people covered by Medicaid may be partially due to this change.
[5]Health insurance questions were redesigned. Increases in estimates of employment-based and military health care coverage may be partially due to questionnaire changes. Overall coverage estimates were not affected.
[6]Data collection method changed from paper and pencil to computer-assisted interviewing.
[7]Implementation of 1990 census population controls.
[8]Implementation of a new CPS ASEC processing system.
. . . = Not available.

Table III-70. Health Insurance Coverage Status and Type of Coverage, by Age, 1987–2004—*Continued*

(Number in thousands, percent.)

Year and age	Total population	Covered by private or government health insurance								Not covered
		Total	Private health insurance			Government health insurance				
			Total	Employment-based	Direct purchase	Total	Medicaid	Medicare	Military health care [1]	

55–64 YEARS

Number

2004	29 532	25 596	22 174	19 872	3 066	5 442	2 036	2 651	1 785	3 936
2003	28 375	24 679	21 569	19 324	2 987	4 893	1 757	2 494	1 471	3 696
2002	27 399	23 879	20 797	18 505	3 071	4 882	1 773	2 392	1 482	3 521
2001	25 874	22 482	19 581	17 521	2 761	4 567	1 807	2 301	1 220	3 392
2000 [2]	24 672	21 312	18 614	16 444	2 936	4 185	1 731	2 159	1 024	3 360
1999 [3]	23 981	20 785	18 335	16 195	2 932	4 033	1 551	2 084	1 053	3 196
1999	23 387	19 992	17 654	15 662	2 763	3 874	1 474	2 024	1 014	3 395
1998	22 909	19 475	17 179	15 210	2 688	3 844	1 415	2 016	1 077	3 434
1997 [4]	22 255	19 065	16 748	14 466	3 052	3 771	1 509	1 794	1 095	3 190
1996	21 475	18 501	16 258	14 031	3 087	3 916	1 577	1 822	1 052	2 974
1995	21 084	18 270	16 124	14 098	3 056	3 790	1 415	1 660	1 231	2 814
1994 [5]	20 755	17 878	15 735	13 496	3 202	3 836	1 295	1 545	1 471	2 877
1993 [6]	20 737	17 957	15 938	13 291	. . .	3 499	1 204	1 536	1 234	2 781
1992 [7]	20 528	17 925	15 876	13 212	. . .	3 540	1 152	1 624	1 242	2 603
1991	21 150	18 520	16 479	13 613	. . .	3 681	1 234	1 589	1 362	2 630
1990	21 345	18 660	16 586	13 691	. . .	3 675	1 178	1 523	1 444	2 685
1989	21 232	18 765	16 693	13 711	. . .	3 715	1 144	1 575	1 490	2 467
1988	21 399	19 052	16 934	13 999	. . .	3 772	1 094	1 597	1 532	2 347
1987 [8]	21 641	19 361	17 423	14 262	. . .	3 726	993	1 528	1 643	2 281

Percent

2004	100.0	86.7	75.1	67.3	10.4	18.4	6.9	9.0	6.0	13.3
2003	100.0	87.0	76.0	68.1	10.5	17.2	6.2	8.8	5.2	13.0
2002	100.0	87.2	75.9	67.5	11.2	17.8	6.5	8.7	5.4	12.8
2001	100.0	86.9	75.7	67.7	10.7	17.7	7.0	8.9	4.7	13.1
2000 [2]	100.0	86.4	75.4	66.7	11.9	17.0	7.0	8.8	4.2	13.6
1999 [3]	100.0	86.7	76.5	67.5	12.2	16.8	6.5	8.7	4.4	13.3
1999	100.0	85.5	75.5	67.0	11.8	16.6	6.3	8.7	4.3	14.5
1998	100.0	85.0	75.0	66.4	11.7	16.8	6.2	8.8	4.7	15.0
1997 [4]	100.0	85.7	75.3	65.0	13.7	16.9	6.8	8.1	4.9	14.3
1996	100.0	86.2	75.7	65.3	14.4	18.2	7.3	8.5	4.9	13.8
1995	100.0	86.7	76.5	66.9	14.5	18.0	6.7	7.9	5.8	13.3
1994 [5]	100.0	86.1	75.8	65.0	15.4	18.5	6.2	7.4	7.1	13.9
1993 [6]	100.0	86.6	76.9	64.1	. . .	16.9	5.8	7.4	6.0	13.4
1992 [7]	100.0	87.3	77.3	64.4	. . .	17.2	5.6	7.9	6.1	12.7
1991	100.0	87.6	77.9	64.4	. . .	17.4	5.8	7.5	6.4	12.4
1990	100.0	87.4	77.7	64.1	. . .	17.2	5.5	7.1	6.8	12.6
1989	100.0	88.4	78.6	64.6	. . .	17.5	5.4	7.4	7.0	11.6
1988	100.0	89.0	79.1	65.4	. . .	17.6	5.1	7.5	7.2	11.0
1987 [8]	100.0	89.5	80.5	65.9	. . .	17.2	4.6	7.1	7.6	10.5

65 YEARS AND OVER

Number

2004	35 213	34 916	21 336	12 505	9 979	33 595	3 297	33 452	2 509	297
2003	34 659	34 373	21 159	12 204	9 962	33 345	3 190	33 257	2 206	286
2002	34 234	33 976	20 685	11 583	10 135	32 813	3 283	32 631	2 259	258
2001	33 769	33 498	20 751	11 645	10 229	32 618	3 270	32 458	2 156	272
2000 [2]	33 566	33 314	20 702	11 278	10 671	32 398	3 339	32 289	1 410	251
1999 [3]	33 377	33 109	20 796	11 584	10 422	32 083	2 956	32 004	1 257	268
1999	32 621	32 199	20 054	11 169	10 049	31 312	2 917	31 231	1 232	422
1998	32 394	32 036	20 171	11 150	10 312	31 167	2 962	31 085	1 186	358
1997 [4]	32 082	31 749	20 687	10 963	10 853	30 942	2 901	30 870	1 125	333
1996	31 877	31 541	21 224	10 948	11 567	30 714	3 215	30 616	998	336
1995	31 658	31 358	21 754	11 137	12 148	30 597	2 820	30 521	1 152	300
1994 [5]	31 267	30 977	21 259	11 071	11 742	30 291	2 875	30 176	1 550	290
1993 [6]	30 779	30 416	20 324	9 947	. . .	29 490	2 709	29 390	1 208	363
1992 [7]	30 430	30 082	20 643	9 944	. . .	29 387	2 869	29 290	1 163	349
1991	30 590	30 301	20 715	10 114	. . .	29 465	2 891	29 377	1 178	289
1990	30 093	29 816	20 566	10 002	. . .	28 898	2 582	28 795	1 151	276
1989	29 566	29 258	20 003	9 448	. . .	28 337	2 576	28 251	1 105	308
1988	29 022	28 747	19 841	9 171	. . .	27 831	2 451	27 724	1 079	275
1987 [8]	28 487	28 181	20 127	8 830	. . .	27 428	2 387	27 333	1 113	306

[1] Includes CHAMPUS (Comprehensive Health and Medical Plan for Uniformed Services)/Tricare, veterans', and military health care.
[2] Implementation of a 28,000 household sample expansion.
[3] Estimates reflect the results of follow-up verification questions and implementation of Census 2000-based population controls.
[4] Beginning with the 1998 CPS ASEC, people with no coverage other than access to Indian Health Service are no longer considered covered by health insurance; instead, they are considered to be uninsured. The effect of this change on the overall estimates of health insurance coverage is negligible; however, the decrease in the number of people covered by Medicaid may be partially due to this change.
[5] Health insurance questions were redesigned. Increases in estimates of employment-based and military health care coverage may be partially due to questionnaire changes. Overall coverage estimates were not affected.
[6] Data collection method changed from paper and pencil to computer-assisted interviewing.
[7] Implementation of 1990 census population controls.
[8] Implementation of a new CPS ASEC processing system.
. . . = Not available.

Table III-70. Health Insurance Coverage Status and Type of Coverage, by Age, 1987–2004—*Continued*

(Number in thousands, percent.)

Year and age	Total population	Covered by private or government health insurance								Not covered
		Total	Private health insurance			Government health insurance				
			Total	Employment-based	Direct purchase	Total	Medicaid	Medicare	Military health care [1]	
Percent										
2004	100.0	99.2	60.6	35.5	28.3	95.4	9.4	95.0	7.1	0.8
2003	100.0	99.2	61.0	35.2	28.7	96.2	9.2	96.0	6.4	0.8
2002	100.0	99.2	60.4	33.8	29.6	95.8	9.6	95.3	6.6	0.8
2001	100.0	99.2	61.5	34.5	30.3	96.6	9.7	96.1	6.4	0.8
2000 [2]	100.0	99.3	61.7	33.6	31.8	96.5	9.9	96.2	4.2	0.7
1999 [3]	100.0	99.2	62.3	34.7	31.2	96.1	8.9	95.9	3.8	0.8
1999	100.0	98.7	61.5	34.2	30.8	96.0	8.9	95.7	3.8	1.3
1998	100.0	98.9	62.3	34.4	31.8	96.2	9.1	96.0	3.7	1.1
1997 [4]	100.0	99.0	64.5	34.2	33.8	96.4	9.0	96.2	3.5	1.0
1996	100.0	98.9	66.6	34.3	36.3	96.4	10.1	96.0	3.1	1.1
1995	100.0	99.1	68.7	35.2	38.4	96.6	8.9	96.4	3.6	0.9
1994 [5]	100.0	99.1	68.0	35.4	37.6	96.9	9.2	96.5	5.0	0.9
1993 [6]	100.0	98.8	66.0	32.3	...	95.8	8.8	95.5	3.9	1.2
1992 [7]	100.0	98.9	67.8	32.7	...	96.6	9.4	96.3	3.8	1.1
1991	100.0	99.1	67.7	33.1	...	96.3	9.5	96.0	3.9	0.9
1990	100.0	99.1	68.3	33.2	...	96.0	8.6	95.7	3.8	0.9
1989	100.0	99.0	67.7	32.0	...	95.8	8.7	95.6	3.7	1.0
1988	100.0	99.1	68.4	31.6	...	95.9	8.4	95.5	3.7	0.9
1987 [8]	100.0	98.9	70.7	31.0	...	96.3	8.4	95.9	3.9	1.1

[1] Includes CHAMPUS (Comprehensive Health and Medical Plan for Uniformed Services)/Tricare, veterans', and military health care.
[2] Implementation of a 28,000 household sample expansion.
[3] Estimates reflect the results of follow-up verification questions and implementation of Census 2000-based population controls.
[4] Beginning with the 1998 CPS ASEC, people with no coverage other than access to Indian Health Service are no longer considered covered by health insurance; instead, they are considered to be uninsured. The effect of this change on the overall estimates of health insurance coverage is negligible; however, the decrease in the number of people covered by Medicaid may be partially due to this change.
[5] Health insurance questions were redesigned. Increases in estimates of employment-based and military health care coverage may be partially due to questionnaire changes. Overall coverage estimates were not affected.
[6] Data collection method changed from paper and pencil to computer-assisted interviewing.
[7] Implementation of 1990 census population controls.
[8] Implementation of a new CPS ASEC processing system.
... = Not available.

CHAPTER IV: MARRIAGE AND DIVORCE

TABLE IV-1. MARRIAGES AND DIVORCES, 2002–2004

The marriage rate fell slightly between 2002 and 2003, dropping from an annual rate of 7.9 per 1,000 total population to 7.6 per 1,000 total population. It remained stable in 2004. Reported divorce rates declined slightly between 2002 and 2004, falling from 3.9 to 3.7 per 1,000 total population annually. Events for nonresidents are included in the marriage and divorce figures (but not in the birth and death data shown in previous chapters). Divorce figures include reported annulments. Marriage data were not completely reported from Oklahoma, while divorce data were not reported from several states. (Non-reporting states changed somewhat each year—see footnote to Table IV-1.) The 12-month divorce rates shown in Table IV-1 were based solely on the combined number of divorces and total population of each reporting state and the District of Columbia. The National Center for Health Statistics (NCHS) does not publish 12-month counts for divorce, because they would be based on less than the full complement of states.

TABLE IV-2. NUMBER AND RATE OF MARRIAGES, BY MONTH, 2003–2004

This table shows monthly aggregate marriage counts and rates for the United States during 2003 and 2004. The marriage rate shown in this table is the annual rate that would have occurred if the observed monthly rate had held steady for 12 months. There was a noticeable increase in marriage counts and rates during the warmer months of the year.

Table IV-1. Marriages and Divorces, 2002–2004

(Number, rate per 1,000 population.)

Item	Number			Annual rate		
	2004	2003	2002	2004	2003	2002
Marriages [1]	2 223 822	2 224 379	2 254 000	7.6	7.6	7.9
Divorces [2]	...	...	...	3.7	3.8	3.9
Population base (in millions)	...	...	...	293.6	291.4	288.4

[1] Marriage rates may be underestimated due to incomplete reporting in Oklahoma.
[2] Divorce rates exclude data for California, Georgia, Hawaii, Indiana, and Louisiana in 2004; California, Hawaii, Indiana, Louisiana, and Oklahoma in 2003; and California, Indiana, Louisiana, and Oklahoma in 2002. Populations for these rates also exclude these states.
... = Not available.

Table IV-2. Number and Rate of Marriages, by Month, 2003–2004

(Number, rate per 1,000 population.)

Year and month	2004		2003	
	Number	Annual rate per 1,000 population [1]	Number	Annual rate per 1,000 population [1]
January	131 000	5.3	126 000	5.1
February	147 000	6.3	149 000	6.7
March	155 000	6.3	164 000	6.6
April	161 000	6.7	170 000	7.1
May	215 000	8.7	216 000	8.8
June	239 000	9.9	242 000	10.1
July	238 000	9.6	220 000	8.9
August	218 000	8.8	241 000	9.7
September	208 000	8.6	200 000	8.3
October	208 000	8.3	199 000	8.0
November	147 000	6.1	151 000	6.3
December	156 000	6.3	147 000	5.9

[1] Marriage rates may be underestimated due to incomplete reporting in Oklahoma.

TABLE IV-3. NUMBER OF MARRIAGES AND DIVORCES FOR EACH STATE, JULY 2003, JANUARY 2004, AND CUMULATIVE FIGURES, 2002–2004

This table shows state-specific counts for marriages and divorces for 2002 through 2004, with special focus on the months of July 2003 and January 2004. Due to incomplete reporting, marriage and divorce counts for Oklahoma were not included. Divorces were not reported from several states. Certain large states, such as California, Florida, New York, Ohio, Texas, and Nevada (a popular wedding destination), experienced declining marriage counts between 2002 and 2003, reflecting the drop in the national rates shown in Table IV-1. However, this pattern was not universal across all states. On average, July was the most popular wedding month, while January was the least popular. This contrast was most pronounced in states with cold winters, but was less noticeable in states with warmer climates, such as Florida and Nevada. Certain warm-weather states, such as Arizona, had peaks in the spring and fall (not shown). Differences in reported divorces by state in July and January did not seem to follow a specific pattern.

Table IV-3. Number of Marriages and Divorces for Each State, July 2003, January 2004, and Cumulative Figures, 2002–2004

(Number.)

State	Marriages Annual number 2004	2003	2002	January 2004	July 2003	Divorces Annual number 2004	2003	2002	January 2004	July 2003
Alabama	42 536	43 139	44 158	1 416	3 404	22 405	23 205	24 059	1 135	1 792
Alaska	5 594	5 237	5 327	75	723	2 829	2 498	2 957	275	211
Arizona [1]	37 882	35 873	36 199	3 383	2 742	24 403	24 248	25 896	1 699	2 129
Arkansas	36 806	36 445	38 721	1 807	3 849	16 874	16 452	16 708	954	1 193
California	172 302	194 914	217 880	21 921	22 525	. . .	. . .	. . .	. . .	. . .
Colorado	33 826	35 204	35 774	2 130	5 420	20 230	19 280	21 055	1 632	1 596
Connecticut	20 240	19 216	19 573	714	1 498	10 942	11 065	11 340	1 005	875
Delaware	5 095	4 924	5 171	230	597	3 108	3 178	2 792	245	553
District of Columbia	2 497	2 927	2 940	102	296	1 043	1 157	1 384	39	41
Florida	156 370	153 023	157 554	10 522	13 551	82 662	85 367	85 181	6 503	7 226
Georgia	68 897	60 252	55 432	4 811	6 781	. . .	27 693	21 308	. . .	2 508
Hawaii	28 843	27 495	25 795	1 457	2 536	. . .	. . .	4 612	. . .	. . .
Idaho	14 997	14 867	14 684	1 127	1 768	6 922	7 082	7 088	578	624
Illinois	77 845	82 076	83 208	3 272	9 085	33 076	34 553	36 854	1 903	3 041
Indiana	48 354	43 974	48 342	4 972	3 281	. . .	. . .	. . .	. . .	. . .
Iowa	20 455	20 371	20 406	1 060	2 282	8 305	8 285	9 113	640	606
Kansas	19 072	18 781	19 783	768	1 928	9 102	8 946	9 645	685	874
Kentucky	36 391	37 345	36 909	3 297	4 914	20 298	20 468	21 086	1 186	1 838
Louisiana	36 282	37 288	36 543	2 967	3 320	. . .	15 230	14 767	. . .	. . .
Maine	11 234	11 005	10 887	163	1 620	5 677	5 776	5 937	. . .	271
Maryland	38 318	38 176	38 877	1 606	4 018	17 802	17 642	18 448	751	1 928
Massachusetts	41 549	36 225	37 738	1 600	3 753	14 148	15 903	16 253	1 783	141
Michigan	61 932	62 911	65 164	1 488	8 738	34 701	35 598	37 836	2 394	2 994
Minnesota	30 359	31 638	32 836	1 049	3 612	14 235	14 991	15 722	1 245	1 291
Mississippi	17 705	17 798	18 360	1 551	2 013	13 077	13 283	14 066	1 471	909
Missouri	40 824	41 295	41 552	2 371	4 262	21 700	22 166	22 593	1 491	1 639
Montana	6 946	6 640	6 511	234	1 044	3 516	3 582	3 634	190	243
Nebraska	12 489	12 240	12 889	777	1 346	5 962	5 940	6 186	502	484
Nevada	145 763	143 600	146 468	11 547	11 363	14 828	16 379	15 478	1 260	1 570
New Hampshire	10 383	10 327	10 564	604	1 220	5 131	5 219	5 483	388	400
New Jersey	50 662	50 228	51 469	3 409	5 258	25 981	27 417	29 191	2 322	1 875
New Mexico [2, 3]	14 067	12 865	14 662	878	1 341	8 829	9 740	8 099	740	644
New York	130 813	130 900	139 682	10 506	9 901	57 830	61 011	65 340	10 030	6 983
North Carolina	62 235	61 932	63 730	7 899	4 973	35 926	35 678	37 049	4 102	3 897
North Dakota	4 424	4 562	4 316	276	628	1 979	1 860	1 873	158	165
Ohio	75 287	76 808	80 373	4 473	8 492	40 770	42 626	45 955	3 879	4 075
Oklahoma	22 812	19 613	17 373	988	. . .	17 146	. . .	. . .	1 220	. . .
Oregon	29 040	25 565	24 979	1 753	2 120	14 774	15 359	16 146	1 335	1 342
Pennsylvania	73 599	72 635	70 269	2 556	7 882	36 692	37 765	38 016	2 241	3 111
Rhode Island	8 243	8 349	8 278	297	904	3 287	3 356	3 388	296	308
South Carolina	34 546	37 183	38 207	601	2 393	13 448	13 602	13 956	543	1 630
South Dakota	6 485	6 428	6 687	273	834	2 364	2 289	2 545	174	239
Tennessee	67 104	69 335	75 909	3 215	8 500	28 858	29 155	29 792	2 026	2 020
Texas	178 512	178 751	181 989	9 779	13 353	81 324	84 316	85 395	8 080	7 871
Utah	23 796	24 087	24 073	450	1 949	9 811	9 517	9 494	500	899
Vermont	5 835	5 988	6 010	423	770	2 442	2 493	2 599	275	287
Virginia	61 990	61 754	62 650	3 238	5 812	29 411	29 718	30 818	2 113	2 388
Washington	40 169	39 622	39 518	3 696	4 854	26 674	26 752	28 023	2 241	2 318
West Virginia	13 621	13 659	14 557	473	1 722	9 148	9 335	9 438	442	568
Wisconsin	34 056	34 220	34 241	1 493	3 893	16 802	17 150	17 471	1 327	1 459
Wyoming	4 740	4 689	4 755	189	629	2 656	2 724	2 712	150	238
Puerto Rico	23 710	25 236	25 645	1 653	2 536	16 061	14 222	16 186	1 069	1 266

[1]Figures for marriages include licenses issued for some counties.
[2]Figures for marriages are marriage licenses issued.
[3]Figures for divorces include estimates for some counties.
. . . = Not available.

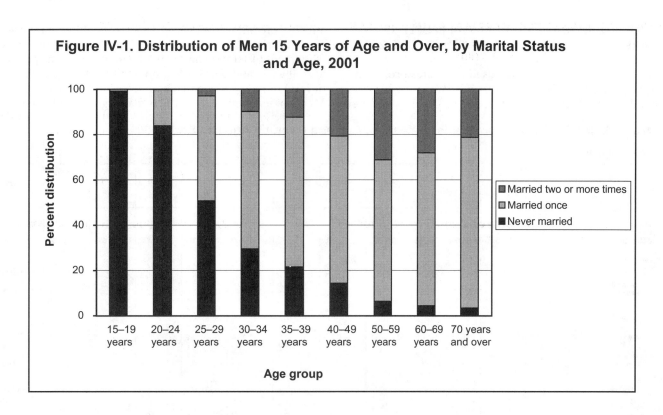

Figure IV-1. Distribution of Men 15 Years of Age and Over, by Marital Status and Age, 2001

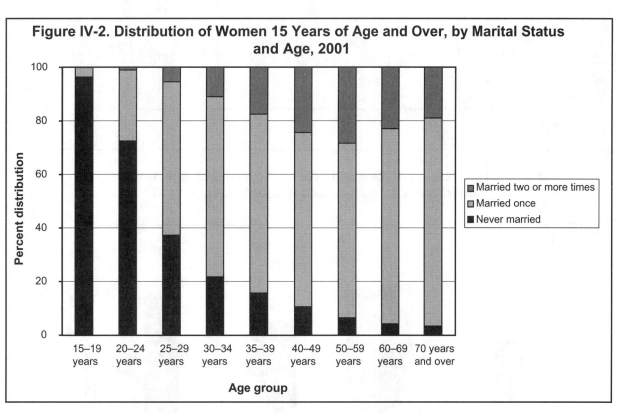

Figure IV-2. Distribution of Women 15 Years of Age and Over, by Marital Status and Age, 2001

TABLE IV-4. MARITAL HISTORY FOR PEOPLE 15 YEARS OF AGE AND OVER, BY AGE AND SEX, 2001

Tables IV-4 through IV-9 are based on figures projected onto U.S. population in 2001 from a survey of 56,574 people (about 30,000 households). In 2001, 31 percent of men

and 25 percent of women age 15 years and over had never been married. Among teenagers, 99 percent of males and 96 percent of females had never been married. For people age 50 years and over, only a small proportion (6 percent or less) of men and women had never been married. Men's older average age at first marriage was reflected in

Table IV-4. Marital History for People 15 Years of Age and Over, by Age and Sex, 2001

(Numbers in thousands, percent.)

Characteristic	Total, 15 years and over		15–19 years	20–24 years	25–29 years	30–34 years	35–39 years	40–49 years	50–59 years	60–69 years	70 years and over
	Estimate	90-percent confidence interval									
Men											
Total (in thousands)	105 850	104 698–107 002	10 186	9 465	9 177	10 069	10 704	21 202	15 694	9 558	9 795
Percent											
Never married	30.9	30.2–31.6	99.1	83.9	50.8	29.5	21.5	14.2	6.3	4.3	3.3
Ever married	69.1	68.4–69.8	0.9	16.1	49.2	70.5	78.5	85.8	93.7	95.7	96.7
Married once	53.4	52.6–54.2	0.9	16.0	46.3	60.8	66.2	65.1	62.6	67.5	75.5
Still married [1]	43.7	42.9–44.5	0.6	14.3	39.6	52.3	53.0	53.1	58.0	58.1	58.1
Married twice	12.5	12.0–13.0	-	0.1	2.8	8.7	10.9	17.1	23.2	21.3	16.5
Still married [1]	9.9	9.4–10.4	-	0.1	2.6	7.4	9.1	13.8	17.6	17.0	12.2
Married 3 or more times	3.2	2.9–3.5	-	-	0.1	1.1	1.4	3.6	8.0	6.8	4.7
Still married [1]	2.4	2.2–2.6	-	-	0.1	0.8	1.2	2.9	5.7	5.1	3.5
Ever divorced	21.0	20.4–21.6	0.1	1.0	7.5	15.4	22.9	29.5	40.8	30.9	18.6
Currently divorced	8.8	8.4–9.2	-	0.8	4.7	7.0	12.5	12.5	16.9	9.7	5.5
Ever widowed	3.6	3.3–3.9	-	-	0.1	0.3	0.5	1.3	2.9	7.6	23.1
Currently widowed	2.4	2.2–2.6	-	-	0.1	-	0.2	0.8	1.8	4.5	16.8
Women											
Total (in thousands)	113 777	112 625–114 929	9 764	9 518	9 239	10 211	11 110	22 036	16 626	10 956	14 318
Percent											
Never married	24.6	24.0–25.2	96.3	72.4	37.3	21.7	15.6	10.5	6.4	4.1	3.3
Ever married	75.4	74.9–76.0	3.7	27.6	62.7	78.3	84.4	89.5	93.6	95.9	96.7
Married once	58.7	58.0–59.4	3.6	26.5	57.3	67.3	66.8	65.1	65.2	72.9	77.8
Still married [1]	40.7	40.0–41.4	3.1	22.6	47.1	56.2	53.0	48.8	46.4	47.5	29.8
Married twice	13.6	13.1–14.1	0.1	1.1	5.1	10.0	15.7	19.8	22.1	17.4	15.5
Still married [1]	9.1	8.7–9.5	0.1	0.8	4.1	7.9	12.0	14.5	15.3	10.6	6.1
Married 3 or more times	3.1	2.8–3.4	-	-	0.3	1.0	1.8	4.6	6.3	5.6	3.5
Still married [1]	1.9	1.7–2.1	-	-	0.2	0.8	1.5	3.3	4.1	3.1	1.1
Ever divorced	23.1	22.5–23.7	0.2	2.6	11.9	18.6	28.1	35.4	38.9	28.4	17.7
Currently divorced	10.8	10.3–11.3	-	1.6	7.4	9.3	13.7	16.8	17.9	12.6	6.5
Ever widowed	11.6	11.1–12.1	-	0.3	0.5	0.6	1.1	3.5	9.5	23.3	56.3
Currently widowed	10.2	9.8–10.6	-	0.3	0.4	0.4	0.6	2.4	7.1	19.7	52.6

[1]Includes those currently separated.
- = Quantity zero or rounds to zero.

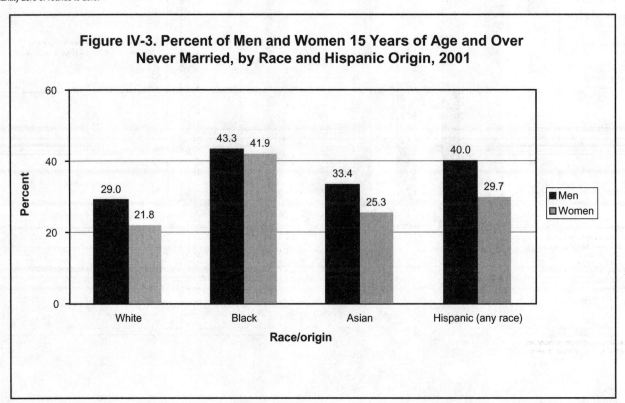

Figure IV-3. Percent of Men and Women 15 Years of Age and Over Never Married, by Race and Hispanic Origin, 2001

the difference between the proportions of married men and women at the ages when most people marry. Among the population age 20 to 24 years, 84 percent of men and 72 percent of women had never been married (a difference of 12 percentage points). For 30- to 34-year-olds, the difference was 8 percentage points; for 40- to 49-year-olds, the difference was only 4 percentage points.

TABLE IV-5. MARITAL HISTORY FOR PEOPLE 15 YEARS OF AGE AND OVER, BY AGE, SEX, RACE, AND HISPANIC ORIGIN, 2001

Black men and women age 25 to 29 years were more likely to have never married than their White counterparts. Among Asians and Pacific Islanders in this age

Table IV-5. Marital History for People 15 Years of Age and Over, by Age, Sex, Race, and Hispanic Origin, 2001

(Numbers in thousands, percent.)

Characteristic	Total, 15 years and over	15–19 years	20–24 years	25–29 years	30–34 years	35–39 years	40–49 years	50–59 years	60–69 years	70 years and over
WHITE										
Men										
Total (in thousands)	88 834	8 139	7 686	7 420	8 295	8 908	17 827	13 456	8 370	8 733
Percent										
Never married	29.0	99.1	83.1	48.0	28.1	19.5	13.0	5.8	3.8	3.3
Ever married	71.0	0.9	16.9	52.0	71.9	80.5	87.0	94.2	96.2	96.7
Married once	54.4	0.8	16.8	48.8	61.4	67.6	65.3	61.6	68.0	75.5
Still married [1]	44.9	0.6	15.1	41.8	53.1	54.0	54.0	49.3	59.2	59.0
Married twice	13.1	-	0.1	3.2	9.2	11.4	18.0	23.9	21.3	16.4
Still married [1]	10.5	-	0.1	2.9	7.8	9.6	14.5	18.7	17.2	12.3
Married 3 or more times	3.5	-	-	0.1	1.3	1.5	3.7	8.7	7.0	4.7
Still married [1]	2.6	-	-	0.1	0.9	1.3	2.9	6.3	5.4	3.5
Ever divorced	21.9	-	1.0	8.3	16.1	24.2	30.5	42.0	30.8	18.1
Currently divorced	8.9	-	0.9	5.1	7.1	13.2	12.7	16.6	9.3	5.2
Ever widowed	3.6	-	-	0.1	0.3	0.4	1.2	2.6	7.2	22.5
Currently widowed	2.4	-	-	0.1	-	0.2	0.8	1.4	4.0	16.1
Women										
Total (in thousands)	93 517	7 711	7 440	7 298	8 052	8 933	17 949	13 999	9 302	12 833
Percent										
Never married	21.8	95.9	70.0	33.1	16.6	12.7	8.0	5.4	3.4	3.0
Ever married	78.2	4.1	30.0	66.9	83.4	87.3	92.0	94.6	96.6	97.0
Married once	60.2	4.1	28.6	60.7	71.2	67.9	65.6	64.5	73.0	78.0
Still married [1]	42.5	3.5	24.3	50.3	59.8	55.2	50.2	47.9	49.8	30.3
Married twice	14.6	-	1.3	5.9	10.9	17.4	21.2	23.4	17.6	15.5
Still married [1]	10.0	-	1.0	4.7	8.5	13.5	15.8	16.4	11.2	6.5
Married 3 or more times	3.4	-	-	0.3	1.3	2.0	5.2	6.8	6.0	3.6
Still married [1]	2.1	-	-	0.3	1.0	1.7	3.6	4.5	3.4	1.2
Ever divorced	24.2	0.1	3.1	13.3	20.4	29.3	37.4	39.5	28.6	17.5
Currently divorced	10.8	0.1	1.9	8.0	10.3	13.4	17.1	17.0	12.2	6.2
Ever widowed	12.1	-	0.3	0.4	0.6	1.2	3.3	9.0	22.0	56.2
Currently widowed	10.6	-	0.3	0.4	0.4	0.7	2.1	6.6	18.2	52.4
WHITE NON-HISPANIC										
Men										
Total (in thousands)	77 085	6 679	5 981	5 811	6 680	7 691	15 781	12 378	7 807	8 277
Percent										
Never married	27.4	99.4	83.7	48.3	28.1	19.0	12.8	5.7	4.0	3.5
Ever married	72.6	0.6	16.3	51.7	71.9	81.0	87.2	94.3	96.0	96.5
Married once	54.8	0.5	16.2	48.0	61.3	67.1	64.5	60.8	67.3	75.1
Still married [1]	45.1	0.3	14.4	41.0	52.7	53.2	52.8	48.9	58.7	59.2
Married twice	14.0	0.1	0.1	3.6	9.3	12.2	18.9	24.4	21.5	16.5
Still married [1]	11.3	0.1	0.1	3.3	7.9	10.2	15.2	19.2	17.3	12.5
Married 3 or more times	3.8	-	-	0.1	1.3	1.6	3.8	9.1	7.3	4.9
Still married [1]	2.9	-	-	0.1	1.0	1.5	3.1	6.7	5.6	3.7
Ever divorced	23.3	0.1	1.1	8.7	16.8	25.7	32.1	42.8	31.3	18.1
Currently divorced	9.4	-	1.0	5.1	7.8	13.8	13.4	16.6	9.5	5.0
Ever widowed	3.8	-	-	0.1	0.3	0.4	1.2	2.5	7.2	22.3
Currently widowed	2.5	-	-	0.1	0.1	0.1	0.7	1.4	4.0	15.7
Women										
Total (in thousands)	82 128	6 310	6 015	5 904	6 696	7 584	15 977	12 880	8 525	12 237
Percent										
Never married	20.7	97.3	70.9	34.1	17.1	12.3	8.1	5.0	2.9	2.9
Ever married	79.3	2.7	29.1	65.9	82.9	87.7	91.9	95.0	97.1	97.1
Married once	60.0	2.7	27.6	59.2	69.6	67.1	64.1	63.8	72.8	78.1
Still married [1]	42.1	2.3	23.4	48.2	58.7	55.0	49.5	48.0	50.2	30.5
Married twice	15.5	-	1.4	6.3	12.0	18.3	22.2	24.1	18.3	15.5
Still married [1]	10.6	-	1.1	5.0	9.5	14.3	16.4	17.0	11.7	6.6
Married 3 or more times	3.7	-	-	0.4	1.4	2.3	5.6	7.1	6.1	3.6
Still married [1]	2.3	-	-	0.3	1.0	2.0	3.9	4.7	3.4	1.2
Ever divorced	25.4	0.1	3.3	14.5	21.9	30.4	38.8	40.4	29.1	17.4
Currently divorced	11.1	0.1	1.9	8.9	10.8	13.5	17.6	17.0	12.1	6.0
Ever widowed	12.9	-	0.2	0.4	0.5	1.2	3.2	8.9	22.2	56.5
Currently widowed	11.3	-	0.2	0.4	0.3	0.7	2.0	6.4	18.4	52.6

[1] Includes those currently separated.
- = Quantity zero or rounds to zero.

group, a much higher proportion of men than women had never married (67 percent versus 39 percent). Relatively few 50- to 59-year-old Whites and Hispanics had never married, with rates ranging between 5 percent and 10 percent. These shares were higher for Blacks, with 12 percent of Black men and 14 percent of Black women in their fifties having never been married.

Table IV-5. Marital History for People 15 Years of Age and Over, by Age, Sex, Race, and Hispanic Origin, 2001—Continued

(Numbers in thousands, percent.)

Characteristic	Total, 15 years and over	15–19 years	20–24 years	25–29 years	30–34 years	35–39 years	40–49 years	50–59 years	60–69 years	70 years and over
BLACK										
Men										
Total (in thousands)	11 554	1 507	1 223	1 088	1 149	1 229	2 314	1 505	844	695
Percent										
Never married	43.3	99.2	89.2	60.6	41.5	34.0	25.1	11.6	10.2	3.1
Ever married	56.7	0.8	10.8	39.4	58.5	66.0	74.9	88.4	89.8	96.9
Married once	44.3	0.8	10.8	38.0	51.6	56.3	57.5	62.0	60.8	72.3
Still married ¹	31.4	0.3	9.9	31.2	39.3	42.5	38.2	41.9	43.6	43.8
Married twice	10.0	-	-	1.4	6.7	8.1	13.6	21.9	21.7	20.0
Still married ¹	7.3	-	-	1.4	5.9	7.0	11.0	13.4	16.5	10.8
Married 3 or more times	2.3	-	-	-	0.1	1.6	3.8	4.5	7.2	4.7
Still married ¹	1.5	-	-	-	0.1	1.3	3.2	2.2	3.5	3.1
Ever divorced	18.8	0.2	-	4.2	13.7	18.2	28.1	40.2	35.1	26.9
Currently divorced	9.2	0.2	-	2.8	7.6	9.5	14.0	21.1	12.9	10.3
Ever widowed	3.7	-	0.3	-	0.2	1.0	1.9	4.2	10.9	30.4
Currently widowed	2.9	-	0.3	-	-	0.6	1.0	3.2	8.6	25.2
Women										
Total (in thousands)	14 284	1 520	1 465	1 358	1 437	1 526	2 804	1 842	1 215	1 117
Percent										
Never married	41.9	97.9	82.6	59.4	49.5	34.0	27.9	14.4	10.4	6.8
Ever married	58.1	2.1	17.4	40.6	50.5	66.0	72.1	85.6	89.6	93.2
Married once	46.9	1.8	17.4	37.7	44.3	55.5	56.0	66.1	67.5	72.4
Still married ¹	25.1	0.9	14.7	26.7	32.2	35.0	31.1	32.1	27.7	17.3
Married twice	9.8	0.3	-	2.8	6.3	9.2	13.7	16.3	19.3	18.1
Still married ¹	5.0	0.3	-	2.3	5.1	5.4	8.1	9.6	7.5	2.7
Married 3 or more times	1.5	-	-	0.2	-	1.2	2.5	3.2	2.8	2.8
Still married ¹	0.8	-	-	-	-	0.6	1.9	1.6	0.9	0.5
Ever divorced	20.1	0.3	0.6	8.4	12.4	24.6	30.4	38.2	30.3	23.7
Currently divorced	11.9	-	0.6	6.1	6.4	16.3	18.5	24.1	15.7	10.4
Ever widowed	10.5	-	0.3	0.8	1.1	0.9	5.1	13.1	32.0	60.7
Currently widowed	9.7	-	0.3	0.5	0.8	0.9	4.1	11.1	30.2	59.1
ASIAN										
Men										
Total (in thousands)	4 311	393	429	514	538	473	834	556	259	315
Percent										
Never married	33.4	99.3	82.6	66.7	24.9	23.1	7.9	5.0	3.7	2.1
Ever married	66.6	0.7	17.4	33.3	75.1	76.9	92.1	95.0	96.3	97.9
Married once	59.7	0.7	16.4	32.4	70.8	71.5	80.5	84.2	81.8	83.9
Still married ¹	54.4	0.7	15.8	30.7	65.4	66.4	75.7	74.6	76.0	65.8
Married twice	6.1	-	1.0	0.8	3.8	5.4	10.2	9.6	13.0	11.3
Still married ¹	4.8	-	1.0	0.8	3.8	3.6	8.8	5.7	8.3	10.7
Married 3 or more times	0.8	-	-	-	0.5	-	1.4	1.3	1.5	2.7
Still married ¹	0.5	-	-	-	0.5	-	0.8	0.5	1.5	1.7
Ever divorced	8.8	-	1.7	1.5	9.0	9.6	15.5	13.9	12.7	10.6
Currently divorced	3.9	-	0.7	0.6	4.7	6.3	4.9	9.1	3.2	1.8
Ever widowed	3.1	-	-	-	-	0.9	0.4	5.8	9.3	22.1
Currently widowed	2.3	-	-	-	-	-	-	4.5	6.2	17.9
Women										
Total (in thousands)	4 645	339	511	501	558	527	1 007	562	334	306
Percent										
Never married	25.3	96.3	75.2	38.6	17.4	7.9	8.0	7.9	0.4	2.3
Ever married	74.7	3.7	24.8	61.4	82.6	92.1	92.0	92.1	99.6	97.7
Married once	67.9	2.7	23.9	61.4	76.7	85.7	80.6	80.0	92.2	87.1
Still married ¹	56.3	2.7	21.8	57.4	73.0	72.2	71.6	58.9	64.7	49.5
Married twice	5.9	1.0	0.8	-	6.0	6.4	10.6	8.1	4.8	10.6
Still married ¹	4.6	1.0	0.8	-	6.0	5.5	8.7	4.6	4.8	5.0
Married 3 or more times	0.8	-	-	-	-	-	0.8	1.6	2.6	-
Still married ¹	0.6	-	-	-	-	-	0.8	3.9	2.6	4.9
Ever divorced	10.4	1.0	0.8	2.5	8.9	16.6	16.1	20.9	9.9	2.3
Currently divorced	5.8	-	-	2.5	2.9	11.1	7.0	14.8	5.9	2.3
Ever widowed	6.7	-	-	0.6	-	-	2.0	7.8	26.5	42.1
Currently widowed	5.4	-	-	0.6	-	-	-	3.5	20.3	38.3

¹Includes those currently separated.
- = Quantity zero or rounds to zero.

Table IV-5. Marital History for People 15 Years of Age and Over, by Age, Sex, Race, and Hispanic Origin, 2001—*Continued*

(Numbers in thousands, percent.)

Characteristic	Total, 15 years and over	15–19 years	20–24 years	25–29 years	30–34 years	35–39 years	40–49 years	50–59 years	60–69 years	70 years and over
HISPANIC [2]										
Men										
Total (in thousands)	13 007	1 603	1 913	1 832	1 751	1 330	2 247	1 210	621	500
Percent										
Never married	40.0	98.1	81.1	46.9	28.2	22.9	14.3	5.8	2.8	1.3
Ever married	60.0	1.9	18.9	53.1	71.8	77.1	85.7	94.2	97.2	98.7
Married once	51.6	1.9	18.8	51.3	61.9	70.3	72.2	70.8	75.1	83.0
Still married [1]	43.2	1.7	17.0	43.9	54.9	57.9	63.2	53.7	63.1	54.3
Married twice	7.1	-	0.1	1.8	8.7	6.3	11.0	18.8	18.9	13.0
Still married [1]	5.8	-	0.1	1.6	7.5	6.0	9.1	13.2	16.8	9.4
Married 3 or more times	1.3	-	-	-	1.1	0.5	2.5	4.6	3.3	2.6
Still married [1]	0.7	-	-	-	0.8	0.2	1.6	1.8	2.5	1.4
Ever divorced	13.0	-	1.0	7.0	13.0	16.0	18.0	34.0	24.0	18.8
Currently divorced	6.0	-	0.7	5.5	4.3	9.8	7.2	17.7	6.3	10.3
Ever widowed	2.1	-	-	-	0.3	0.4	1.6	4.6	6.9	25.4
Currently widowed	1.6	-	-	-	-	0.4	1.4	3.1	4.4	21.8
Women										
Total (in thousands)	12 545	1 539	1 527	1 577	1 513	1 457	2 213	1 260	826	633
Percent										
Never married	29.7	89.9	66.3	28.0	15.8	15.0	8.6	10.4	8.8	6.1
Ever married	70.3	10.1	33.7	72.0	84.2	85.0	91.4	89.6	91.2	93.9
Married once	61.0	10.1	32.9	67.5	77.2	72.6	76.4	71.0	76.2	76.5
Still married [1]	44.4	9.1	28.4	57.2	63.0	55.6	54.4	46.1	44.3	27.4
Married twice	8.0	-	0.8	4.4	5.9	12.0	13.2	15.4	10.2	14.1
Still married [1]	5.6	-	0.5	3.8	4.5	8.9	10.5	10.1	6.3	4.5
Married 3 or more times	1.3	-	-	-	1.0	0.3	1.8	3.2	4.8	3.3
Still married [1]	0.8	-	-	-	0.8	0.1	1.5	1.6	3.3	1.2
Ever divorced	16.0	-	3.0	9.0	13.0	23.0	26.0	30.0	24.0	20.2
Currently divorced	9.0	-	2.0	5.0	7.0	13.0	14.0	17.0	13.0	11.1
Ever widowed	5.9	-	0.7	0.3	0.6	1.3	4.3	11.0	19.4	48.7
Currently widowed	5.3	-	0.7	0.3	0.6	0.8	3.3	9.1	16.8	47.3

[1]Includes those currently separated.
[2]May be of any race.
- = Quantity zero or rounds to zero.

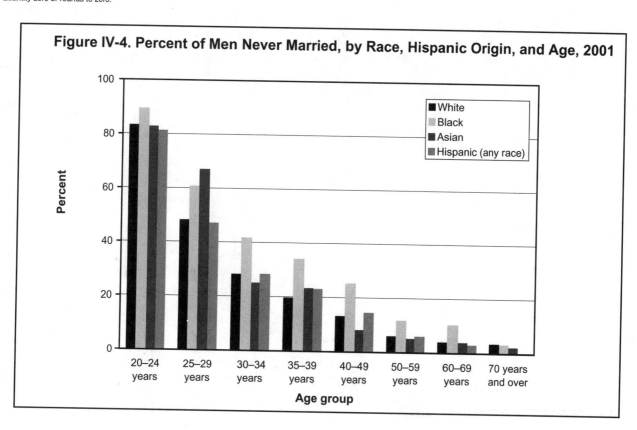

Figure IV-4. Percent of Men Never Married, by Race, Hispanic Origin, and Age, 2001

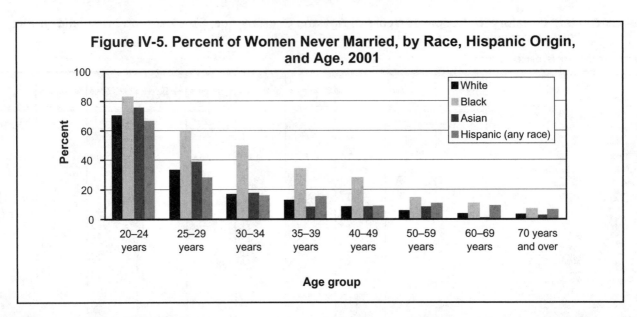

Figure IV-5. Percent of Women Never Married, by Race, Hispanic Origin, and Age, 2001

TABLE IV-6. MARITAL HISTORY BY SEX FOR SELECTED BIRTH COHORTS, 2001

Because people born during a specific period of time ("birth cohort") experience similar historical circumstances during their life cycles, it is useful to compare trends in marital patterns by birth cohort. There have been delays in age of marriage and increases in divorce rates during the period of time covered by this table, which begins with the 1935–1939 birth cohort. Since this data was collected in 2001, the 1965–1969 birth cohort was the most recent cohort that had lived long enough to allow an examination of delays in marriage (percent married by age 30). The increase in divorce rates also indicated a higher percentage of persons in more recent cohorts who were able to marry more than once during their lifetimes.

Table IV-6. Marital History by Sex for Selected Birth Cohorts, 2001

(Numbers in thousands, percent.)

Characteristic	1935–1939	1940–1944	1945–1949	1950–1954	1955–1959	1960–1964	1965–1969	1970–1974	1975–1979
MEN (in thousands)	4 907	6 442	8 146	9 752	10 770	11 262	10 087	9 504	9 070
Percent Ever Married by:									
20 years	20.9	24.1	20.4	23.0	17.6	15.8	13.0	11.0	8.1
25 years	66.6	70.0	66.6	59.2	49.9	45.0	40.6	39.4	X
30 years	85.3	85.3	79.7	74.0	68.8	65.6	65.2	X	X
35 years	89.4	89.6	86.2	81.7	78.5	76.6	X	X	X
40 years	91.0	91.4	89.6	85.9	83.6	X	X	X	X
45 years	92.8	92.7	91.5	88.2	X	X	X	X	X
50 years	94.1	94.0	93.1	X	X	X	X	X	X
Percent Ever Divorced by:									
20 years	0.7	0.6	0.6	1.3	1.0	0.6	1.1	1.0	0.5
25 years	4.0	5.9	5.8	7.2	5.4	6.1	7.0	5.8	X
30 years	8.5	13.3	15.6	17.8	14.7	13.8	13.1	X	X
35 years	15.2	21.9	25.3	26.2	20.8	19.9	X	X	X
40 years	22.7	27.4	31.0	31.4	26.2	X	X	X	X
45 years	27.4	31.5	36.3	34.7	X	X	X	X	X
50 years	30.2	34.7	39.7	X	X	X	X	X	X
55 years	32.0	37.3	X	X	X	X	X	X	X
Percent Married Two Times or More by:									
25 years	1.7	2.3	1.8	2.5	2.0	1.8	3.0	1.9	X
30 years	5.5	6.9	8.1	8.4	6.0	6.7	7.5	X	X
35 years	11.0	13.0	15.0	17.0	12.0	11.0	X	X	X
40 years	15.5	19.7	22.4	21.7	16.8	X	X	X	X
45 years	21.7	24.2	26.4	25.4	X	X	X	X	X
50 years	26.0	27.2	29.5	X	X	X	X	X	X
55 years	28.8	30.2	X	X	X	X	X	X	X
WOMEN (in thousands)	5 718	6 914	8 600	10 289	11 181	11 468	10 153	9 837	9 091
Percent Ever Married by:									
20 years	51.3	46.2	44.8	40.5	36.6	30.2	24.6	21.9	17.5
25 years	82.5	79.0	78.7	70.1	66.0	59.5	54.8	53.4	X
30 years	88.7	87.6	85.4	80.7	78.1	74.4	74.3	X	X
35 years	91.1	90.5	88.3	86.2	84.5	83.0	X	X	X
40 years	92.2	92.2	90.9	89.1	87.7	X	X	X	X
45 years	93.8	93.9	92.1	90.6	X	X	X	X	X
50 years	94.5	94.6	93.0	X	X	X	X	X	X
Percent Ever Divorced by:									
20 years	2.5	1.9	1.7	2.1	3.0	2.7	1.8	2.1	1.1
25 years	5.8	7.0	9.4	10.8	11.8	11.5	9.9	9.7	X
30 years	11.6	14.1	18.9	21.6	21.3	19.4	16.9	X	X
35 years	16.9	21.6	27.9	28.9	27.3	26.0	X	X	X
40 years	22.7	26.9	33.2	35.2	31.7	X	X	X	X
45 years	25.4	29.9	36.7	38.8	X	X	X	X	X
50 years	27.2	32.6	39.0	X	X	X	X	X	X
55 years	28.9	34.1	X	X	X	X	X	X	X
Percent Married Two Times or More by:									
25 years	3.4	3.9	3.8	3.8	5.0	4.2	4.4	3.7	X
30 years	6.4	7.8	10.3	11.1	11.7	10.8	9.8	X	X
35 years	11.5	12.9	16.6	17.4	17.7	16.1	X	X	X
40 years	15.2	16.9	22.3	23.1	21.7	X	X	X	X
45 years	18.7	20.7	25.4	26.6	X	X	X	X	X
50 years	21.1	23.2	28.5	X	X	X	X	X	X
55 years	22.8	24.9	X	X	X	X	X	X	X

X = Not applicable. Cohort had not lived to stated age at the time of the survey.

TABLE IV-7. PERCENT REACHING STATED ANNIVERSARY, BY MARRIAGE COHORT AND SEX, FOR FIRST AND SECOND MARRIAGES, 2001

The proportions of both men and women reaching various anniversaries declined from marriages begun in the mid-1950s to marriages begun in the early 1990s. For example, 87 percent of women who first married in the 1955–1959 period reached their 10th anniversary, compared with only 75 percent of those who first married in the 1985–1989 period. This reflected a rapid increase in the likelihood of divorce during the last half of the twentieth century.

TABLE IV-8. MEDIAN AGE AT MARITAL EVENT FOR PEOPLE 15 YEARS OF AGE AND OVER, BY SEX, RACE, AND HISPANIC ORIGIN, 2001

This table shows the median age for marital events associated with first and second marriages. In 2001, the median age for first marriage was roughly between 21 and 22 years old for non-Hispanic White, Hispanic, and Black women. Women's median age at separation from first marriage ranged from 28 to 31 years old, and the median age at divorce from first marriage was between 29 and 33 years old. For men, the corresponding ages were roughly two years older. Differences indicated in this table may be partly explained by different age distributions in specific population subgroups, in addition to actual variation in age-specific marital behavior.

Table IV-7. Percent Reaching Stated Anniversary, by Marriage Cohort and Sex, for First and Second Marriages, 2001

(Numbers in thousands, percent.)

Sex and year of marriage	Number of marriages (thousands)	Anniversary [1]							
		5th	10th	15th	20th	25th	30th	35th	40th
FIRST MARRIAGES									
Men									
1990–1994	7 718	90.1	X	X	X	X	X	X	X
1985–1989	8 048	87.6	74.7	X	X	X	X	X	X
1980–1984	7 606	89.8	74.5	66.2	X	X	X	X	X
1975–1979	7 109	89.3	72.2	63.4	58.4	X	X	X	X
1970–1974	7 436	90.4	72.5	61.3	55.8	52.9	X	X	X
1965–1969	6 357	93.0	78.3	67.8	62.1	58.0	54.8	X	X
1960–1964	5 033	94.0	81.6	71.1	66.1	62.3	60.3	57.7	X
1955–1959	4 100	96.1	89.5	82.2	76.2	72.3	68.7	66.1	63.5
Women									
1990–1994	7 967	86.9	X	X	X	X	X	X	X
1985–1989	8 299	86.6	74.7	X	X	X	X	X	X
1980–1984	8 448	87.3	71.5	64.2	X	X	X	X	X
1975–1979	7 852	84.7	67.7	58.5	52.6	X	X	X	X
1970–1974	8 176	87.8	70.2	60.3	54.1	49.1	X	X	X
1965–1969	7 138	91.3	77.9	65.7	59.2	55.5	51.9	X	X
1960–1964	5 714	93.8	84.0	72.9	66.9	60.9	57.0	53.1	X
1955–1959	5 162	94.0	86.8	78.6	73.1	67.0	64.1	58.9	54.4
SECOND MARRIAGES									
Men									
1990–1994	2 834	88.8	X	X	X	X	X	X	X
1985–1989	2 881	90.0	72.2	X	X	X	X	X	X
1980–1984	2 544	90.9	71.8	54.9	X	X	X	X	X
1975–1979	1 985	90.8	81.0	57.6	49.0	X	X	X	X
Women									
1990–1994	3 126	86.8	X	X	X	X	X	X	X
1985–1989	3 008	86.9	67.8	X	X	X	X	X	X
1980–1984	2 703	89.2	71.0	54.6	X	X	X	X	X
1975–1979	2 187	86.3	75.9	55.9	47.2	X	X	X	X

[1]Persons reaching stated anniversary for specified marital order.
X = Not applicable.

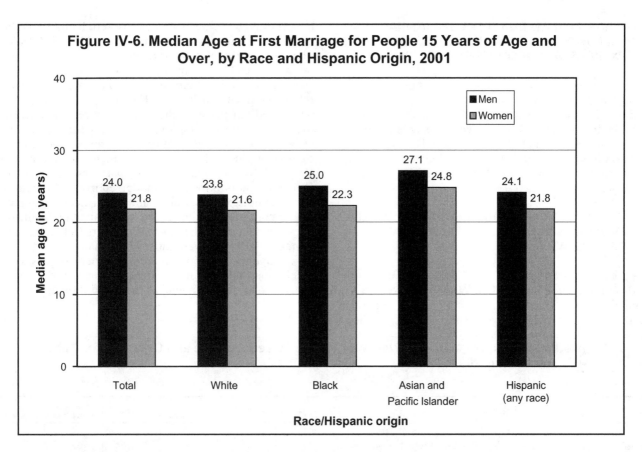

Figure IV-6. Median Age at First Marriage for People 15 Years of Age and Over, by Race and Hispanic Origin, 2001

Table IV-8. Median Age at Marital Event for People 15 Years of Age and Over, by Sex, Race, and Hispanic Origin, 2001

(Median age in years for those who experienced the specified event.)

Sex and year of marriage	Total	White	White non-Hispanic	Black	Asian and Pacific Islander	Hispanic (of any race)
MEN						
Total Population	41.3	42.0	43.5	38.4	37.7	33.1
First Marriage						
Age when married	24.0	23.8	23.8	25.0	27.1	24.1
Age when separated [1]	30.3	30.2	30.3	30.9	30.3	29.3
Age when divorced	31.5	31.3	31.4	32.5	31.5	30.7
Age when widowed	59.4	60.3	60.8	B	B	57.4
Second Marriage						
Age when married	35.1	35.0	35.0	B	35.3	34.6
Age when separated [1]	38.8	38.7	38.8	B	B	38.5
Age when divorced	42.2	42.0	42.2	B	B	39.8
Age when widowed	63.4	63.5	B	B	B	B
WOMEN						
Total Population	43.0	44.0	45.2	39.4	39.1	35.5
First Marriage						
Age when married	21.8	21.6	21.5	22.3	24.8	21.8
Age when separated [1]	28.0	27.8	27.8	28.8	31.2	28.6
Age when divorced	29.4	29.2	29.1	31.1	32.5	29.9
Age when widowed	58.6	59.3	59.8	B	52.0	50.7
Second Marriage						
Age when married	32.7	32.4	32.3	34.3	35.8	33.3
Age when separated [1]	35.6	35.3	35.2	B	B	35.9
Age when divorced	38.4	38.1	38.0	B	B	39.8
Age when widowed	57.3	58.1	58.0	B	B	B

[1] For those who divorced.
B = Base less than 200,000. Median not calculated.

TABLE IV-9. MEDIAN DURATION OF MARRIAGE EVENTS FOR PEOPLE 15 YEARS OF AGE AND OVER, BY SEX, RACE, AND HISPANIC ORIGIN, 2001

The median length of a first marriage that ended in divorce was about 8 years for both men and women. The median time from marriage to separation was about 7 years. Half the men and women who remarried after divorce did so within about 3 to 4 years. The median duration of second marriages that ended in divorce, as compared to first marriages that ended in divorce, was roughly equal for women but longer for men.

TABLE IV-10. MARRIED-COUPLE AND UNMARRIED-PARTNER HOUSEHOLDS, BY METROPOLITAN RESIDENCE STATUS, 2000

The 2000 census enumerated 105.5 million total households in the United States, about 60 million of which were maintained by couples. Of these, 54.5 million (52 percent) were shared by married couples. There were 5.5 million

households shared by couples who were living together but remained unmarried, up from 3.2 million in 1990. These unmarried-partner households were self-identified on the census form as being maintained by people who were sharing living quarters and had a close personal relationship with each other. The majority of these unmarried-partner households were shared by partners of the opposite sex (4.9 million), but about 1 in 9 (594,000) were shared by partners of the same sex. Of the unmarried-partner households shared by members of the same sex, 301,000 were shared by male partners and 293,000 by female partners. Substantial underreporting of the number of same-sex households cannot be ruled out, in part due to continued prejudice and discrimination against homosexual people. Unmarried partners (and especially same-sex partners) were more likely than married couples to live in metropolitan areas. Married couples were much more likely than unmarried partners of the opposite sex to identify the man as the "householder."

Table IV-9. Median Duration of Marriage Events for People 15 Years of Age and Over, by Sex, Race, and Hispanic Origin, 2001

(Duration in years.)

Subject	Total	White	White non-Hispanic	Black	Asian and Pacific Islander	Hispanic (of any race)
Duration of First Marriage for Those Whose First Marriage Ended in Divorce						
Men	8.2	8.1	8.2	8.9	8.3	7.8
Women	7.9	7.8	7.8	8.4	9.0	8.1
Duration Between First Marriage and First Separation for Those Who Separated						
Men	6.9	6.8	6.8	7.3	6.8	6.3
Women	6.7	6.7	6.6	6.6	7.7	6.8
Duration Between First Separation and First Divorce for Those Who Divorced						
Men	0.9	0.8	0.8	1.1	0.9	0.8
Women	0.8	0.8	0.8	1.2	0.7	0.8
Duration Between First Divorce and Remarriage for Those Whose First Marriages Ended in Divorce and Who Had Remarried						
Men	3.3	3.3	3.3	3.8	3.1	3.2
Women	3.5	3.3	3.3	4.3	3.7	3.6
Duration of Second Marriage for Those Whose Second Marriage Ended in Divorce						
Men	9.2	9.2	9.3	8.7	B	6.4
Women	8.1	8.0	8.0	8.4	B	9.1

B = Base less than 200,000. Median not calculated.

Table IV-10. Married-Couple and Unmarried-Partner Households, by Metropolitan Residence Status, 2000

(Number, percent.)

Household type and sex of householder	Total	In a metropolitan area						Not in a metropolitan area	
		Total		In central city		Not in central city			
		Number	Percent of all households	Number	Percent of all households	Number	Percent of all households	Number	Percent of all households
TOTAL HOUSEHOLDS [1]	105 480 101	84 304 885	79.9	32 753 918	31.1	51 550 967	48.9	21 175 216	20.1
Total Coupled Households [2]	59 969 000	47 214 481	78.7	15 189 744	25.3	32 024 737	53.4	12 754 519	21.3
Married-couple households	54 493 232	42 757 993	78.5	13 232 903	24.3	29 525 090	54.2	11 735 239	21.5
Male householder	47 449 405	36 968 706	77.9	11 101 326	23.4	25 867 380	54.5	10 480 699	22.1
Female householder	7 043 827	5 789 287	82.2	2 131 577	30.3	3 657 710	51.9	1 254 540	17.8
Unmarried-partner households	5 475 768	4 456 488	81.4	1 956 841	35.7	2 499 647	45.6	1 019 280	18.6
Opposite-sex partners	4 881 377	3 949 743	80.9	1 709 317	35.0	2 240 426	45.9	931 634	19.1
Male householder	2 615 119	2 083 069	79.7	849 082	32.5	1 233 987	47.2	532 050	20.3
Female householder	2 266 258	1 866 674	82.4	860 235	38.0	1 006 439	44.4	399 584	17.6
Same-sex partners	594 391	506 745	85.3	247 524	41.6	259 221	43.6	87 646	14.7
Male householder	301 026	259 807	86.3	135 546	45.0	124 261	41.3	41 219	13.7
Female householder	293 365	246 938	84.2	111 978	38.2	134 960	46.0	46 427	15.8

[1]Total includes other types of households, including family and nonfamily households which do not contain either spouses or unmarried partners.
[2]Coupled households represent the total number of married-couple and unmarried-partner households.

TABLE IV-11. MARRIED-COUPLE AND UNMARRIED-PARTNER HOUSEHOLDS, BY REGION AND STATE, 2000

Table IV-11 shows that the West and Midwest had the highest proportions (58 percent each) of households maintained by couples, while the Northeast had the lowest proportion (55 percent). Overall, 9 percent of all coupled households were unmarried-partner households, with the West having the highest percentage (10 percent) and the South having the lowest percentage (8 percent).

Large clusters of unmarried-partner households were found in: 1) the southwestern states of Colorado, New Mexico, and Arizona, extending up the Pacific coast into Alaska; 2) New York and New England; 3) Maryland, Delaware, and the District of Columbia; 4) the lower Mississippi Valley (not shown separately); and 5) southern Florida. The proportion of coupled households maintained by same-sex partners ranged from 0.7 percent in the Midwest to 1.2 percent in the West. Among the states, California had the highest percentage of unmarried-partner households shared by members of the same sex, with

Table IV-11. Married-Couple and Unmarried-Partner Households, by Region and State, 2000

(Number, percent.)

Area	Total households	Total coupled households [1] Number	Total coupled households [1] Percent of all households	Married-couple households	Total unmarried-partner households Number	Total unmarried-partner households Percent of coupled households	Opposite-sex unmarried partners Number	Opposite-sex unmarried partners Percent of coupled households	Same-sex unmarried partners Total Number	Same-sex unmarried partners Total Percent of coupled households	Sex of partners Male partners	Sex of partners Female partners
UNITED STATES	105 480 101	59 969 000	56.9	54 493 232	5 475 768	9.1	4 881 377	8.1	594 391	1.0	301 026	293 365
Region												
Northwest	20 285 622	11 205 641	55.2	10 127 653	1 077 988	9.6	958 742	8.6	119 246	1.1	59 328	59 918
Midwest	24 734 532	14 222 533	57.5	12 963 564	1 258 969	8.9	1 153 219	8.1	105 750	0.7	52 142	53 608
South	38 015 214	21 549 582	56.7	19 740 328	1 809 254	8.4	1 599 512	7.4	209 742	1.0	107 636	102 106
West	22 444 733	12 991 244	57.9	11 661 687	1 329 557	10.2	1 169 904	9.0	159 653	1.2	81 920	77 733
State												
Alabama	1 737 080	965 453	55.6	906 916	58 537	6.1	50 428	5.2	8 109	0.8	3 980	4 129
Alaska	221 600	132 886	60.0	116 318	16 568	12.5	15 388	11.6	1 180	0.9	483	697
Arizona	1 901 327	1 104 499	58.1	986 303	118 196	10.7	105 864	9.6	12 332	1.1	6 278	6 054
Arkansas	1 042 696	606 944	58.2	566 401	40 543	6.7	36 120	6.0	4 423	0.7	2 176	2 247
California	11 502 870	6 560 600	57.0	5 877 084	683 516	10.4	591 378	9.0	92 138	1.4	49 614	42 524
Colorado	1 658 238	949 895	57.3	858 671	91 224	9.6	81 179	8.5	10 045	1.1	4 640	5 405
Connecticut	1 301 670	745 340	57.3	676 467	68 873	9.2	61 487	8.2	7 386	1.0	3 559	3 827
Delaware	298 736	171 434	57.4	153 136	18 298	10.7	16 430	9.6	1 868	1.1	979	889
District of Columbia	248 338	71 517	28.8	56 631	14 886	20.8	11 208	15.7	3 678	5.1	2 693	985
Florida	6 337 929	3 561 888	56.2	3 192 266	369 622	10.4	328 574	9.2	41 048	1.2	22 988	18 060
Georgia	3 006 369	1 694 543	56.4	1 548 800	145 743	8.6	126 455	7.5	19 288	1.1	10 251	9 037
Hawaii	403 240	239 593	59.4	216 077	23 516	9.8	21 127	8.8	2 389	1.0	1 234	1 155
Idaho	469 645	299 075	63.7	276 511	22 564	7.5	20 691	6.9	1 873	0.6	902	971
Illinois	4 591 779	2 573 438	56.0	2 353 892	219 546	8.5	196 659	7.6	22 887	0.9	12 155	10 732
Indiana	2 336 306	1 376 309	58.9	1 251 458	124 851	9.1	114 632	8.3	10 219	0.7	5 054	5 165
Iowa	1 149 276	690 076	60.0	633 254	56 822	8.2	53 124	7.7	3 698	0.5	1 789	1 909
Kansas	1 037 891	610 223	58.8	567 924	42 299	6.9	38 326	6.3	3 973	0.7	1 888	2 085
Kentucky	1 590 647	929 210	58.4	857 944	71 266	7.7	64 152	6.9	7 114	0.8	3 310	3 804
Louisiana	1 656 053	893 061	53.9	809 498	83 563	9.4	74 755	8.4	8 808	1.0	4 180	4 628
Maine	518 200	310 033	59.8	272 152	37 881	12.2	34 487	11.1	3 394	1.1	1 493	1 901
Maryland	1 980 859	1 104 884	55.8	994 549	110 335	10.0	99 092	9.0	11 243	1.0	5 230	6 013
Massachusetts	2 443 580	1 328 836	54.4	1 197 917	130 919	9.9	113 820	8.6	17 099	1.3	7 943	9 156
Michigan	3 785 661	2 149 930	56.8	1 947 710	202 220	9.4	186 852	8.7	15 368	0.7	7 293	8 075
Minnesota	1 895 127	1 118 603	59.0	1 018 245	100 358	9.0	91 211	8.2	9 147	0.8	4 290	4 857
Mississippi	1 046 434	567 582	54.2	520 844	46 738	8.2	41 964	7.4	4 774	0.8	2 251	2 523
Missouri	2 194 594	1 251 876	57.0	1 140 866	111 010	8.9	101 582	8.1	9 428	0.8	4 684	4 744
Montana	358 667	210 008	58.6	192 067	17 941	8.5	16 723	8.0	1 218	0.6	554	664
Nebraska	666 184	390 533	58.6	360 996	29 537	7.6	27 205	7.0	2 332	0.6	1 112	1 220
Nevada	751 165	427 103	56.9	373 201	53 902	12.6	48 929	11.5	4 973	1.2	2 739	2 234
New Hampshire	474 606	294 998	62.2	262 438	32 560	11.0	29 857	10.1	2 703	0.9	1 156	1 547
New Jersey	3 064 645	1 789 640	58.4	1 638 322	151 318	8.5	134 714	7.5	16 604	0.9	8 257	8 347
New Mexico	677 971	385 360	56.8	341 818	43 542	11.3	39 046	10.1	4 496	1.2	1 901	2 595
New York	7 056 860	3 667 070	52.0	3 289 514	377 556	10.3	331 066	9.0	46 490	1.3	24 494	21 996
North Carolina	3 132 013	1 789 026	57.1	1 645 346	143 680	8.0	127 482	7.1	16 198	0.9	7 849	8 349
North Dakota	257 152	148 812	57.9	137 433	11 379	7.6	10 676	7.2	703	0.5	360	343
Ohio	4 445 773	2 514 887	56.6	2 285 798	229 089	9.1	210 152	8.4	18 937	0.8	9 266	9 671
Oklahoma	1 342 293	770 918	57.4	717 611	53 307	6.9	47 544	6.2	5 763	0.7	2 811	2 952
Oregon	1 333 723	777 166	58.3	692 532	84 634	10.9	75 702	9.7	8 932	1.1	3 846	5 086
Pennsylvania	4 777 003	2 705 295	56.6	2 467 673	237 622	8.8	216 456	8.0	21 166	0.8	10 492	10 674
Rhode Island	408 424	219 937	53.9	196 757	23 180	10.5	20 709	9.4	2 471	1.1	1 172	1 299
South Carolina	1 533 854	853 564	55.6	783 142	70 422	8.3	62 813	7.4	7 609	0.9	3 561	4 048
South Dakota	290 245	171 282	59.0	157 391	13 891	8.1	13 065	7.6	826	0.5	389	437
Tennessee	2 232 905	1 267 908	56.8	1 173 960	93 948	7.4	83 759	6.6	10 189	0.8	5 090	5 099
Texas	7 393 354	4 316 987	58.4	3 989 741	327 246	7.6	284 334	6.6	42 912	1.0	21 740	21 172
Utah	701 281	467 035	66.6	442 931	24 104	5.2	20 734	4.4	3 370	0.7	1 665	1 705
Vermont	240 634	144 492	60.0	126 413	18 079	12.5	16 146	11.2	1 933	1.3	762	1 171
Virginia	2 699 173	1 552 409	57.5	1 426 044	126 365	8.1	112 563	7.3	13 802	0.9	7 053	6 749
Washington	2 271 398	1 321 464	58.2	1 181 995	139 469	10.6	123 569	9.4	15 900	1.2	7 652	8 248
West Virginia	736 481	432 254	58.7	397 499	34 755	8.0	31 839	7.4	2 916	0.7	1 494	1 422
Wisconsin	2 084 544	1 226 564	58.8	1 108 597	117 967	9.6	109 735	8.9	8 232	0.7	3 862	4 370
Wyoming	193 608	116 560	60.2	106 179	10 381	8.9	9 574	8.2	807	0.7	412	395
Puerto Rico	1 261 325	723 042	57.3	682 804	40 238	5.6	33 420	4.6	6 818	0.9	3 122	3 696

[1]Coupled households represent the total number of married-couple and unmarried-partner households.

1.4 percent. This was closely followed by Massachusetts, Vermont, and New York, each with 1.3 percent. The lowest proportions were found in Iowa, South Dakota, and North Dakota (each with 0.5 percent).

TABLE IV-12. SELECTED HOUSEHOLD AND FAMILY CHARACTERISTICS OF MARRIED-COUPLE AND UNMARRIED-PARTNER HOUSEHOLDS, BY REGION AND STATE, 2000

The 2000 census asked respondents to designate one household member as the "householder." Table IV-4 shows that only 13 percent of married-couple households had a female householder, but nearly half (46 percent) of all unmarried-partner households shared by members of the opposite sex had this designation. For married couples (who tended to co-own their home), this trend most likely reflected a norm of a male "head of household," whereas for unmarried couples, the "householder" may

Table IV-12. Selected Household and Family Characteristics of Married-Couple and Unmarried-Partner Households, by Region and State, 2000

(Percent.)

Area	Percent of householders female		Percent of householders with children under 18 years						
				Unmarried-partner households					
				Opposite-sex partners		Male partners		Female partners	
	Married-couple households	Opposite-sex, unmarried-partner households	Married-couple households [1]	Own children [1]	Own and/or unrelated children [2]	Own children [1]	Own and/or unrelated children [2]	Own children [1]	Own and/or unrelated children [2]
UNITED STATES	12.9	46.4	45.6	38.9	43.1	21.8	22.3	32.7	34.3
Region									
Northwest	15.4	48.4	45.2	37.4	40.9	21.3	21.7	31.2	32.6
Midwest	11.1	45.8	45.1	38.7	43.9	22.3	22.9	32.8	34.7
South	12.6	46.7	44.4	39.7	44.0	22.1	23.9	34.4	36.1
West	13.4	45.0	48.5	39.2	42.7	20.6	21.1	31.5	33.1
State									
Alabama	11.7	48.2	43.1	41.6	46.1	27.8	28.3	36.8	38.1
Alaska	15.0	43.8	54.4	40.6	45.1	36.2	37.1	37.0	38.6
Arizona	12.7	44.6	43.5	40.5	44.3	22.5	23.0	33.1	35.0
Arkansas	9.9	44.4	41.9	41.8	47.6	26.1	26.7	36.2	38.2
California	14.0	45.3	50.9	41.4	44.4	19.6	20.2	32.8	34.3
Colorado	13.8	45.7	47.2	31.3	34.6	19.9	20.5	26.1	27.8
Connecticut	17.2	50.7	45.4	35.6	38.7	21.9	22.2	30.2	31.6
Delaware	14.5	48.6	42.8	39.9	44.1	18.4	18.9	29.4	31.8
District of Columbia	24.9	56.6	36.6	31.8	32.8	4.8	5.0	23.4	24.5
Florida	14.4	46.5	38.1	35.5	39.2	17.4	17.8	29.3	31.0
Georgia	14.1	48.9	47.3	42.2	46.1	21.1	21.6	34.4	36.2
Hawaii	13.9	45.2	44.8	35.8	39.0	20.7	21.3	30.6	32.6
Idaho	10.0	42.3	47.8	37.6	43.0	30.3	30.8	35.7	37.9
Illinois	11.9	46.2	47.3	38.3	42.5	23.5	24.0	35.6	37.0
Indiana	10.3	44.0	44.4	40.5	47.0	22.8	23.5	33.6	36.3
Iowa	10.0	44.6	43.4	37.5	43.0	24.9	25.4	33.8	35.5
Kansas	10.1	44.8	45.9	39.1	44.1	28.3	29.0	36.5	38.1
Kentucky	11.4	46.1	43.7	40.1	46.0	23.5	24.4	33.0	34.9
Louisiana	12.1	47.7	46.2	44.4	48.5	25.9	26.3	38.5	39.8
Maine	15.1	45.2	41.4	35.7	40.9	18.7	19.0	25.2	27.1
Maryland	15.0	49.5	46.4	38.1	42.1	23.3	24.0	31.7	33.3
Massachusetts	16.6	49.8	45.8	32.8	35.9	18.1	18.6	27.7	29.0
Michigan	11.3	46.9	44.8	40.1	45.3	22.8	23.6	33.2	35.3
Minnesota	11.4	45.7	46.9	35.4	40.2	17.2	17.9	26.8	28.5
Mississippi	12.2	48.9	45.0	49.2	53.4	30.7	31.1	42.0	43.8
Missouri	10.3	45.5	43.6	39.9	45.7	20.9	21.5	31.7	33.7
Montana	11.7	44.0	42.9	35.1	39.3	28.7	29.6	34.2	35.5
Nebraska	9.8	44.6	45.9	36.4	41.5	24.7	25.7	32.7	34.4
Nevada	13.9	41.9	44.5	36.1	40.2	24.7	25.3	35.4	37.5
New Hampshire	15.3	43.7	45.9	33.0	38.1	22.3	22.9	27.2	29.0
New Jersey	14.7	48.0	47.4	38.1	40.9	25.4	25.8	33.6	34.7
New Mexico	12.0	44.2	46.1	48.4	51.7	27.4	27.9	31.0	32.2
New York	17.5	50.1	46.4	39.2	42.2	21.3	21.7	33.1	34.3
North Carolina	12.3	46.1	43.0	38.4	42.9	25.2	25.9	33.3	34.7
North Dakota	8.8	43.0	45.1	36.9	41.5	21.4	21.7	34.4	34.7
Ohio	12.4	46.9	43.6	40.2	45.3	20.9	21.6	31.8	34.0
Oklahoma	10.6	45.1	43.4	42.1	47.2	26.7	27.3	35.0	36.9
Oregon	13.7	45.6	42.8	33.9	38.4	18.9	19.5	26.3	28.1
Pennsylvania	11.6	45.6	42.3	38.5	42.8	20.9	21.3	31.5	33.2
Rhode Island	16.6	50.4	43.6	37.1	40.1	20.5	20.6	27.3	28.6
South Carolina	14.2	47.8	42.6	41.9	45.7	26.8	27.2	37.1	38.8
South Dakota	9.9	44.2	45.2	42.1	47.4	33.2	33.9	41.4	42.3
Tennessee	11.3	46.3	42.5	39.1	44.3	23.9	24.7	33.4	35.4
Texas	11.5	45.2	50.2	42.9	46.8	26.7	27.3	39.2	40.9
Utah	8.9	41.9	55.5	42.2	47.2	29.7	30.2	40.6	42.3
Vermont	16.5	46.2	44.2	33.8	38.3	19.9	20.6	26.7	28.9
Virginia	12.6	46.5	45.3	35.0	39.6	19.8	20.3	31.2	32.7
Washington	13.3	45.9	45.8	35.1	39.7	18.1	18.6	26.7	28.2
West Virginia	9.9	43.7	39.5	40.2	45.6	27.6	27.9	34.9	36.4
Wisconsin	10.5	45.4	44.5	34.9	40.5	21.7	22.4	30.6	32.4
Wyoming	10.9	41.2	44.3	36.0	41.8	28.2	29.9	35.7	37.5
Puerto Rico	14.1	54.4	49.4	56.5	56.7	39.2	39.2	42.2	42.5

[1] Refers to own sons/daughters of the householder.
[2] Refers to own sons/daughters of the householder and other children not related to the householder.

have been more likely to be the sole homeowner. Furthermore, research has shown that unmarried partners of the opposite sex tended to share household activities more equally than married couples. Regionally, the Northeast had the highest and the Midwest had the lowest percentage of married-couple householders who were women (15 percent and 11 percent, respectively). The Northeast had the highest proportion of women householders in unmarried-partner households, and the West

had the lowest proportion (48 percent and 45 percent, respectively).

Nationally, 46 percent of married-couple households had at least one son or daughter living in the household (defined as an "own child" of the householder). The proportion of unmarried households with children was 43 percent for partners of the opposite sex, 22 percent for male partners, and 34 percent for female partners. Households

Table IV-13. Selected Race and Hispanic Origin Characteristics of Married-Couple and Unmarried-Partner Households, by Region and State, 2000

(Percent.)

Area	Percent of households with partners of different races				Percent of households with only one partner of Hispanic origin[1]				Percent of households with partners of different races or origins			
	Married-couple households	Unmarried-partner households			Married-couple households	Unmarried-partner households			Married-couple households	Unmarried-partner households		
		Opposite-sex partners	Male partners	Female partners		Opposite-sex partners	Male partners	Female partners		Opposite-sex partners	Male partners	Female partners
UNITED STATES	5.7	12.2	11.5	10.0	3.1	6.4	6.9	5.4	7.4	15.0	15.3	12.6
Region												
Northwest	4.3	10.3	10.7	8.5	2.1	5.2	5.9	4.3	5.7	12.8	14.2	10.8
Midwest	3.5	9.4	8.2	7.4	1.7	4.0	3.8	3.0	4.5	11.2	10.3	8.9
South	4.9	10.3	8.7	8.0	2.7	5.2	5.8	4.3	6.5	12.8	12.4	10.3
West	10.6	19.3	17.7	15.7	6.1	11.2	11.1	9.2	13.7	23.7	23.2	19.7
State												
Alabama	2.8	6.7	4.5	4.6	0.9	1.9	1.5	1.2	3.3	7.5	5.4	5.3
Alaska	15.4	26.0	17.4	19.4	3.6	4.9	5.4	6.0	17.1	27.7	19.3	22.1
Arizona	8.0	15.7	12.2	13.0	6.6	12.3	10.7	10.3	11.5	20.9	17.7	17.6
Arkansas	3.6	8.4	6.1	6.5	1.2	2.7	2.1	1.8	4.2	9.6	7.0	7.4
California	12.0	21.0	19.8	17.3	7.2	12.7	12.8	10.5	15.6	26.0	26.2	21.8
Colorado	7.8	15.0	13.6	11.6	6.2	11.5	11.5	9.1	11.2	20.1	19.5	15.6
Connecticut	4.2	11.8	8.4	8.1	2.3	6.6	5.2	3.9	5.7	14.6	11.6	10.2
Delaware	4.1	10.5	9.8	7.1	1.7	3.9	4.0	3.5	5.1	12.2	12.5	9.0
District of Columbia	7.8	10.4	16.0	13.3	2.9	3.9	9.4	4.1	9.6	12.6	22.5	15.0
Florida	5.2	10.4	8.6	8.4	4.1	7.3	8.5	6.7	8.3	14.9	15.0	12.8
Georgia	3.7	8.2	7.6	6.4	1.6	3.1	3.8	2.6	4.6	9.5	10.0	7.8
Hawaii	34.7	55.6	43.8	40.9	6.2	12.6	7.9	8.9	36.1	57.6	46.1	42.3
Idaho	5.3	11.0	8.0	8.1	3.0	6.7	4.9	5.4	6.8	13.8	10.4	10.2
Illinois	4.3	10.0	11.0	8.6	2.6	5.7	6.7	4.3	5.8	12.6	14.7	10.8
Indiana	2.9	8.2	5.8	6.0	1.5	3.4	2.5	2.3	3.8	9.7	7.4	7.1
Iowa	2.3	7.7	5.5	6.4	1.2	3.6	2.2	2.7	3.0	9.2	6.8	8.0
Kansas	5.4	14.5	8.4	9.2	2.8	6.9	3.7	4.2	6.8	17.1	10.2	11.1
Kentucky	2.3	7.3	4.6	5.6	0.8	1.8	1.6	1.6	2.8	8.1	5.7	6.4
Louisiana	3.3	7.2	6.5	5.2	1.8	2.9	3.7	2.9	4.5	8.8	8.8	6.9
Maine	2.3	4.9	4.2	4.0	0.7	1.1	1.5	1.5	2.8	5.6	5.4	4.9
Maryland	5.1	9.6	9.7	8.6	1.9	2.9	3.5	3.2	6.3	11.0	11.9	10.6
Massachusetts	4.1	10.3	9.9	8.1	1.5	4.4	4.6	3.5	5.1	12.3	12.7	9.9
Michigan	4.1	9.7	8.5	7.4	1.8	4.2	3.5	2.8	5.2	11.7	10.4	8.7
Minnesota	3.4	10.6	9.1	8.0	1.2	3.3	3.4	2.6	4.1	12.0	10.8	8.9
Mississippi	2.1	5.1	3.7	3.2	0.8	1.5	1.7	1.1	2.6	5.8	4.8	3.8
Missouri	3.5	8.8	7.3	7.5	1.4	2.7	2.7	2.9	4.3	10.0	8.9	9.1
Montana	5.3	11.2	8.8	8.4	1.9	4.3	4.0	3.3	6.4	13.3	11.6	10.5
Nebraska	3.4	11.2	5.7	8.3	2.0	5.9	3.1	4.4	4.4	13.5	7.3	10.5
Nevada	10.9	18.9	14.9	15.2	6.2	10.7	9.1	8.3	14.3	23.7	19.5	19.2
New Hampshire	2.6	5.2	5.3	4.2	1.0	2.0	2.1	2.3	3.3	6.3	6.7	5.4
New Jersey	5.1	12.0	11.2	8.8	3.1	7.5	6.6	5.2	7.2	15.8	14.9	11.7
New Mexico	10.8	18.6	15.8	16.4	11.2	18.4	17.6	14.7	16.9	26.3	25.4	23.2
New York	5.7	12.3	13.7	10.9	3.0	6.7	8.0	6.0	7.6	15.6	18.4	14.1
North Carolina	3.6	9.6	6.9	6.5	1.4	3.0	2.1	2.2	4.3	10.7	8.0	7.5
North Dakota	3.1	9.3	4.4	6.4	0.8	2.3	0.6	1.7	3.6	10.4	4.7	7.6
Ohio	2.9	8.5	6.9	6.7	1.2	2.9	2.4	2.0	3.6	9.8	8.4	7.7
Oklahoma	14.8	24.6	17.6	18.2	2.6	5.8	3.3	4.5	16.0	26.5	18.8	19.9
Oregon	7.4	14.1	12.4	11.7	3.0	6.4	5.6	4.6	8.9	16.7	15.0	13.5
Pennsylvania	2.4	7.5	7.1	5.6	1.1	3.2	3.1	2.2	3.1	8.9	8.8	6.8
Rhode Island	4.4	11.1	9.0	8.0	1.5	4.3	3.9	2.8	5.2	13.0	10.6	9.6
South Carolina	2.9	7.3	5.4	4.8	1.1	2.3	1.4	1.7	3.5	8.3	6.2	5.7
South Dakota	3.6	10.9	5.7	7.3	1.0	2.8	1.8	0.9	4.1	12.1	6.7	7.6
Tennessee	2.7	7.4	5.2	5.7	1.0	2.2	1.8	1.8	3.3	8.4	6.3	6.6
Texas	6.8	14.1	11.5	10.7	5.4	11.2	10.7	8.0	9.8	19.0	17.4	14.6
Utah	5.4	14.6	9.2	9.6	3.8	10.0	6.4	6.5	7.3	18.8	12.5	12.8
Vermont	2.6	4.7	4.7	4.5	0.9	1.4	1.7	0.9	3.2	5.5	5.9	5.2
Virginia	5.3	11.3	10.4	8.3	2.1	3.6	4.2	3.5	6.5	12.9	12.8	10.1
Washington	9.2	17.3	14.8	13.6	3.2	6.6	5.9	5.4	10.8	19.8	17.6	16.1
West Virginia	1.8	5.6	3.6	3.2	0.5	1.0	0.9	0.9	2.2	6.1	4.4	3.8
Wisconsin	2.9	8.7	7.2	6.8	1.4	3.9	3.3	3.0	3.7	10.4	8.9	8.2
Wyoming	5.3	10.8	7.5	7.6	4.0	8.7	5.6	5.8	7.4	14.9	10.7	10.9
Puerto Rico	12.5	18.5	13.7	13.8	1.3	1.7	1.7	1.7	13.5	19.7	14.7	15.0

[1]May be of any race.

in three states (Mississippi, New Mexico, and West Virginia) were more likely to have children in unmarried-partner households than in married-couple households. Variation between states in the presence of children in same-sex, unmarried-partner households may be influenced by geographical differences in fertility patterns of previously married partners before they entered a same-sex relationship, as well as by state laws related to child custody placements and adoption by same-sex couples.

TABLE IV-13. SELECTED RACE AND HISPANIC ORIGIN CHARACTERISTICS OF MARRIED-COUPLE AND UNMARRIED-PARTNER HOUSEHOLDS, BY REGION AND STATE, 2000

Nationally, in 6 percent of married-couple households, the householder and the spouse were of different races. Three to five percent of married couples in the Midwest, the Northeast, and the South had spouses of different races, compared with 11 percent in the West. The highest proportion was found in Hawaii (35 percent), followed by Alaska and Oklahoma (15 percent each). All three states have high proportions of native populations.

Unmarried-partner households had consistently higher percentages of partners of different races at the national, regional, and state levels than married-couple households. For unmarried-partner households shared by members of the opposite sex, the West recorded the highest percentage of mixed-race partnerships (19 percent), and the Midwest recorded the lowest percentage (9 percent).

The New England states of Maine, New Hampshire, and Vermont, which have very low proportions of minority populations, had the lowest proportions of mixed-race partnerships for all four household types (approximately 5 percent or less). Mississippi, Alabama, and West Virginia also had comparatively low percentages of mixed-race partnerships for all four household types. Nationally, 3 percent of married couples had one Hispanic partner and one non-Hispanic partner, compared with about 6 percent of all unmarried partners. The highest percentages of mixed-Hispanic households for all four household types were found in the western states.

TABLE IV-14. AVERAGE AGE OF PARTNERS IN MARRIED-COUPLE AND UNMARRIED-PARTNER HOUSEHOLDS, BY REGION AND STATE, 2000

The average ages of partners in households shared by unmarried partners of the opposite sex, many of whom will ultimately marry each other, were about 12 years younger than the average ages of their married-couple counterparts. Nationally, the average age of husbands was 49 years old, 2.4 years older than the average age of their wives. Unmarried partners of the opposite sex were only slightly closer in age: male partners were 36.8 years old on average, 2.1 years older than their female counterparts. Overall, married couples who lived in the Northeast were the oldest, while those living in the West were the youngest. Among the individual states, the oldest husbands and wives were in Florida (53 years and 50 years, respectively), while the youngest lived in Alaska and

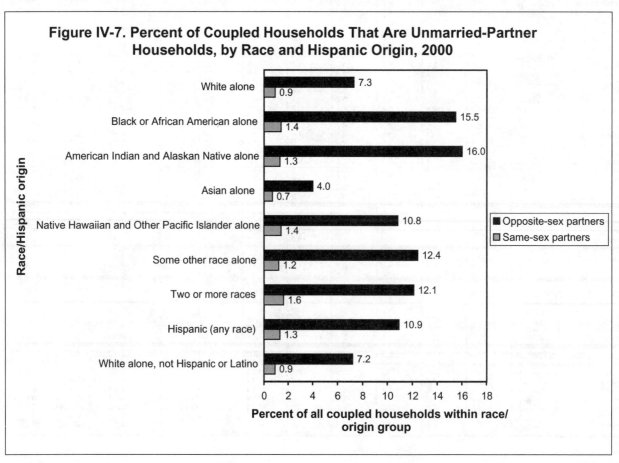

Figure IV-7. Percent of Coupled Households That Are Unmarried-Partner Households, by Race and Hispanic Origin, 2000

Utah (about 46 years and 43 years, respectively, for both states). On average, the youngest unmarried partners of the opposite sex lived in the Midwest. The Great Plains states of Kansas, Nebraska, South Dakota, and North Dakota tended to have both partners below 35 years of age. While the lowest average ages for unmarried partners of the opposite sex were in Utah (34 years for men and 32 years for women), the oldest were in Florida (39 years and 37 years). Partners of the same sex were, on average, in their early forties, falling between the average ages of married couples and unmarried partners of the opposite sex. For same-sex couples, an age comparison can be made between the householder and the partner. In male unmarried-partner households, the householder was about two years older, while in female unmarried-partner households, the householder was just over one year older. The average age of partners of the same sex was lowest in the West and highest in the Northeast for both types of households.

Table IV-14. Average Age of Partners in Married-Couple and Unmarried-Partner Households, by Region and State, 2000

(Number.)

Area	Married-couple households		Unmarried-partner households					
			Opposite-sex partners		Male partners		Female partners	
	Age of husband	Age of wife	Age of male partner	Age of female partner	Age of male partner	Age of partner	Age of householder	Age of partner
UNITED STATES	49.0	46.6	36.8	34.7	44.5	42.4	43.4	42.2
Region								
Northwest	50.0	47.5	37.8	35.5	45.2	43.3	44.3	43.2
Midwest	49.2	46.8	35.8	33.7	44.8	42.8	43.1	42.0
South	48.8	46.3	36.8	34.7	44.5	42.5	43.4	42.1
West	48.4	45.9	37.1	35.2	43.9	41.5	42.7	41.6
State								
Alabama	48.8	46.2	36.5	34.3	46.8	44.6	45.0	43.6
Alaska	45.5	43.0	36.9	34.6	43.9	41.7	40.8	39.9
Arizona	49.8	47.3	37.0	35.1	43.5	41.3	42.7	41.5
Arkansas	49.3	46.6	36.3	34.0	46.2	44.5	44.8	43.3
California	48.2	45.6	37.6	35.6	44.0	41.5	42.9	41.7
Colorado	47.4	45.2	35.5	33.7	41.9	39.9	41.3	40.2
Connecticut	50.1	47.7	37.6	35.5	45.7	44.0	44.4	43.5
Delaware	49.7	47.4	37.2	35.1	45.4	43.1	43.7	42.7
District of Columbia	50.8	48.0	38.6	36.2	42.4	39.8	42.4	41.3
Florida	52.5	49.6	39.2	36.9	46.1	44.0	45.1	43.8
Georgia	47.1	44.7	35.8	33.8	41.8	40.1	41.7	40.4
Hawaii	50.6	47.8	38.5	36.2	47.9	45.0	46.6	44.8
Idaho	48.1	45.6	36.1	34.0	46.4	43.9	43.5	42.4
Illinois	48.7	46.3	36.5	34.4	43.8	41.6	42.9	41.8
Indiana	48.7	46.4	35.5	33.4	44.5	42.4	42.4	41.3
Iowa	50.0	47.8	34.8	32.8	46.7	44.7	43.6	42.5
Kansas	48.8	46.6	34.5	32.5	44.4	42.4	42.8	41.6
Kentucky	48.1	45.6	35.9	33.6	45.7	43.6	43.8	42.3
Louisiana	48.5	45.9	36.7	34.2	45.5	43.1	44.2	42.5
Maine	50.2	47.8	37.2	34.8	46.4	44.9	43.5	42.7
Maryland	49.0	46.6	37.8	35.6	44.6	42.7	42.8	41.6
Massachusetts	49.7	47.4	37.3	35.2	44.4	42.7	43.4	42.6
Michigan	49.3	46.9	36.2	34.0	45.5	43.5	43.9	42.6
Minnesota	48.9	46.6	35.5	33.5	44.0	42.0	42.7	41.5
Mississippi	48.5	45.9	36.6	34.2	46.8	44.6	44.7	43.3
Missouri	49.4	47.0	36.1	33.9	45.2	43.3	42.6	41.5
Montana	50.2	47.5	36.4	34.1	46.2	44.1	45.2	44.1
Nebraska	49.2	47.0	34.6	32.6	45.7	43.5	44.1	43.0
Nevada	48.5	45.7	38.2	36.1	42.9	40.8	42.2	40.6
New Hampshire	49.0	46.7	37.3	35.1	45.2	43.8	43.7	42.6
New Jersey	49.6	47.1	38.7	36.4	45.3	43.5	44.5	43.3
New Mexico	49.2	46.7	36.3	34.4	45.2	42.9	43.8	42.8
New York	49.9	47.2	38.3	35.9	44.7	42.6	44.4	43.1
North Carolina	48.2	45.9	35.6	33.6	43.9	42.2	43.2	42.0
North Dakota	50.0	47.5	33.9	31.7	52.3	50.5	47.2	46.4
Ohio	49.4	47.1	35.8	33.7	45.2	43.3	43.5	42.3
Oklahoma	48.9	46.4	35.5	33.4	45.2	43.1	43.2	41.8
Oregon	49.6	47.1	36.9	34.9	44.9	42.5	42.5	41.7
Pennsylvania	50.6	48.3	37.3	35.0	46.8	44.9	45.2	44.0
Rhode Island	50.2	47.8	36.8	34.6	44.9	43.2	43.5	42.6
South Carolina	48.9	46.5	36.2	34.1	45.7	43.7	44.2	42.9
South Dakota	49.9	47.5	35.0	32.6	46.7	45.1	44.4	42.6
Tennessee	48.4	45.9	36.4	34.2	44.8	42.7	43.1	41.8
Texas	47.1	44.6	35.6	33.6	42.9	40.6	42.1	40.6
Utah	45.5	43.2	34.2	32.1	41.7	39.6	41.5	40.0
Vermont	49.9	47.4	37.4	35.0	45.7	43.9	43.3	43.1
Virginia	48.4	46.0	36.5	34.5	44.5	42.5	43.3	42.0
Washington	48.6	46.2	36.6	34.7	43.3	41.2	42.3	41.3
West Virginia	50.0	47.2	36.9	34.4	47.8	45.5	46.0	44.3
Wisconsin	49.5	47.2	35.6	33.5	44.7	43.0	42.8	42.0
Wyoming	49.0	46.5	36.4	34.1	48.2	45.6	44.1	42.9
Puerto Rico	48.2	45.1	40.9	38.5	47.4	45.4	47.4	45.6

SOURCES AND DEFINITIONS

This section provides sources for the data used in this book, along with some additional reference of related interest. A brief glossary follows the section.

INTRODUCTION:

Data for Tables A-1 and A-2 were obtained from *Health, United States, 2005,* an annual report on trends in health statistics by the National Center of Health Statistics, a component of the Centers for Disease Control and Prevention (CDC) [Trend tables 25 and 26]. See: Centers for Disease Control and Prevention. National Center for Health Statistics. 2005. *Health, United States, 2005, with Chartbook on Trends in the Health of Americans.* (Hyattsville, MD: National Center for Health Statistics.) <http://www.cdc.gov/nchs/data/hus/hus05.pdf>. (Accessed Feb. 27, 2006.)

Table A-3 was adapted from two tables (A5 and A12) contained in the *Global Population Profile* prepared by the U.S. Census Bureau in 2002. See: U.S. Census Bureau. 2004. *International Population Reports, WP/02.* (Washington, DC: U.S. Government Printing Office) < http://www.census.gov/ipc/prod/wp02/wp-02.pdf >. (Accessed Feb. 27, 2006.)

Data contained in Table A5 can be found at <http://www.census.gov/ipc/prod/wp02/tabA-05.pdf>, and data for Table A12 is located at <http://www.census.gov/ipc/prod/wp02/tabA-12.pdf>. (Both accessed Feb. 17, 2006.)

CHAPTER I: BIRTHS

Most of the tables in Chapter I were obtained from: Martin, Joyce A., Brady E. Hamilton, et al. 2005. Births: Final data for 2003. *National Vital Statistics Reports* 54 (2): 1-116. (Hyattsville, MD: National Center for Health Statistics.) <http://www.cdc.gov/nchs/data/nvsr/nvsr54/nvsr54_02.pdf>. (Accessed Feb. 17, 2006.)

The following tables were obtained from the text tables from "Births: Final Data for 2003": I-10A (C in the text), I-18A (D in the text), I-33A (E in the text), I-44B (G in the text), I-44C (H in the text), and I-50B (J in the text).

In addition, some preliminary data were available for 2004. These were presented in: Hamilton, Brady E., Stephanie A.Ventura, et al. 2005. Births: Preliminary data for 2004. *National Vital Statistics Reports* 54 (8). (Hyattsville, MD: National Center for Health Statistics.). <http://www.cdc.gov/nchs/data/nvsr/nvsr54/nvsr54_08.pdf>. (Accessed Feb. 17, 2006.)

The preliminary tables in Chapter I are: I-1A, I-2A, I-4A, and I-17A.

The data for Table I-50A were not shown in Births: Final

Data for 2003, but were available in: Martin, Joyce A., Brady E. Hamilton, et al. 2003. Births: Final data for 2002. *National Vital Statistics Reports* 52 (10): 1-116. <http://www.cdc.gov/nchs/data/nvsr/nvsr52/nvsr52_10.pdf>. (Accessed Feb. 27, 2006.)

Some tables (Tables I-19A, I-21A, I-34A, I-44A, I-50A, I-51, I-52, and I-53) were obtained from *Health, United States, 2005,* which included 156 trend tables. See: Centers for Disease Control and Prevention. National Center for Health Statistics. 2005. Fertility and natality. *Health United States, 2005, with Chartbook on Trends in the Health of Americans.* (Hyattsville, MD: National Center for Health Statistics.) <http://www.cdc.gov/nchs/data/hus/hus05.pdf>. (Accessed Feb. 16, 2006.)

Data for all other tables are from "Births: Final Data for 2003."

Since 1985, the data shown in the tables (with the exception of the preliminary data) have been based on 100 percent of the birth certificates registered in the 50 states and the District of Columbia. Some additional data are shown for U.S. territories.

Since 1980, tabulations of birth data have been by race of mother; for earlier years, they were by race of child. Race and Hispanic origin are reported independently on the birth certificate. While Hispanics can belong to any race, the majority of Hispanic origin births have been reported as White; the bulk of the remainder have been reported as Black. The tables in Chapter I usually show data for these categories: White total, non-Hispanic White, Black total, non-Hispanic Black, and Hispanic. Data for American Indians and Asian or Pacific Islanders (API) are also included. Some data are presented for Hispanic and API subgroups by country of origin.

To calculate birth and fertility rates, the underlying populations must be calculated. For 2003, these were estimated by using counts from the 2000 census, after adjusting them to their July 1, 2003, level. This census included an option for persons to report more than one race. Since birth certificates collected only one race for the mother, the census data had to be "bridged" to return the data to estimates of single race categories. These procedures are discussed in: Ingram, D.D., J.D. Parker, et al. 2003. U.S. Census 2000 population with bridged race categories. *Vital and Health Statistics* 2 (135): III-55. <http://www.cdc.gov/nchs/data/series/sr_02/sr02_135.pdf>. (Accessed Feb. 16, 2006.)

Also see: Schenker, N., J.D. Parker. 2003. From single race reporting to multiple race reporting: Using imputation methods to bridge the transition. *Statistics in Medicine* 22: 1571-1587.

Birth certificates provide nearly complete coverage of

most of the requested characteristics. Reports with missing characteristics were subtracted from the total for 2003, and the percentages in the tables reflected the distributions of respondents. The proportions of "not stated" data were generally quite small, but they exceeded 5 percent for maternal weight gain during pregnancy and 10 percent for information about fathers. Table 1 in the technical notes to "Births: Final Data for 2003," by the National Center for Health Statistics, gives detailed data on the extent of missing information.

CHAPTER II: MORTALITY

Four publications were used for the mortality data:

For Tables II-1A, II-2 through II-9, II-10A, II-11 through II-29, II-30A, II-31C, II-32, II-33, and II-34: Kochanek, Kenneth D., Sherry L. Murphy, et al. 2004. Deaths: Final data for 2002. *National Vital Statistics Reports* 53 (5): 1-116. (Hyattsville, MD: National Center for Health Statistics.)
<http://www.cdc.gov/nchs/data/nvsr/nvsr53/nvsr53_05.pdf>.
(Accessed Feb. 17, 2006.)

In addition, three text tables from this document were reproduced: Tables II-9A (C in the text), II-30B (D in the text), and II-31A (E in the text).

For Tables II-1B, II-9C, II-10, II-29A, II-31B, and II-31D: Hoyert, Donna L., Hsiang-Ching Kung, et al. 2005. Deaths: Preliminary data for 2003. *National Vital Statistics Reports* 53 (15): 1-48. (Hyattsville, MD: National Center for Health Statistics.)
<http://www.cdc.gov/nchs/data/nvsr/nvsr53/nvsr53_15.pdf >.
(Accessed Feb. 17, 2006.)

For Tables II-1, II-9B, II-30 and II-31: Hoyert, Donna L., Melonie Heron, et al. 2006. Deaths: Final data for 2003. *Health E-Stats.* (Hyattsville, MD: National Center for Health Statistics.)
<http://www.cdc.gov/nchs/products/pubs/pubd/hestats/ finaldeaths03/finaldeaths03.htm>. (Accessed Feb. 27, 2006.)

For Table II-30A: MacDorman, Marian F., Joyce A. Martin, et al. 2005. Explaining the 2001–02 infant mortality increase: Data from the linked birth/infant death data set. *National Vital Statistics Reports* 53 (12): 1-24. (Hyattsville, MD: National Center for Health Statistics.)
<http://www.cdc.gov/nchs/data/nvsr/nvsr53/nvsr53_12.pdf >.
(Accessed Feb. 27, 2006.)

For Tables II-18 and II-18A: Miniño, Arialdi, Robert Anderson, et al. 2006. Deaths: Injuries, 2002. *National Vital Statistics Reports* 54 (10): 1-128. (Hyattsville, MD: National Center for Health Statistics.)
<http://www.cdc.gov/nchs/data/nvrs/nvrs54/nvrs54_10.pdf>.

(Accessed Feb. 27, 2006.)
Final data are based on information from all resident death certificates filed in the 50 states and the District of Columbia. It is believed that more than 99 percent of all deaths that occur in the United States are registered. Tables showing data by states also include information for Puerto Rico and other U.S. territories. Cause of death statistics are classified in accordance with the *International Classification of Diseases, Tenth Revision (ICD-10).*

To obtain death rates for 2002 and 2003, population data were used in the denominator. In contrast to the actual counts of deaths, estimates were based on the 2000 census and adjusted to July 1st of the year in question. As discussed in the section for births, data were also adjusted to "bridge" entries for multiple-race persons back to the earlier single race categories.

All of the data excluded fetal deaths. Many death certificates were multiple-cause coded, but the statistics derived by NCHS were based solely on the underlying cause of death. This cause is defined as the disease or injury which initiated the events that led directly to the death. Computer software was used to input the multiple-cause codes, and to employ the World Health Organization rules for selecting the underlying cause.

Persons classified as members of a minority group in the 2000 census were sometimes misclassified as White on death certificates. Persons may have also been erroneously reported as White on the census. Estimates of approximate percentages of appropriate corrections in death rates were as follows: White, -1.0 percent; Black, -5.0 percent; American Indian, +20.6 percent; Asian/Pacific Islander, +10.7 percent; Hispanics, +1.6 percent. (Rosenberg, H.M., J. D. Maurer, et al. 1999. Quality of death rates by race and Hispanic origin: A summary of current research. *Vital and Health Statistics* 2 [128]: 1-13. <http://www.cdc.gov/nchs/data/series/sr_02/sr02_128.pdf>. [Accessed Feb. 17, 2006.])

Cause of death data, as shown in the principal tables in this text, can also be classified by alternative frameworks. For instance, in Tables II-9 to II-17, injury mortality data are categorized by intent, such as suicide and homicide. However, these deaths can also be classified by mechanism, such as deaths by firearms or poisoning, as shown in Tables II-18 to II-24. In addition, the CDC occasionally estimates of the number of deaths caused by behavioral risk factors or causal agents of fatal diseases, such as tobacco, poor diet and physical inactivity, pollutants and asbestos, etc.

The Current Population Survey, conducted by the U.S. Census Bureau, is the source of population estimates by marital status, educational attainment, and country of origin (for Hispanics).

There is a tendency for preliminary data to slightly underestimate rates for causes of death in which the cause was pending investigation, such as homicide, suicide, accidents, and sudden infant death syndrome (SIDS). Rates due to highly seasonal conditions, such as influenza and pneumonia and chronic lower respiratory diseases, may also be misestimated.

In general, death rates are on an annual basis per 1,000 or per 100,000 of the estimated population residing in the specified area. Infant mortality rates are per 1,000 or 100,000 live births.

CHAPTER III: HEALTH

The principal source for data presented in the Health chapter is the CDC's *Health, United States, 2005* and its 156 trend tables, which were produced by the National Center for Health Statistics. See: Centers for Disease Control and Prevention. National Center for Health Statistics. 2005. *Health, United States, 2005, with Chartbook on Trends in the Health of Americans.* (Hyattsville, MD: National Center for Health Statistics.) <http://www.cdc.gov/nchs/data/hus/hus05.pdf>. (Accessed Feb. 27, 2006.)

Most of the 71 tables in the Health chapter were obtained from the 156 trend tables in *Health, United States, 2005*, as cited in the previous paragraph.

The original compiler of the data for several of the medical personnel tables included in this text had copyright protections. Permission to reproduce the data shown in Tables III-58, III-59, III-60, and III-62 was obtained from the American Medical Association (AMA).

Health, United States, 2005 contains a section called "Chartbook on Trends in the Health of Americans." This was the source for the data contained in Table III-8: Selected Chronic Health Conditions Causing Limitation of Activity Among Working-Age Adults, by Age, 2002–2003. This table is shown on pages 50–52 and page 109 of *Health, United States, 2005*.

Table III-26, Cocaine-Related Emergency Department Episodes, According to Age, Sex, Race, and Hispanic Origin, Selected Years, 1990–2002, was derived from: Centers for Disease Control and Prevention. National Center for Health Statistics. 2004. Trend table 65. *Health, United States, 2004, with Chartbook on Trends in the Health of Americans.* (Hyattsville, MD: National Center for Health Statistics). <http://www.cdc.gov/nchs/data/hus/hus04.pdf>. (Accessed Feb. 27, 2006.)

The source for data on health insurance is from the U.S. Census Bureau. See: DeNavas-Walt, Carmen, Bernadette D. Proctor, and Cheryl Hill Lee. 2005. *Income, Poverty,*

and Health Insurance Coverage in the United States: 2004 (Current Population Report P60-229). (Washington, DC: U.S. Government Printing Office.) <http://www.census.gov/prod/2005pubs/p60-229.pdf >. (Accessed Feb. 16, 2006.)

Table 7 from *Income, Poverty, and Health Insurance Coverage in the United States: 2004* is shown here as Table III-67, Table 11 is shown as Table III-68, Table C1 is shown as Table III-69, and Table C2 is shown as Table III-70.

CHAPTER IV: MARRIAGE AND DIVORCE

Information on the total number and the rates of marriages and divorces at the national and state levels are published by NCHS in the agency's National Vital Statistics Reports. The collection of detailed data was suspended beginning in January 1996, due to limitations on the information collected by the states and budgetary considerations. Occasionally, more comprehensive analyses of marriage and divorce rates became available; these are used in this text for Tables IV-4 to IV-14.

Table IV-1 was adapted from two sources:

Munson, M.L., and P.D. Sutton. 2005. Table A. Births, marriages, divorces, and deaths: Provisional data for 2004. *National Vital Statistics Reports* 53 (21): 1-7. (Hyattsville, MD: National Center for Health Statistics.) <http://www.cdc.gov/nchs/data/nvsr/nvsr53/nvsr53_21.pdf>. (Accessed Feb. 27, 2006.)

Munson, M.L., and P.D. Sutton. 2004. Table A. Births, marriages, divorces, and deaths: Provisional data for 2003. *National Vital Statistics Reports* 52 (22): 1-7. (Hyattsville, MD: National Center for Health Statistics.) <http://www.cdc.gov/nchs/data/nvsr/nvsr52/nvsr52_22.pdf >. (Accessed Feb. 27, 2006.)

Table IV-2 was adapted from:

Munson, M.L., and P.D. Sutton. 2005. Table B. Births, marriages, divorces, and deaths: Provisional data for 2004. *National Vital Statistics Reports* 53 (21):1-7. (Hyattsville, MD: National Center for Health Statistics.) <http://www.cdc.gov/nchs/data/nvsr/nvsr53/nvsr53_21.pdf>. (Accessed Feb. 27, 2006.)

Table IV-3 was adapted from three sources:

Munson, M.L., and P.D. Sutton. 2005. Table 3. Births, marriages, divorces, and deaths: Provisional data for 2004. *National Vital Statistics Reports* 53 (21): 1-7. (Hyattsville, MD: National Center for Health Statistics.) <http://www.cdc.gov/nchs/data/nvsr/nvsr53/nvsr53_21.pdf>. (Accessed Feb. 27, 2006.)

For the July 2003 columns: Sutton, P.D., and M.L. Munson. 2005. Table 3. Births, marriages, divorces, and deaths: Provisional data for July 2004. *National Vital Statistics Reports* 53 (13): 1-7. (Hyattsville, MD: National Center for Health Statistics.) <http://www.cdc.gov/nchs/data/nvsr/nvsr53/nvsr53_13.pdf>. (Accessed Feb. 27, 2006.)

For the January 2004 columns: Sutton, P.D., and M.L. Munson. 2005. Table 3. Births, marriages, divorces, and deaths: Provisional data for January 2005. *National Vital Statistics Reports* 54 (1): 1-6. (Hyattsville, MD: National Center for Health Statistics.) <http://www.cdc.gov/nchs/data/nvsr/nvsr54/nvsr54_01.pdf>. (Accessed Feb. 27, 2006.)

Tables IV-4 and IV-6 through IV-9 derived from (and Figures IV-1 through IV-3 and IV-6 adapted from):

Kreider, Rose M. 2005. *Number, Timing, and Duration of Marriages and Divorces: 2001* (Current Population Report, P70-97). (Washington, DC: U.S. Census Bureau.) <http://www.census.gov/prod/2005pubs/p70-97.pdf>. (Accessed Feb. 8, 2006.)

Table IV-5 derived from (and Figures IV-4 and IV-5 adapted from):

U.S. Census Bureau. Survey of Income and Program Participation (SIPP). 2001 Panel. Wave 2 Topical Module. Table 1: Marital History for People 15 Years and Over, by Age, Sex, Race, and Hispanic Origin: 2001. (Feb. 10, 2005.) <http://www.census.gov/population/socdemo/marital-hist/p70-97/tab01.pdf>. (Accessed Feb. 27, 2006.)

Tables IV-10 through IV-14 derived from (and Figure IV-7 adapted from):

Simmons, Tavia, and Martin O'Connell. 2003. *Married-Couple and Unmarried-Partner Households: 2000.*(Census 2000 Special Reports: CENSR-5) (Washington, DC: U.S. Census Bureau.) <http://www.census.gov/prod/2003pubs/censr-5.pdf>. (Accessed Feb. 27, 2006.)

GLOSSARY

ADL — See **Limitations of activity.**

Age-adjusted death rate — Age-adjusted rates are computed by applying the age-specific rates in a population of interest to a standardized age distribution, in order to eliminate the differences in observed rates caused by age differences in population composition. This concept can be illustrated by an example: Suppose a standard population has been selected in a country. (This selection is arbitrary, but it must be the same across years and regions. In the United States, the population from the year 2000 was selected.) In the example, the standard population consists of 10,000 younger persons and 5,000 older persons. Thus, the younger persons have a weight of 2/3 and the older persons have a weight of 1/3. In this population, there is a specific population subset with a larger proportion of elderly people. It consists of 1,000 younger persons, who experienced 1 death during the year, and 1,000 older persons, with 2 deaths during the year. The death rate for the specific population is 3 divided by 2,000, or 1.5 per 1,000.

For age adjustment, the death rate in the specific population must be determined as if it had the same age distribution as the standard population. To get the answer, the weights of the age distribution from the standard population are applied. The 1 death per 1,000 gets a weight of 2/3 and the 2 deaths per 1,000 get a weight of 1/3. When combining these two terms, we obtain 1x2/3 plus 2x1/3, or 4/3, which is 1.33. Thus, the crude death rate of 1.5 has been adjusted to 1.33. In this example, the high death rate of the older age group is applied, after age adjustment, to a relatively smaller population, thereby reducing the adjusted death rate.

Birth cohort — All persons born within a given period of time, such as a calendar year.

Birth rate — The birth rate, generally stated as number of live births per 1,000 population, relates the number of live births in a year to the midyear resident population in a specified group; this population could be females in a certain age group, or it could be the total population of the United States. The **fertility rate** shows live births per 1,000 women of childbearing age (defined as women age 15–44 years). While **birth rates and fertility rates** usually describe events during a single year, **total fertility rates** show the number of children that a representative woman could expect to have during her lifetime, should current fertility rates in each age group remain constant.

Birthweight — **Low birthweight** is defined as less than 2,500 grams (5lb 8oz). **Very low birthweight** is defined as less than 1,500 grams (3lb 4oz).

BMI (body mass index) — BMI is a measure that adjusts body weight for height. It is calculated as weight in kilograms divided by height in meters squared. **Healthy weight** for adults is defined as a BMI of 18.5 to less than 25; **overweight** is greater than or equal to a BMI of 25; **obesity** is greater than or equal to a BMI of 30. These guidelines were developed by the Department of Agriculture.

Cause of death — In these data, every death is attributed to one underlying condition, based on information from the death certificate and the World Health Organization. The underlying cause is the disease or injury that initiated the train of events leading directly to the death. Generally, more medical information than the underlying cause of death is reported on death certificates, thus requiring analytic approaches when studying this data.

Fertility rate — See **Birth rate.**

Health insurance coverage — The term "health insurance" is broadly defined to include both public and private payers who cover medical expenditures incurred by a defined population in a variety of settings.

Hispanic origin — This is an ethnic classification. Hispanics may be of any race, but most of them classify themselves as White. Hispanic Blacks rank second.

Hypertension — A person is considered to have hypertension if his or her systolic blood pressure is 140 mmHg or more, if his or her diastolic pressure is 90 mmHg or more, or if he or she is currently taking antihypertensive medication.

IADL — See **Limitations of activity.**

Infant mortality — This measures the rate of infant deaths, per 1,000 live births, of children under 1 year old. The **neonatal mortality rate** measures deaths of infants less than 28 days old, and the **postneonatal rate** measures deaths of infants from 28 days old to 1 year old.

Life expectancy — This term defines the expected life span at birth—or the remaining life span at a later age—if current mortality rates in each age bracket were to remain unchanged.

Limitations of activity— These represent a reduction in performance of activities usually associated with a person's age group, due to chronic physical or mental conditions. Stringent limitations are categorized as **ADLs** (activities of daily living), which include needing help for bathing, dressing, or eating. Limitations of activity can also be classified as **IADLs** (instrumental activities of daily living), which include requiring assistance for preparing meals, shopping, and using a telephone.

Notifiable diseases — A disease that, when diagnosed, health providers are required (usually by law) to report to state or local public health officials. Notifiable diseases are those of public interest due to their contagiousness, severity, or frequency.

Nulliparous — Nulliparous women are those who have had no live births, and **parous** women are those who have given birth to at least one baby.

Perinatal mortality rate — This rate is the sum of late fetal deaths plus infant deaths within 7 days of birth, divided by the sum of live births plus late fetal deaths (per 1,000 live births), plus late fetal deaths. (**Perinatal** relates to the period surrounding the birth event. Rates and ratios are based on events reported in a calendar year.)

Period of gestation — A period of gestation under 37 weeks is classified as **preterm**. If less than 32 weeks of gestation are completed, the label **very preterm** is applied. A period of gestation of 37 to 41 weeks is labeled, and if the pregnancy lasts 42 weeks or more, it is considered to be **postterm**.

Poverty level — Poverty statistics are based on definitions originally developed by the Social Security Administration. These include a set of money income thresholds that vary by family size and composition. Families or individuals with income below their appropriate thresholds are classified as below the poverty level. These thresholds are updated annually by the U.S. Census Bureau to reflect changes in the Consumer Price Index for all urban consumers (CPI-U). For example, the average poverty threshold for a family of four was $17,603 in 2000 and $13,359 in 1990.

Short-stay hospital — These are hospitals that provide general (rather than specialized) care, and have an average length of stay of less than 30 days.

INDEX